# Pharmacotherapy Casebook

## NOTICE

# Pharmacotherapy Casebook

## A Patient-Focused Approach

**Eighth Edition**

*Edited by*

**Terry L. Schwinghammer, PharmD, FCCP, FASHP, FAPhA, BCPS**

Professor and Chair
Department of Clinical Pharmacy
West Virginia University
School of Pharmacy
Morgantown, West Virginia

**Julia M. Koehler, PharmD, FCCP**

Associate Professor and Chair
Department of Pharmacy Practice
Butler University
College of Pharmacy and Health Sciences
and
Clinical Pharmacist in Family Medicine
Methodist Hospital and the Indiana University-Methodist Family Practice Center
Clarian Health Partners
Indianapolis, Indiana

A companion workbook for: *Pharmacotherapy: A Pathophysiologic Approach, 8th ed.*
*DiPiro JT, Talbert RL, Yee GC, Matzke GR, Wells BG, Posey ML, eds. New York, NY: McGraw-Hill, 2011.*

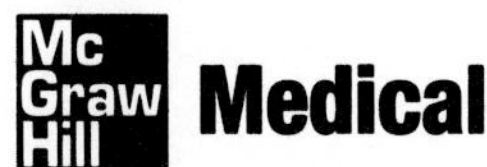


New York Chicago San Francisco Lisbon London Madrid Mexico City
Milan New Delhi San Juan Seoul Singapore Sydney Toronto

**Pharmacotherapy Casebook: A Patient-Focused Approach, Eighth Edition**



1 2 3 4 5 6 7 8 9 0 QDB/QDB 15 14 13 12 11

ISBN 978-0-07-174626-7
MHID 0-07-174626-9

This book was set in Minion by Thomson Digital.
The editors were Michael Weitz and Peter J. Boyle.
The production supervisor was Sherri Souffrance.
Project management was provided by Anand Kumar, Thomson Digital.
The designer was Alan Barnett; cover design by The Gazillion Group with photo by David Mack/Photo researchers, Inc.
Quad/Graphics was the printer and binder.

This book is printed on acid-free paper.

**Library of Congress Cataloging-in-Publication Data**

Pharmacotherapy casebook : a patient-focused approach / edited by Terry L. Schwinghammer, Julia M. Koehler.—8th ed.
p. ; cm.
A companion workbook for: Pharmacotherapy: a pathophysiologic approach / editors, Joseph T. DiPiro ... [et al.]. 8th ed. c2011.
Includes bibliographical references and index.
ISBN 978-0-07-174626-7 (pbk.)
1. Chemotherapy—Case studies. 2. Physiology, Pathological—Case studies. I. Schwinghammer, Terry L. II. Koehler, Julia M. III. Pharmacotherapy.
[DNLM: 1. Drug Therapy. 2. Case Reports. 3. Disease Management. 4. Examination Questions. 5. Patient-Centered Care. WB 18.2]
RM263.P56 2011
615.5'8—dc23
2011013040

# CONTENTS

## SECTION 3

### Respiratory Disorders



## SECTION 4

### Gastrointestinal Disorders



## SECTION 5

### Renal Disorders



## SECTION 6

### Neurologic Disorders

## SECTION 7

## Psychiatric Disorders



## SECTION 8

## Endocrinologic Disorders



## SECTION 9

## Women's Health (Gynecologic Disorders)



## SECTION 10

## Urologic Disorders

## SECTION 11
### Immunologic Disorders



## SECTION 12
### Bone and Joint Disorders



## SECTION 13
### Disorders of the Eyes, Ears, Nose, and Throat



## SECTION 14
### Dermatologic Disorders



## SECTION 15
### Hematologic Disorders



## SECTION 16
### Infectious Diseases

## SECTION 17

## Oncologic Disorders



## SECTION 18

## Nutrition and Nutritional Disorders



## SECTION 19

# CONTRIBUTORS

**Marie A. Abate, BS, PharmD**

Professor and Director, West Virginia Center for Drug and Health Information, Department of Clinical Pharmacy; Director of Programmatic Assessment, School of Pharmacy, West Virginia University, Morgantown, West Virginia

**Cesar Alaniz, PharmD**

Clinical Associate Professor of Pharmacy, Department of Clinical Sciences, College of Pharmacy; Clinical Pharmacist, Adult Medicine Intensive Care Unit, University of Michigan Health Systems, University of Michigan, Ann Arbor, Michigan

**Nicole Paolini Albanese, PharmD, CDE**

Clinical Assistant Professor, School of Pharmacy and Pharmaceutical Sciences, State University of New York at Buffalo, Buffalo, New York

**Kwadwo Amankwa, PharmD**

Assistant Professor, Clinical and Administrative Sciences, School of Pharmacy, College of Notre Dame of Maryland, Baltimore, Maryland

**Jarrett R. Amsden, PharmD, BCPS**

Assistant Professor, Butler University College of Pharmacy and Health Sciences; Infective Diseases Clinical Specialist, Community Health Network Hospitals, Indianapolis, Indiana

**Laurel Andrews, PharmD**

Assistant Professor, Department of Clinical and Administrative Sciences, College of Pharmacy, University of Louisiana at Monroe, Monroe, Louisiana

**Alexander J. Ansara, PharmD, BCPS**

Clinical Pharmacy Specialist, Internal Medicine, Clarian Health/ Methodist Hospital; Associate Professor of Pharmacy Practice, Butler University College of Pharmacy and Health Sciences, Indianapolis, Indiana

**Edward P. Armstrong, PharmD**

Professor, Department of Pharmacy Practice and Science, University of Arizona College of Pharmacy, Tucson, Arizona

**Kendra M. Atkinson, PharmD**

Assistant Professor of Pharmacy Practice, Butler University College of Pharmacy and Health Sciences, Indianapolis, Indiana

**Jacquelyn L. Bainbridge, PharmD, FCCP**

Professor, Department of Clinical Pharmacy, School of Pharmacy, and Department of Neurology, School of Medicine, University of Colorado, Aurora, Colorado

**Chad M. Barnett, PharmD, BCOP**

Clinical Pharmacy Specialist—Breast Oncology, University of Texas MD Anderson Cancer Center, Houston, Texas

**Scott Bergman, PharmD, BCPS**

Assistant Professor, Department of Pharmacy Practice and School of Medicine, Division of Infectious Diseases, Southern Illinois University Edwardsville School of Pharmacy, Springfield, Illinois

**Lisa R. Biondo, PharmD**

Clinical Pharmacy Specialist, Pediatric Hematology/Oncology, West Virginia University Hospitals, Ruby Memorial, Morgantown, West Virginia

**Scott Bolesta, PharmD, BCPS**

Assistant Professor, Department of Pharmacy Practice, Nesbitt College of Pharmacy and Nursing, Wilkes University; Clinical Pharmacist, Internal Medicine/Critical Care, Mercy Hospital, Wilkes-Barre, Pennsylvania

**Bonnie Lin Boster, PharmD, BCOP**

Clinical Pharmacy Specialist—Breast Medical Oncology, Division of Pharmacy, University of Texas MD Anderson Cancer Center, Houston, Texas

**Jessica Helmer Brady, PharmD, BCPS**

Clinical Assistant Professor, Department of Clinical and Administrative Sciences, College of Pharmacy, University of Louisiana at Monroe, Monroe, Louisiana

**Kelsey Briggs, PharmD**

Pediatric Clinical Specialist, West Virginia University Hospitals, Morgantown, West Virginia

**Gretchen M. Brophy, PharmD, BCPS, FCCP, FCCM**

Professor, Department of Pharmacotherapy and Outcome Sciences, and Department of Neurosurgery, Virginia Commonwealth University, Medical College of Virginia Campus, Richmond, Virginia

**Rodrigo M. Burgos, PharmD, AAHIVE**

Clinical Assistant Professor, Section of Infectious Diseases Pharmacotherapy, College of Pharmacy, University of Illinois at Chicago, Chicago, Illinois

**Karim Anton Calis, PharmD, MPH, FASHP, FCCP**

Senior Clinical Investigator, Eunice Kennedy Shriver National Institute of Child Health and Human Development and National Institute of Diabetes and Digestive and Kidney Diseases, National Institutes of Health, Bethesda, Maryland; Clinical Professor, University of Maryland School of Pharmacy, Baltimore, Maryland; Professor, Virginia Commonwealth University School of Pharmacy, Richmond, Virginia

**Bruce R. Canaday, PharmD, FASHP, FAPhA**
Professor and Chair, University of the Sciences in Philadelphia, Philadelphia, Pennsylvania

**Gina M. Carbonara Baugh, PharmD**
Clinical Assistant Professor, School of Pharmacy, West Virginia University, Morgantown, West Virginia

**Katie E. Cardone, PharmD**
Assistant Professor, Department of Pharmacy Practice, Albany College of Pharmacy and Health Sciences, Albany, New York

**Diana Hey Cauley, PharmD, BCOP**
Clinical Pharmacy Specialist, Genitourinary Medical Oncology, Division of Pharmacy, University of Texas MD Anderson Cancer Center, Houston, Texas

**Juliana Chan, PharmD**
Assistant Director, Pharmacy Clinical Services; Clinical Assistant Professor, Department of Pharmacy Practice, College of Pharmacy and Department of Medicine, Sections of Digestive Diseases and Nutrition and Section of Hepatology, University of Illinois at Chicago, Chicago, Illinois

**Amber Nicole Chiplinski, PharmD**
Assistant Professor of Clinical Pharmacy, Internal Medicine, West Virginia University School of Pharmacy, Martinsburg, West Virginia

**Kevin W. Cleveland, PharmD, ANP**
Associate Professor, Department of Pharmacy Practice, Idaho State University, College of Pharmacy, Pocatello, Idaho

**Antoinette B. Coe, PharmD**
Clinical Instructor, Department of Pharmacy, School of Pharmacy, Virginia Commonwealth University, Richmond, Virginia

**Lawrence J. Cohen, PharmD, BCPP, FASHP, FCCP**
Professor, Department of Pharmacotherapy, College of Pharmacy, Washington State University; Assistant Director for Psychopharmacology Research and Training, Washington Institute for Mental Health Research and Training, Spokane, Washington

**Jennifer Confer, PharmD, BCPS**
Critical Care Clinical Specialist, Cabell Huntington Hospital, Huntington, West Virginia; Clinical Assistant Professor, West Virginia University, Morgantown, West Virginia

**John R. Corboy, MD**
Professor, Department of Neurology, University of Colorado Denver School of Medicine, Aurora, Colorado

**Elizabeth A. Coyle, PharmD, FCCM, BCPS**
Clinical Associate Professor, University of Houston College of Pharmacy, Houston, Texas

**James D. Coyle, PharmD**
Associate Professor of Clinical Pharmacy and Clinical Family Medicine, College of Pharmacy and Department of Family Medicine, College of Medicine, Ohio State University; Director, Collaborative Antithrombotic Management Program, Rardin Family Practice Center, Columbus, Ohio

**Brian L. Crabtree, PharmD, BCPP**
Associate Professor of Pharmacy Practice, University of Mississippi School of Pharmacy; Clinical Associate Professor of Psychiatry, University of Mississippi Medical Center; Psychopharmacologist, Mississippi State Hospital, Jackson, Mississippi

**Nicole S. Culhane, PharmD, FCCP, BCPS**
Director of Experiential Education, Associate Professor, Clinical and Administrative Sciences, College of Notre Dame of Maryland, School of Pharmacy, Baltimore, Maryland

**Aaron Cumpston, PharmD**
Clinical Pharmacy Specialist—BMT/Hematological Malignancy Program, West Virginia University Hospitals, Morgantown, West Virginia

**Lisa E. Davis, PharmD, FCCP, BCPS, BCOP**
Associate Professor of Clinical Pharmacy, Department of Pharmacy Practice and Pharmacy Administration, Philadelphia College of Pharmacy, University of the Sciences in Philadelphia, Philadelphia, Pennsylvania

**Christopher M. Degenkolb, PharmD, BCPS**
Clinical Pharmacy Specialist, Internal Medicine, Richard L. Roudebush VA Medical Center, Indianapolis, Indiana

**Marcy T. DelMonte, PharmD**
Clinical Instructor, Eshelman School of Pharmacy, University of North Carolina, Chapel Hill, North Carolina

**Paulina Deming, PharmD**
Assistant Professor, University of New Mexico College of Pharmacy, Project ECHO Hepatitis C Community Clinic, Albuquerque, New Mexico

**Margarita V. DiVall, PharmD**
Associate Clinical Professor, School of Pharmacy, Bouvé College of Health Sciences, Northeastern University, Boston, Massachusetts

**Holly S. Divine, PharmD, CGP, CDE**
Associate Professor, Department of Pharmacy Practice and Science, University of Kentucky College of Pharmacy, Lexington, Kentucky

**Jennifer A. Donaldson, PharmD**
Clinical Pharmacist, Riley Hospital for Children; Adjunct Assistant Professor of Pharmacy Practice, Butler University; Affiliate Assistant Professor of Clinical Pharmacy, Purdue University, Indianapolis, Indiana

**Victor G. Dostrow, MD**
Clinical Associate Professor, Department of Neurology, University of Mississippi School of Medicine; Adjunct Associate Professor, University of Mississippi School of Pharmacy, Jackson, Mississippi

**Scott R. Drab, PharmD, CDE, BC-ADM**
Assistant Professor of Pharmacy and Therapeutics, University of Pittsburgh School of Pharmacy; Director, University Diabetes Care Associates, Pittsburgh, Pennsylvania

**Michael D. Egeberg, PharmD**
Clinical Research Fellow—Neurology, University of Colorado Denver School of Pharmacy, Aurora, Colorado

**Sharon M. Erdman, PharmD**
Clinical Associate Professor of Pharmacy Practice, Purdue University College of Pharmacy; Infectious Diseases Clinical Pharmacist, Wishard Health Services, Indianapolis, Indiana

**Brian L. Erstad, PharmD, FCCP, FCCM, FASHP**
Professor, Department of Pharmacy Practice and Science, University of Arizona College of Pharmacy, Tucson, Arizona

**John S. Esterly, PharmD, BCPS**
Assistant Professor, Pharmacy Practice, Chicago State University College of Pharmacy; Infectious Diseases Pharmacist, Northwestern Memorial Hospital, Chicago, Illinois

**Jeffery D. Evans, PharmD**
Assistant Professor of Pharmacy Practice, University of Louisiana College of Pharmacy; Gratis Assistant Professor of Family Medicine and Comprehensive Care, Louisiana State University Health Science Center-Shreveport College of Medicine, Shreveport, Louisiana

**Patrick J. Fahey, MD**
Professor of Family Medicine, Department of Family Medicine, The Ohio State University College of Medicine, Columbus, Ohio

**Virginia H. Fleming, PharmD**
Clinical Assistant Professor, Department of Clinical and Administrative Pharmacy, University of Georgia College of Pharmacy, Athens, Georgia

**Michelle Fravel, PharmD, BCPS**
Assistant Clinical Professor, Department of Pharmacy Practice and Science, University of Iowa College of Pharmacy, Iowa City, Iowa

**Allan D. Friedman, MD, MPH**
Professor and Chair, Division of General Pediatrics, Virginia Commonwealth University, Richmond, Virginia

**Michelle D. Furler, BSc Pharm, PhD**
Pharmacist, Kingston, Ontario, Canada

**William R. Garnett, PharmD, FCCP, FAPHA**
Professor of Pharmacy and Neurology, Virginia Commonwealth University, Medical College of Virginia, Richmond, Virginia

**Sharon B.S. Gatewood, PharmD**
Assistant Professor, Department of Pharmacy, School of Pharmacy, Virginia Commonwealth University, Richmond, Virginia

**Amanda Geist, PharmD**
Clinical Assistant Professor, West Virginia University School of Pharmacy; Clinical Pharmacy Specialist, Pediatric Intensive Care Unit, Charleston Area Medical Center Women and Children's Hospital, Charleston, West Virginia

**Jane Gervasio, PharmD, BCNSP, FCCP**
Vice Chair and Associate Professor of Pharmacy Practice, Butler University College of Pharmacy and Health Science; Nutrition Support Clinical Pharmacist, Clarian Health Partners, Indianapolis, Indiana

**Michael J. Gonyeau, BPharm, PharmD, BCPS**
Associate Clinical Professor, Northeastern University School of Pharmacy; Internal Medicine Clinical Pharmacist, Brigham and Women's Hospital, Boston, Massachusetts

**Jean-Venable "Kelly" R. Goode, PharmD, BCPS, FAPhA, FCCP**
Professor and Director, Community Pharmacy Practice and Residency Programs, Department of Pharmacotherapy and Outcomes Science, School of Pharmacy, Virginia Commonwealth University, Richmond, Virginia

**Wayne P. Gulliver, MD**
Professor of Medicine and Dermatology, Chair, Discipline of Medicine, Faculty of Medicine, Memorial University of Newfoundland, St. John's, Newfoundland, Canada

**John G. Gums, PharmD, FCCP**
Professor of Pharmacy and Medicine; Associate Chair, Departments of Pharmacotherapy and Translational Research and Community Health and Family Medicine; Associate Chair for Clinical Programs, University of Florida, Gainesville, Florida

**Deanne L. Hall, PharmD, CDE**
Assistant Professor, Department of Pharmacy and Therapeutics, School of Pharmacy, University of Pittsburgh, Pittsburgh, Pennsylvania

**Larissa N. Hall, PharmD, BCPS**
Assistant Professor, Department of Pharmacy Practice, Bill Gatton College of Pharmacy, East Tennessee State University, Johnson City, Tennessee

**Shawn R. Hansen, PharmD**
Clinical Lead Pharmacist, Cardiology and Internal Medicine, Ministry Saint Joseph's Hospital, Marshfield, Wisconsin; Clinical Instructor, University of Wisconsin School of Pharmacy, Madison, Wisconsin

**Deborah A. Hass, PharmD, BCOP**
Assistant Professor, Midwestern University Chicago College of Pharmacy; Hematology/Oncology Clinical Pharmacist, Rush University Hospital, Chicago, Illinois

**Keith A. Hecht, PharmD, BCOP**
Clinical Associate Professor of Pharmacy Practice, Clinical Pharmacy Specialist, Hematology/Oncology, Southern Illinois University School of Pharmacy, Edwardsville, Illinois

**Brian A. Hemstreet, PharmD, BCPS**
Department of Clinical Pharmacy, University of Colorado Denver School of Pharmacy, Aurora, Colorado

**Richard N. Herrier, PharmD, FAPhA, CAPT, USPHS (Ret)**
Clinical Professor, Department of Pharmacy Practice and Science, College of Pharmacy, University of Arizona, Tucson, Arizona

**Catherine A. Heyneman-Cashmore, PharmD, MS, ANP, FASCP**
Associate Professor of Pharmacy Practice, Idaho State University College of Pharmacy, Pocatello, Idaho

**Lisa M. Holle, PharmD, BCOP**
Director, Medical Writing, Syntaxx Communications, Inc; Instructional Assistant, Department of Pharmacy Practice, University of Connecticut School of Pharmacy, Storrs, Connecticut

**Michael R. Holowatyj, PharmD, BCPS**

Assistant Professor of Pharmacy Practice, Butler University College of Pharmacy and Health Sciences; Clinical Pharmacist, Internal Medicine, St. Vincent Health, Indianapolis, Indiana

**Denise L. Howrie, PharmD**

Associate Professor of Pharmacy and Pediatrics, Schools of Pharmacy and Medicine, University of Pittsburgh; Clinical Pharmacy Specialist, Hematology–Oncology, Children's Hospital of Pittsburgh of UPMC, Pittsburgh, Pennsylvania

**Timothy J. Ives, PharmD, MPH**

Professor of Pharmacy and Medicine, Eshelman School of Pharmacy, University of North Carolina, Chapel Hill, North Carolina

**Carrie L. Johnson, PharmD, CDE**

Assistant Professor, Department of Pharmacy Practice and Science, University of Kentucky College of Pharmacy, Lexington, Kentucky

**Leticia K. Jones, PharmD, BCPP**

Assistant Professor of Pharmacy Practice, College of Pharmacy and Health Sciences, Butler University, Indianapolis, Indiana; Clinical Pharmacy Specialist, Psychiatry, Logansport State Hospital, Logansport, Indiana

**Laura L. Jung, BS Pharm, PharmD**

Syntaxx Communications, Inc, Duluth, Georgia

**Michael D. Katz, PharmD**

Associate Professor, Department of Pharmacy Practice and Science, University of Arizona College of Pharmacy, Tucson, Arizona

**Michael B. Kays, PharmD, FCCP**

Associate Professor, Department of Pharmacy Practice, Purdue University College of Pharmacy, West Lafayette, Indiana

**Tien T. Kiat-Winarko, PharmD, BSC**

Clinical Assistant Professor of Ophthalmology, Department of Ophthalmology, University of Southern California Keck School of Medicine, Los Angeles, California

**Patrick J. Kiel, PharmD, BCPS, BCOP**

Clinical Pharmacy Specialist, Hematology/Stem Cell Transplant, Indiana University Simon Cancer Center, Indianapolis, Indiana

**Cynthia K. Kirkwood, PharmD, BCPP**

Associate Professor and Vice Chair for Education, Department of Pharmacotherapy and Outcome Science, School of Pharmacy, Virginia Commonwealth University, Richmond, Virginia

**Joseph J. Kishel, PharmD**

Clinical Scientific Director, Cubist Pharmaceuticals, Inc, Lexington, Massachusetts

**Julie C. Kissack, PharmD, BCPP**

Professor and Chair, Department of Pharmacy Practice, College of Pharmacy, Harding University, Searcy, Arkansas

**Jonathan M. Kline, PharmD, CACP, BCPS**

Clinical Assistant Professor, Department of Clinical Pharmacy, Eastern Division, School of Pharmacy, West Virginia University, Martinsburg, West Virginia

**Julia M. Koehler, PharmD, FCCP**

Associate Professor and Chair, Department of Pharmacy Practice, Butler University College of Pharmacy and Health Sciences; Clinical Pharmacist in Family Medicine, Methodist Hospital and the Indiana University-Methodist Family Practice Center, Clarian Health Partners, Indianapolis, Indiana

**Cynthia P. Koh-Knox, PharmD, RPh**

Clinical Associate Professor, Pharmacy Practice, Purdue University School of Pharmacy and Pharmaceutical Sciences, West Lafayette, Indiana

**Michael D. Kraft, PharmD, BCNSP**

Clinical Associate Professor, University of Michigan College of Pharmacy; Clinical Coordinator, University of Michigan Health System, Ann Arbor, Michigan

**Connie Kraus, PharmD, BCPS**

Clinical Professor and Director of the Office of Global Health, School of Pharmacy, University of Wisconsin School of Pharmacy, Madison, Wisconsin

**Poh Gin Kwa, MD, FRCP**

Clinical Assistant Professor, Faculty of Medicine, Memorial University of Newfoundland; Pediatrician, Eastern Health, St. John's, Newfoundland and Labrador, Canada

**Ninh M. La-Beck, PharmD**

Department of Pharmacotherapy and Experimental Therapies, UNC Eshelman School of Pharmacy, University of North Carolina at Chapel Hill, Chapel Hill, North Carolina

**Rebecca M. Law, PharmD**

Associate Professor, School of Pharmacy and Faculty of Medicine, Memorial University of Newfoundland, St. John's, Newfoundland and Labrador, Canada

**W. Greg Leader, PharmD†**

Interim Dean and Professor of Clinical Pharmacy Practice, College of Pharmacy, University of Louisiana, Monroe, Louisiana

**Mary W.L. Lee, PharmD, BCPS, FCCP**

Vice President and Chief Academic Officer, Pharmacy and Health Science Education, Midwestern University, Downers Grove, Illinois

**Cara Liday, PharmD, BCPS, CDE**

Associate Professor, Department of Pharmacy Practice and Administrative Sciences, Idaho State University; Clinical Pharmacist, Intermountain Medical Clinic, Pocatello, Idaho

**John L. Lock, PharmD, BCPS**

Adult Infectious Disease Clinical Specialist, St. Vincent Health, Indianapolis, Indiana

**Kristen L. Longstreth, PharmD, BCPS**

Clinical Pharmacy Specialist, Internal Medicine, St. Elizabeth Health Center, Youngstown, Ohio; Assistant Professor of Pharmacy Practice, Northwestern Ohio University College of Pharmacy, Rootstown, Ohio

**Sherry Luedtke, PharmD**

Associate Professor, Pharmacy Practice, Texas Tech University Health Sciences Center, School of Pharmacy, Amarillo, Texas

---

†Deceased.

**Amy M. Lugo, PharmD, BCPS, BC-ADM**
Clinical Pharmacy Specialist, Department of Defense Pharmacoeconomic Center, Fort Sam Houston, San Antonio, Texas

**Cheen T. Lum, PharmD, BCPP**
Clinical Pharmacist, Behavioral Care Services, Community Hospital North, Indianapolis, Indiana

**Robert MacLaren, BSc, PharmD, FCCM, FCCP**
Associate Professor, Department of Clinical Pharmacy, University of Colorado School of Pharmacy, Aurora, Colorado

**Carrie Maffeo, PharmD, BCPS, CDE**
Director, Health Education Center, Assistant Professor of Pharmacy Practice, Butler University College of Pharmacy and Health Sciences, Indianapolis, Indiana

**Erik D. Maki, PharmD, BCPS**
Assistant Professor, Drake University College of Pharmacy and Health Sciences, Des Moines, Iowa

**Robert M. Malone, PharmD, CDE, CPP**
Clinical Associate Professor of Medicine, School of Medicine; Adjunct Associate Professor of Pharmacy, Eshelman School of Pharmacy, University of North Carolina at Chapel Hill, Chapel Hill, North Carolina

**Margery H. Mark, MD**
Associate Professor of Neurology and Psychiatry, UMDNJ-Robert Wood Johnson Medical School, New Brunswick, New Jersey

**Joel C. Marrs, PharmD, BCPS, CLS**
Assistant Professor, Department of Clinical Pharmacy, School of Pharmacy, University of Colorado, Aurora, Colorado

**Jay L. Martello, PharmD**
Clinical Assistant Professor, West Virginia University Hospitals and School of Pharmacy, Morgantown, West Virginia

**Lena M. Maynor, PharmD, BCPS**
Clinical Assistant Professor, Department of Clinical Pharmacy, West Virginia University School of Pharmacy, Morgantown, West Virginia

**James W. McAuley, PhD, FAPhA**
Associate Professor of Pharmacy Practice and Neurology, Director of Teaching and Learning, Division of Pharmacy Practice and Administration, The Ohio State University College of Pharmacy, Columbus, Ohio

**William McGhee, PharmD**
Clinical Pharmacy Specialist, Children's Hospital of Pittsburgh; Adjunct Clinical Assistant Professor, University of Pittsburgh School of Pharmacy, Pittsburgh, Pennsylvania

**Cydney E. McQueen, PharmD**
Clinical Associate Professor, Pharmacy Practice and Administration, University of Missouri-Kansas City School of Pharmacy, Kansas City, Missouri

**Sarah T. Melton, PharmD, BCPP, CGP**
Director of Addiction Outreach, Associate Professor of Pharmacy Practice, Appalachian College of Pharmacy, Oakwood, Virginia

**Renee-Claude Mercier, PharmD, BCPS**
Associate Professor of Pharmacy and Medicine, University of New Mexico College of Pharmacy, Albuquerque, New Mexico

**Brice Labruzzo Mohundro, PharmD**
Assistant Professor of Clinical Pharmacy Practice, College of Pharmacy, University of Louisiana at Monroe, Baton Rouge Campus; Clinical Pharmacist, Baton Rouge General Family Medicine Residency Program, Baton Rouge, Louisiana

**Scott Mueller, PharmD, BCPS**
Department of Clinical Pharmacy, University of Colorado School of Pharmacy, University of Colorado Hospital, Aurora, Colorado

**Pamela J. Murray, MD, MHP**
Professor and Vice Chair, Department of Pediatrics, General Pediatrics and Adolescent Medicine, West Virginia University Health Sciences Center, Morgantown, West Virginia

**James J. Nawarskas, PharmD, BCPS**
Associate Professor of Pharmacy, University of New Mexico College of Pharmacy, Albuquerque, New Mexico

**Michael Newton, PharmD, BCOP**
Clinical Assistant Professor, West Virginia University School of Pharmacy; West Virginia University Mary Babb Randolph Cancer, Center, Morgantown, West Virginia

**Sarah A. Nisly, PharmD, BCPS**
Assistant Professor, Department of Pharmacy Practice, Butler University College of Pharmacy and Health Sciences; Clinical Pharmacy Specialist, Internal Medicine, Clarian Health Partners, Methodist Hospital, Indianapolis, Indiana

**Kimberly J. Novak, PharmD, BCPS**
Clinical Assistant Professor, Ohio State University College of Pharmacy; Clinical Pharmacy Specialist—Pediatric Pulmonary Medicine, Nationwide Children's Hospital, Columbus, Ohio

**Kelly Nystrom, PharmD, BCOP**
Associate Professor of Pharmacy Practice, Creighton University School of Pharmacy and Health Professions; Clinical Pharmacist, Alegent Health Bergan Mercy Medical Center, Omaha, Nebraska

**Cindy L. O'Bryant, PharmD, BCOP**
Associate Professor, University of Colorado School of Pharmacy; Clinical Oncology Pharmacist, University of Colorado Cancer Center, Aurora, Colorado

**Dannielle O'Donnell, PharmD, BCPS**
Adjunct Clinical Assistant Professor, Division of Pharmacy Practice, College of Pharmacy, University of Texas at Austin, Austin, Texas

**Christine O'Neil**
Professor, Pharmacy Practice, Duquesne University Mylan School of Pharmacy, Pittsburgh, Pennsylvania

**Megan Ose, PharmD**
Clinical Pharmacist, Ministry Saint Joseph's Hospital, Marshfield, Wisconsin

**Carol A. Ott, PharmD, BCPP**
Clinical Assistant Professor of Pharmacy Practice, Purdue University College of Pharmacy, West Lafayette, Indiana

**Manjunath P. Pai, PharmD**
Associate Professor, Department of Pharmacy Practice, Albany College of Pharmacy and Health Sciences, Albany, New York

**Laura M. Panko, MD**
Visiting Instructor of Pediatrics, Children's Hospital of Pittsburgh of UPMC, University of Pittsburgh School of Medicine, Pittsburgh, Pennsylvania

**Emily Farthing Papineau, PharmD, BCPS**
Assistant Professor of Pharmacy Practice, Butler University College of Pharmacy and Health Sciences; Clinical Pharmacy Specialist, Community Family Medicine Center, Indianapolis, Indiana

**Dennis Parker, Jr., PharmD**
Assistant Professor, Eugene Applebaum College of Pharmacy, Wayne State University; Clinical Specialist, NeuroCritical Care, Detroit Receiving Hospital, Detroit, Michigan

**Robert B. Parker, PharmD, FCCP**
Professor, Department of Clinical Pharmacy, College of Pharmacy, University of Tennessee, Memphis, Tennessee

**Beth Bryles Phillips, PharmD, FCCP, BCPS**
Clinical Associate Professor, University of Georgia College of Pharmacy, Athens, Georgia

**Bradley G. Phillips, PharmD, BCPS, FCCP**
Millikan-Reeve Professor and Head, Department of Clinical and Administrative Pharmacy, University of Georgia College of Pharmacy, Athens, Georgia

**Amy M. Pick, PharmD, BCOP**
Assistant Professor of Pharmacy Practice, Creighton University School of Pharmacy and Health Professions, Omaha, Nebraska

**Melissa Pleva, PharmD, BCPS, BCNSP**
Clinical Pharmacist, Surgical Critical Care/Nutrition Support, University of Michigan Hospitals and Health Centers; Adjunct Clinical Instructor, University of Michigan College of Pharmacy, Ann Arbor, Michigan

**Charles D. Ponte, PharmD, BC-ADM, BCPS, CDE, CPE, DPNAP, FAPhA, FASHP, FCCP**
Professor of Clinical Pharmacy and Family Medicine, Robert C. Byrd Health Sciences Center, Schools of Pharmacy and Medicine, West Virginia University, Morgantown, West Virginia

**Darin C. Ramsey, PharmD, BCPS**
Assistant Professor of Pharmacy Practice, Butler University College of Pharmacy and Health Sciences; Clinical Pharmacy Specialist, Primary Care, Richard L. Roudebush VA Medical Center, Indianapolis, Indiana

**Randolph E. Regal, BS, PharmD**
Clinical Associate Professor, Adult Internal Medicine, University of Michigan Hospitals and College of Pharmacy, Ann Arbor, Michigan

**Denise H. Rhoney, PharmD, FCCP, FCCM**
Associate Professor, Eugene Applebaum College of Pharmacy and Health Sciences, Wayne State University, Detroit, Michigan

**Michelle L. Rockey, PharmD, BCOP**
Clinical Pharmacist, Oncology; Director, Oncology Pharmacy Residency Program, University of Cincinnati Health-University Hospital; Adjunct Assistant Professor of Pharmacy Practice, James L. Winkle College of Pharmacy, University of Cincinnati, Cincinnati, Ohio

**Juliana V.F. Roddy, PharmD, BCOP**
Specialty Practice Pharmacist, Hematology/Oncology, Arthur G. James Cancer Hospital and Richard J. Solove Research Institute, Ohio State University, Columbus, Ohio

**Keith A. Rodvold, PharmD, FCCP, FIDSA**
Professor of Pharmacy Practice and Medicine, Colleges of Pharmacy and Medicine, University of Illinois at Chicago, Chicago, Illinois

**Kelly C. Rogers, PharmD**
Associate Professor, Department of Clinical Pharmacy, University of Tennessee College of Pharmacy; Cardiology Clinical Specialist, VA Medical Center, Memphis, Tennessee

**Carol J. Rollins, MS, RD, PharmD, BCNSP**
Coordinator, Nutrition Support Team and Interim Assistant Director, Clinical Pharmacy, University Medical Center; Clinical Associate Professor, Department of Pharmacy Practice and Science, College of Pharmacy, University of Arizona, Tucson, Arizona

**Rochelle Rubin, PharmD**
Assistant Professor, Midwestern University Chicago College of Pharmacy; Clinical Pharmacist, Dreyer Medical Clinic, Downers Grove, Illinois

**Amy W. Rudenko, PharmD**
Assistant Professor, Department of Pharmacotherapy and Outcomes Science, School of Pharmacy, Virginia Commonwealth University, Richmond, Virginia

**Laura Ruekert, PharmD, BCPP**
Assistant Professor of Pharmacy Practice, Butler University College of Pharmacy and Health Sciences; Clinical Pharmacist Specialist, Psychiatry, Community Hospital North, Indianapolis, Indiana

**Laurajo Ryan, PharmD, MSc, BCPS, CDE**
Clinical Assistant Professor, University of Texas at Austin College of Pharmacy, University of Texas Health Science Center; Pharmacotherapy Education Research Center, Department of Medicine, San Antonio, Texas

**Elizabeth J. Scharman, PharmD, DABAT, BCPS, FAACT**
Director, West Virginia Poison Center; Professor, Department of Clinical Pharmacy, West Virginia University School of Pharmacy, Charleston, West Virginia

**Marc H. Scheetz, PharmD, Makes, BCPS**
Assistant Professor of Pharmacy Practice, Midwestern University Chicago College of Pharmacy, Downers Grove, Illinois; Infectious Diseases Pharmacist, Northwestern Memorial Hospital, Chicago, Illinois

**Kristine S. Schonder, PharmD**
Assistant Professor, Department of Pharmacy and Therapeutics, University of Pittsburgh School of Pharmacy; Clinical Pharmacist, Thomas E. Starzl Transplantation Institute, Pittsburgh, Pennsylvania

**Terry L. Schwinghammer, PharmD, FCCP, FASHP, FAPhA, BCPS**
Professor and Chair, Department of Clinical Pharmacy, West Virginia University School of Pharmacy, Morgantown, West Virginia

**Christopher M. Scott, PharmD, BCPS, FCCM**
Director of Pharmacy Services, Wishard Health Services, Indianapolis, Indiana

**Mollie Ashe Scott, PharmD, BCPS, CPP**
Director of Pharmacotherapy, Mountain Area Health Education Center, Asheville, North Carolina; Clinical Associate Professor, University of North Carolina Eshelman School of Pharmacy and UNC School of Medicine, Chapel Hill, North Carolina

**Brian C. Sedam, PharmD, BCPS**
Clinical Pharmacist, Family Medicine, Jackson Memorial Hospital, Miami, Florida

**Roohollah Sharifi, MD, FACS**
Professor, Department of Surgery, University of Illinois at Chicago College of Medicine, Chicago, Illinois

**Amy Heck Sheehan, PharmD**
Associate Professor, Department of Pharmacy Practice, Purdue University College of Pharmacy, Indianapolis, Indiana

**Justin J. Sherman, MCS, PharmD**
Associate Professor, Department of Pharmacy Practice, School of Pharmacy, University of Mississippi, Jackson, Mississippi

**Brigitte L. Sicat, PharmD, BCPS, BC-ADM**
Assistant Professor, Department of Pharmacotherapy and Outcomes Science, Virginia Commonwealth University School of Pharmacy, Richmond, Virginia

**Carrie A. Sincak, PharmD, BCPS**
Associate Professor and Vice Chair, Acute Care, Department of Pharmacy Practice, Midwestern University Chicago College of Pharmacy, Downers Grove, Illinois

**Douglas Slain, PharmD, BCPS, FCCP**
Associate Professor, Infectious Diseases Clinical Specialist, School of Pharmacy, West Virginia University, Morgantown, West Virginia

**Curtis L. Smith, PharmD**
Professor, Department of Pharmacy Practice, College of Pharmacy, Ferris State University; Clinical Pharmacy Specialist, Sparrow Health System, Lansing, Michigan

**Steven M. Smith, PharmD**
Postdoctoral Fellow, Departments of Pharmacotherapy and Translational Research and Community Health and Family Medicine, Colleges of Pharmacy and Medicine, University of Florida, Gainesville, Florida

**Denise R. Sokos, PharmD, BCPS**
Adjunct Assistant Professor, University of Pittsburgh School of Pharmacy, Pittsburgh, Pennsylvania

**Suellyn J. Sorensen, PharmD, BCPS**
Clinical Pharmacist, Infectious Diseases and Clinical Pharmacy Manager, Health Director, Midwest AIDS Training and Education Center, Indiana University Hospital, Indianapolis, Indiana

**Mikayla L. Spangler, PharmD, BCPS**
Assistant Professor, Department of Pharmacy Practice and Family Medicine, Creighton University, Omaha, Nebraska

**William J. Spruill, PharmD, FCCP, FASHP**
Professor, Department of Clinical and Administrative Pharmacy, College of Pharmacy, University of Georgia, Athens, Georgia

**Tracy L. Sprunger, PharmD, BCPS**
Assistant Professor, Pharmacy Practice, Butler College of Pharmacy and Health Sciences, Indianapolis, Indiana

**Mary K. Stamatakis, PharmD**
Associate Dean for Academic Affairs and Educational Innovation, Associate Professor of Clinical Pharmacy, West Virginia University School of Pharmacy, Morgantown, West Virginia

**Jennifer L. Swank, PharmD, BCOP**
Clinical Pharmacist, Medical Oncology, H. Lee Moffitt Cancer Center, Tampa, Florida

**Lynne M. Sylvia, PharmD**
Clinical Pharmacy Specialist, Department of Pharmacy, Tufts Medical Center; Adjunct Clinical Professor, Northeastern University, School of Pharmacy, Boston, Massachusetts

**Colleen M. Terriff, PharmD, BCPS**
Clinical Associate Professor, Department of Pharmacotherapy, Washington State University College of Pharmacy, Deaconess Medical Center, Spokane, Washington

**James E. Tisdale, PharmD**
Professor, College of Pharmacy, Purdue University; Adjunct Professor, School of Medicine, Indiana University, Indianapolis, Indiana

**Trent G. Towne, PharmD, BCPS**
Assistant Professor of Clinical Pharmacy, Department of Pharmacy Practice/Pharmacy Administration, Philadelphia College of Pharmacy, Philadelphia, Pennsylvania

**Sharon M. Tramonte, PharmD**
Clinical Pharmacist, San Antonio State Supported Living Center, Texas Department of Aging and Disability Services; Clinical Assistant Professor, Department of Pharmacology, University of Texas Health Sciences Center at San Antonio, San Antonio, Texas

**Tate N. Trujillo, PharmD, BCPS, FCCM**
Director of Pharmacy, Methodist Hospital, Clarian Health, Indianapolis, Indiana

**Kevin M. Tuohy, PharmD, BCPS**
Assistant Professor of Pharmacy Practice, Butler University College of Pharmacy and Health Sciences; Clinical Pharmacy Specialist, Internal Medicine, Methodist Hospital of Indiana, Indianapolis, Indiana

**Joseph P. Vande Griend, PharmD, BCPS**
Assistant Professor, University of Colorado at Denver School of Pharmacy, Aurora, Colorado

**Ashley H. Vincent, PharmD, BCPS**
Assistant Clinical Professor, Department of Pharmacy Practice, College of Pharmacy, Purdue University; Clinical Pharmacy Specialist, Ambulatory Care, Clarian Health Partners, Inc, Indianapolis, Indiana

**J. Michael Vozniak, PharmD, BCOP**
Oncology Clinical Pharmacy Specialist, Hospital of the University of Pennsylvania, Philadelphia, Pennsylvania

**William E. Wade, PharmD, FASHP, FCCP**
Professor, Department of Clinical and Administrative Pharmacy, College of Pharmacy, University of Georgia, Athens, Georgia

**Mary L. Wagner, PharmD, MS**
Associate Professor, Department of Pharmacy Practice, Ernest Mario School of Pharmacy, Rutgers, State University of New Jersey, Piscataway, New Jersey

**Christine M. Walko, PharmD, BCOP**
Assistant Professor, Division of Pharmacotherapy and Experimental Therapeutics, Institute of Pharmacogenomics and Individualized Therapy, University of North Carolina Eshelman School of Pharmacy, Chapel Hill, North Carolina

**Mark D. Walsh, PharmD**
Translational Oncology and Drug Development Fellow, University of North Carolina Eshelman School of Pharmacy, Chapel Hill, North Carolina

**Alison M. Walton, PharmD, BCPS**
Assistant Professor of Pharmacy Practice, Butler University College of Pharmacy and Health Sciences; Primary Care Clinical Pharmacy Specialist, St. Vincent Health, Indianapolis, Indiana

**Zachary A. Weber, PharmD, BCPS**
Assistant Clinical Professor, Department of Pharmacy Practice, Purdue University School of Pharmacy and Pharmaceutical Sciences, Indianapolis, Indiana

**Laurie M. Whalin, BS, PharmD**
Clinical Manager, Pharmacy Department, New Hanover Regional Medical Center, Wilmington, North Carolina

**Jon P. Wietholter, PharmD, BCPS**
Clinical Assistant Professor, West Virginia University School of Pharmacy, Morgantown, West Virginia; Internal Medicine Clinical Pharmacist, Cabell Huntington Hospital, Huntington, West Virginia

**Craig Williams, PharmD, FNLA**
Associate Professor of Pharmacy Practice, Oregon State University College of Pharmacy and Oregon Health Sciences University Medical Center, Portland, Oregon

**Susan R. Winkler, PharmD, BCPS**
Professor and Chair, Department of Pharmacy Practice, Midwestern University Chicago College of Pharmacy, Downers Grove, Illinois

**Mark J. Wrobel, PharmD**
Clinical Assistant Professor, Department of Pharmacy Practice, State University of New York at Buffalo School of Pharmacy and Pharmaceutical Sciences, Buffalo, New York

**Nancy S. Yunker, PharmD, BCPS**
Assistant Professor, Department of Pharmacotherapy and Outcome Science, Virginia Commonwealth University School of Pharmacy, Medical College of Virginia Campus, Richmond, Virginia

**William C. Zamboni, PharmD, PhD**
Associate Professor, Director of UNC GLP Bioanalytical Facility, Director of Translational Oncology and Drug Development Initiative Lab, UNC Eshelman School of Pharmacy, UNC Lineberger Comprehensive Cancer Center, University of North Carolina, Chapel Hill, North Carolina

**Dustin G. Zeigler, PharmD, BCPS**
Clinical Pharmacist, Moses Cone Memorial Hospital, Greensboro, North Carolina

# PREFACE

The purpose of the *Pharmacotherapy Casebook* is to help students in the health professions and practicing clinicians develop and refine the skills required to identify and resolve drug therapy problems by using case studies. Case studies can actively involve students in the learning process, engender self-confidence, and promote the development of skills in independent self-study, problem analysis, decision making, oral communication, and teamwork. Patient case studies can also be used as the focal point of discussions about pathophysiology, medicinal chemistry, pharmacology, and the pharmacotherapy of individual diseases. By integrating the biomedical and pharmaceutical sciences with pharmacotherapeutics, case studies can help students appreciate the relevance and importance of a sound scientific foundation in preparation for practice.

The patient cases in this book are intended to complement the scientific information presented in the eighth edition of *Pharmacotherapy: A Pathophysiologic Approach*. This edition of the casebook contains 157 unique patient cases, 42 more than the first edition. The case chapters are organized into organ system sections that correspond to those of the *Pharmacotherapy* textbook. Students should read the relevant textbook chapter to become thoroughly familiar with the pathophysiology and pharmacotherapy of each disease state before attempting to make "decisions" about the care of patients described in this casebook. The *Pharmacotherapy* textbook, *Casebook*, and other useful learning resources are also available on *AccessPharmacy.com* (subscription required). By using these realistic cases to practice creating, defending, and implementing pharmacotherapeutic care plans, students can begin to develop the skills and self-confidence that will be necessary to make the real decisions required in professional practice.

The knowledge and clinical experience required to answer the questions associated with each patient presentation vary from case to case. Some cases deal with a single disease state, whereas others have multiple diseases and drug therapy problems. As a guide for instructors, each case is identified as being one of three complexity levels; this classification system is described in more detail in Chapter 1.

The eighth edition has a new introductory section called Principles of Patient-Focused Therapy that contains 11 chapters.

Chapter 1 describes the format of case presentations and the means by which students and instructors can maximize the usefulness of the casebook. A systematic approach is consistently applied to each case. The steps involved in this approach include:

1. Identifying real or potential drug therapy problems;
2. Determining the desired therapeutic outcome(s);
3. Evaluating therapeutic alternatives;
4. Designing an optimal individualized pharmacotherapeutic plan;
5. Developing methods to evaluate the therapeutic outcome;
6. Providing patient education;
7. Communicating and implementing the pharmacotherapeutic plan.

In Chapter 2, the philosophy and implementation of active learning strategies are presented. This chapter sets the tone for the casebook by describing how these approaches can enhance student learning. The chapter offers a number of useful active learning strategies for instructors and provides advice to students on how to maximize their learning opportunities in active learning environments.

Chapter 3 presents an efficient method of patient counseling developed by the Indian Health Service. The information can be used as the basis for simulated counseling sessions related to the patient cases.

Chapter 4 describes the pharmaceutical care process and delineates the steps necessary to create pharmaceutical care plans that can help to ensure that the drug-related needs of patients are met. A blank care plan form is included at the end of the chapter. Students should be encouraged to practice using this form (or a similar one) when completing the case studies in this casebook.

Chapter 5 describes two methods for documenting clinical interventions and communicating recommendations to other health care providers. These include the traditional SOAP note and the more pharmacy-specific FARM note. Student preparation of SOAP or FARM notes for the patient cases in this book will be excellent practice for future documentation in actual patient records.

New to this edition are three case-based chapters in the section "Foundation Issues" related to pediatrics, geriatrics, and palliative care. The patient cases on clinical toxicology (acetaminophen overdose) and emergency preparedness (cyanide exposure, chemical exposure) were also moved to this section of the casebook.

An important change in this edition is a redesigned section on Complementary and Alternative Therapies (Section 19). The editors gratefully acknowledge Cydney McQueen, PharmD, for the quality of her work on this section. The section contains patient vignettes that are directly related to patient cases that were presented earlier in this casebook. Each scenario involves the potential use of one or more dietary supplements. Additional follow-up questions are then asked to help the reader gain the scientific and clinical knowledge required to provide an evidence-based recommendation about use of the supplement in that particular patient. Fourteen different dietary supplements are discussed: garlic, fish oil (omega-3 fatty acids), *Ginkgo biloba*, St. John's wort, black cohosh, soy, α-lipoic acid, coenzyme Q10 (Co-Q10), kava, American ginseng, saw palmetto, pygeum, butterbur, and feverfew.

It should be emphasized that the focus of classroom discussions about these cases should be on the process of solving patient problems as much as it is on finding the actual answers to the questions themselves. Isolated scientific facts learned today may be obsolete or incorrect tomorrow. Health care providers who can identify patient problems and solve them using a reasoned approach will be able to adapt to the continual evolution in the body of scientific knowledge and contribute in a meaningful way to improving the quality of patients' lives.

We are grateful for the broad acceptance that previous editions of the casebook have received. In particular, it has been adopted by many schools of pharmacy and nurse practitioner programs. It has also been used in institutional staff development efforts and by individual pharmacists wishing to upgrade their pharmacotherapy skills. It is our hope that this new edition will be even more valuable in assisting health care practitioners to meet society's need for safe and effective drug therapy.

# ACKNOWLEDGMENTS

We would like to thank the 197 case and chapter authors from 87 schools of pharmacy, health care systems, and other institutions in the United States and Canada who contributed their scholarly efforts to this casebook. We especially appreciate their diligence in meeting deadlines, adhering to the unique format of the casebook, and providing the most current drug therapy information available. The next generation of health care practitioners will benefit from the willingness of these clinicians to share their expertise.

We would also like to thank all of the individuals at McGraw-Hill Professional whose cooperation, advice, and commitment were instrumental in maintaining the high standards of this publication: in particular, James Shanahan, Michael Weitz, Peter Boyle, and Laura Libretti. We appreciate the meticulous attention to composition detail provided by Thomson Digital. Finally, we are grateful to our spouses, Donna Schwinghammer and Brad Bowman, for their understanding, support, and encouragement during the preparation of this new edition.

This edition is dedicated to the memory of W. Greg Leader, PharmD—author, colleague, and friend.

*Terry L. Schwinghammer, PharmD, FCCP, FASHP, FAPhA, BCPS*
*Julia M. Koehler, PharmD, FCCP*

SECTION 1
# PRINCIPLES OF PATIENT-FOCUSED THERAPY

CHAPTER 1

# Introduction: How to Use This Casebook

TERRY L. SCHWINGHAMMER, PHARMD, FCCP, FASHP, FAPHA, BCPS

## USING CASE STUDIES TO ENHANCE STUDENT LEARNING

The case method is used primarily to develop the skills of self-learning, critical thinking, problem identification, and decision making. When case studies from this casebook are used in the curricula of the health care professions or for independent study by practitioners, the focus of attention should be on learning the process of solving drug therapy problems, rather than simply on finding the scientific answers to the problems themselves. Students do learn scientific facts during the resolution of case study problems, but they usually learn more of them from their own independent study and from discussions with their peers than they do from the instructor. Working on subsequent cases with similar problems reinforces information recall. Traditional programs in the health care professions that rely heavily on the lecture format tend to concentrate on scientific content and the rote memorization of facts rather than the development of higher-order thinking skills.

Case studies in the health sciences provide the personal history of an individual patient and information about one or more health problems that must be solved. The learner's job is to work through the facts of the case, analyze the available data, gather more information, develop hypotheses, consider possible solutions, arrive at the optimal solution, and consider the consequences of the learner's decisions.[1] The role of the teacher is to serve as coach and facilitator rather than as the source of "the answer." In fact, in many cases there is more than one acceptable answer to a given question. Because instructors do not necessarily need to possess the correct answer, they need not be experts in the field being discussed. Rather, the students become teachers and learn from each other through thoughtful discussion of the case.

## FORMAT OF THE CASEBOOK

### BACKGROUND READING

The patient cases in this casebook should be used as the focal point for independent self-learning by individual students and for in-class problem-solving discussions by student groups and their instructors. If meaningful learning and discussion are to occur, students must come to discussion sessions prepared to discuss the case material rationally, to propose reasonable solutions, and to defend their pharmacotherapeutic plans. This requires a strong commitment to independent self-study prior to the session. The cases in this book were prepared to correspond with the scientific information contained in the eighth edition of *Pharmacotherapy: A Pathophysiologic Approach*.[2] For this reason, thorough understanding of the corresponding textbook chapter is recommended as the principal method of student preparation. The online learning center *AccessPharmacy* (www.AccessPharmacy.com, subscription required) contains the *Pharmacotherapy* textbook and many other resources that will be beneficial in answering case questions. The cases in the casebook can also be used with the textbook *Pharmacotherapy Principles & Practice*, 2nd ed.,[3] or other therapeutics texts. Primary literature should also be consulted as necessary to supplement textbook readings.

Most of the cases in the casebook represent common diseases likely to be encountered by generalist practitioners. As a result, not all of the *Pharmacotherapy* textbook chapters have an associated patient case in the casebook. On the other hand, some of the textbook chapters that discuss multiple disease entities have several corresponding cases in the casebook.

### LEVELS OF CASE COMPLEXITY

Each case is identified at the top of the first page as being one of the three levels of complexity. Instructors may use this classification system to select cases for discussion that correspond to the experience level of the student learners. These levels are defined as follows:

*Level I*—An uncomplicated case; only a single textbook chapter is required to complete the case questions. Little prior knowledge of the disease state or clinical experience is needed.

*Level II*—An intermediate-level case; several textbook chapters or other reference sources may be required to complete the case. Prior clinical experience may be helpful in resolving all of the issues presented.

*Level III*—A complicated case; multiple textbook chapters, additional readings, and substantial clinical experience may be required to solve all of the patient's drug therapy problems.

### USING LEARNING OBJECTIVES

Learning objectives are included at the beginning of each case for student reflection. The focus of these outcomes is on achieving competency in the clinical arena, not simply on learning isolated scientific facts. These items reflect some of the knowledge, skills, and abilities that students should possess after reading the textbook chapter, studying the case, preparing a pharmacotherapeutic plan, and defending their recommendations.

The learning objectives provided are meant to serve as a starting point to stimulate student thinking, but they are not intended to be all-inclusive. In fact, students should also generate their own personal ability outcome statements and learning objectives for each case. By so doing, students take greater control of their own learning, which serves to improve personal motivation and the desire to learn.

## PATIENT PRESENTATION

The format and organization of cases reflect those usually seen in actual clinical settings. The patient's medical history and physical examination findings are provided in the following standardized outline format.

### CHIEF COMPLAINT

The chief complaint is a brief statement of the reason why the patient consulted the physician, stated in the patient's own words. In order to convey the patient's symptoms accurately, medical terms and diagnoses are generally not used. The appropriate medical terminology is used after an appropriate evaluation (i.e., medical history, physical examination, laboratory and other testing) leads to a medical diagnosis.

### HPI

The history of present illness is a more complete description of the patient's symptom(s). Usually included in the HPI are:

- Date of onset
- Precise location
- Nature of onset, severity, and duration
- Presence of exacerbations and remissions
- Effect of any treatment given
- Relationship to other symptoms, bodily functions, or activities (e.g., activity, meals)
- Degree of interference with daily activities

### PMH

The past medical history includes serious illnesses, surgical procedures, and injuries the patient has experienced previously. Minor complaints (e.g., influenza, colds) are usually omitted unless they might have a bearing on the current medical situation.

### FH

The family history includes the age and health of parents, siblings, and children. For deceased relatives, the age and cause of death are recorded. In particular, heritable diseases and those with a hereditary tendency are noted (e.g., diabetes mellitus, cardiovascular disease, malignancy, rheumatoid arthritis, obesity).

### SH

The social history includes the social characteristics of the patient as well as the environmental factors and behaviors that may contribute to the development of disease. Items that may be listed are the patient's marital status; number of children; educational background; occupation; physical activity; hobbies; dietary habits; and use of tobacco, alcohol, or other drugs.

### MEDS

The medication history should include an accurate record of the patient's current use of prescription medications, nonprescription products, and dietary supplements. Because there are thousands of prescription and nonprescription products available, it is important to obtain a complete medication history that includes the names, doses, routes of administration, schedules, and duration of therapy for all medications, including dietary supplements and other alternative therapies.

### ALL

Allergies to drugs, food, pets, and environmental factors (e.g., grass, dust, pollen) are recorded. An accurate description of the reaction that occurred should also be included. Care should be taken to distinguish adverse drug effects ("upset stomach") from true allergies ("hives").

### ROS

In the review of systems, the examiner questions the patient about the presence of symptoms related to each body system. In many cases, only the pertinent positive and negative findings are recorded. In a complete ROS, body systems are generally listed starting from the head and working toward the feet and may include the skin, head, eyes, ears, nose, mouth and throat, neck, cardiovascular, respiratory, gastrointestinal, genitourinary, endocrine, musculoskeletal, and neuropsychiatric systems. The purpose of the ROS is to evaluate the status of each body system and to prevent the omission of pertinent information. Information that was included in the HPI is generally not repeated in the ROS.

### PHYSICAL EXAMINATION

The exact procedures performed during the physical examination vary depending on the chief complaint and the patient's medical history. In some practice settings, only a limited and focused physical examination is performed. In psychiatric practice, greater emphasis is usually placed on the type and severity of the patient's symptoms than on physical findings. A suitable physical assessment textbook should be consulted for the specific procedures that may be conducted for each body system. The general sections for the PE are outlined as follows:

Gen (general appearance).

VS (vital signs)—blood pressure, pulse, respiratory rate, and temperature. In hospital settings, the presence and severity of pain is included as "the fifth vital sign." For ease of use and consistency in this casebook, weight and height are included in the vital signs section, but they are not technically considered to be vital signs.

Skin (integumentary).

HEENT (head, eyes, ears, nose, and throat).

Lungs/Thorax (pulmonary).

Cor or CV (cardiovascular).

Abd (abdomen).

Genit/Rect (genitalia/rectal).

MS/Ext (musculoskeletal and extremities).

Neuro (neurologic).

## LABS

The results of laboratory tests are included with most cases in this casebook. **Appendix A** contains a number of commonly used conversion factors and anthropometric information that will be helpful in solving many case answers. Normal (reference) ranges for the laboratory tests used throughout the casebook are included in **Appendix B**. Values are provided in both traditional units and SI units (*le système International d'Unités*). The normal range for a given laboratory test is generally determined from a representative sample of the general population. The upper and lower limits of the range usually encompass two standard deviations from the population mean, which includes a range within which about 95% of healthy persons would fall. The term *normal range* may therefore be misleading, because a test result may be abnormal for a given individual even if it falls within the "normal" range. Furthermore, given the statistical methods used to calculate the range, about 1 in 20 normal, healthy individuals may have a value for a test that lies outside the range. For these reasons, the term *reference range* is preferred over normal range. Reference ranges differ among laboratories, so the values given in Appendix B should be considered only as a general guide. Institution-specific reference ranges should be used in actual clinical settings.

All of the cases include some physical examination and laboratory findings that are within normal limits. For example, a description of the cardiovascular examination may include a statement that the point of maximal impulse is at the fifth intercostal space; laboratory evaluation may include a serum sodium level of 140 mEq/L. The presentation of actual findings (rather than simple statements that the heart examination and the serum sodium were normal) reflects what will be seen in actual clinical practice. More importantly, listing both normal and abnormal findings requires students to carefully assess the complete database and identify the pertinent positive and negative findings for themselves. A valuable portion of the learning process is lost if students are only provided with findings that are abnormal and are known to be associated with the disease being discussed.

The patients described in this casebook have fictitious names in order to humanize the situations and to encourage students to remember that they will one day be caring for patients, not treating disease states. However, in the actual clinical setting, patient confidentiality is of utmost importance, and real patient names should not be used during group discussions in patient care areas unless absolutely necessary. To develop student sensitivity to this issue, instructors may wish to avoid using these fictitious patient names during class discussions. In this casebook, patient names are usually given only in the initial presentation; they are seldom used in subsequent questions or other portions of the case.

The issues of race, ethnicity, and gender also deserve thoughtful consideration. The traditional format for case presentations usually begins with a description of the patient's age, race, and gender, as in: "The patient is a 65-year-old white male. . . ." Single-word racial labels such as "black" or "white" are actually of limited value in many cases and may actually be misleading in some instances.[4] For this reason, racial descriptors are usually excluded from the opening line of each presentation. When ethnicity is pertinent to the case, this information is presented in the social history or physical examination. Patients in this casebook are referred to as men or women, rather than males or females, to promote sensitivity to human dignity.

The patient cases in this casebook include medical abbreviations and drug brand names, just as medical records do in actual practice. Although these customs are sometimes the source of clinical problems, the intent of their inclusion is to make the cases as realistic as possible. **Appendix C** lists the medical abbreviations used in the casebook. This list is limited to commonly accepted abbreviations; thousands more exist, which makes it difficult for the novice practitioner to efficiently assess patient databases. Most health care institutions have an approved list of accepted abbreviations; these lists should be consulted in practice to facilitate one's understanding and to avoid using abbreviations in the medical record that are not on the official approved list. Appendix C also lists abbreviations and designations that should be avoided. Given the immense human toll resulting from medical errors, this section should be considered "must" reading for all students.

The casebook also contains some photographs of commercial drug products. These illustrations are provided as examples only and are not intended to imply endorsement of those particular products.

## PHARMACEUTICAL CARE AND DRUG THERAPY PROBLEMS

Modern drug therapy plays a crucial role in improving the health of people by enhancing quality of life and extending life expectancy. The advent of biotechnology has led to the introduction of unique compounds for the prevention and treatment of disease that were unimagined just a decade ago. Each year the US Food and Drug Administration approves approximately two dozen new drug products that contain active substances that have never before been marketed in the United States. Although the cost of new therapeutic agents has received intense scrutiny in recent years, drug therapy actually accounts for a relatively small proportion of overall health care expenditures. Appropriate drug therapy is cost-effective and may actually serve to reduce total expenditures by decreasing the need for surgery, preventing hospital admissions, and shortening hospital stays.

Several studies have indicated that improper use of prescription medications is a frequent and serious problem. Based on a decision analytic model, one study estimated that the cost of drug-related morbidity and mortality was more than $177 billion in 2000. Hospital admissions accounted for almost 70% ($121.5 billion) of total costs; long-term care admissions were responsible for 18% of costs ($32.8 billion).[5] In 1999, the Institute of Medicine estimated that 7,000 patients die each year from medication errors that occur both within and outside hospitals. A societal need for better use of medications clearly exists. Widespread implementation of pharmaceutical care has the potential to positively impact this situation by the design, implementation, and monitoring of rational therapeutic plans to produce defined outcomes that improve the quality of patients' lives.[6]

The mission of the pharmacy profession is to render pharmaceutical care. Schools of pharmacy have implemented innovative instructional strategies and curricula that have an increased emphasis on patient-centered care, including more experiential training, especially in ambulatory settings. Many programs are structured to promote self-directed learning, develop problem-solving and communication skills, and instill the desire for lifelong learning.

In its broadest sense, pharmaceutical care involves the identification, resolution, and prevention of actual or potential drug therapy problems. A drug therapy problem has been defined as "any undesirable event experienced by a patient which involves, or is suspected to involve, drug therapy and that interferes with achieving the desired goals of therapy."[6] Seven distinct types of drug therapy problems have been identified that may potentially lead to an undesirable event that has physiologic, psychological, social, or economic ramifications.[7] These problems can be placed into four categories that include:

1. *Inappropriate indication* for drug use:
   a. The patient requires additional drug therapy.
   b. The patient is taking unnecessary drug therapy.

2. *Ineffective* drug therapy:
    a. The patient is taking a drug that is not effective for his or her situation.
    b. The medication dose is too low.
3. *Unsafe* drug therapy:
    a. The patient is experiencing an adverse drug reaction.
    b. The medication dose is too high.
4. *Inappropriate adherence* or *compliance*:
    a. The patient is unable or unwilling to take the medication as prescribed.

These drug therapy problems are discussed in more detail in **Chapter 4** of the casebook. Because this casebook is intended to be used in conjunction with the *Pharmacotherapy* textbook, one of its purposes is to serve as a tool for learning about the pharmacotherapy of disease states. For this reason, the primary problem to be identified and addressed for most of the patients in the casebook is the need for additional drug treatment for a specific medical indication (**problem 1.a.**, above). Other actual or potential drug therapy problems may coexist during the initial presentation or may develop during the clinical course of the disease.

## PATIENT-FOCUSED APPROACH TO CASE PROBLEMS

In this casebook, each patient presentation is followed by a set of patient-centered questions that are similar for each case. These questions are applied consistently from case to case to demonstrate that a systematic patient care process can be successfully applied regardless of the underlying disease state(s). The questions are designed to enable students to identify and resolve problems related to pharmacotherapy. They help students recognize what they know and what they do not know, thereby guiding them in determining what information must be learned to satisfactorily resolve the patient's problems.[8] A description of each of the steps involved in solving drug therapy problems is included in the following paragraphs.

### 1. Identification of real or potential drug therapy problems

The first step in the patient-focused approach is to collect pertinent patient information, interpret it properly, and determine whether drug therapy problems exist. Some authors prefer to divide this process into two or more separate steps because of the difficulty that inexperienced students may have in performing these complex tasks simultaneously.[9] This step is analogous to documenting the subjective and objective patient findings in the Subjective, Objective, Assessment, Plan (SOAP) format. It is important to differentiate the process of identifying the patient's drug therapy problems from making a disease-related medical diagnosis. In fact, the medical diagnosis is known for most patients seen by pharmacists. However, pharmacists must be capable of assessing the patient's database to determine whether drug therapy problems exist that warrant a change in drug therapy. In the case of preexisting chronic diseases, such as asthma or rheumatoid arthritis, one must be able to assess information that may indicate a change in severity of the disease. This process involves reviewing the patient's symptoms, the signs of disease present on physical examination, and the results of laboratory and other diagnostic tests. Some of the cases require the student to develop complete patient problem lists. Potential sources for this information in actual practice include the patient or his or her advocate, the patient's physician or other health care professionals, and the patient's medical chart or other records.

After the drug therapy problems are identified, the clinician should determine which ones are amenable to pharmacotherapy. Alternatively, one must also consider whether any of the problems could have been caused by drug therapy. In some cases (both in the casebook and in real life), not all of the information needed to make these decisions is available. In that situation, providing precise recommendations for obtaining additional information needed to satisfactorily assess the patient's problems can be a valuable contribution to the patient's care.

### 2. Determination of the desired therapeutic outcome

After pertinent patient-specific information has been gathered and the patient's drug therapy problems have been identified, the next step is to define the specific goals of pharmacotherapy. The primary therapeutic outcomes include:

- Cure of disease (e.g., bacterial infection)
- Reduction or elimination of symptoms (e.g., pain from cancer)
- Arresting or slowing of the progression of disease (e.g., rheumatoid arthritis, HIV infection)
- Preventing a disease or symptom (e.g., coronary heart disease)

Other important outcomes of pharmacotherapy include:

- Not complicating or aggravating other existing disease states
- Avoiding or minimizing adverse effects of treatment
- Providing cost-effective therapy
- Maintaining the patient's quality of life

Sources of information for this step may include the patient or his or her advocate, the patient's physician or other health care professionals, medical records, and the *Pharmacotherapy* textbook or other literature references.

### 3. Determination of therapeutic alternatives

After the intended outcome has been defined, attention can be directed toward identifying the types of treatments that might be beneficial in achieving that outcome. The clinician should ensure that all feasible pharmacotherapeutic alternatives available for achieving the predefined therapeutic outcome(s) are considered before choosing a particular therapeutic regimen. Nondrug therapies (e.g., diet, exercise, psychotherapy) that might be useful should be included in the list of therapeutic alternatives when appropriate. Useful sources of information on therapeutic alternatives include the *Pharmacotherapy* textbook and other references, as well as the clinical experience of the health care provider and other involved health care professionals.

There has been a resurgence of interest in dietary supplements and other alternative therapies in recent years. The public spends billions of dollars each year on supplements to treat diseases for which there is little scientific evidence of efficacy. Furthermore, some products are hazardous, and others may interact with a patient's prescription medications or aggravate concurrent disease states. On the other hand, scientific evidence of efficacy does exist for some dietary supplements (e.g., glucosamine for osteoarthritis). Health care providers must be knowledgeable about these products and prepared to answer patient questions regarding their efficacy and safety. The casebook contains a separate section devoted to this important topic (**Section 19**). This portion of the casebook contains a number of fictitious patient vignettes that are directly related to patient cases that were presented earlier in this casebook. Each scenario involves the potential use of one or more dietary supplements by the patient. Additional follow-up questions are then asked to help the reader gain the scientific and clinical knowledge required to provide an evidence-based recommendation about use of the supplement in that particular patient. Fourteen different dietary supplements are included in this section: garlic, fish oil (omega-3 fatty acids), *Ginkgo biloba*, St. John's wort, black cohosh, soy, alpha-lipoic acid, coenzyme Q10 (Co-Q10), kava, American ginseng, saw palmetto, pygeum, butterbur, and feverfew.

## 4. Design of an optimal individualized pharmacotherapeutic plan

The purpose of this step is to determine the drug, dosage form, dose, schedule, and duration of therapy that are best suited for a given patient. Individual patient characteristics should be taken into consideration when weighing the risks and benefits of each available therapeutic alternative. For example, an asthma patient who requires new drug therapy for hypertension might better tolerate treatment with a thiazide diuretic rather than a β-blocker. On the other hand, a hypertensive patient with gout may be better served by use of a β-blocker rather than by use of a thiazide diuretic.

Students should state the reasons for avoiding specific drugs in their therapeutic plans. Some potential reasons for drug avoidance include drug allergy, drug–drug or drug–disease interactions, patient age, renal or hepatic impairment, adverse effects, poor compliance, pregnancy, and high treatment cost.

The specific dose selected may depend on the indication for the drug. For example, the dose of aspirin used to treat rheumatoid arthritis is much higher than that used to prevent myocardial infarction. The likelihood of adherence with the regimen and patient tolerance come into play in the selection of dosage forms. The economic, psychosocial, and ethical factors that are applicable to the patient should also be given due consideration in designing the pharmacotherapeutic regimen. An alternative plan should also be in place that would be appropriate if the initial therapy fails or cannot be used.

## 5. Identification of parameters to evaluate the outcome

Students must identify the clinical and laboratory parameters necessary to assess the therapy for achievement of the desired therapeutic outcome and for detection and prevention of adverse effects. The outcome parameters selected should be specific, measurable, achievable, directly related to the therapeutic goals, and have a defined endpoint. As a means of remembering these points, the acronym SMART has been used (*S*pecific, *M*easurable, *A*chievable, *R*elated, and *T*ime bound). If the goal is to cure bacterial pneumonia, students should outline the subjective and objective clinical parameters (e.g., relief of chest discomfort, cough, and fever), laboratory tests (e.g., normalization of white blood cell count and differential), and other procedures (e.g., resolution of infiltrate on chest x-ray) that provide sufficient evidence of bacterial eradication and clinical cure of the disease. The intervals at which data should be collected are dependent on the outcome parameters selected and should be established prospectively. It should be noted that expensive or invasive procedures may not be repeated after the initial diagnosis is made.

Adverse effect parameters must also be well defined and measurable. For example, it is insufficient to state that one will monitor for potential drug-induced "blood dyscrasias." Rather, one should identify the likely specific hematologic abnormality (e.g., anemia, leukopenia, or thrombocytopenia) and outline a prospective schedule for obtaining the appropriate parameters (e.g., obtain monthly hemoglobin/hematocrit, white blood cell count, or platelet count).

Monitoring for adverse events should be directed toward preventing or identifying serious adverse effects that have a reasonable likelihood of occurrence. For example, it is not cost-effective to obtain periodic liver function tests in all patients taking a drug that causes mild abnormalities in liver injury tests only rarely, such as omeprazole. On the other hand, serious patient harm may be averted by outlining a specific screening schedule for drugs associated more frequently with hepatic abnormalities, such as methotrexate for rheumatoid arthritis.

## 6. Provision of patient education

The concept of pharmaceutical care is based on the existence of a covenantal relationship between the patient and the provider of care. Patients are our partners in health care, and our efforts may be for naught without their informed participation in the process. For chronic diseases such as diabetes mellitus, hypertension, and asthma, patients may have a greater role in managing their diseases than do health care professionals. Self-care is becoming widespread as increasing numbers of prescription medications receive over-the-counter status. For these reasons, patients must be provided with sufficient information to enhance compliance, ensure successful therapy, and minimize adverse effects. **Chapter 3** describes patient interview techniques that can be used efficiently to determine the patient's level of knowledge. Additional information can then be provided as necessary to fill in knowledge gaps. In the questions posed with individual cases, students are asked to provide the kind of information that should be given to the patient who has limited knowledge of his or her disease. Under the Omnibus Budget Reconciliation Act (OBRA) of 1990, for patients who accept the offer of counseling, pharmacists should consider including the following items:

- Name and description of the medication (which may include the indication)
- Dosage, dosage form, route of administration, and duration of therapy
- Special directions or procedures for preparation, administration, and use
- Common and severe adverse effects, interactions, and contraindications (with the action required should they occur)
- Techniques for self-monitoring
- Proper storage
- Prescription refill information
- Action to be taken in the event of missed doses

Instructors may wish to have simulated patient-interviewing sessions for new and refill prescriptions during case discussions to practice medication education skills. Factual information should be provided as concisely as possible to enhance memory retention. One source for information on individual drugs is *Detailed Drug Information for the Consumer™—Drug Information in Lay Language*. Available through *Micromedex Healthcare Series*, this subscription-based electronic product provides drug information written for patients at the 12th grade literacy level.[10] MedlinePlus is the National Institute of Health's free Web site for consumers that contains information on prescription and nonprescription drugs, dietary supplements, medical conditions, wellness, diagnostic tests, and other medical information.[11]

## 7. Communication and implementation of the pharmacotherapeutic plan

The most well-conceived plan is worthless if it languishes without implementation because of inadequate communication with prescribers or other health care providers. Permanent, written documentation of significant recommendations in the medical record is important to ensure accurate communication among practitioners. Oral communication alone can be misinterpreted or transferred inaccurately to others. This is especially true because there are many drugs that sound alike when spoken but that have different therapeutic uses.

The SOAP format has been used by clinicians for many years to assess patient problems and to communicate findings and plans in the medical record. However, writing SOAP notes may not be the optimal process for learning to solve drug therapy problems because several important steps taken by experienced clinicians are not always apparent and may be overlooked. For example, the precise therapeutic outcome desired is often unstated in SOAP notes, leaving others to presume what the desired treatment goals are. Health care professionals using the SOAP format also commonly move directly from an assessment of the patient (diagnosis) to outlining a diagnostic or therapeutic plan, without necessarily conveying whether careful consideration has been given to all available feasible diagnostic or therapeutic alternatives. The plan itself as outlined in SOAP notes may also give short shrift to the monitoring parameters that are required to ensure successful therapy and to detect and prevent adverse drug effects. Finally, there is often little suggestion provided as to the treatment information that should be conveyed to the most important individual involved: the patient. If SOAP notes are used for documenting drug therapy problems, consideration should be given to including each of these components.

In **Chapter 5** of this casebook, the FARM note (*F*indings, *A*ssessment, *R*ecommendations, *M*onitoring) is presented as a useful method of consistently documenting therapeutic recommendations and implementing plans.[12] This method can be used by students as an alternative to the SOAP note to practice communicating pharmacotherapeutic plans to other members of the health care team. Although preparation of written communication notes is not included in written form with each set of case questions, instructors are encouraged to include the composition of a SOAP or FARM note as one of the requirements for successfully completing each case study assignment.

In addition to communicating with other health care professionals, practitioners of pharmaceutical care must also develop a personal record of each patient's drug therapy problems and the health care provider's plan for resolving them, interventions made, and actual therapeutic outcomes achieved. A pharmaceutical care plan is a well-conceived and scientifically sound method of documenting these activities. **Chapter 4** of this casebook discusses the philosophy of care planning and describes their creation and use. A sample care plan document is included in that chapter for use by students as they work through the cases in this book.

## CLINICAL COURSE

The process of pharmaceutical care entails an assessment of the patient's progress in order to ensure achievement of the desired therapeutic outcomes. A description of the patient's clinical course is included with many of the cases in this book to reflect this process. Some cases follow the progression of the patient's disease over months to years and include both inpatient and outpatient treatment. Follow-up questions directed toward ongoing evaluation and problem solving are included after presentation of the clinical course.

## SELF-STUDY ASSIGNMENTS

Each case concludes with several study assignments related to the patient case or the disease state that may be used as independent study projects for students to complete outside class. These assignments generally require students to obtain additional information that is not contained in the corresponding *Pharmacotherapy* textbook chapter.

## LITERATURE REFERENCES AND INTERNET SITES

Selected literature references that are specific to the case at hand are included at the end of the cases. References selected for inclusion were those thought to be useful to students for answering the questions posed. The citations are generally limited to major clinical trials or meta-analyses, authoritative review articles, and clinical practice guidelines. The *Pharmacotherapy* textbook contains a more comprehensive list of references pertinent to each disease state.

Some cases list Internet sites as sources of drug therapy information. The sites listed are recognized as authoritative sources of information, such as the Food and Drug Administration (*www.fda.gov*) and the Centers for Disease Control and Prevention (*www.cdc.gov*). Students should be advised to be wary of information posted on the Internet that is not from highly regarded health care organizations or publications. The uniform resource locators (URLs) for Internet sites sometimes change, and it is possible that not all sites listed in the casebook will remain available for viewing.

## DEVELOPING ANSWERS TO CASE QUESTIONS

The use of case studies for independent learning and in-class discussion may be unfamiliar to many students. For this reason, students may find it difficult at first to devise complete answers to the case questions. **Appendix D** contains the answers to three cases in order to demonstrate how case responses might be prepared and presented. The authors of the cases contributed the recommended answers provided in the appendix, but they should not be considered the sole "right" answer. Thoughtful students who have prepared well for the discussion sessions may arrive at additional or alternative answers that are also appropriate.

With diligent self-study, practice, and the guidance of instructors, students will gradually acquire the knowledge, skills, and self-confidence to develop and implement pharmaceutical care plans for their own future patients. The goal of the casebook is to help students progress along this path of lifelong learning.

## REFERENCES

1. Herreid CF. Case studies in science: a novel method of science education. J Coll Sci Teach 1994;23:221–229.
2. DiPiro JT, Talbert RL, Yee GC, et al., eds. Pharmacotherapy: A Pathophysiologic Approach, 8th ed. New York, McGraw-Hill, 2011.
3. Chisholm-Burns MA, Schwinghammer TL, Wells BG, Malone PM, Kolesar JM, DiPiro JT. Pharmacotherapy Principles & Practice, 2nd ed. New York, McGraw-Hill, 2010.
4. Caldwell SH, Popenoe R. Perceptions and misperceptions of skin color. Ann Intern Med 1995;122:614–617.
5. Ernst FR, Grizzle AJ. Drug-related morbidity and mortality: updating the cost-of-illness model. J Am Pharm Assoc 2001;41:192–199.
6. Cipolle RJ, Strand LM, Morley PC. Pharmaceutical Care Practice: The Clinician's Guide, 2nd ed. New York, McGraw-Hill, 2004.
7. Strand LM, Morley PC, Cipolle RJ, et al. Drug-related problems: their structure and function. Drug Intell Clin Pharm 1990;24: 1093–1097.

8. Delafuente JC, Munyer TO, Angaran DM, et al. A problem-solving active-learning course in pharmacotherapy. Am J Pharm Educ 1994;58:61–64.
9. Winslade N. Large-group problem-based learning: a revision from traditional to pharmaceutical care-based therapeutics. Am J Pharm Educ 1994;58:64–73.
10. Detailed Drug Information for the Consumer. Micromedex® Healthcare Series [Internet database]. Greenwood Village, CO, Thomson Reuters (Healthcare) Inc. 2010. Updated periodically. Available at: *http://www.micromedex.com/products/ddic/*. Accessed Aug 17, 2010.
11. MedlinePlus: Trusted Health Information for You. A Service of the U.S. National Library of Medicine. Bethesda, MD, National Institutes of Health, 2010. Available at: *http://www.nlm.nih.gov/medlineplus/*. Accessed Aug 17, 2010.
12. Canaday BR, Yarborough PC. Documenting pharmaceutical care: creating a standard. Ann Pharmacother 1994;28:1292–1296.

CHAPTER 2

# Active Learning Strategies

BRIGITTE L. SICAT, PHARMD, BCPS
GRETCHEN M. BROPHY, PHARMD, BCPS, FCCP, FCCM
CYNTHIA K. KIRKWOOD, PHARMD, BCPP

Health care providers today are faced with situations daily that require the use of effective problem solving, critical thinking, and communication skills. Therefore, providing students with knowledge alone is insufficient to equip them with the tools needed to be valuable contributors to patient care. Students must understand that it is imperative to provide more than just drug information, which is readily obtained by using personal digital devices (e.g., PDAs), computers, and other references in today's world. They must be able to evaluate, analyze, and synthesize information and apply their knowledge to prevent and resolve drug-related problems. As clinicians, they will be required to call upon previous experiences with similar situations, ask appropriate questions, integrate information, and develop action plans.

Students who finish their formal training in health care must recognize that learning is a lifelong process. Scores of new drugs are approved every year, drug use practices change, and innovative research alters the way that diseases are treated. Students can develop these skills, attitudes, and abilities by using case studies. Actively developing recommendations and drug therapy plans in oral and written formats can increase student confidence in addressing drug-related problems in practice.

Warren identified several traits that prepare students for future careers: analytic thinking, polite assertiveness, tolerance, communication skills, understanding of one's own physical well-being, and the ability to continue to teach oneself after graduation.[1] To prepare students to become health care professionals who are essential members of the health care team, many health care educators are using active learning strategies in the classroom.[2,3]

## ACTIVE LEARNING VERSUS TRADITIONAL TEACHING

Active learning has numerous definitions, and various methods are described in the educational literature. Simply put, ***active learning is the process of having students engage in activities that require reflection on ideas and how students use them.***[3] Most proponents agree that compared with passively receiving lectures, active engagement of students promotes deeper learning, enhances critical thinking skills, provides feedback to students and instructors, and promotes social development. Learning is reinforced when students actually apply their knowledge to new situations.[3] Active learning is learner-focused.

In contrast, traditional teaching involves a teacher-centered approach. At the beginning of the course, students are given a massive course syllabus packet that contains "everything they need to know" for the semester. In class, the teacher lectures on a predetermined subject that does not require student preparation. Students are passive recipients of information, and the testing method is usually a written examination that employs a multiple-choice or short-answer format. With this method, students are tested primarily on their ability to recall isolated facts that the teacher has identified as being important. They do not learn to apply their knowledge to situations that they will ultimately encounter in practice. The reward is an external one (i.e., exam or course grade) that may or may not reflect a student's actual ability to use knowledge to improve patient care.

To teach students to be lifelong learners, it is essential to stimulate them to be inquisitive and actively involved with the learning that takes place in the classroom. This requires that teachers move away from more comfortable teaching methods and learn new techniques that will help students "learn to learn." In classes with active learning formats, students are involved in much more than listening. The transmission of information is deemphasized and replaced with the development of skills. Active learning shifts the control of learning from the teacher to the students; this provides an opportunity for students to become active participants in their own learning.

## ACTIVE LEARNING STRATEGIES

Teachers implement active learning exercises into classes in a variety of ways. Some of the active learning strategies give students the opportunity to pause and recall information, cooperate and collaborate in groups, solve problems, and generate questions.[4] More advanced methods include the use of simulation, role playing, debates, peer teaching, problem-based learning (PBL), case studies, and team-based learning.[5,6] Technology is increasingly used in active learning in numerous ways to maximize the use of class time for higher-order thinking tasks such as analysis, synthesis, and evaluation.[7–10] The following are examples of active learning strategies that involve students in the learning process.

### EXERCISES FOR INDIVIDUAL STUDENTS

These exercises can complement lectures and are easily implemented. A technique for assessing student understanding or reaction to material is to ask them to write a "minute paper" or "half-sheet response" to a question or issue raised in class.[11] Writing helps students identify knowledge deficits, clarify understanding of the material, and organize thoughts in a logical manner. One question might be, "What was the main point of today's class session?" or "What was the muddiest point of today's class session?" Students can also be asked to finish a sentence beginning with, "I was surprised that ...." Tests and quizzes are effective tools to help students review reading assignments or class presentations. Quizzes given at the beginning of class on pre-class readings help stimulate students to review information they did not know and listen for clarification during class lectures. Quizzes can also be administered several times during class (e.g., using electronic audience response systems [ARS]) and may or may not be graded. ARS can help instructors quickly assess prior knowledge, identify and address misunderstandings or misperceptions, and stimulate discussion.[8] Quizzes at the end of the class session allow students to use their problem-solving skills by applying what they have just learned to a patient case or problem. The "quick-thinks" technique allows students to quickly process the information they have learned (e.g., complete a sentence presented by the teacher on the treatment of a disease state, contrast drug treatments for a specific patient, draw conclusions on the best treatment strategies for a disease state, identify and correct errors in a case).[12]

## QUESTIONS AND ANSWERS

Active learning strategies that involve questions and answers can increase student involvement and comprehension. "Wait time" is a method whereby the instructor poses a question and asks students to think about it.[13] After a brief pause, the instructor can ask for volunteers or randomly call on a student to answer the question. This wait time forces every student to think about the question rather than relying on those students who immediately raise their hands to answer questions. With the "fish bowl" method, students are asked to write questions related to the course material for discussion at the end of class or at the beginning of the next class session.[13] Instructors then draw several questions out of the "fish bowl" to discuss or ask the class to answer. In classes that use active learning, much of the learning will come from class discussion. However, many students may not pay attention to their classmates, but rather wait for instructors to either repeat or clarify what one of their classmates has said. To promote active listening, after one student has volunteered to answer a question, instructors could ask another student to summarize the first student's response.

## THINK–PAIR–SHARE

The "think–pair–share" exercise involves providing students with a question or problem to solve.[14] After working on the assignment individually (think) for 2–5 minutes, they discuss their ideas for 3–5 minutes with the student sitting next to them (pair). Finally, student pairs are chosen to share their ideas with the whole class (share). This method provides immediate feedback. The "shared paragraph" exercise requires students to write a paragraph at the end of class summarizing the major ideas that were presented.[5] The paragraph is then shared with a partner to clarify the material and receive feedback. The "pause procedure" is designed to enhance student comprehension and retention of material.[15] It involves 15- to 20-minute mini-lectures with 2- to 3-minute pauses for students to rework their notes, discuss the material with their peers for clarification, and develop questions.[16] This procedure is particularly useful after presenting a difficult concept and may help improve students' note-taking skills and ability to identify important learning points. It is also a useful method for classes that require retention of factual information.[5] Once students see the value in supplementing their own note-taking with others, they may continue this practice outside of class.

## PROBLEM-BASED LEARNING

Problem-solving skills can be developed during a class period by applying knowledge of pharmacotherapy to a patient case. Application reinforces the previously learned material and helps students understand the importance of the topic in a real-life situation. PBL is a teaching and learning method in which a problem is used as the stimulus for developing critical thinking and problem-solving skills for acquiring new knowledge. The process of PBL starts with the student identifying the problem in a case. The student spends time either alone or in a group exploring and analyzing the case and identifying learning resources needed to solve the problem. After acquiring the knowledge, the student applies it to solve the problem.[17] Small or large groups can be established for case discussions to help students develop communication skills, respect for other students' opinions, satisfaction for contributing to the discussion, and the ability to give and accept criticism.[17] Interactive PBL computer tools and the use of real patients also stimulate learning both outside and inside the classroom.[18,19] Computer technology can be used creatively in PBL cases as a tool for problem solving.[20]

## COOPERATIVE OR COLLABORATIVE LEARNING

Cooperative or collaborative learning strategies involve students in the generation of knowledge.[5] Students are randomly assigned to groups of four to six at the beginning of the school term. Several times during the term, each group is given a patient case and a group leader is selected. Each student in the group volunteers to work on a certain portion of the case. The case is discussed in class, and each member receives the same grade. After students have finished working in their small groups or during large group sessions, the teacher serves as a facilitator of the discussion rather than as a lecturer. The students actively participate in the identification and resolution of the problem. The integration of this technique helps with development of skills in decision making, conflict management, and communication.[4] Group discussions help students develop concepts from the material presented, clarify ideas, and develop new strategies for clinical problem solving. These skills are essential for lifelong learning and will be used by the students throughout their careers.

## TEAM-BASED LEARNING

Team-based learning is an instructional strategy for use during the entire semester. The course is structured around the activity of teams of five to seven students that apply course content, assess student learning on both individual and team levels, and use peer assessment. Teams are formed in the classroom, students are held accountable for individual and team work, assignments are applications of course content performed during class time, and students receive frequent, prompt feedback.[6,21,22]

## CASE STUDIES

Case studies are used by a number of professional schools to teach pharmacotherapy.[1,18,23–25] They are a written description of a real-life problem or situation. Only the facts are provided, usually in chronologic sequence similar to what would be encountered in a patient care setting. Many times, as in real life, the information given is incomplete, or important details are not available. When working through a case, the student must distinguish between relevant and irrelevant facts and become accustomed to the fact that there is no single "correct" answer. The use of cases actively involves the student in the analysis of facts and details of the case, selection of a solution to the problem, and defense of his or her solution through discussion of the case.[26] In case-based learning, students use their recall of previously learned information to solve clinical cases.[27]

During class, active participation is essential for the maximum learning benefit to be achieved. Because of their various backgrounds, students learn different perspectives when dealing with patient problems. Some general steps proposed by McDade[26] for students when preparing cases for class discussion include:

- Skim the text quickly to establish the broad issues of the case and the types of information presented for analysis.
- Reread the case very carefully, underlining key facts as you go.
- Note on scratch paper the key issues and problems. Next, go through the case again and sort out the relevant considerations and decisions for each problem.
- Prioritize problems and alternatives.
- Develop a set of recommendations to address the problems.
- Evaluate your decisions.

## ADVICE ON ACTIVE LEARNING FOR STUDENTS AND INSTRUCTORS

Active learning provides students with an opportunity to take a dynamic role in the learning process. Willing students, innovative teachers, and administrative support within the school are required for active learning to be successful.[27–28]

### ADVICE FOR STUDENTS

Students may have concerns about active learning. Some students may be accustomed to passively receiving information and feel uncomfortable with participating in the learning process. Taking initiative is the key to deriving the benefits of active learning. It is crucial to recognize the three largest squelchers of initiative: laziness, fear of change, and force of habit.[29]

***Prepare for class.*** Assigned readings and homework must be completed before class in order to use class time efficiently for questions that are not answered in other reference material. Time management is important. Use time between classes wisely, identify the times of day when you are most productive, and focus on the results rather than the time to complete an activity.[1] When reading assignments, take notes and summarize the information using tables or charts. Alternatively, make lists of questions from class or readings to discuss with your colleagues or faculty or try to answer them on your own.

***Seek to understand versus memorize.*** To develop appropriate therapeutic recommendations or answers to a question, you may have to look beyond the reading materials provided by the teacher. You may need to go back to review notes from previous courses or perform literature searches and use the library or Internet to retrieve additional information. It is important that you understand "why" and "how" and not just memorize "what." Memorizing results in short-term retention of knowledge, whereas understanding results in long-term retention and will enable you to better justify your clinical recommendations. In active learning, much of what you learn you will learn on your own. You will probably find that you read more, but you will gain understanding from reading. At the same time, you are developing a critical lifelong learning skill. Your reading will become more "depth processing" in which you focus on:

- The intent of the reading;
- Actively integrating what you read with previous parts of the text or previous courses;
- Using your own ability to make a logical construction;
- Thinking about the functional role of the different parts of an argument.

***During class, take an active role in the learning process.*** Be an active participant in class or group discussions; lively debates about pharmacotherapy issues allow more therapeutic options to be discussed.[30] Discussing material helps you to apply your knowledge, verbalize the medical and pharmacologic terminology, engage in active listening, think critically, and develop interpersonal skills. When working in groups, all members should participate in problem solving. Teaching others is an excellent way to learn the subject matter.[1] Listen carefully to and be respectful of the thoughts and opinions of classmates. Writing about a topic develops critical thinking, communication, and organization skills. Stopping to write allows you to reflect on the information you have just heard and reinforces learning. While taking notes in class, leave a wide margin on the left to write down questions that you generate later when reviewing the notes.[14] By talking about what you are learning, writing about it, relating it to previous patient cases, and applying it to the current case, you repeatedly manipulate the information until it becomes a part of you.

### ADVICE FOR INSTRUCTORS

Instructors may also have concerns about incorporating active learning strategies. They may feel as though their class is too large to accommodate active learning, have concerns that they will not be able to cover all the content or that it will take too much time to change their course, or even have fears that students may be resistant to active learning strategies. Some of the hesitation may lie in the belief that active learning is an alternative to lecture. Rather, active learning strategies can easily be incorporated into didactic lectures to enhance lectures. Several strategies can be used to increase the successful implementation of active learning strategies.

***Discuss course expectations.*** Take time to describe teaching, learning, and assessment methods and how students can be successful in the course. Help students to understand the benefits of active learning.[31]

***Consider slowly implementing a change in the classroom.*** To implement active learning strategies, teachers must overcome the anxiety that change often creates. Experiment with simple active learning methods (i.e., the pause technique) and slowly implement active learning methods.

***Consider techniques to maximize student discussion.*** Allowing students to discuss content in pairs or small groups before asking them to share their ideas with the entire class can help minimize student anxiety about engaging in classroom discussions. Use of a wireless microphone is helpful in encouraging student participation in large classrooms. Consider moving around the room during discussions, if possible, and make an effort to learn the names of all students.

***Take a stepwise approach.*** Learners become self-directed in stages, not in one single moment of transformation. Sequence activities and assignments that gradually develop all three stages: learning, intellectual development, and interpersonal skills.[32]

***Have a preconceived plan for how the learning session will go and stick to it.*** Determine what learning objectives you would like to achieve during the session. Consider developing a "schedule" for the learning session, estimating the time that will be spent on each active learning activity.

## USING THE CASEBOOK

The casebook was prepared to assist in the development of each student's understanding of a disease and its management as well as problem-solving skills. It is important for students to realize that learning and understanding the material is guided through problem solving. Students are encouraged to solve each of the cases individually or with others in a study group before discussion of the case and topic in class. These cases can be used as an active learning strategy by allowing time for students to work on the cases during class as an application exercise for TBL.[21] Teams can then report verbally on the questions and debate various treatment options. These exercises can be completed for a team grade.

## SUMMARY

The use of case studies and other active learning strategies will enhance the development of essential skills necessary to practice in any setting, including community, ambulatory care, primary care, health systems, long-term care, home health care, managed care, and the pharmaceutical industry. The role of the health care professional is constantly changing; thus, it is important for students to acquire the knowledge, skills, and attitudes to develop the lifetime skills required for continued learning. Teachers who incorporate active learning strategies into the classroom are facilitating the development of lifelong learners who will be able to adapt to change that occurs in their profession.

## REFERENCES

1. Warren G. Carpe Diem: A Student Guide to Active Learning. Landover, MD, University Press of America, 1996.
2. Brandt BF. Effective teaching and learning strategies. Pharmacotherapy 2000;20:307S–316S.
3. Michael J. Where's the evidence that active learning works? Adv Physiol Educ 2006;30:159–167.
4. Bonwell CC, Eison JA. Active Learning: Creating Excitement in the Classroom. Washington, DC, George Washington University, School of Education and Human Development, 1991. ASHE-ERIC Higher Education Report no. 1.
5. Shakarian DC. Beyond lecture: active learning strategies that work. JOPERD May–June 1995;21–24.
6. Michaelson LK, Knight AB, Fink LD. Team-Based Learning: A Transformative Use of Small Groups in College Teaching. Sterling, VA, Stylus Publishing, 2002.
7. Moore AH, Fowler SB, Watson CE. Active learning and technology: designing change for faculty, students, and institutions. EDUCAUSE Rev 2007;42:42–61.
8. Slain D, Abate M, Hodges BM, Stamatakis MK, Wolak S. An interactive response system to promote active learning in the doctor of pharmacy curriculum. Am J Pharm Educ 2004;68(5):1–9.
9. Blouin RA, Joyner PU, Pollack GM. Preparing for a renaissance in pharmacy education: the need, opportunity, and capacity for change. Am J Pharm Educ 2008;72(2):1–3.
10. Poirier TI, O'Neil CK. Use of web technology and active learning strategies in a quality assessment methods course. Am J Pharm Educ 2000;64:289–298.
11. McKeachie WJ. Teaching large classes (you can still get active learning!). In: McKeachie WJ, ed. Teaching Tips: Strategies, Research, Theory for College and University Teachers, 10th ed. Boston, Houghton Mifflin, 1999:209–215.
12. Johnson SP, Cooper J. Quick-thinks: active-thinking tasks in lecture classes and televised instruction. Coop Learn Coll Teach 1997;8:2–6.
13. Paulson DR, Faust JL. Active Learning for the College Classroom. Available at: *http://www. Calstatela.edu/dept/chem./chem2/active.* Accessed January 28, 2010.
14. Elliot DD. Promoting critical thinking in the classroom. Nurs Educator 1996;21:49–52.
15. Ruhl KL, Hughs CA, Schloss PJ. Using the pause procedure to enhance lecture recall. Teach Educ Spec Educ 1987;10:14–18.
16. Rowe MB. Pausing principles and their effects on reasoning in science. New Dir Community Coll 1980;8:27–34.
17. Walton HJ, Matthews MB. Essentials of problem-based learning. Med Educ 1989;23:542–558.
18. Raman-Wilms L. Innovative enabling strategies in self-directed, problem-based therapeutics: enhancing student preparedness for pharmaceutical care. Am J Pharm Educ 2001;65:56–64.
19. Dammers J, Spencer J, Thomas M. Using real patients in problem-based learning: students' comments on the value of using real, as opposed to paper cases, in a problem-based learning module in general practice. Med Educ 2001;35:27–34.
20. Lowther DL, Morrison GR. Integrating computers into the problem-solving protocol. New Dir Teach Learn 2003;95:33–38.
21. Letassy NA, Fugate SE, Medina MS, Stroup JS, Britton ML. Using team-based learning in an endocrine module taught across two campuses. Am J Pharm Educ 2008;72(5): Article 103.
22. Thompson BM, Schneider VF, Haidet P, et al. Team-based learning at ten medical schools: two years later. Med Educ 2007;41:250–257.
23. Winslade N. Large-group problem-based learning: a revision from traditional to pharmaceutical care-based therapeutics. Am J Pharm Educ 1994;58:64–73.
24. Hartzema AG. Teaching therapeutic reasoning through the case-study approach: adding the probabilistic dimension. Am J Pharm Educ 1994;58:436–440.
25. Delafuente JC, Munyer TO, Angaran DM, et al. A problem-solving active-learning course in pharmacotherapy. Am J Pharm Educ 1994;58:61–64.
26. McDade SA. An Introduction to the Case Study Method: Preparation, Analysis, Participation. New York, Teachers College Press, 1988.
27. Williams B. Case-based learning—a review of the literature: is there scope for this educational paradigm in prehospital education? Emerg Med J 2005;22:577–581.
28. Rangachari PK. Active learning: in context. Adv Physiol Educ 1995;13:S75–S80.
29. Robbins A. Awaken the Giant Within. New York, Simon & Schuster, 1991.
30. Chickering AW, Gamson ZF, Barsi LM. Seven Principles for Good Practice in Undergraduate Education. Racine, WI, The Johnson Foundation, 1989.
31. Prince M. Does active learning work? A review of the research. J Eng Educ 2004;93:223–231.
32. Weimer ME. Learner-Centered Teaching, 1st ed. San Francisco, CA, Jossey-Bass, 2002:167–183.

# CHAPTER 3 Case Studies in Patient Communication

RICHARD N. HERRIER, PHARMD

Delivering quality pharmaceutical care requires both strong technical and people skills. While all pharmacists are well versed in the technical aspects of the profession, many are not well prepared regarding interpersonal communication within the clinical context. In contemporary pharmacy practice, good communication skills are critical for achieving optimal patient outcomes and increasing pharmacists' satisfaction with their professional roles. The focus of this chapter is limited to the essential skills needed for symptom assessment, medication consultation, and strategies to improve compliance and monitor clinical progress. Readers are encouraged to review aspects of basic communication skills in other sources.[1–5]

## THE IMPORTANCE OF ASKING OPEN-ENDED QUESTIONS IN HEALTH CARE SETTINGS

One of the most important techniques to effectively communicate with patients is the primary use of open-ended questions. Open-ended questions are ones that start with *who, what, where, when, why,* and *how.* Closed-ended questions can be answered with either a simple yes or no answer and start with *can, do, did, are, would,* or *could.* Open-ended questions have numerous advantages compared to closed-ended questions. They markedly increase the comprehensiveness and accuracy of patient responses compared to closed-ended questions. Open-ended questions help readily identify patients with special needs requiring interventions, including patients with cognitive impairment, hearing loss, or lack of fluency in English or other primary language. Closed-ended questions allow patients with special needs to go undetected by hiding behind their yes or no answers. Open-ended questions minimize the need for the professional to speak, maximizing opportunities for listening for patient understanding and symptom-defining answers. Finally, they force the patient to answer with something other than yes or no, encouraging dialogue or further conversation with the patient. Closed-ended questions are perceived by patients as discouraging further response and are used to bring closure to conversations. Whether collecting information regarding a patient's symptoms or verifying that patients understand how to take their medication during medication counseling, the use of open-ended questions is the most effective communication technique and is therefore emphasized in this chapter.

## BASIC MEDICATION CONSULTATION SKILLS

Consultation on prescription medication use is a fundamental and important activity of the pharmacist and is mandated by both state and federal law or regulation.[6] The primary goal of traditional methods of medication counseling is to provide information: the pharmacist "tells" and the patient "listens." Pharmacists may try and check for patient understanding by asking ineffective closed-ended questions such as, "Do you understand?" or "Do you have any questions?" This traditional approach never verifies that the patient understands how to properly use his or her medication, which can lead to poor outcomes. Given the low level of patient health literacy in the United States, reliance on written patient handouts may also lead to a similar level of poor patient outcomes.[7] Using a modification of the effective educational approach, the "teach back" method, the Indian Health Service Pharmacy program developed a needs-based interactive medication counseling technique, *with the goal of verifying patient understanding.*

Using open-ended questions to initiate dialogue negates the disadvantages of the traditional lecture format. Retention of information is superior because patients forget 90% of *what you tell them* within 60 minutes, but they remember nearly 90% of *what they said* 24 hours later.[1] Using open-ended questions helps temporarily refocus the patient's attention, preventing the tendency to multitask and lose focus after 45–60 seconds. Finally, the consultation is quicker, and you maintain the patient's attention span because you are not repeating boring facts the patient already knows.

Two sets of open-ended questions are used in the consultation. One is for new prescriptions (*prime questions*), and the other is for refill prescriptions (*show-and-tell questions*), as shown in Table 3-1. These open-ended questions make the patient an active participant in the learning process. They provide an organized approach to ascertain what the patient already knows about the medication. Using a systematic approach has been associated with improved recall of prescription instructions.[8] The pharmacist can praise the patient for correct information recalled, clarify points misunderstood, and add new information as needed. It spares the pharmacist from repeating information already known by the patient, which is an inefficient use of time. The steps in the consultation process are described next.

## OPEN THE CONSULTATION

When the patient is called for counseling, introduce yourself by name and state the purpose of the consultation. Next, verify the patient's identity, either by asking for identification or at least by asking, "And you are…?" If the patient is non-English speaking, hard of hearing, or otherwise unable to provide his or her name, or answers inappropriately to a question, you have identified a barrier in the consultation that must be overcome before discussing the medication.

Use of a private space is required for patients who have hearing problems or those needing extra privacy, such as patients receiv-

**TABLE 3-1 Indian Health Service Medication Counseling Technique**

**Prime questions**

1. What did your doctor tell you the medication is for?
   *or*
   What were you told the medication is for?
   What problem or symptom is it supposed to help?
   What is it supposed to do?
2. How did your doctor tell you to take the medication?
   *or*
   How were you told to take the medication?
   How often did your doctor say to take it?
   How much are you supposed to take?
   What did your doctor say to do when you miss a dose?
   How did your doctor tell you to use it?
   What does three times a day mean to you?
3. What did your doctor tell you to expect?
   *or*
   What were you told to expect?
   What good effects are you supposed to expect?
   What bad effects did your doctor tell you to watch for?
   What should you do if a bad reaction occurs or if the medication does not work?

**Show-and-tell questions**

1. What do you take the medication for?
2. How do you take it?
3. What kind of problems are you having?

ing vaginal creams or those with AIDS. Sit facing the patient, and maintain the appropriate interpersonal distance (1.5–2 ft) during the consultation.

## CONDUCT THE COUNSELING SESSION FOR NEW PRESCRIPTIONS

Begin by asking the *prime questions* if the prescription is a new one. The *prime questions* are a series of three structured questions that probe the patient's understanding of proper medication use. If the patient knows the answer to a question, the pharmacist moves on to the next question. If there are gaps in the patient's understanding, the pharmacist "fills in the gap" by providing the missing information before moving on to the next prime question. If the patient is able to tell you what the medication is for (the first question), move to the next question. If the patient does not know what the medication is for, or if the patient says, "Don't you know?" you should ask why the patient visited the physician. The patient may describe symptoms of a condition known to be treatable with the medication in question.

After verifying that the patient knows what the medication is for, ask the second prime question. Often, patients are unaware of the dosage instructions or indicate, "It's on the label, isn't it?" Be aware of the optimal dosing instructions because the patient may correctly respond "twice a day," but you may need to ask about exact timing, or whether to take the drug with meals. Other questions to include under the second prime question are related to the following areas of concern: (a) how long to take the medication; (b) exactly how much or how often to take the medication when it is prescribed as needed; (c) what to do when a dose is missed; and (d) how to store the medication. Rather than providing facts, consider asking the patient, "What did the doctor say about how long to take this medication?" or "What will you do if you miss a dose?" Asking a question of the patient prompts the patient's attention, whereas "telling" the information is less effective, and the patient may not listen as well. Keep the information you provide brief and to the point.

After verifying patient understanding about how to take the medication, proceed to the third prime question. This question verifies that the patient understands the beneficial effects that are expected and what to do if the medication does not work. In addition, the question verifies the patient's understanding of potential common and uncommon (but serious) adverse effects plus what to do if a bad effect occurs.

For example, for angiotensin-converting enzyme (ACE) inhibitors, the pharmacist should warn about mild cough (talk with your physician) and any sudden swelling in the face, mouth, or tongue (get to an emergency room), which may represent the uncommon but potentially serious adverse effect of angioedema. Research shows that patients want information about their medications, especially adverse effects, and that providing such information does not lead to the development of those reactions.[9–11] If the patient does not know a specific item of information, first probe with focused open-ended question such as "What side effects were you warned about?" or "What were you told to do if that happened?" before "filling in the gaps."

The manner in which the consultation is closed is extremely important. Most consultations are a combination of the patient knowing some information and the pharmacist "filling in the gaps" by providing additional information as the prime questions are reviewed. Because of this, it is important to close the consultation with the *final verification*. Think of the final verification as asking the patient to "play back" everything learned so the pharmacist can verify that the patient's understanding is complete and accurate. Say to the patient, "Just to make sure I didn't leave anything out, please go over with me how you are going to use the medication." Avoid saying "Just to make sure you've got this…" because the patient may feel embarrassed if he or she does not recall important facts. At this point, the patient should describe correct use of the medication. Any errors can be corrected and any omissions clarified. Then ask the patient if there is anything else he or she needs and offer assistance as required.

## CONDUCT THE COUNSELING SESSION FOR REFILL PRESCRIPTIONS

A similar process is used for refill prescriptions. The *show-and-tell questions* verify patient understanding of proper use of chronic medications or medications that the patient has used in the past. The pharmacist begins the process by showing the medication to the patient, that is, by opening the bottle and displaying the contents. Then, the patient tells the pharmacist how he or she uses the medication by answering the questions listed in Table 3-1. Note that the doctor is omitted as a reference because the patient should have been counseled properly by the pharmacist before this and should have all information needed for proper medication usage. The show-and-tell technique enables the pharmacist to detect problems with compliance or unwanted drug effects. If the patient answers incorrectly to the second question, the patient may be noncompliant, or the physician may have changed the dosage. The pharmacist will need to further define the reason for the discrepancy. The second show-and-tell question also allows the pharmacist to ask the patient to demonstrate proper use of an inhaler, ophthalmic solution, or how to measure liquid doses to assure proper usage.

Some pharmacists have difficulty asking the third question, fearing that they may arouse suspicion in the patient. However, research discounts this notion, as previously discussed. If potential adverse effects were discussed when the patient was initially counseled, it seems natural, and certainly relevant and important, to query the patient about adverse effects at the refill visit. If new symptoms are present, explore this further using the *Chief Complaint history taking*. Because it is important to evaluate new symptoms critically, we will describe this in detail next.

## EXPLORING SYMPTOMS

At the prescription counter, over the telephone, at a bedside visit, or in requesting assistance with self-care via nonprescription products, the patient may mention symptoms that could be related to drug therapy or to an illness. Knowing how to explore the patient's symptoms and how to evaluate their relationship to either an acute disease or a chronic disease and its treatment or complications is a key assessment skill. The first step is to get the patient to reveal more information about the symptom. An introductory statement such as "Tell me more about it" encourages the patient to provide more specific details. After this, the *Basic 7 Questions* should be used. These seven focused, open-ended questions, based on *Chief Complaint history-taking* techniques, seek specifics that will help to define whether the symptom is related to drug therapy or to a specific disease that may require referral or be suitable for self-care with nonprescription products.[12] The *Basic 7 Questions* are as follows:

1. *Location:* Where is it located? Where does it hurt the worst?
2. *Quality:* What do you bring up when you cough? How would you describe the pain? What does it feel like?
3. *Severity:* How bad is it?
4. *Context:* How did it happen? When do you notice it?
5. *Timing:* When did it start? *or* How long have you had it? How frequently does it happen?
6. *Modifying factors:* What makes it better? *or* What have you done about it? What makes it worse?
7. *Associated symptoms:* What other symptoms are you having?

Finally *summarize* what the patient has told you, allowing the patient to verify your understanding and correct any misinformation collected or add information omitted during initial questioning.

Without proper attention to detail, many pharmacists assume that the symptom expressed is caused by a disease state and do not adequately address it. Or they may jump to conclusions about the cause of the symptom and recommend a treatment without knowing the true cause. For example, a patient taking a nonsteroidal anti-inflammatory drug who complains of fatigue might be recommended a vitamin if the pharmacist thinks the patient is tired because of inadequate nutrition. Probing the symptom of fatigue with the questions listed above may reveal that the fatigue started after the medication was begun and is accompanied by gastric distress, suggesting anemia from GI blood loss as a possible cause for the fatigue.

The *Basic 7 Questions* are also important when there is a tendency to attribute every symptom to a medication, as patients are sometimes inclined to do. For instance, a pharmacy student reviewed the chart of a patient with bipolar illness, seizures, and parkinsonism. The patient was receiving several medications, including carbamazepine and carbidopa/levodopa. She complained of blurred vision and insomnia, which the student initially felt were caused by the medications. However, using all of the *Basic 7 Questions* disclosed that the patient had blurred vision only out of the left eye and that she had insomnia "since the day I was born." Her answers suggested that the symptoms were unlikely to be related to her drug therapy. The most important point in addressing symptoms is to obtain enough information to make an informed clinical judgment. This is accomplished by using the *Basic 7 Questions*.

## BARRIERS DURING CLINICAL COMMUNICATION

The clinical skills described are easily applied in situations where there are few or no barriers in communication between patient and pharmacist. In reality, there are often obstacles to overcome in the environment or within the pharmacist or patient. Examples of problems within the pharmacy environment that deter optimal patient communication include lack of privacy, interruptions, high workload, and insufficient staff. Barriers present within the pharmacist include lack of desire or skills to adequately counsel patients, stereotyping patients and problems, and difficulty maintaining concentration, especially when stress is a factor. A detailed analysis of these barriers is beyond the scope of this discussion but can be found in the references.[3] The structured approach for patient consultation and exploring symptoms can be likened to knowing the road on which you are traveling. However, unforeseen events happen on every path and may arise at any time. Just as one must remove or negotiate around the obstacle on the highway, the pharmacist must recognize and manage barriers brought by the patient during the encounter for the consultation to reach the desired end.

*Functional barriers* include problems with hearing and vision that make it difficult for the patient to absorb information during the consultation. Language barriers and illiteracy are formidable obstacles to proper consultation. Language problems become apparent early in the counseling process when you use open-ended questions that require more than a yes/no answer. Strategies specific to each barrier are needed when these problems are identified. It is important to use translators, show picture diagrams, and involve English-speaking caregivers when language problems exist.

*Emotional barriers* are common in everyday pharmacist–patient interactions. When not handled properly, they give rise to further aggravation and break down communication, inhibiting effective consultation or history taking. Patients may express anger, hostility, sadness, depression, fear, anxiety, or embarrassment directly or indirectly during consultation with the pharmacist. They may also give the attitude of a "know-it-all," be suspicious of medications, or seem unmotivated or uninterested.

Unlike seeing the patient with a white cane and knowing that a vision problem exists, emotional barriers can be more difficult to discern. Because most patients will not say, "I'm angry and frustrated about feeling so ill," or "I'm upset that my doctor didn't spend much time with me," their feelings surface in statements such as, "I don't know why it takes all day to put a few pills in the bottle!" or "I don't know why I have to take this stupid medicine… nothing seems to help anyway." Unfortunately, we usually respond to the content of the message (e.g., "I'll have this ready for you as soon as I can") without recognizing that there may be other issues behind the statement, issues that will interfere with the effectiveness of counseling or interviewing and, more important, impact the patient's decision to comply with therapy.

## OVERCOMING BARRIERS WITH REFLECTIVE RESPONSES

*Reflective responding*, also known as active listening or empathetic responding, is a skill that can be practiced to listen beyond just the words spoken. When we respond with a reflection of what the patient is saying, thinking, or feeling, we let the person know we are truly listening and give the person the opportunity to admit to feelings, clarify thoughts, and bring forth information. Making a reflective response is not natural for us because most of us have not been trained to use these skills. Reflective responding attempts to reflect in words what the patient is saying or feeling. The reflection may be based on the content or thought expressed by the patient, and/or the feelings associated with it that are often not outwardly expressed. Reflective responses are especially called for when the patient is demonstrating emotions. Angry looks, pounding fists, averted eye contact, and head drooping all convey certain emotional states. Hesitating gestures or remarks such as, "Well... I guess I could try it," call for reflective responses to bring concerns to light. Also, reflective responding calms the patient down and puts him or her in a better mental state for answering questions or receiving counseling.

The first step in effective reflective responding is to identify and label the emotional state. The four basic emotional states are mad, sad, glad, and scared. As you observe the patient during consultation, certain nonverbal or verbal signs (e.g., hesitating words) may suggest one of the four feeling states. The second step is to put the word describing the feeling state into a sentence to use as a response to the patient. Some basic structures for sentences include, "It sounds as if you are (frustrated, mad, happy)," or "I can see that you are (happy, confused, mad)." These remarks indicate to patients that you are truly attempting to understand their concerns; thus, the patient and his or her concerns remain the focus of the encounter.

To the patient who remarked, "I don't know why I have to take this... nothing helps anyway," the pharmacist might determine that the nonverbal tone of voice and choice of words indicate that the patient is disappointed with results of his or her therapy. Alternatively, the patient may be feeling hopeless about getting better. One reflective response is, "It sounds as if you have been frustrated with the things you have tried." This statement neither judges nor advises. It gives the patient an opportunity to open discussion of a difficult topic, if the patient so chooses. Contrast this with, "This is a good medicine, Joe, and I really think it will help." Although this may be true, maintaining the communication on a technical, information-providing level avoids dealing with the underlying issues of the patient's fears and markedly decreases the efficacy of the pharmacist's communication with the patient.

Emotional barriers can occur at any time throughout the consultation, and they must be dealt with first in order to put the patient in a receptive frame of mind. Embarrassment is a factor when vaginal preparations, condom use, and similar topics are the subject of the consultation. Observe for signs of embarrassment such as averted gaze or fidgeting, and respond with, "This can be hard to talk about, but it's important that we discuss...." Also, be matter-of-fact, move to a private space, and speak in a normal tone of voice to help alleviate the embarrassment.

When faced with patients' emotional outbursts, acknowledge their expressed feelings before continuing with the consultation or the interview. The initial use of reflective responses will allow the consultation or interview to proceed with both parties devoting attention to the primary issues of drug therapy and usage, rather than to interpersonal difficulties. Remember, though, that reflective responses will not work in every situation nor with every type of patient.

## MEDICATION ADHERENCE AND DISEASE MONITORING

In no other situation is the pharmacist's role in monitoring and managing medication usage more vital than in the case of patients requiring chronic drug therapy, especially for diseases that are asymptomatic. Contemporary pharmacy practice continues to evolve into more direct patient care roles. The monitoring and management of common chronic diseases such as hypertension, asthma, and diabetes are now being done in partnership between pharmacists and medical professionals. Models of community pharmacy practice now include private consultations and advanced practice techniques that were formerly limited to sites such as the Indian Health Service and the Department of Veterans Affairs. A majority of states now have regulations that allow pharmacists to assess and prescribe.[13]

## WHOSE DISEASE IS IT ANYWAY?

A common misperception held by health care professionals regarding a patient with a chronic disease is that the professional manages the patient's disease. Nothing could be further from the truth, and this medical myth is probably a major contributor to compliance problems among patients with chronic diseases. In the traditional medical care model, health care professionals perceive their roles to be in the diagnosis, treatment, and management of disease. As drug therapy managers, pharmacists focus on blood levels, kinetic dosage calculations, and drug interactions. Guided by this focus on technical aspects of patient care, health care professionals often become frustrated and angry when patients do not follow instructions or, despite the provider's best efforts, achieve only partial results. In reality, the only time the professional manages the treatment is during an office visit or while the patient is institutionalized in a hospital or long-term care facility. Almost all of the time, the patient controls the treatment of his or her disease, especially those that require continuous medication. Failure to recognize this basic truth has created: (a) considerable tension in patient–provider relationships; (b) provider frustration and anger; (c) poor communication; (d) negative provider attitudes toward individual patients; (e) poor patient outcomes; (f) patient distrust of providers; and (g) legal consequences that have been a major contributor to rising health care costs.

One author strongly suggests that noncompliance in diabetes mellitus is due in large part to the failure of providers to recognize that their goal is not to treat the disease, but to *help the patient to treat the disease.*[14] That contention is supported by current medical literature on compliance that links good communication and a partnership style of provider–patient relationship to increased satisfaction, compliance, and better patient outcomes.[15,16]

To be successful in assisting patients to achieve good outcomes, the provider and pharmacist must adopt a partnership approach, with health professionals acting as facilitators to help patients manage their disease. That is, it is patients' disease; the providers' job is *to help them manage it.*

## GO SLOW/USE INTERACTIVE TECHNIQUES

Patients can absorb only a limited amount of new information at each encounter. In an attempt to do a thorough job, health care professionals often overwhelm the patient with information at or near the time of diagnosis or treatment initiation. Patients' active listening abilities last less than a minute during a monologue presentation, and they retain only a few pieces of information from a prolonged discussion and may miss key facts. In addition, a large volume of technical information may confuse or frighten patients, leading to the poor outcome that educational efforts are intended to prevent.[15] Also, newly diagnosed patients may not have accepted their diagnosis or the need for treatment.

Successful patient educators do three things: (a) they give patients information in small manageable increments, (b) they actively involve the patient in the educational process by creating an interactive dialogue and using other hands-on approaches that are consistent with adult learning principles,[16] and (c) they understand patient readiness for information. For the pharmacist dispensing the initial prescription, this entails verifying that the patient understands how to take the medicine and its most common side effects. For example, with hydrochlorothiazide

25 mg daily for hypertension, the pharmacist should verify that the patient knows what it is for, knows to take it once daily in the morning to prevent nighttime voiding, knows that it takes a while before any changes in blood pressure occur, and knows that there will be a noticeable increase in urination the first week, which should lessen thereafter. Discussions about diet, exercise, and related issues can wait until later visits. Giving the patient a handout on hypertension and diuretics is appropriate and can lead to questions and subsequent education at later visits or during a follow-up phone call.

## SET THE STAGE FOR FUTURE ENCOUNTERS

Many providers explain to patients what follow-up visits will entail so that patients view subsequent laboratory tests and examinations as a normal part of their care. However, few providers follow a similar process regarding medication compliance. Patients then perceive questions about compliance to be intrusive and, fearing parental-type sanctions from the provider, lie about being compliant. Using specific strategies during the *initial* patient visit when follow-up care is discussed can prevent this all-too-common problem. Explain that compliance is very important to successful outcomes, but that you know how hard it is to remember to take medication every day. Tell the patient that you expect that he or she will be like all patients and experience some difficulty remembering to take the medication. Ask the patient to keep track of those instances if possible, and further explain that you will be asking at each visit about the problems the patient has had with the medication so you can assist the patient to better remember to take the medication. It may be necessary to probe into his or her daily habits and to help him or her find a way to tie medication taking into a particular activity. For instance, if the patient always makes coffee in the morning, having the medication nearby may be a sufficient reminder to promote compliance. Be sure to use a partnership approach. Additional compliance-enhancing skills are discussed in the next section.

## MONITORING PATIENT PROGRESS AT RETURN VISITS

Regardless of practice setting, there are opportunities to provide value-added services to patients with chronic diseases managed primarily by pharmacotherapy. From disease management programs with pharmacist prescriptive authority to a typical busy community practice environment, where opportunities to monitor patient progress may be limited by time and physical plant availability, there is a simple common approach for dealing with patients with chronic diseases during a return visit or when patients pick up refills. One simple way to look at all patients returning for follow-up of chronic diseases is to use the "Three Cs": *control, compliance,* and *complications* (Fig. 3-1). To evaluate the *control* of the chronic disease, couple objective findings (e.g., blood pressure or range of motion) with subjective findings from the consultation (e.g., reports of dizziness, nocturnal voiding, or degree of morning joint stiffness). *Complications* can occur from both disease progression and drug effects. As with the control parameters, a combination of subjective findings (e.g., symptoms) and objective findings from the health record or patient profile can disclose the presence of potential complications. For example, a patient with hypertension, diabetes mellitus, and osteoarthritis who takes lisinopril, glyburide, and ibuprofen can be queried about the presence of cough, difficulty sleeping, and exercise tolerance. These questions are primarily directed at detecting congestive heart failure or renal failure caused by hypertension and/or diabetes, but they also will help detect drug-related problems such as cough caused by the ACE inhibitor and renal effects from

### Collecting Subjective Information as a Primary Care Provider

1. How have things been going with your __________ since your last visit? *(Control)*
2. What kind of problems have you had remembering to take your medication? *(Compliance)*
   - Tell me about the last time it happened.
   - How many times has it happened since your last visit?
3. What kind of changes have you noticed since your last visit? *(Complications)*
   - What problems are you having with your medication?
   - In order to make sure you aren't having any problems, are you experiencing:
     e.g., Drowsiness? Yes ❑ No ❑
     Dizziness? Yes ❑ No ❑

   *Note:* In this situation, using closed-ended questions covering major potential problems or complications is an efficient method.
4. If any problems are noted, shift gears to *Chief Complaint History Taking* and begin with:
   - Tell me more about it.
5. Follow with the *Basic 7 Questions* as needed.

**FIGURE 3-1.** Example form for collecting subjective information as a primary care provider. General approach to interviewing patients returning for chronic disease follow-up.

ibuprofen. Checking recent laboratory values for serum creatinine, electrolytes, and blood glucose will help assess diabetes and hypertension control and complications such as NSAID-induced renal impairment, excessive glyburide dosage, and ACE inhibitor–induced hyperkalemia. Collecting subjective information at each visit can be organized by integrating the "Three Cs" with broad open-ended questions similar to the *Basic 7 Questions*.

To identify potential compliance problems, review the health record or patient profile for objective evidence of potential noncompliance before talking with the patient. During profile review, three items should alert the pharmacist to potential compliance problems. The first and most common item is a discrepancy between the number of doses that should have been taken and the number of doses dispensed. Second, patients with incomplete refill requests (e.g., only one or two of multiple chronic medications due at the same time) raise suspicion for noncompliance. Third, the prescribing of a new medication for the same condition or one that may unknowingly be prescribed to offset adverse effects from another medication may indicate compliance problems. Patients often present to medical providers with new complaints. If the provider does not make the connection between the new symptom and the side effect, compliance or therapeutic problems may eventually occur. If patients taking ACE inhibitors present with new or repeat prescriptions for cough suppressants, the pharmacist should consider the potential for ACE inhibitor–induced cough.

Potential compliance problems found during profile or chart review call for further exploration before a definite compliance problem can be ascertained. There may be rational explanations for the objective findings. Gaps in refills may be a result of patients obtaining refills at another location, or the doctor may have told the patient to change the dosage schedule or to stop the drug altogether.

Begin the consultation using the *show-and-tell* technique for refill prescriptions when the profile indicates potential noncompliance.

The patient may provide one or more clues during consultation to confirm your suspicions. Patients who tell the pharmacist during the *show-and-tell* questioning that they are taking their medication differently than prescribed are providing evidence of a potential compliance problem. Some clues are obvious, such as when a patient asks, "Why do I have to keep taking this medicine?" This is a "red flag" because it is clear that the patient wishes not to take the prescription. However, many statements are more subtle. Examples of these vague clues, called "pink flags," include: "My doctor says I *should* take it…," "My doctor *wants* me to…," or "I'm *supposed* to be taking…." These are usually detected when the pharmacist asks the first two *show-and-tell* questions. "What kinds of problems are you having with the medication?" may prompt the following "pink flag" responses: "Well… none, really," or a hesitation before saying "No, none." Reflective responses discussed earlier in this chapter are appropriate in this situation. Responses include, "It seems as if you are not too sure about taking that," or "It sounds as if you think the medicine is causing a problem." These responses open the dialogue in a nonthreatening manner and focus on the patient's perceptions or suggestion that a problem exists.

A *supportive compliance probe* is a more direct approach that must be initiated if the profile review reveals potential problems but the consultation does not confirm suspicions. This is a specific type of statement that uses "I" language to describe what the profile shows and to probe the discrepancy. For example, "I noticed when I reviewed your profile that you hadn't had your prednisone refilled in about 2 weeks. I was concerned that there might have been some changes that I'm not aware of." This combination of "I noticed… and I'm concerned…" can be very effective in getting a dialogue started in a nonthreatening manner. The *universal statement* is another useful approach, such as, "Most of my patients have problems remembering to take every dose of their medication. What kinds of problems are you having?" Open the discussion of compliance problems with nonthreatening language, and there is a greater likelihood that the patient will disclose problems.

Patients may ask, "Does this medicine have any side effects?" or "What kind of side effects does this have?" or "Is this anything like (another specific drug)?" More often than not, pharmacists simply answer the question without really listening to the underlying concern. "Why do you ask?" is an appropriate response, especially if the patient looks hesitant or the intonation of the question suggests doubt about taking the medication. When the author uses this question, patients often disclose that a relative had it (or a similar medication) or the media has reported problems with the drug. These indirect experiences create enough doubt such that the patient wavers about taking the medication.

Compliance problems can be categorized into three groups. The first is a *knowledge* deficit. In these cases, patients have insufficient information or skills or misinformation that prevents compliance. An example is the patient who was never been shown or has forgotten how to use an inhaler. The second group involves *practical impediments* or barriers, such as complex drug regimens involving multiple drugs and/or different dosage schedules, difficulty in developing routines that facilitate medication compliance, difficulty in opening containers, or insufficient mental aptitude to comply. The final category is *attitudinal barriers*. Among the most difficult to identify and manage, these include patient beliefs about health, disease, and/or treatment that are inconsistent with the prescribed regimen. Once the specific cause is identified, a specific strategy to manage that problem can be attempted. Most knowledge and skill deficiencies can be successfully corrected with education and/or training. Practical impediments respond well to specific measures such as simplifying regimens, use of easy-open containers, and enlisting the aid of a spouse or caregiver. Attitudinal issues tend to be the most complex and difficult to solve.

## CONCLUSIONS

Contemporary pharmacy practice is changing at a very rapid pace. Pharmaceutical care, which focuses on the outcomes of drug therapy, is the founding principle for today's practitioners. The delivery of quality pharmaceutical care involves the skills and techniques discussed in this chapter and many others that support the pharmacist–patient interaction and medication use process. As direct patient contact and responsibility for drug therapy outcomes become the main task for pharmacists, the skills of interpersonal communication, medication history taking, patient consultation, plus compliance monitoring and enhancement become the "tools of the trade." The consistent application of a high level of interpersonal and applied clinical skills by pharmacists will lead to optimal outcomes for patients.

## REFERENCES


1. Bolton R. People Skills. New York, Simon & Schuster, 1986.
2. Gardner M, Herrier RN, Meldrum H, Gourley DR. Pharmacist–Patient Consultation Program, Unit 1: An Interactive Approach to Verify Patient Understanding. New York, Pfizer, 2003.
3. Pharmacist–Patient Consultation Program, Unit 2: Counseling Patients in Challenging Situations. New York, Pfizer, 1993.
4. Meldrum H. Interpersonal Communication in Pharmaceutical Care. New York, Haworth Press, 1994.
5. Muldary TW. Interpersonal Relations for Health Professionals: A Social Skills Approach. New York, Macmillan, 1983.
6. Meade V. OBRA '90: how has pharmacy reacted? Am Pharm 1995;NS35:12–16.
7. Parker RM, Williams MV, Weiss BD, et al. Health literacy: report of the council on scientific affairs. JAMA 1999;281:552–557.
8. Gardner M, Hurd PD, Slack M. Effect of information organization on recall of medication instructions. J Clin Pharm Ther 1989;14:1–7.
9. Lamb GC, Green SS, Heron J. Can physicians warn patients of potential side effects without fear of causing those side effects? Arch Intern Med 1994;154:2753–2756.
10. Howland JS, Baker MG, Poe T. Does patient education cause side effects? A controlled trial. J Fam Pract 1990;31:62–64.
11. Meldrum H, Hardy M. Challenges in communicating about risk. In: Communicating Risk to Patients: Proceedings of the Conference. Rockville, MD; United States Pharmacopeial Convention, 1995: 36–49.
12. Boyce RW, Herrier RN. Obtaining and using patient data. Am Pharm 1991;NS31:65–71.
13. Hammond RW, Schwartz AH, Campbell MJ, et al. Collaborative drug therapy management. Pharmacotherapy 2003;23:1210–1225.
14. Anderson RM. Is the problem of noncompliance all in our heads? Diabetes Educ 1985;11:31–34.
15. Herrier RN. Medication compliance in the elderly. J Pharm Pract 1995;8(5):232–244.
16. Eraker SA, Kirscht JP, Becker MH. Understanding and improving patient compliance. Ann Intern Med 1984;100:258–268.


## PATIENT CASES

This section includes three scenarios with patient profiles and prescriptions that require education. First, review the profile and prescription and think about issues that may arise during the consultation. Then provide written answers to the questions asked. Use concepts from the preceding material on education strategies, as well as any other techniques you think are useful or have been found to be useful through your own experience or by observing others in practice.

**Patient Medication Profile**

| Name: | Sally M. Johnson | Known Diseases | | Allergies and Sensitivities | | Additional Information | |
|---|---|---|---|---|---|---|---|
| Address: | 1862 Briar Court<br>Lansdale, PA 18018 | S/P hysterectomy 9/00 with estrogen replacement<br>S/P surgery, CA breast 12/2010 | | Sulfa: rash | | | |
| Telephone: | 832-7358 | | | | | | |
| Date of Birth: | 4/15/48 | | | | | | |
| **Date** | **Rx No.** | **Medication** | **Strength** | **Quantity** | **Dosage Regimen** | **R.Ph.** | **Physician** |
| 07/18/10 | 83104 | Premarin | 0.625 mg | #100 | 1 QD | JD | Hepler |
| 10/25/10 | 89436 | Premarin | 0.625 mg | #100 | 1 QD | HV | Hepler |
| 12/04/10 | 145922 | Tylox | | #30 | 1–2 Q 4 h PRN | JD | Cavanaugh |
| 12/04/10 | 145923 | Dicloxacillin | 250 mg | #40 | 2 QID | JD | Cavanaugh |

CA, cancer; S/P, status post.

## CASE NO. 1: SALLY M. JOHNSON

| NAME | **Johnson, Sally M.** | DATE 2/20/11 |
|---|---|---|
| ADDRESS | 1862 Briar Court<br>Lansdale, PA 18018 | AGE IF CHILD |
| $R_x$ | FULL DIRECTIONS FOR USE | Rx No. 148647 |
| | | Date filled |
| | Anastrozole 1 mg | Cost |
| | #30 | Fee |
| | Sig: 1 po daily | Total Price<br>❑ Do not refill<br>No. of refills authorized: 6 |
| ❑ IDENTIFY CONTENTS ON LABEL UNLESS CHECKED | | |
| ❑ NONPROPRIETARY EQUIVALENT UNLESS CHECKED | | |
| | | S. Mayer M.D. |

Sally comes to the pharmacy alone to pick up an anastrozole prescription. You have reviewed the profile and are ready to educate her on the medication.

1. Before talking with the patient, what functional and emotional barriers would you expect during the consultation? What else would you like to know about your patient?
2. How are you going to begin the consultation?
3. Listed below are three different responses by the patient to the first *prime question*. For each statement, consider what each statement reveals about what the patient knows or feels, and state what should happen next in the consultation.

   Patient Response A[1]: *"He gave it to me after my surgery."*

   Patient Response B: *"I just had surgery for breast cancer."*

   Patient Response C: *"I know what it's for."*

4. Listed below are three different responses to the second *prime question*. Consider what each tells you, and state what you would do next in the consultation.

   Patient Response A: *"I'm going to take it twice a day."*

   Patient Response B: *"It's on the label, isn't it?"*

   Patient Response C: *"I don't remember. He didn't tell me."*

5. Listed below are three different responses to the third *prime question*. Consider what each tells you, and state what you would do next in the consultation.

   Patient Response A: *"I hope it will keep my cancer in check."*

   Patient Response B: *"The doctor says things look good, but I thought I heard something about uterine cancer?"*

   Patient Response C: *"Nothing. I'm not sure anything is going to help me now."*

[1]Patient statements A, B, and C do not necessarily correspond throughout the consultation.

## CASE NO. 2: THOMAS GORDON

| NAME | **Gordon, Thomas** | DATE 2/15/11 |
|---|---|---|
| ADDRESS | 38 Main Street<br>Muncie, IL 82695 | AGE IF CHILD |
| $R_x$ | FULL DIRECTIONS FOR USE | Rx No. 148647 |
| | | Date filled |
| | Cephalexin 500 mg | Cost |
| | #40 | Fee |
| | Sig: 1 po QID | Total Price<br>❑ Do not refill<br>No. of refills authorized: 0 |
| ❑ IDENTIFY CONTENTS ON LABEL UNLESS CHECKED | | |
| ❑ NONPROPRIETARY EQUIVALENT UNLESS CHECKED | | |
| | | B. Higley M.D. |

Tom is a 53-year-old man with type 2 diabetes mellitus who is picking up an antibiotic for an infected cut on his arm. He owns his own construction company and is always "on the go." You are ready to counsel him about his antibiotic prescription.

1. What concerns do you have based on review of the patient's medication profile? What else would you like to know about your patient? Before talking with the patient, what functional and emotional barriers would you expect during education? What are the goals of the education?
2. How are you going to begin the consultation?
3. Listed below are Tom's responses to the *prime questions*. Consider what each response reveals about what the patient knows or feels, and state how you would address any concerns you detect.

   Pharmacist: "What did the doctor tell you the medication was for?"

   Tom: "He said he was giving me an antibiotic for this infection on my arm. It started as just a scratch, but it's gotten really bad."

   Pharmacist: "How did the doctor tell you to take the medicine?"

| Patient Medication Profile | | | | | | | |
|---|---|---|---|---|---|---|---|
| Name: | Thomas Gordon | **Known Diseases** | | **Allergies and Sensitivities** | | **Additional Information** | |
| Address: | 38 Main Street<br>Muncie, IL 82695 | Diabetes since 1997 | | NKA | | | |
| Telephone: | 542-5016 | | | | | | |
| Date of Birth: | 01/10/52 | | | | | | |
| **Date** | **Rx No.** | **Medication** | **Strength** | **Quantity** | **Dosage Regimen** | **R.Ph.** | **Physician** |
| 01/10/10 | 75243 | Glipizide | 10 mg | 100 | 1 Q AM | EM | B. Higley |
| 06/20/10 | 75243R | Glipizide | 10 mg | 100 | 1 Q AM | EM | B. Higley |
| 10/28/10 | 75243R | Glipizide | 10 mg | 100 | 1 Q AM | JR | B. Higley |

NKA, no known allergies.

Tom: "I don't know. He said it was on the label. I know I'm supposed to take it all."

Pharmacist: "What did the doctor tell you to expect?"

Tom: "I guess it will kill the infection and make the scratch heal."

4. When you ask about glipizide, Tom's answer to your inquiry is listed below. Consider what the statement reveals, and state how you would address his concerns.

   Tom: "Yeah, well, I'm really busy with my business and it's hard to remember to take it."

## CASE NO. 3: WILLIAM HODGES

| | | |
|---|---|---|
| NAME | **Hodges, William** | DATE 7/12/11 |
| ADDRESS | 4212 W. Mission Lane<br>Albuquerque, NM 87546 | AGE IF CHILD |
| $R_x$ | FULL DIRECTIONS FOR USE | Rx No. 148647 |
| | 1. Warfarin 5 mg #45 | Date filled |
| | Sig: 1 tab po Q AM on Sat M W F | Cost |
| | 2 tabs po Q AM on Tues Thurs Sun | Fee |
| | | Total Price |
| | | ❑ Do not refill |
| | | No. of refills authorized: 0 |
| ❑ IDENTIFY CONTENTS ON LABEL UNLESS CHECKED | | |
| ❑ NONPROPRIETARY EQUIVALENT UNLESS CHECKED | | |
| | | K. Jones Drew PharmD |

Bill is a 71-year-old man with an 8-year history of atrial fibrillation with congestive heart failure. He is a regular in your pharmacy-based anticoagulation clinic. In addition to his prescription medications, he takes aspirin 81 mg daily to prevent re-infarction.

Bill is here for his regular visit with you and wants refills of furosemide, K Tabs, and amlodipine, but not his enalapril, which was added to his existing medications because his blood pressure and CHF are still not under control. His INR is 1.8 today. It has been frustrating because his INR has been on the low end of normal or just below normal since you began changing his regimen 12 months ago. You have steadily increased the dose due to poor response with limited success. Today you plan to increase his weekly dose by one pill by changing the regimen to two tablets on Sunday, Tuesday, and Thursday with one tablet daily on other days.

1. Review the patient's profile. What concerns do you have based on your review of the patient profile? What are the goals of the visit?
2. How are you going to begin the visit?
3. Listed below are Bill's responses to the primary care visit model. What do you notice?

   Pharmacist: "How have things been going with your warfarin since the last visit?"

   Bill: "Great; I'm not bruising as easily and have had no other bleeding problems."

   Pharmacist: "What kind of problems have you had remembering to take your warfarin?"

   Bill: "Uhh ... none I guess."
4. What should the pharmacist do next?

   After the pharmacist's response, Bill says on many days he has had trouble remembering to take the second pill. Moving on....

   Pharmacist: "What kind of changes have you noticed since your last visit?"

   Bill: "I've been feeling kind of funny."
5. What should the pharmacist say next?

   In response to the pharmacist's inquiry, Bill tells you that enalapril made him feel funny when he first started taking it.
6. What should be your next response, and what technique should you now use?

   The patient's response to your questions was:

   a. "I felt real dizzy."

   b. "It started about 24 hours after I started taking it."

   c. "It was bad enough that I saw spots and almost fell."

   d. "It happened primarily when I got up out of bed or from a chair."

   e. "I tried getting up slowly and it only helped some, so I stopped it for a day and it went away. Yesterday, I started back at one in the morning only and the dizziness started again in the morning, but it is not as bad and getting up slowly helps keep me from passing out."
7. What clinical assessment do you make from these responses?
8. Before taking action to correct the problem, what should you do now?
9. What about the problem with his warfarin?
10. You need to call Dr Ames. How would you phrase your comments to Dr Ames regarding the two problems you detected?
11. What would you do next?

**Patient Medication Profile**

| | | | | | | | |
|---|---|---|---|---|---|---|---|
| Name: | William Hodges | **Known Diseases** | | **Allergies and Sensitivities** | | **Additional Information** | |
| Address: | 4212 W. Mission Ln. | S/P CABG 1999 | | Penicillin | | | |
| | Albuquerque, NM 87546 | Angina, AFib | | | | | |
| Telephone: | 505/425-7219 | CHF | | | | | |
| Date of Birth: | 3/22/39 | | | | | | |

| Date | Rx No. | Medication | Strength | Quantity | Dosage Regimen | R.Ph. | Physician |
|---|---|---|---|---|---|---|---|
| 04/20/10 | 18590 | Metoprolol | 50 mg | 60 | 1 po BID | BR | Ames |
| 04/20/10 | 18591 | Warfarin | 5 mg | 36 | 1 Sat M T W F/2 Sun Th | BR | Jones-Drew |
| 04/20/10 | 18592 | K Tabs | 10 mEq | 60 | 2 QD | BR | Ames |
| 04/20/10 | 18593 | Furosemide | 40 mg | 15 | 1/2 tab QD | BR | Ames |
| 04/20/10 | 18594 | Amlodipine | 5 mg | 30 | 1 q AM | BR | Ames |
| 05/15/10 | 18590 | Metoprolol | 0.125 mg | 45 | | JC | Ames |
| 05/15/10 | 18592 | K Tabs | 10 mEq | 120[a] | 2 QD | JC | Ames |
| 05/15/10 | 18593 | Furosemide | 40 mg | 30[a] | 1/2 tab QD | JC | Ames |
| 05/15/10 | 18594 | Amlodipine | 5 mg | 60[a] | 1 q AM | JC | Ames |
| 6/16/10 | 18591 | Warfarin | 5 mg | 36 | 1 Sat M T W F/2 Sun Th | DT | Jones-Drew |
| 6/16/10 | 18592 | K Tabs | 10 mEq | 60 | 2 QD | DT | Ames |
| 6/16/10 | 18593 | Furosemide | 40 mg | 15 | 1/2 tab QD | DT | Ames |
| 6/16/10 | 24276 | Enalapril | 20 mg | 60 | 1 BID | DT | |

BID, twice daily; CABG, coronary artery bypass graft; CHF, congestive heart failure; QD, every day; S/P, status post.
[a]Vacation supply.

CHAPTER 4

# Pharmaceutical Care Planning: A Component of the Patient Care Process

TERRY L. SCHWINGHAMMER, PHARMD, FCCP, FASHP, FAPHA, BCPS

## THE PATIENT CARE PROCESS

The *patient care process* is a systematic and comprehensive method for interacting with patients that must be applied consistently to every patient seen by the health care provider. The process may vary among health care practitioners who have different purposes and goals. For pharmacists, the primary purpose of the patient care process is to identify, solve, and prevent drug therapy problems.[1] A drug therapy problem is "any undesirable event experienced by a patient which involves, or is suspected to involve, drug therapy and that interferes with achieving the desired goals of therapy."[1] The pharmacist's patient care process includes three essential elements: (1) assessment of the patient's drug-related needs; (2) creation of a pharmaceutical care plan to meet those needs; and (3) follow-up evaluation to determine whether positive outcomes were achieved. Consequently, development of a pharmaceutical care plan is only one component of the overall patient care process. Before developing a patient-specific pharmaceutical care plan, it is important for the clinician to understand the comprehensive nature of the patient care process. This process offers a logical and consistent framework that can be most useful in pharmaceutical care planning and serves as the framework for this chapter.

## ASSESSMENT OF DRUG-RELATED NEEDS

The first step in assessment is to identify the patient's drug-related needs by collecting, organizing, and integrating pertinent patient, drug, and disease information. In the patient care process, as with all direct patient care services, the patient is the primary source of information. This involves asking patients what they *want* (expectations) and what they *do not want* (concerns) and determining how well they understand their drug therapies. For example, the clinician may ask, "How may I help you today?" or "What concerns do you have that I may address for you today?" In addition to speaking with the patient, data can also be obtained from: (1) family members or caretakers when appropriate; (2) the patient's current and past medical records; and (3) discussions with other health care providers. The types of information that may be relevant are described below.[1,2]

### Patient Information

- Demographics and background information: age, gender, race, height, and weight.
- Social history: living arrangements, occupation, and special needs (e.g., physical abilities, cultural traits, drug administration devices).
- Family history: relevant health histories of parents and siblings.
- Insurance/administrative information: name of health plan and primary care physician.

### Disease Information

- Past medical history.
- Current medical problems.
- History of present illness.
- Pertinent information from the review of systems, physical examination, laboratory results, and x-ray/imaging results.
- Medical diagnoses.

### Drug Information

- Allergies and side effects (include the name of the medication and the reaction that occurred).
- Current prescription medications:
  - ✓ How the medication was prescribed.
  - ✓ How the patient is actually taking the medication.
  - ✓ Effectiveness and side effects of current medications.
  - ✓ Questions or concerns about current medications.
- Current nonprescription medications, vitamins, dietary supplements, and other alternative/complementary therapies.
- Past prescription and nonprescription medications (i.e., those discontinued within the past 6 months).

The information obtained is then organized, analyzed, and integrated to: (1) determine whether the patient's drug therapy is appropriate, effective, safe, and convenient for the patient; (2) identify drug therapy problems that may interfere with goals of therapy; and (3) identify potential drug therapy problems that require prevention. One method of organizing and integrating this information with appropriate pharmacotherapeutic knowledge has been described as the Pharmacotherapy Workup© (copyright 2003, the Peters Institute of Pharmaceutical Care).[1]

Drug therapy problems are uncovered through careful assessment of the patient, drug, and disease information to determine the appropriateness of each medication regimen. This process involves a logical sequence of steps. It begins with evaluating each medication regimen for appropriateness of indication, then optimizing the drug and dosage regimen to ensure maximum effectiveness, and finally, individualizing drug therapy to make it as safe as possible for the patient. After completing these three steps, the practitioner considers other issues such as cost, compliance, and convenience.

**TABLE 4-1** Drug Therapy Problems to Be Resolved or Prevented

| Assessment | Drug Therapy Problem |
|---|---|
| **Indication** | **Unnecessary drug therapy** |
| | No medical indication |
| | Duplicate therapy |
| | Nondrug therapy indicated |
| | Treating avoidable adverse drug reaction |
| | Addictive/recreational use |
| | **Needs additional drug therapy** |
| | Untreated condition |
| | Preventive/prophylactic |
| | Synergistic/potentiating |
| **Effectiveness** | **Needs different drug product** |
| | More effective drug available |
| | Condition refractory to drug |
| | Dosage form inappropriate |
| | Not effective for condition |
| | **Dosage too low** |
| | Wrong dose |
| | Frequency too long |
| | Duration too short |
| | Drug interaction |
| | Incorrect administration |
| **Safety** | **Adverse drug reaction** |
| | Undesirable effect |
| | Unsafe drug for patient |
| | Drug interaction |
| | Dose administered or changed too rapidly |
| | Allergic reaction |
| | Contraindications present |
| | **Dosage too high** |
| | Wrong dose |
| | Frequency too short |
| | Duration too long |
| | Drug interaction |
| | Incorrect administration |
| **Compliance** | **Nonadherence** |
| | Directions not understood |
| | Patient prefers not to take |
| | Patient forgets to take |
| | Drug product too expensive |
| | Cannot swallow or administer |
| | Drug product not available |

*Adapted with permission from Cipolle RJ, Strand LM, Morley PC. Pharmaceutical Care Practice: A Clinician's Guide, 2nd ed. New York, McGraw-Hill, 2004:168.*

Drug therapy problems can be placed into distinct categories, as summarized below. See Table 4-1 for a useful checklist that can be used in actual practice situations.[1]

1. *Inappropriate indication* for drug use:
   a. The patient requires additional drug therapy.
   b. The patient is taking unnecessary drug therapy.
2. *Ineffective* drug therapy:
   a. The patient is taking a drug that is not effective for his or her situation.
   b. The medication dose is too low.
3. *Unsafe* drug therapy:
   a. The patient is experiencing an adverse drug reaction.
   b. The medication dose is too high.
4. Inappropriate *adherence* or *compliance*:
   a. The patient is unable or unwilling to take the medication as prescribed.

**TABLE 4-2** Causes of Drug Therapy Problems

| Drug Therapy Problem | Possible Causes of Drug Therapy Problems |
|---|---|
| **Unnecessary drug therapy** | No valid medication indication for the drug at this time.<br>Multiple drug products are used when only single-drug therapy is required.<br>The condition is better treated with nondrug therapy.<br>Drug therapy is used to treat an avoidable adverse drug reaction associated with another medication.<br>The medical problem is caused by drug abuse, alcohol use, or smoking. |
| **Need for additional drug therapy** | A medical condition exists that requires initiation of new drug therapy.<br>Preventive therapy is needed to reduce the risk of developing a new condition.<br>A medical condition requires combination therapy to achieve synergism or additive effects. |
| **Ineffective drug** | The drug is not the most effective one for the medical problem.<br>The drug product is not effective for the medical condition.<br>The condition is refractory to the drug product being used.<br>The dosage form is inappropriate. |
| **Dosage too low** | The dose is too low to produce the desired outcome.<br>The dosage interval is too infrequent.<br>A drug interaction reduces the amount of active drug available.<br>The duration of therapy is too short. |
| **Adverse drug reaction** | The drug product causes an undesirable reaction that is not dose-related.<br>A safer drug is needed because of patient risk factors.<br>A drug interaction causes an undesirable reaction that is not dose-related.<br>The regimen was administered or changed too rapidly.<br>The product causes an allergic reaction.<br>The drug is contraindicated because of patient risk factors. |
| **Dosage too high** | The dose is too high for the patient.<br>The dosing frequency is too short. The duration of therapy is too long.<br>A drug interaction causes a toxic reaction to the drug product.<br>The dose was administered too rapidly. |
| **Noncompliance** | The patient does not understand the instructions.<br>The patient prefers not to take the medication.<br>The patient forgets to take the medication.<br>Drug product is too expensive.<br>The patient cannot swallow or self-administer the medication properly.<br>The drug product is not available for the patient. |

*Adapted with permission from Cipolle RJ, Strand LM, Morley PC. Pharmaceutical Care Practice: A Clinician's Guide, 2nd ed. New York, McGraw-Hill, 2004:178–179.*

A drug therapy problem can be resolved or prevented only when the cause of the problem is clearly understood. Therefore, it is necessary to identify and categorize both the drug therapy problem and its cause (Table 4-2).[1]

## CREATION OF A PHARMACEUTICAL CARE PLAN

Care plan development is a cooperative effort that should involve the patient as an active participant. It may also involve an interdisciplinary team of care providers and the patient's family. Care planning involves establishing therapeutic goals and determining appropriate interventions to:

1. Resolve all existing drug therapy problems.
2. Achieve the goals of therapy intended for each active medical problem.
3. Prevent future drug therapy problems that have a potential to develop.

Although care plans have been a standard component of the practice of other health professionals (e.g., nurses, physical therapists, respiratory therapists) for many years, there is still no standard, widely accepted method of care planning in pharmacy. In 1995, the Joint Commission on Accreditation of Healthcare Organizations (JCAHO) made pharmaceutical care planning a requirement for accreditation in all settings that it accredits. This requirement mandates that pharmaceutical care planning be included in the overall plan of care for the patient.[3] Implementation of a systematic care planning process serves to organize the pharmacist's practice, to communicate activities to other health care professionals, and to provide a record of drug therapy interventions in the event that questions arise regarding the standard of care provided to a patient.

It cannot be overemphasized that a plan of care is not merely a document; rather, it is a systematic, ongoing process of planning, action, and documentation. It is a dynamic instrument that reflects the continuing care that is modified according to the patient's changing needs.[4] The most essential element to remember is that the needs of the patient drive the plan, regardless of the care planning format used. In short, the plan must be tailored to the needs of each unique patient. All care providers and the patient should agree on the care plan because each participant has a responsibility for implementing a portion of the plan. In the ambulatory care setting, the patient often assumes much of the responsibility for plan implementation.

Organization of a care plan is important, and each medical problem should be addressed separately and in its entirety so that the drug therapy problems associated with each condition and the plans for intervention are logically organized and implemented. The elements of a care plan include:

- *Medical condition:* List the disease state for which the patient has drug-related needs.
- *Drug therapy problems:* State the drug therapy problems by including the patient's problem or condition, the drug therapy involved, and the association between the drug(s) and the patient's condition(s).
- *Goals of therapy:* State the goals in the future tense. Goals should be realistic, measurable and/or observable, specific, and associated with a definite time frame.
- *Interventions:* In collaboration with the patient, the practitioner develops and prioritizes a list of activities to address the patient's drug-related needs. The patient's input is important because the plan should adequately address the patient's unique concerns, needs, and preferences. The list of activities may be stated in the past, present, or future tense. Include the recommendations made to the patient, the caregiver on the patient's behalf, or the prescriber to resolve (or prevent) the patient's drug therapy problems.
- *Follow-up plan:* Determine when the patient should return for follow-up and what will occur at that subsequent visit.

An example of how each of these components might be incorporated into a care plan is given in the following case vignette:

*Patrick Murphy is a 73-year-old man who underwent coronary artery bypass grafting 2 months ago and was started on simvastatin 10 mg by mouth (po) once daily 6 weeks ago for dyslipidemia. The results of this week's fasting lipid profile revealed total cholesterol 230 mg/dL, low-density lipoprotein (LDL) cholesterol 141 mg/dL, high-density lipoprotein cholesterol 45 mg/dL, and triglycerides 220 mg/dL. He continues to smoke 1.5 packs of cigarettes per day.*

- *Medical condition:* Dyslipidemia.
- *Drug therapy problems:* Dyslipidemia treated with an inadequate dose of a lipid-lowering agent.
- *Goals of therapy:* The patient's LDL cholesterol will be lowered to <100 mg/dL within 6 weeks. (*Note*: Because the patient has known coronary artery disease, his goal LDL cholesterol is <100 mg/dL, with an optional goal of 70 mg/dL.[5])
- *Interventions:* The maximum dose of simvastatin is 80 mg, so the dose should be increased in an attempt to achieve the target LDL level. Increase simvastatin to 20 mg po once daily; #30 dispensed. Reviewed possible side effects of simvastatin with patient (constipation, rare muscle weakness) and monitored for liver injury (serum alanine aminotransferase measurements). Recommended that the patient consider stopping smoking—advised to keep a log of smoking habits, including number of cigarettes, time of day, and trigger events.
- *Follow-up plan:* Patient will return to clinic in 6 weeks for a repeat fasting lipid profile, questioning about potential adverse effects, and discussion of a plan for smoking cessation.

## FOLLOW-UP EVALUATION

The purpose of a follow-up evaluation is to evaluate the positive and negative impact of the care plan on the patient, to uncover new drug therapy problems, and to take appropriate action to address new problems or adjust previous therapies as needed. Follow-up evaluation requires direct contact with the patient to obtain feedback about the benefits of therapy achieved, the occurrence of problems such as side effects, and patient concerns about the treatment. Additionally, relevant data are gathered from current clinical assessments, laboratory tests, radiographs, and other procedures. The practitioner evaluates and documents the patient's progress in achieving the goals of therapy.

The evaluation involves comparing goals of therapy with the patient's current status. Cipolle et al. developed terminology to describe the patient's status, the medical conditions, and the

| Status | Definition |
|---|---|
| Resolved | Therapeutic goals achieved for the acute condition; discontinue therapy |
| Stable | Therapeutic goals achieved; continue the same therapy for chronic disease management |
| Improved | Progress is being made in achieving goals; continue the same therapy because more time is required to assess the full benefit of therapy |
| Partial improvement | Progress is being made, but minor adjustments in therapy are required to fully achieve the therapeutic goals before the next assessment |
| Unimproved | Little or no progress has been made, but continue the same therapy to allow additional time for benefit to be observed |
| Worsened | A decline in health is observed despite an adequate duration using the optimal drug; modify drug therapy (e.g., increase the dose of the current medication, add a second agent with additive or synergistic effects) |
| Failure | Therapeutic goals have not been achieved despite an adequate dose and duration of therapy; discontinue current medication(s) and start new therapy |
| Expired | The patient died while receiving drug therapy; document possible contributing factors, especially if they may be drug related |

comparative evaluation of that status with the previously determined therapeutic goals.[1] These terms also describe the actions taken as a result of the follow-up evaluation:

Example: If the patient Mr Murphy described above returns in 6 weeks with a repeat fasting LDL cholesterol of 120 mg/dL without complaints of side effects, the outcome status of this patient would be partial improvement. Another adjustment in therapy is indicated to further reduce his LDL cholesterol (e.g., increase the simvastatin dose to 40 mg po once daily).

## EXAMPLE OF PHARMACEUTICAL CARE PLAN DOCUMENTATION

Each step in the patient care process must be documented. Documentation should take place on an ongoing basis to provide an updated record of the patient's current and changing needs, care activities in response to those needs, the patient's progress, and plans for future care and follow-up evaluation. This document provides a means for communication among health care providers and is now required for accreditation by JCAHO. What JCAHO requires is not merely a list of the patient's current medications but a document that reflects the systematic and dynamic process of patient care. The example provided in Figure 4-1 is intended to demonstrate to students how a pharmaceutical care plan might be created.

A blank care plan form is also included at the end of this chapter for use by students who are completing the cases for this casebook (see Appendix A). Students may practice using this form when completing the case studies in this casebook. The vast amount of medical information available and the widespread computerization of patient records make the use of electronic pharmaceutical care records virtually mandatory. Consequently, use of this relatively simple hard-copy form should be considered only the first step in developing the student's ability to electronically organize and manage large volumes of complex medical information.

On the electronic resource *AccessPharmacy* (www.AccessPharmacy.com, subscription required), care plans from the casebook can be completed electronically and e-mailed to course instructors for grading. The patient cases from this casebook are also available on *AccessPharmacy*, providing a seamless resource for creating and evaluating the patient care plans written by students.

*Example Case Vignette: Donald Bennett is a 64-year-old man with osteoarthritis currently treated with nabumetone. He has been diagnosed with hypertension based on the average of two blood pressure (BP) readings taken at three previous clinic visits.[6] The hypertension is presently untreated. What information must be included in the patient's pharmaceutical care plan?*

## PATIENT INFORMATION

- *The patient's name* is essential to identify the patient to whom the record belongs. The name, Donald Bennett, should be the first information placed on the chart. Although this guideline seems logical, it sometimes does not happen. When in a hurry, a care provider may grab a blank form and begin to make notes with the intention of placing the patient's personal information on it later, and in the midst of distractions, the name is not recorded.
- *Current address and phone number* are necessary for future contact and follow-up evaluation. The information should be complete (621 E. Greene Street, Washington, PA 15301), and the telephone number should include the area code (412-555-1950).
- *Insurance* information should include the name of the insurance plan and policy number (Metro United Health Plan #1234789) to ensure accurate billing of services.
- *Demographic* information including *age (birth date), gender, race, height, and weight* should be recorded for the purpose of individualizing drug therapy. Mr Bennett is a 64-year-old Caucasian man who is 5′11″ tall and weighs 177 lb. Include weight information in both pounds and kilograms. The equation for converting pounds to kilograms is as follows: weight in pounds/2.2 = weight in kilograms. Mr Bennett weighs 177 lb or 80.4 kg (177/2.2 = 80.4). This information is used to determine the appropriate drug and dosage regimens for treatment. *Ideal body weight (IBW)* is necessary for calculating appropriate dosage for medications that do not distribute into fatty tissues. IBW is calculated as follows: for men, IBW = 50 kg + (2.3 × [height in inches above 5 ft]); for women, IBW = 45.5 kg + (2.3 × [height in inches above 5 ft]). For Mr Bennett, 50 kg + (2.3 × 11) = 75.3 kg.
- *Allergies and adverse drug reactions* should be documented with specific descriptions of the reactions that occurred. Reactions should be clearly identified as allergies or side effects. Mr Bennett has an allergic reaction to penicillin that resulted in hives. He also has experienced dyspepsia, a well-documented side effect of ibuprofen. This information is critical to avoiding patient harm. Allergies are distinct from side effects. An allergy is an immune-mediated reaction that often precludes future use of the medication except in rare cases in which the benefit of using the drug outweighs the risk of the reaction. However, a side effect may sometimes be self-limiting with continued use, or it may be successfully managed with adjustments in the dosage regimen or administration. For example, a drug that is taken once daily and causes drowsiness may be administered at bedtime. A drug that causes GI upset may be successfully managed by taking it with meals.
- *Tobacco/alcohol/substance use* information is important for appropriate drug selection, dosing calculation, and patient education. Include the name of the substance, the amount, and frequency, when possible. Mr Bennett occasionally smokes approximately three cigars each week and drinks 1 oz of whiskey with each cigar. It is important to record pertinent negatives for substance use. For example, caffeine may increase BP acutely, although tolerance to this effect develops quickly. Nevertheless, caffeine use may be relevant to this patient and should be recorded. Alcohol and tobacco may affect the metabolism of certain drugs and potentiate or counteract the benefits of other drugs. For example, tobacco enhances the metabolism of theophylline. Therefore, smokers generally require higher doses of theophylline to achieve therapeutic benefits. Substances such as cocaine, caffeine, or tobacco may enhance the sympathomimetic effect of some drugs while counteracting the sympatholytic effects of others, such as some antihypertensive medications.
- *Medical conditions* should be listed to offer a general overview of the patient's medical problems. The care plan is also organized according to the medical condition whereby all drug therapy problems associated with each medical condition are addressed separately and in their entirety.

## MEDICATION RECORD

- The list of medications should include the date each was started; the indication for use; and the drug name, strength, and regimen that the patient is actually taking. The *actual* regimen may differ from the *prescribed* regimen because patients

## PHARMACEUTICAL CARE PATIENT RECORD

| | |
|---|---|
| **Patient Name:** Donald Benferardo | **Gender:** M |
| **Address:** 621 E. Greene St., Washington PA 15301 | **Race:** W |
| **Telephone:** 412-555-1950 **Age:** 64 | **Actual Weight:** 177 lb (80 kg) |
| **Insurance:** Metro United Health Plan #1234789 | **Ideal Weight:** 166 lb (75.3 kg) |
| **Medical Conditions:** Osteoarthritis left knee (stable) | **Allergies:** Penicillin ⟶ hives |
| **Tobacco/Alcohol/Substance Use:** Occasional cigar 3×/wk; EtOH 3×/wk; no caffeine | **Adverse Reactions:** Ibuprofen ⟶ dyspepsia |

### Medication Record

| Start Date | Stop Date | Indication | Drug Name | Actual Strength | Regimen | Clinical Impressions |
|---|---|---|---|---|---|---|
| 12/14/05 | | Osteoarthritis | Nabumetone | 750 mg | 2 tablet po once daily | Tolerating well minor knee pain |
| 5/03/08 | 5/17/08 | HTN | Hydrochlorothiazide | 25 mg | 1 tablet po once daily | 5/17/08: D/C due to hypokalemia |
| 5/17/08 | | HTN | Triamterene/ Hydrochlorothiazide | 37.25/25 mg | 1 tablet po once daily | 5/31/08: $K^+$ WNL; HTN partially improved |
| 5/31/08 | | HTN | Atenolol | 50 mg | 1 tablet po once daily | |
| | | | | | | |

### Assessment, Plan, and Follow-Up Evaluation

| Date | Medical Condition | Drug-Therapy Problem | Goal | Current Status | Interventions | Follow-Up Plan |
|---|---|---|---|---|---|---|
| 5/3/08 | HTN | Untreated HTN | Lower BP to 110–138/70–88 within 4 wks | Untreated (BP 160/104) | Start hydrochlorothiazide 25 mg po once daily × 4 wks | Return for BP check & serum K+ in 2 wks |
| 5/17/08 | HTN | Hypokalemia secondary to hydrochlorothiazide | K+ 3.5–5.0 mEq/L | Untreated (K+ 3.2 mEq/L) | Discontinue HCT Start triamterene/HCT 3.75/25 mg po once daily | Recheck $K^+$ in 2 wks |
| 5/17/08 | HTN | HTN inadequately treated with hydrochlorothiazide | BP 110–138/70–88 | Partial improvement (BP 150/92) | Change to triamterene/HCT as above | Return in 2 wks for BP & K+ check |
| 5/31/08 | HTN | Hypokalemia requiring drug therapy | K+ 3.5–5.0 mEq/L | Stable (K+ 3.6 mEq/L) | Continue current therapy | Check symptoms of ↓K+ in 1 mo |
| 5/31/08 | HTN | HTN inadequately treated with hydrochlorothiazide | Same as above | Partial improvement (BP 146/92) | Add atenolol 50 mg po once daily × 4 wks | Return for BP check in 1 mo |
| | | | | | | |
| | | | | | | |
| | | | | | | |
| | | | | | | |

**FIGURE 4-1.** Sample pharmaceutical care patient record. (BP, blood pressure; HTN, hypertension; WNL, within normal limits; $K^+$, potassium; HCT, hydrochlorothiazide.)

do not always take medications as directed. Assessment of therapy must be made based on the actual therapy the patient is receiving. Mr Bennett is currently taking nabumetone two 750-mg tablets po daily. A stop date should be recorded for medications that have been discontinued.

- Relevant clinical impressions or comments can also be recorded, for example: "Discontinued ibuprofen secondary to dyspepsia that occurred even when taken with food." Also note the antihypertensive regimen, which was initiated with hydrochlorothiazide 25 mg po once daily and subsequently changed to triamterene/hydrochlorothiazide 37.5/25 mg po once daily. Atenolol 50 mg po once daily was added later because only partial improvement in hypertension was achieved with diuretic therapy.

## ASSESSMENT, PLAN, AND FOLLOW-UP EVALUATION

This section of the patient's record provides a record of therapeutic interventions and the patient's responses to them. Information is documented as events occur, providing a "flow chart" of the patient's progress to date. The historical information contained in this chart is important to incorporate in therapeutic decision making.

- *The date* should be recorded in the far left column to document when each encounter occurred. Mr Bennett's chart shows that he has been seen three times: on May 3, May 17, and May 31, 2011.
- The next column, *medical condition*, specifies the medical diagnosis for which the medications are indicated. On May 3, Mr Bennett was diagnosed with hypertension; his subsequent visits also were for evaluation of hypertension.
- The *drug therapy problem* is recorded in the next column to indicate the drug therapy problem(s) associated with each medical diagnosis. Each medical diagnosis may have one or more drug therapy problems associated with it. On May 3, Mr Bennett had one drug therapy problem—untreated hypertension. That is, he had an indication for drug therapy but was not receiving treatment. On May 17 and May 31, the dates were recorded twice because on these days he had two drug therapy problems that were being addressed. Each drug therapy problem should be recorded in a separate row. Although he had only one active diagnosis (hypertension), he had two drug therapy problems associated with that diagnosis as shown on May 17 and May 31. He had hypokalemia possibly secondary to hydrochlorothiazide and hypertension inadequately treated with hydrochlorothiazide.
- The *goal* of therapy is recorded in the next column. Using the SMART acronym, therapy goals should be ***Specific***, ***Measurable*** (or observable), and ***Achievable***. The goal should also be directly ***Related*** to the drug therapy problem. In this case, the systolic BP goal should be less than 140 mm Hg with a diastolic pressure of less than 90 mm Hg. Treatment to lower levels may be useful if tolerated by the patient. For example, the clinician may establish an acceptable range of BP control, such as systolic BP between 110 and 138 mm Hg and diastolic BP between 70 and 88 mm Hg. The ***Timeline*** to achieve the goal should also be specified. For example, his BP should be reduced to within the indicated range within 4 weeks of therapy.
- The *current status* includes the patient's actual BP at each encounter. In this case, Mr Bennett's BP was 160/104 mm Hg on May 3 prior to starting drug therapy. Notice that his BP continues to decline with treatment. On May 17 and May 31, his BPs were 150/92 and 146/92 mm Hg, respectively. The status on May 31 (4 weeks after treatment) is considered partially improved because the BP did decrease with treatment, but an adjustment in treatment is still required to achieve the BP goal.
- *Interventions* that were implemented must be recorded. The drug name, dose, route, frequency, and duration of therapy should be documented. On May 3, hydrochlorothiazide was started at a dose of 25 mg orally once a day. As you look down this column, you can see that the therapy was adjusted on May 17 and May 31. These interventions were made in response to the patient's BP as recorded in the previous column. By looking across the row, you can see the supportive evidence for the intervention: a clearly documented problem (hypertension) and the patient's status measured objectively (BP). Looking down the columns, one can see what interventions have been made and also how the patient has responded over time.
- The *follow-up plan* specifies details of how the outcome of therapy will be assessed. This column should contain information about who will do what and when they will do it. The plan made on May 3 indicated that Mr Bennett was to return to the clinic in 2 weeks to have his BP and serum potassium level measured. This flow chart provides an easy way to see whether the patient is appearing for the follow-up visits. Mr Bennett did return for follow-up in 2 weeks (May 17) according to the plan. There should continue to be a follow-up plan as long as a person is receiving drug therapy. After the patient's condition is stabilized, the follow-up intervals may be much longer, such as every 6 months or once a year. However, the assessment, plan, and follow-up must continue for the duration of drug therapy. In this case, after Mr Bennett's BP is stabilized, he may be responsible for monitoring his own BP and assessing the side effects by self-monitoring while keeping a twice-yearly appointments for a more formal evaluation at the clinic. The patient's care plan remains active and represents the ongoing and dynamic process of providing pharmaceutical care.

## PATIENT SUMMARY

Based on the information documented in the care plan, the practitioner providing care to this patient and other health care professionals who have access to this information should be able to extract the following summary of this patient's past and present status regarding hypertension treatment and response:

*Mr Bennett is a 64-year-old man diagnosed with osteoarthritis and hypertension. He was seen on May 3, 2011, at which time his BP was 160/104 mm Hg. His goal BP range was set as systolic BP of 110–138 mm Hg and diastolic BP of 70–88 mm Hg. This was the standard against which future BP measurements would be compared. He was started on hydrochlorothiazide 25 mg orally once daily for 2 weeks and was to return to clinic for a follow-up BP check and serum potassium level 2 weeks later. He returned according to the plan, but the BP reading of 152/98 mm Hg indicated only a partial improvement. The BP reduction had not yet reached the goal level; it may take 4 weeks for the full effect of diuretic therapy to be manifested. Consequently, no adjustment in therapy was made pending an adequate trial of single-agent diuretic therapy. However, the low serum potassium value of 3.2 mEq/L (reference range 3.5–5.0 mEq/L) indicated hypokalemia that required treatment. Because the hypokalemia may have resulted from the thiazide diuretic, hydrochlorothiazide 25 mg was discontinued and a combination product containing triamterene 37.5 mg + hydrochlorothiazide 25 mg, one tablet orally once daily, was begun. He returned 2 weeks later as planned and his BP continued to show improvement (148/96 mm Hg), but it was not at the therapeutic goal that had been established 4 weeks earlier. This indicated partial improvement requiring further adjustment of his antihypertensive therapy. However, his potassium level had risen to within the normal range. Therefore, atenolol 50 mg orally once daily was added to the regimen. The patient was scheduled to return for a follow-up visit in 1 month.*

## CONCLUSIONS

Implementation of a care planning process is necessary for providing consistent pharmaceutical care and for documenting the outcomes of that care. It is also essential for obtaining compensation for care provided. Care planning captures past and current events occurring in a dynamic patient care process that is provided in response to changing patient needs. This process should be incorporated into the practice of each provider of pharmaceutical care, regardless of the practice setting.

## REFERENCES


1. Cipolle RJ, Strand LM, Morley PC. Pharmaceutical Care Practice: The Clinician's Guide, 2nd ed. New York, McGraw-Hill, 2004.
2. ASHP Council on Professional Affairs. ASHP guidelines on a standard method for pharmaceutical care. Am J Hosp Pharm 1996;53:1713–1716.
3. Rich DS. JCAHO's pharmaceutical care plan requirements. Hosp Pharm 1995;30(4):315–319.
4. McCallian DJ, Carlstedt BC, Rupp MT. Elements of a pharmaceutical care plan. Am J Pharm Assoc 1999;39(1):82–83.
5. Expert Panel on Detection, Evaluation, and Treatment of High Blood Cholesterol in Adults. Executive summary of the third report of the National Cholesterol Education Program (NCEP) Expert Panel on Detection, Evaluation, and Treatment of High Blood Cholesterol in Adults (Adult Treatment Panel III). JAMA 2001;285:2486–2497.
6. Chobaman AV, Bakris GL, Black HR, et al. The seventh report of the Joint National Committee on Prevention, Detection, Evaluation, and Treatment of High Blood Pressure: the JNC 7 report. JAMA 2003;289(19):2560–2572.

## APPENDIX A

Sample Pharmaceutical Care Patient Record for Creating a Care Plan

| PHARMACEUTICAL CARE PATIENT RECORD | | |
|---|---|---|
| **Patient Name:** | | **Gender:** |
| **Address:** | | **Race:** |
| **Telephone:** | **Age:** | **Actual Weight:** |
| **Insurance:** | | **Ideal Weight:** |
| **Medical Conditions:** | | **Allergies:** |
| **Tobacco/Alcohol/Substance Use:** | | **Adverse Reactions:** |

**Medication Record**

| Start Date | Stop Date | Indication | Drug Name | Actual Strength | Regimen | Clinical Impressions |
|---|---|---|---|---|---|---|
| | | | | | | |
| | | | | | | |
| | | | | | | |
| | | | | | | |
| | | | | | | |
| | | | | | | |
| | | | | | | |
| | | | | | | |
| | | | | | | |
| | | | | | | |

**Assessment, Plan, and Follow-Up Evaluation**

| Date | Medical Condition | Drug-Therapy Problem | Goal | Current Status | Interventions | Follow-Up Plan |
|---|---|---|---|---|---|---|
| | | | | | | |
| | | | | | | |
| | | | | | | |
| | | | | | | |
| | | | | | | |
| | | | | | | |
| | | | | | | |
| | | | | | | |
| | | | | | | |

CHAPTER

# 5 Documentation of Pharmacotherapy Interventions

BRUCE R. CANADAY, PHARMD, FASHP, FAPhA
ROBERT M. MALONE, PHARMD, CDE, CPP
LAURIE M. WHALIN, PHARMD
TIMOTHY J. IVES, PHARMD, MPH, BCPS, FCCP, FASHP, CPP

If there is no documentation, then it did not happen! This philosophy is the standard in all health care settings as physicians, nurses, respiratory therapists, physical therapists, social workers, and other health care providers generate and maintain detailed notes regarding the patient's condition and their efforts to achieve the best possible outcomes for the patient. Documentation chronologically outlines the care the patient received and serves as a form of communication among health care practitioners, an important element that contributes to the quality of care provided. Each practitioner involved knows what evaluation has occurred, what the patient's treatment plan is, and who will provide it. Furthermore, third-party payers may require reasonable documentation from practitioners that assures that the services provided are consistent with the insurance coverage.[1] General components of documentation include:

- A complete and legible record;
- Documentation for each encounter with a rationale for the encounter, physical findings, prior test results, assessment, clinical impression (or diagnosis), and plan for care;
- Identified health risk factors, and an easily inferred rationale for ordering diagnostic tests or ancillary services; and
- The patient's progress, response to and changes in treatment, and revision of the original diagnosis/assessment.

Traditionally, this documentation was paper based. These records are often inaccessible at the point of patient care, not easily transferable or transportable, illegible, poorly organized, and often may be missing key information. Due to these limitations, many academic centers and health care systems have developed and implemented electronic health records (EHRs). Further, *Crossing the Quality Chasm* was published in 2001 by the Institute of Medicine. This report identified the EHR as a key component to improve access to medical information, facilitate decision support and collection of data, and reduce medical errors.[2] The EHR may also assist in improved documentation, with reduced clinical variation and better provision of quality preventative and chronic care.[3–5] Furthermore, use of EHR features in primary care is associated with higher performance on certain quality measures.[6]

## PRINCIPLES OF DOCUMENTATION

Documentation in the record is required to record pertinent facts, findings, and observations about a patient's health history, including past and present illnesses, examinations, tests, treatments, and outcomes. Particularly in an era of evolution of electronic databases,[7] it also facilitates:

- The ability of providers to evaluate and plan the patient's immediate treatment and monitor his or her health care over time;
- Communication and continuity of care among providers involved in the patient's care;
- Accurate and timely claims review and payment;
- Appropriate utilization review and quality of care evaluations;
- Collection of data that may be useful for research and education; and
- Appropriate coding (i.e., Current Procedural Terminology [CPT] and International Statistical Classification of Diseases and Related Health Problems, Tenth Revision, Clinical Modification [ICD-10-CM], from the World Health Organization) for use on health insurance claim forms should be supported by documentation in the patient record.

Much of this documentation is derived from a systematic patient care process of evaluation that is standardized within each discipline. For example, physicians are taught to perform a history and physical examination based on a standardized review of body systems and to document their results using a universally accepted, standardized, and systematic process.

Several evaluation/documentation systems have been suggested for health care professionals. More than 30 years ago, the use of a Problem-Oriented Medical Record was proposed,[8] and most, if not all, physicians, nurse practitioners, physician associates, and other health care practitioners have been taught to write progress notes using the Subjective, Objective, Assessment, Plan (SOAP) format. The example elements of SOAP are as follows:

**S** = Subjective: Chief complaint; history of present illness; why the patient is being seen;

**O** = Objective: Physical findings and measurable data such as laboratory values, drug levels, and imaging studies.

**A** = Assessment: Analysis or conclusion about the patient's current status/behavior, evidence of progress, response to intervention or medication, and change in functional status;

**P** = Plan: Interventions or actions taken in response to assessment, collaboration with others, plan for follow-up, change in diagnosis, and documentation that the patient was informed of changes in interventions and/or medications.

Institutional consultant notes often use an abbreviated version of the SOAP format. This abbreviated version usually includes Findings (i.e., subjective and objective information), Assessment (or Impression), and Diagnosis (or Recommendations). In most cases, the EHR has embraced many of the key components of the above formats. EHR documentation is tailored to documenting medical encounters and history and also to maximize billing by meeting requirements established by the federal Centers for Medicare & Medicaid Services. Traditionally this documentation has been performed by dictation and transcription. Most EHRs use templates to accept automated insertion of clinical data and fields with "copy and paste" capabilities, both of which facilitate documentation.

Historically, pharmacy has not had a corresponding standardized approach to the evaluation and documentation of the patient's pharmacotherapy that is applicable to all types of pharmacy practice settings. Thus, pharmacy has not been as active as other disciplines in documenting its contributions to patient care.

## EVOLUTION OF PHARMACIST-PROVIDED CARE AND THE IMPORTANCE OF DOCUMENTATION

Pharmacist-provided care has gone through a long evolutionary process that, like all evolutionary processes, continues to bring change. Early descriptors such as *clinical pharmacy* continue to hold meaning[9] but have also spawned terms such as *pharmaceutical care* and, most recently, *medication therapy management* (MTM).

### PHARMACEUTICAL CARE

Pharmaceutical care uses a process through which a pharmacist cooperates with a patient and other health care professionals in designing, implementing, and monitoring a therapeutic plan that will produce specific therapeutic outcomes for the patient.[10] This process involves three major functions:

1. Identifying potential and actual drug-related problems;
2. Resolving actual drug-related problems;
3. Preventing potential drug-related problems.

These functions aid in the provision of patient care through the identification of medication-related problems, development of a pharmacotherapeutic plan to address the problems, and the ultimate resolution or prevention of those problems.

As described in **Chapter 1**, a systematic approach is used in this casebook to identify and resolve the medication-related problems of patients. The steps can be summarized as follows:

1. Identification of real or potential medication therapy problems;
2. Determination of desired therapeutic outcomes and therapeutic endpoints;
3. Determination of therapeutic alternatives;
4. Design of an optimal pharmacotherapeutic plan for the patient;
5. Identification of parameters to evaluate the outcome;
6. Provision of patient education;
7. Communication and implementation of the pharmacotherapeutic plan.

Step 7 is crucial; the tenets of pharmaceutical care suggest that pharmacists should document, at the very least, the actual or potential drug therapy problems identified, as well as the associated interventions that they desire to implement or have implemented. Pharmacists must adequately communicate their recommendations and actions to nonpharmacy health care practitioners (e.g., physicians, nurses), the patient or caregiver (e.g., parents), or other pharmacists. The goal is to provide a clear, concise record of the actual/potential problem,[11,12] the thought process that led the pharmacist to select an intervention, and the intervention itself. Additionally, the ability to receive remuneration for services provided also necessitates an acceptable documentation strategy.

### MEDICATION THERAPY MANAGEMENT

MTM has been defined as a distinct service or group of services that optimize therapeutic outcomes for individual patients.[13] MTM services are independent of, but can occur in conjunction with, the provision of a medication product. MTM encompasses a broad range of professional activities and responsibilities within the scope of practice of the licensed pharmacist or other qualified health care providers. These services include, but are not limited to, the following activities according to the individual needs of the patient:

1. Performing or obtaining necessary assessments of the patient's health status;
2. Formulating a medication treatment plan;
3. Selecting, initiating, modifying, or administering medication therapy;
4. Monitoring and evaluating the patient's response to therapy, including safety and effectiveness;
5. Performing a comprehensive medication review to identify, resolve, and prevent medication-related problems, including adverse drug events;
6. Documenting the care delivered and communicating essential information to the patient's other primary care providers;
7. Providing verbal education and training designed to enhance patient understanding and appropriate use of his or her medications;
8. Providing information, support services, and resources designed to enhance patient adherence with his or her therapeutic regimens;
9. Coordinating and integrating MTM services within the broader health care management services being provided to the patient.

In concert with this definition, patients, providers, payers, and health information technology system vendors have been encouraged to develop a documentation format that meets individual and customer needs.[14] This documentation format, while not a standard, can be useful in achieving the goals of the process. The white paper notes that the pharmacist is responsible for documenting services in a manner appropriate for evaluating patient progress and sufficient for billing purposes, and that the use of core documentation elements will help to create consistency in professional documentation and information sharing among members of the health care team, while facilitating practitioner, organization, or regional variations.[13] Documentation of MTM services includes the following information categories:

- Patient demographics;
- Known allergies, diseases (e.g., heart failure), or conditions (e.g., pregnancy);
- A record of all medications, including prescription, nonprescription, herbal, and other dietary supplement products;
- Assessment of medication therapy problems and plans for resolution;
- Therapeutic monitoring performed;
- Interventions or referrals made;
- Education provided to the patient;
- Schedule and plan for follow-up appointment;
- Amount of time spent with the patient;
- Feedback provided to providers or patients.

While the precise format may not be critical at this point, standardization of documentation must and will evolve to provide for clarity in the history and plan, timely feedback, consistent follow-up, and enhanced continuity of care.

## THE SOAP NOTE FORMAT FOR DOCUMENTATION

As noted above, in the SOAP note format subjective (S) and objective (O) data are recorded and then assessed (A) to formulate a plan (P). Subjective data include patient symptoms (e.g., pain), clinician observations (e.g., agitation), or information obtained about the patient (e.g., history of smoking). By its nature, subjective information is descriptive and generally cannot be confirmed by diagnostic tests or procedures. Much of the subjective information is obtained by speaking with the patient while obtaining the medical history, as described in **Chapter 1** (i.e., chief complaint, history of present illness, past medical history, family history, social history, medications, allergies, and review of systems). Important subjective information may also be obtained by direct interview with the patient after the initial medical history has been performed (e.g., a description of an adverse drug effect, rating of pain severity using standard scales).

A primary source of objective information (O) is the physical examination. Other relevant objective information includes laboratory values, serum drug concentrations (along with the target therapeutic range for each level), and the results of other diagnostic tests (e.g., electrocardiogram [ECG], x-rays, culture and sensitivity tests). Risk factors that may predispose the patient to a particular problem should also be considered for inclusion. The communication note should include only the pertinent positive and negative findings. Pertinent negative findings are signs and symptoms of the disease or problem that are not present in the particular patient being evaluated.

The assessment (A) section outlines what the practitioner thinks the patient's problem is, based on the subjective and objective information acquired. This assessment often takes the form of a diagnosis or differential diagnosis. This portion of the SOAP note should include all of the reasons for the clinician's assessment. This helps other health care providers reading the note to understand how the clinician arrived at his or her particular assessment of the problem.

The plan (P) may include ordering additional diagnostic tests or initiating, revising, or discontinuing treatment. If the plan includes changes in pharmacotherapy, the rationale for the specific changes recommended should be described. The drug, dose, dosage form, schedule, route of administration, and duration of therapy should be included. The plan should be directed toward achieving a specific, measurable goal or endpoint, which should be clearly stated in the note. The plan should also outline the efficacy and toxicity parameters that will be used to determine whether the desired therapeutic outcome is being achieved and to detect or prevent drug-related adverse events. Ideally, information about the therapy that should be communicated to the patient should also be included in the plan. The plan should be reviewed and referred to in the note as often as necessary.

## THE "FARM" NOTE FOR DOCUMENTING DRUG THERAPY PROBLEMS AND PLANS

There is a pharmacist equivalent of a physician's progress note in a systematized approach for the construction and maintenance of a record reflecting the pharmacist's contributions to care.[15] This process includes provisions for the identification and assessment of actual or potential medication-related problems, description of a therapeutic plan, and appropriate follow-up monitoring of the problems. Although there is no current uniform documentation system for the profession of pharmacy, students are encouraged to try this system as they learn to document patient interventions and compare its effectiveness with the SOAP format. In this system, problems that have been identified are addressed systematically in a pharmacist's note under the headings Findings, Assessment, Resolution, and Monitoring. The sections of the pharmacist's note can be easily recalled with the mnemonic F-A-R-M.

## IDENTIFICATION OF DRUG THERAPY PROBLEMS

The first step in the construction of a FARM note is to clearly state the nature of the drug-related problem(s). Each problem in the FARM note should be addressed separately and assigned a sequential number. Understanding the types of problems that may occur facilitates identification of pharmacotherapy problems. Several classifications of problems have been suggested. Cipolle et al. suggested seven types of medication-related problems (see **Chapter 1**)[16]:

1. Unnecessary drug therapy
2. Needs additional drug therapy
3. Ineffective drug
4. Dosage too low
5. Adverse drug reaction
6. Dosage too high
7. Noncompliance

Roth et al.[17] suggested eight categories of drug therapy problems:

1. Suboptimal drug
2. Suboptimal dosing or duration
3. Adverse drug events
4. Nonadherence
5. Drug not cost effective
6. Undertreatment
7. Inadequate medication monitoring
8. Other (potential medical or drug therapy problem)

Use of classification systems such as these for the various types of medication-related problems offers at least two advantages. First, it presents a framework, applicable in any practice setting, to assure that the pharmacist has considered each possible type of problem. Second, categorization allows optimal data analysis and retrieval capabilities. Thus, problems as well as the interventions to resolve them can be stored in a standardized format in a computer. When an analysis of this information is needed at a later date, such as determining how much money was saved through an intervention, how outcomes were improved by the pharmacist, or how many problems of a certain type have occurred, the problems and interventions can be reviewed by groups rather than individually.

## DOCUMENTATION OF FINDINGS

Each statement of a drug-related problem should be followed by documentation of the pertinent findings (F) indicating that the problem may (potential) or does (actual) exist. Information included in this section should include a summary of the pertinent information obtained after collection and thorough assessment of the available patient information. Demographic data that may be reported include a patient identifier (e.g., name, initials, or medical record number), age, race (if pertinent), and gender. As noted earlier in the section "The SOAP Note Format for Documentation," medical information included in the note should include both subjective and objective findings that indicate a drug-related problem.

## ASSESSMENT OF PROBLEMS

The assessment (A) section of the FARM note includes the pharmacist's evaluation of the current situation (i.e., the nature, extent, type, and clinical significance of the problem). This part of the note should delineate the thought process that led to the conclusion that a problem did or did not exist and that an active intervention either was or was not necessary. If additional information is required to satisfactorily assess the problem and make recommendations, these data should be stated along with their source (e.g., the patient, pharmacist, physician). The severity or urgency of the problem should be indicated by stating whether the interventions that follow should be made immediately or within 1 day, 1 week, 1 month, or longer. The desired therapeutic endpoint or outcome should be stated. This may include both short-term goals (e.g., lower blood pressure to <140/90 mm Hg in a patient with primary hypertension [therapeutic endpoint]) and long-term goals (e.g., prevent cardiovascular complications in that patient [therapeutic outcome]).

## PROBLEM RESOLUTION

The resolution (R) section should reflect the actions proposed (or already performed) to resolve the drug-related problem based on the preceding analysis. The note should convey that, after consideration of all appropriate therapeutic options, the option(s) considered to be the most beneficial was either carried out or suggested to someone else (e.g., the physician, patient, or caregiver). Recommendations may include nonpharmacologic therapy, such as dietary modification or assistive devices (e.g., canes, walkers); the rationale for this method of treatment should be described. If pharmacotherapy is recommended, a specific drug, dose, route, schedule, and duration of therapy should be specified. It is not sufficient to simply provide a list of choices for the prescriber. Importantly, the rationale for selecting the particular regimen(s) should be stated. It is reasonable to include alternative regimens that would be satisfactory if the patient is unable to complete treatment with the initial regimen because of adverse effects, allergy, cost, or other reasons. If patient education is recommended, the information that will be included in the session should be described. Conversely, if certain types of information will be withheld from the patient, the reasons for doing so should be stated. If no action is recommended or was taken, that should be documented as well. In this situation, the note serves as a record of the pharmacist's involvement in the patient's care. The pharmacist then has documentation that patient care activities were performed.

## MONITORING FOR ENDPOINTS AND OUTCOMES

It is not enough, however, to only provide a clear, concise record of the nature of a problem, the assessment that led to the conclusion that a problem exists, and the selection of a plan for resolution of the problem. To truly "close the loop" of patient care, we must follow up on our resolution plan to assure that the intended outcome was achieved. A plan for follow-up monitoring (M) of the patient must be documented and adequately implemented. This process is likely to include questioning the patient, gathering laboratory data, and performing the ongoing physical assessments necessary to determine the effect of the plan that was implemented to assure that it results in an optimal outcome for the patient.

Monitoring parameters to assess efficacy generally include improvement in or resolution of the signs, symptoms, and laboratory abnormalities that were initially assessed. The monitoring parameters used to detect or prevent adverse reactions are determined by the most common and most serious events known to be associated with the therapeutic intervention. Potential adverse reactions should be precisely described along with the method of monitoring. For example, rather than stating "monitor for GI complaints," the recommendation may be to "question the patient about the presence of dyspepsia, diarrhea, or constipation." The frequency, duration, and target endpoint for each monitoring parameter should be identified. The points at which changes in the plan may be warranted should be included. For example, in the case of a patient with dyslipidemia, one may recommend to "obtain fasting high density lipoprotein, low density lipoprotein (LDL), total cholesterol, and triglycerides after 3 months of treatment. If the goal LDL of <100 mg/dL is not achieved with good compliance at 3 months, increase simvastatin to 40 mg by mouth (po) once daily. If goal LDL is achieved, maintain simvastatin 20 mg po once daily and repeat fasting lipoprotein profile annually."

## SUMMARY

A SOAP or FARM progress note constructed in the manner described identifies each drug-related problem and states the pharmacist's Findings observed, an Assessment of the findings, the actual or proposed Resolution of the problem based on the analysis, and the parameters and timing of follow-up Monitoring. Either form of note should provide a clear, concise record of process, activity, and projected follow-up. When written for each medication-related problem, these notes should provide data in a standardized, logical system.

Based on recommendations from organizations such as the Institute of Medicine, Centers for Medicare & Medicaid Services, and those who focus on the provision of quality of care, EHRs will proliferate and may change the way pharmacists and other health care providers document encounters. Documentation may occur by transcription, voice recognition, or direct provider entry. Although the format of the documentation may not strictly follow the SOAP or FARM format, the common principles of documentation will remain.

## SAMPLE CASE PRESENTATION

The following case presentation illustrates how such a system can be used in practice.

Geraldine Johns is a 70-year-old woman seen Monday morning in clinic for her first visit.

### CHIEF COMPLAINT

"I get a little short of breath working around the house sometimes."

### HISTORY OF PRESENT ILLNESS

She states that she has mild heart failure and had a heart attack 4 years ago. She lives alone and has generally maintained a good level of activity and self-care, although she complains of some fatigue and shortness of breath lately while cleaning her house or when climbing stairs.

### PAST MEDICAL HISTORY

She has just moved to town to be near her son following the death of her husband. In addition to her CHF and MI history, she has a history of atrial fibrillation and type 2 diabetes mellitus. She is maintained on metformin 500 mg po BID, omeprazole 20 mg po daily, digoxin 0.125 mg po Q AM, warfarin 5 mg po Q AM, aspirin 81 mg po Q AM, furosemide 80 mg po daily, and metoprolol XL 100 mg po Q AM.

## FAMILY HISTORY

Her husband died recently. She has one son alive and well living in the area and one son who committed suicide 8 years ago.

## SOCIAL HISTORY

She denies illicit drugs and quite smoking 15 years ago. She has a 35 pack-year history. She drinks alcohol rarely on social occasions and denies excessive use.

## PHYSICAL EXAMINATION

### VS

B/P 169/88, P 68 and regular, RR 13, T 99°F; Wt 100 lb, Ht 5′2″

### HEENT

Slight AV nicking, otherwise unremarkable

### Skin

No rashes

### Cardiac

No murmurs or rubs. (+) $S_3$ gallop; PMI in the sixth intercostal space 3 cm distal to the midclavicular line. (+) Hepatojugular reflux. Mild neck vein distention at 45°.

### Chest

Slight crackles at the right and left bases; no rales, e-to-a changes, or tactile fremitus

### Ext

1–2+ pedal edema bilaterally. Ankle brachial index (ABI) = 1.02 (negative).
Strength 5/5

### GI and GU

Unremarkable

### Neuro

Cranial nerves II–XII grossly intact bilaterally
Semmes–Weinstein monofilament is unremarkable
Deep tendon reflexes brisk and 3/4

### Laboratory Values Are Unremarkable with the Following Exceptions

INR 3.5
FBG 198 mg/dL
A1C 9.5% = eAG of 226 mg/dL
Serum creatinine 1.3 mg/dL
Digoxin level 1.0 ng/mL

### Imaging

Chest x-ray demonstrates some diffuse patchiness at the bases. Enlarged cardiac silhouette. Decreased density of the vertebrae, consistent with mild osteoporosis.

Echo suggests no valvular abnormalities and an ejection fraction of 40%.

### ECG

Normal sinus rhythm. Changes consistent with left ventricular hypertrophy.

### Medical Assessment

1. Mild, Class II–III heart failure with pedal edema and mild pulmonary congestion on digoxin, furosemide, and metoprolol.
2. Type 2 DM, not optimally controlled on metformin.
3. Hypertension not optimally managed on metoprolol.
4. Atrial fibrillation, currently rate-controlled on digoxin and metoprolol. Warfarin anticoagulation per guidelines above target (target INR 2–3).
5. Moderate renal insufficiency stage 3: SCr 1.3, estimated CLcr = 29 mL/min, GFR MDRD[18] = 43 mL/min.
6. Possible dyslipidemia, as suggested by history of MI.
7. Suggestion of osteoporosis based on chest radiographs.
8. S/P MI on aspirin and metoprolol; lipid status unknown.

## MEDICAL PLAN

1. Clinic appointment in 2 weeks.
2. Consult Cardiology for evaluation of CHF.
3. Consult nephrology for evaluation of renal dysfunction.
4. Consult diabetes teaching nurse for education and review of injection technique should insulin become necessary.
5. Obtain pharmacotherapy consultation for optimization of medications and patient education.
6. Meds till seen by pharmacotherapy:
   Hold warfarin tomorrow, and then resume at current dose.
   Continue digoxin, metformin, and aspirin.
   Increase furosemide to 80 mg po BID.
   Begin vitamin D 400 mg po daily.

## CONSTRUCTION OF A SOAP OR FARM NOTE

*Note: The Subjective and Objective findings of the SOAP note are combined into Findings for a FARM note. The Plan of the SOAP note is split into Recommendations/Resolution and Monitoring/Follow-Up in the FARM note.*

### Findings

**Subjective** A 70-year-old woman recently moved here after the death of her husband. Patient complains of slight shortness of breath when walking up stairs and long distances. She voices no other complaints. She has a history of atrial fibrillation, type 2 diabetes, mild–moderate heart failure, and S/P MI 4 years ago. She lives alone and maintains a good level of activity and self-care, although lately she complains of some fatigue and shortness of breath while cleaning her house or when climbing stairs. She reports that she takes metformin, omeprazole, digoxin, warfarin, aspirin, furosemide, and metoprolol. She states that she takes her medications as prescribed, but she has some difficulty describing precisely how she takes them and is not certain what each medication does for her.

**Objective**

VS: BP 169/88, P 68 and regular, RR 13, T 99°F; Wt 100 lb, Ht 5′2″
Cardiac: $S_3$ gallop, PMI in the sixth intercostal space 3 cm distal to the midclavicular line
Chest: Slight crackles at the right and left bases
Extremities: 1–2+ pedal edema bilaterally, ABI negative

HEENT: Slight AV nicking, otherwise unremarkable

Medications (per labels on vials):

- Metformin 500 mg po BID
- Omeprazole 20 mg po daily
- Digoxin 0.125 mg po Q AM
- Warfarin 5 mg po Q AM
- EC Aspirin 81 mg po Q AM
- Furosemide 80 mg po BID
- Metoprolol XL 100 mg po QAM

Labs:

- INR 3.5
- Fasting blood glucose 198 mg/dL
- A1C 9.5% (eAG 226 mg/dL)
- Serum creatinine 1.3 mg/dL
- Serum digoxin 1.0 ng/mL

Chest x-ray: Diffuse patchiness at the bases. Enlarged cardiac silhouette. Decreased density of the vertebrae consistent with mild osteoporosis.

ECG: LVH

### *Assessment*

1. Possible nonadherence/nonconcordance and lack of knowledge about medications.
2. Mild heart failure, Class II, as suggested by pedal edema, DOE, symptoms on engaging in ordinary activities, cardiomegaly on chest x-ray, and diminished EF. Maintained on a β-blocker and digoxin (level within target range) and is not currently prescribed an ACE inhibitor.
3. Type 2 diabetes mellitus, not optimally controlled on current metformin dose. A1C above goal of <7%. Not prescribed either an ACE inhibitor or an ARB for renal protective effects.
4. Hypertension, not optimally controlled on metoprolol, as suggested by increased BP, elevated serum creatinine, and AV nicking. The renal and ophthalmic findings are suggestive of significant, sustained hypertension. Repeated measurements will be necessary to confirm this assessment. Addition of ACE inhibitor may improve control as well.
5. Atrial fibrillation:
   a. Rate control: Rate currently under control with metoprolol and digoxin. Digoxin level acceptable. No adjustment indicated.
   b. Anticoagulation: INR above target range of 2.0–3.0, without clinical complications at this time. No cause could be identified; although a change in diet associated with recent life events is possible, the patient provides no information to substantiate that idea. Decreased warfarin dose may be appropriate.
6. Possible moderate renal insufficiency as indicated by increased SCr/decreased GFR by MDRD. Renal dose adjustments evaluated. No changes necessary at this time. Addition of ACE inhibitor therapy may be beneficial to slow rate of GFR decline.
7. S/P MI on low-dose aspirin and metoprolol.
8. R/O osteoporosis: Chest radiography suggestive of osteoporosis. Her petite frame and age are consistent with postmenopausal osteoporosis.
9. Adverse medication effects: Although metoprolol may be considered appropriate for both the post-MI and CHF indications and is a $\beta_1$-selective β-blocker, its $\beta_2$-blocking properties may contribute to worsening CHF due to negative inotropic effects.
10. Medication without indication (omeprazole): On further questioning, the patient recalls being started on it while hospitalized for MI 4 years ago. She was given a prescription for it when she left the hospital. She has no complaints related to GERD or PUD. No need for omeprazole can be identified.

### *Plan (Recommendations/Resolution)*

1. Assess and reinforce adherence/concordance with recommended therapy. Educate on purpose of each medication.
2. Mild heart failure: Continue both the β-blocker metoprolol and digoxin, pending evaluation by the Cardiology Service to determine appropriateness. Suggest initiation of an ACE inhibitor, enalapril 5 mg daily titrating to 10 mg twice daily as tolerated, and increasing furosemide to 100 mg po twice daily until her return next week because of persistent pedal edema and pulmonary congestion. No added dietary salt.
3. Type 2 diabetes mellitus:
   a. Medication: Suggest initiation of an ACE inhibitor (enalapril 5 mg daily as noted above) per current ADA guidelines. Suggest icreasing metformin to 1,000 mg BID to improve control. Continue to follow serum creatinine. Monitor blood glucose readings and, if indicated, may supplement with insulin lispro for elevated premeal BG, based on an estimated insulin sensitivity of 1 unit per 30–40 mg/dL.
   b. Diet: Suggest three meals and bedtime snack, with no concentrated carbohydrate (CHO) choices. Limit CHO intake per meal to 60 g; snacks 15–20 g CHO. No added salt. Check blood glucose AC and HS.
4. Hypertension: Suggest initiation of an ACE inhibitor (enalapril 5 mg daily as above), started at low doses. If repeated measurements confirm the diagnosis of hypertension, they may be titrated to maintain blood pressure control (and improve CHF symptoms—goal 10 mg BID). Blood pressure goal is <130/80 mm Hg in patients with compelling indications. Currently, the patient is stage 2, ≥160/100 mm Hg.
5. Atrial fibrillation:
   a. Rate control: Suggest continuing metoprolol and digoxin unless Cardiology recommends otherwise. No adjustment indicated at this time.
   b. Anticoagulation: INR is above target range of 2.0–3.0. Recommend warfarin 2.5 mg today and then resume 5 mg po daily Monday–Saturday and 2.5 mg on Sunday; dose to be adjusted as needed to maintain INR between 2.0 and 3.0.
6. Renal insufficiency: Repeat serum creatinine. No medication dosage adjustments are indicated currently. Begin low-dose ACE inhibitor (enalapril 5mg daily as above) for renal protective effects with diabetes to slow rate of GFR decline.
7. S/P MI: Recommend continuation of aspirin 81 mg po Q AM. Suggest initiation of ACE inhibitor as noted above, and a statin (e.g., pravastatin 10 mg po at bedtime). Continue metoprolol, if acceptable to Cardiology.
8. Possible dyslipidemia: Treat based on lipid panel; goal LDL is <100 mg/dL in patients with existing CAD or diabetes; this patient has both. Optional goal of <70 mg/dL since patient considered high risk per current NCEP guidelines.
9. Possible osteoporosis: If DXA scan indicates osteoporosis, begin a bisphosphonate (e.g., alendronate 70 mg po weekly), vitamin $D_3$ 1,000 mg daily, and calcium 1,500 mg daily.

10. Adverse medication effects: As noted above, will await Cardiology opinion on need for/appropriateness of β-blocker and digoxin to manage CHF.
11. Medication without indication: Suggest discontinuing omeprazole.

### *Monitoring/Follow-Up*

1. RTC in 1 week.
2. Prior to RTC:
   a. Laboratory (slips given):
      i. Baseline electrolytes (K, Na, Ca, and Mg levels in light of unopposed furosemide therapy of unknown duration and use of digoxin) today;
      ii. Serum creatinine today;
      iii. Fasting lipid panel next week prior to RTC;
      iv. INR next week prior to RTC.
   b. DXA scan.
   c. Cardiology education. Appointment made with Dr Welford's office.
3. Patient instructed to monitor blood glucose AC and HS and bring information on RTC.
4. Prescribed medication after this visit:

   Enalapril 5 mg po daily for CHF, hypertension, and type 2 DM.

   Metformin 1,000 mg po BID for type 2 DM.

   Insulin lispro, as indicated.

   Digoxin 0.125 mg po Q AM for CHF symptoms and rate control.

   Furosemide 100 mg po BID for CHF.

   Warfarin 5 mg po Q AM Monday–Saturday, 2.5 mg on Sunday for S/P MI and CVA prevention.

   EC aspirin 81 mg po daily for secondary cardiovascular prevention.

   Metoprolol XL 100 mg po Q AM for S/P MI and rate control.

   Pravastatin 10 mg po at bedtime for post-MI prophylaxis. Await results of lipid panel.

   D/C Prilosec 20 mg po daily.

## REFERENCES


1. Evaluation & Management Services Guide. Washington, DC, Centers for Medicare & Medicaid Services, July 2009. Available at: *http://www.cms.hhs.gov/MLNProducts/Downloads/eval_mgmt_serv_guide.pdf.* Accessed March 3, 2010.
2. Institute of Medicine. Crossing the Quality Chasm: A New Health System for the 21st Century. Washington DC, National Academy Press, 2001.
3. O'Conner PJ, Crain AL, Rush WA, et al. Impact of an electronic medical record on diabetes quality of care. Ann Fam Med 2005;3:300–306.
4. Asch SM, McGlynn EA, Hogan MM, et al. Comparison of quality of care for patients in the Veterans Health Administration and patients in a national sample. Ann Intern Med 2004;141:938–945.
5. Schnipper JL, Hamann C, Ndumele CD, et al. Effect of an electronic medication reconciliation application and process redesign on potential adverse drug events: a cluster-randomized trial. Arch Intern Med. 2009;169:771–780.
6. Poon EG, Wright A, Simon SR, et al. Relationship between use of electronic health record features and health care quality: results of a statewide survey. Med Care 2010;48:203–209.
7. Shortliffe EH. The evolution of electronic medical records. Acad Med 1999;74:414–419.
8. Weed LL. Medical records that guide and teach. N Engl J Med 1968;278:593–600, 652–657.
9. Hepler CD. Clinical pharmacy, pharmaceutical care, and the quality of drug therapy. Pharmacotherapy 2004;24:1491–1498.
10. Hepler CD, Strand LM. Opportunities and responsibilities in pharmaceutical care. Am J Hosp Pharm 1990;47:533–543.
11. Donnelly WJ. The language of medical case histories. Ann Intern Med 1997;127:1045–1048.
12. Voytovich AE. Reduction of medical verbiage. Ann Intern Med 1999;131:146–147.
13. Bluml BM. Definition of medication therapy management: Development of professionwide consensus. J Am Pharm Assoc 2005;45:566–572.
14. American Pharmacists Association, National Association of Chain Drug Stores Foundation. Medication therapy management in pharmacy practice: core elements of an MTM service model (version 2.0). J Am Pharm Assoc 2008;48(3):341–353.
15. Canaday BR, Yarborough PC. Documenting pharmaceutical care: creating a standard. Ann Pharmacother 1994;28:1292–1296.
16. Cipolle RJ, Strand LM, Morley PC. Pharmaceutical Care Practice: The Clinician's Guide, 2nd ed. New York, McGraw-Hill, 2004.
17. Roth MT, Moore CG, Ivey JL, Esserman DA, Campbell WH, Weinberger M. The quality of medication use in older adults: methods of a longitudinal study. Am J Geriatr Pharmacother 2008;6:220–223.
18. Levey AS, Bosch JP, Lewis JB, et al. A more accurate method to estimate glomerular filtration rate from serum creatinine: a new prediction equation. Modification of Diet in Renal Disease Study Group. *Ann Intern Med* 1999;130:461–470.

# 6

# PEDIATRICS

Children are Not Just Little Adults. . . . . . . . . . Level III

Amanda Geist, PharmD

## LEARNING OBJECTIVES

After completing this case study, the reader should be able to:

- Determine the role that the rate and extent of organ development plays in the variation of absorption, distribution, metabolism, and elimination of medications in the pediatric population.
- Compare and contrast the pharmacokinetic and pharmacodynamic differences between pediatric and adult patients, as well as among various pediatric age groups.
- Identify and manage challenges in pediatric pain management.
- Identify and manage challenges in pediatric drug formulation and administration.

## PATIENT PRESENTATION

### Chief Complaint

Nursing reports of new-onset fever and hypotension, increased number of apnea episodes, and "infant acting different"

### HPI

Alexander Halstrom is a premature 730-g male infant born at 25 4/7 weeks, now day of life 22, who is currently intubated, sedated, on vasopressors and parenteral nutrition with new-onset fever, increased number of apnea episodes, and a 1-day history of "acting different" according to nursing reports.

### PMH

Prematurity: born at 25 4/7 weeks with APGARs of 1, 4, and 6
Extremely low birth weight (ELBW) = 760 g
Respiratory distress syndrome (RDS)
Anemia
Apnea of prematurity
At risk for retinopathy of prematurity
Cholestasis
Diaper dermatitis
Grade II intraventricular hemorrhage (IVH)
Hypotension
Microcephaly, head circumference below 10th percentile
Newborn sepsis
NPO, receiving nutritional support
Patent ductus arteriosus (PDA)—small with left-to-right shunt
Pulmonary hemorrhage
Immunizations up-to-date

### FH

Infant born to a 24-year-old G2 P0 AB1 mother secondary to polyhydramnios, nonreassuring fetal status, and premature onset of labor.

Maternal labs: HBsAg (–), rubella (–), VDRL (–), and HIV (–) with unknown GBS status who received partial penicillin prophylaxis prior to delivery and indomethacin for tocolysis.

Mother denies drug and alcohol use during pregnancy.

### SH

Noncontributory

### Current Meds

Ampicillin 73 mg IV every 12 hours (200 mg/kg per day)
Gentamicin 1.8 mg IV every 8 hours (7.5 mg/kg per day)
Caffeine 3.7 mg IV every 24 hours (5 mg/kg per day)
Phenobarbital 3.7 mg IV every 24 hours (5 mg/kg per day)
Vitamin A 5,000 international units IM MWF × 12 doses
Dopamine continuous infusion 10 mcg/kg/min
Morphine continuous infusion 10 mcg/kg/h
Midazolam continuous infusion 0.05 mg/kg/h
TPN at total fluid volume of 150 mL/kg per day
Nystatin 100,000 U/g cream one application to affected area PRN
Aquaphor one application to affected area PRN
Glycerin suppository one suppository PR every 24 hours PRN constipation
Acetaminophen 7.3 mg PO/PR every 6 hours PRN pain/fever (10 mg/kg/dose)

### All

NKDA

### Physical Examination

*Gen*

Intubated, sedated, premature infant in an incubator with hypotension who requires intensive cardiac and respiratory monitoring and continuous vital sign assessment

*VS*

BP 43/23, HR 178, RR 73, current temperature: 38.7°C, $O_2$ saturation: 92%

*HEENT*

Anterior fontanelle soft, open, flat

*Neck*

Supple, nontender, no masses, no lymphadenopathy

*Lungs*

Tachypneic; positive crackles and rhonchi; equal breath sounds

*CV*

Tachycardic, regular rhythm, 3/6 systolic murmur; normal pulses

*Abd*

Soft, nontender, nondistended; no masses or organomegaly; (+) bowel sounds

*Genit*

Normal male external genitalia; rectal exam deferred

*Ext*

No deformities noted; normal range of motion in all extremities

*Skin*

Skin is thin and vascular; no rashes, vesicles, or other lesions are noted.

*Neuro*

Sedated on morphine and midazolam; normal tone and activity for gestational age

*Laboratory Values*

| | | |
|---|---|---|
| Na 138 mEq/L | Hgb 11.5 g/dL | Calcium 9.8 mg/dL |
| K 3.5 mEq/L | Hct 35% | Magnesium 2 mEq/L |
| Cl 99 mEq/L | Plt 170 × $10^3$/mm$^3$ | Albumin 1.9 g/dL |
| $CO_2$ 28 mEq/L | WBC 22.5 × $10^3$/mm$^3$ | Triglyceride 103 mg/dL |
| BUN 12 mg/dL | Neutrophils 73% | CRP 14.8 mg/dL |
| SCr 0.2 mg/dL | Bands 17% | Meconium drug screen at birth (MDS) (–) |
| Glu 87 mg/dL | Lymphs 6% | |
| | Monos 4% | |

*Culture and Sensitivity Data*

| Source | Sensitivities |
|---|---|
| Blood, central line | Pending |
| Blood, peripheral | Pending |
| Urine, catheter | No growth to date |
| Tracheal aspirate | Gram-negative bacilli |
| CSF | No growth to date |
| HSV PCR | Pending |

■ Assessment

Premature infant in an incubator who is intubated and sedated with microcephaly, RDS, apnea of prematurity, grade II IVH, cholestasis, anemia, PDA, hypotension, receiving nutritional and hemodynamic support, now with new late-onset sepsis

## QUESTIONS

### Problem Identification

1.a. What is Alexander's gestational age, postnatal age, and postmenstrual age?

1.b. What influence, if any, do gestational and postmenstrual ages have on pediatric pharmacotherapy?

1.c. What information indicates the presence of infection in this neonate?

1.d. Compare and contrast the clinical findings required to make the diagnosis of sepsis in a child with those required to make the diagnosis in an adult.

## ■ CLINICAL COURSE

Several days later, the final culture and sensitivity data were reported as follows:

| Source | Organism(s)/Sensitivity |
|---|---|
| **Blood, central line** | ***Staphylococcus aureus***<br>Ampicillin–R<br>Ampicillin/sulbactam–R<br>Cefuroxime–R<br>Ceftazidime–R<br>Cefepime–R<br>Clindamycin–S<br>Erythromycin–R<br>Levofloxacin–S<br>Oxacillin–R<br>Linezolid–S<br>Sulfamethoxazole/trimethoprim–S<br>Vancomycin–S |
| **Blood, peripheral** | ***S. aureus***<br>Ampicillin–R<br>Ampicillin/sulbactam–R<br>Cefuroxime–R<br>Ceftazidime–R<br>Cefepime–R<br>Clindamycin–S<br>Erythromycin–R<br>Levofloxacin–S<br>Oxacillin–R<br>Linezolid–S<br>Sulfamethoxazole/trimethoprim–S<br>Vancomycin–S |
| **Urine, catheter** | **No growth** |
| **Tracheal aspirate** | ***Stenotrophomonas maltophilia***<br>Aztreonam–S<br>Ceftazidime–R<br>Ticarcillin/clavulanate–R<br>Levofloxacin–S<br>Sulfamethoxazole/trimethoprim–S |
| **CSF** | **No growth** |
| **HSV PCR** | **Negative** |

*(continued)*

R, resistant; S, sensitive; I, intermediate; HSV, herpes simplex virus.

The medical resident on the NICU team asks you for the appropriate dose of sulfamethoxazole/trimethoprim because he is unable to find it in any of the drug information sources he has used. He plans to start the patient on sulfamethoxazole/trimethoprim for the treatment of both *Stenotrophomonas maltophilia* and methicillin-resistant *Staphylococcus* aureus (MRSA).

### Desired Outcome

2. What are the goals of pharmacotherapy for this infant?

### Therapeutic Alternatives

3.a. What therapeutic alternatives are available for the empiric treatment of neonatal sepsis?

3.b. Was the empiric gentamicin dose appropriate for this patient? If not, recommend an alternative dose and frequency and provide the rationale for your choice.

3.c. What therapeutic alternatives are available for the treatment of *S. maltophilia* in this neonate?

3.d. What therapeutic alternatives are available for the treatment of MRSA bacteremia in this neonate?

### Optimal Plan

4.a. Recommend an appropriate pharmacotherapy regimen for the empiric treatment of neonatal sepsis in this patient on his initial presentation.

4.b. Based on the final culture results, provide an appropriate pharmacotherapy regimen for subsequent treatment of this neonate's infections.

### Outcome Evaluation

5. What clinical and laboratory parameters should be monitored to evaluate efficacy and to prevent adverse drug effects for the therapeutic regimen you recommended?

## Patient Education

6. Alexander's mother is concerned about her child receiving a morphine drip. She has read on the Internet that babies his size are too small and underdeveloped to feel pain, and she is concerned that the physicians are prescribing a medication that is unnecessary and will cause him to be "addicted to drugs." What information and counseling would you provide to this mother to explain the use of morphine in this patient?

## Additional Case Questions

1. What pharmaceutical concerns must be considered when using sulfamethoxazole/trimethoprim in neonates?

## ■ SELF-STUDY ASSIGNMENTS

1. In addition to sulfamethoxazole/trimethoprim, what other medications can cause neonatal gasping syndrome?
2. Which patient populations are most likely to be affected by infection with *S. maltophilia*?
3. In addition to sulfamethoxazole/trimethoprim, what other medications have the potential to cause Stevens–Johnson syndrome?
4. Compare and contrast the differences in morphine metabolism between neonates and adults.

## CLINICAL PEARL

Term and preterm infants can experience alterations in the function of cells involved in the response to infection, which can decrease their ability to fight infection and increase their risk for sepsis. For example, chemotaxis is abnormal at birth, premature infants can have decreased amounts of immunoglobulin, and stressors such as respiratory distress can lead to decreased ability to phagocytose gram-negative bacteria.

## REFERENCES


1. Kearns GL, Abdel-Rahman SM, Alander SE, Blowey DL, Leeder JS, Kauffman RE. Developmental pharmacology: drug disposition, action, and therapy in infants and children. N Engl J Med 2003;349:1157–1167.
2. Goldstein B, Giroir B, Randolph A, et al. International pediatric sepsis consensus conference: definitions for sepsis and organ dysfunction in pediatrics. Pediatr Crit Care Med 2005;6:2–8.
3. Bone RC, Balk RA, Cerra FB, et al. Definitions for sepsis and organ failure and guidelines for the use of innovative therapies in sepsis. The ACCP/SCCM consensus conference committee. Chest 1992;101:1644–1655.
4. Pacifici GM. Clinical pharmacokinetics of aminoglycosides in the neonate: a review. Eur J Clin Pharmacol 2009;65:419–427.
5. Anand KJS, Aranda JV, Berde CB, et al. Summary proceedings from the neonatal pain-control group. Pediatrics 2006;117:S9–S22.
6. Anand KJS. Consensus statement for the prevention and management of pain in the newborn. Arch Pediatr Adolesc Med 2001;155:173–180.


# 7

# GERIATRICS

Falling Frannie ........................ Level II

**Amy M. Lugo, PharmD, BCPS, BC-ADM**

## LEARNING OBJECTIVES

After completing this case study, the reader should be able to:

- Identify medications listed as Beers List drugs, and describe the reason they may be inappropriate in older adults.
- Discuss common geriatric syndromes, including falls, dizziness, syncope, and urinary incontinence, and identify ways to prevent exacerbations of these conditions.
- Establish goals for the treatment of pain, urinary incontinence, and allergic rhinitis in older adults based on patient-specific characteristics and comorbid disease states.
- Describe ways to prevent falls in older adults.
- Provide appropriate patient counseling to help seniors minimize the cost of their medications.

## PATIENT PRESENTATION

### ■ Chief Complaint

"I get so dizzy when I stand up, and I don't have control of my bladder."

### ■ HPI

Fran Jones is an 87-year-old woman who presents to your Pharmacotherapy Clinic today reporting dizziness and urinary incontinence. She was referred by her PCP for a polypharmacy consult and an adverse drug event review. She reports having fallen last night after getting out of the bed to use the bathroom. She states that her hip is hurting where she fell on it. She admits to being "very blue" often and has crying spells when she discusses her husband who passed away last year.

### ■ PMH

Osteoporosis
Atrial fibrillation, no h/o VTE
Seasonal allergic rhinitis
Early onset Alzheimer's dementia diagnosed 2 years ago

### ■ PSH

One cesarean section

### ■ FH

Noncontributory

■ SH

Mrs Jones reports having just started taking *Ginkgo biloba* to help with memory and taking "lots" of Tylenol since her fall. She does not remember the other meds she is taking, and her daughter fills her pill box. She denies using any tobacco or alcohol. She has lived alone since her husband passed away 6 months ago. Mrs Jones is very concerned about paying for medications. She says the last time she was at the pharmacy, the pharmacist said something about being in a "donut hole." She has a Medicare Part D plan.

■ Meds

Warfarin 2 mg Mon–Wed–Fri–Sat and 4 mg Tue–Thu–Sat
Alendronate 70 mg po once weekly
Diphenhydramine 25 mg po TID for allergies
Propoxyphene/APAP 1–2 po Q 6 h PRN pain
Acetaminophen OTC Extra Strength 1–2 po PRN pain
Metoprolol succinate 50 mg po every morning
Donepezil 5 mg po every morning
*G. biloba* po every morning

■ All

NKDA

■ ROS

Reports occasional bladder incontinence and hip pain where she fell as well as a runny nose from allergies; denies heartburn, chest pain, or shortness of breath

■ Physical Examination

*Gen*

WDWN Caucasian female who appears her stated age; NAD

*VS*

BP 118/72 mm Hg sitting, 100/60 mm Hg standing; HR 76 bpm (irregularly irregular), RR 18/min, T 98.4°F, Ht 5′4″, Wt 55 kg, G3P3

*HEENT*

NCAT; PERRL, EOMI, fundi benign; TMs intact; mild sinus drainage

*Neck*

Neck supple without thyromegaly or LAD

*Lungs*

Lung fields CTA bilaterally

*Heart*

Rhythm is irregularly irregular; no murmurs or bruits

*Abd*

Soft, NT/ND; no masses, bruits, or organomegaly; normal BS

*Genit/Rect*

Deferred

*Ext*

No CCE, normal ROM

*Neuro*

Motor, sensory, CNs, cerebellar, and gait normal. Folstein MMSE score 17/30, compared to a score of 17/30 and 19/30 last year and at the initial diagnosis, respectively. Disoriented to month, date, and day of week. Good registration but impaired attention and very poor short-term memory. Able to remember only one of three items after 3 minutes. Able to follow commands. Displayed apathy during MMSE.

■ Labs

| | | | |
|---|---|---|---|
| Na 139 mEq/L | Hgb 13.5 g/dL | T. bili 0.9 mg/dL | Ca 9.7 mg/dL |
| K 3.7 mEq/L | Hct 39.0% | D. bili 0.3 mg/dL | Phos 4.5 mg/dL |
| Cl 108 mEq/L | AST 25 IU/L | T. prot 7.5 g/dL | TSH 3.8 mIU/L |
| $CO_2$ 25.5 mEq/L | ALT 24 IU/L | Alb 4.5 g/dL | T4 5.9 ng/dL |
| BUN 16 mg/dL | Alk phos 81 IU/L | Chol 212 mg/dL | UA 6.8 mg/dL |
| SCr 1.1 mg/dL | GGT 22 IU/L | INR 3.1 | 25-OH vitamin D 21 ng/mL |
| Glu 102 mg/dL | LDH 85 IU/L | | |

■ Radiology

CT scan (head, 2 years ago): Mild to moderate generalized cerebral atrophy

Bone mineral density (last year): T-score −2.6

■ ECG

Atrial fibrillation, rate controlled

■ Assessment

1. Falls, secondary to multiple factors including medications
2. Urinary incontinence
3. Atrial fibrillation, rate controlled
4. Allergic rhinitis
5. Osteoporosis
6. Self-pay for medications, Medicare Part D "donut hole"

# QUESTIONS

## Problem Identification

1.a. Create a list of this patient's drug-related problems, including any medications that may be contributing to the patient's falls and incontinence. Which of her medications are Beers Criteria drugs?

1.b. What are the patient's known risk factors for falls?

## Desired Outcome

2. List the goals of treatment for this patient.

## Therapeutic Alternatives

3.a. What nonpharmacologic therapies should be implemented to prevent falls and other adverse drug events?

3.b. What pharmacotherapeutic options are available for controlling this patient's pain, allergic rhinitis, and urinary incontinence?

3.c. What comorbidities and individual patient considerations should be taken into account when selecting pharmacologic therapy for her?

## Optimal Plan

4.a. Outline specific lifestyle modifications for this patient as well as preventive health measures.

4.b. Outline a specific and appropriate pharmacotherapeutic regimen for this patient including drug(s), dose(s), dosage form(s), and schedule(s). Consider her out-of-pocket costs for medications.

## Outcome Evaluation

5. Based on your recommendations, what parameters should be monitored after initiating this regimen and throughout the treatment course? At what time intervals should these parameters be monitored?

## Patient Education

6. Based on your recommendations, provide appropriate education to this patient.

## SELF-STUDY ASSIGNMENTS

1. Review the Beers Criteria for potentially inappropriate use of medications in older adults, and consider your first-line recommendations for optimal treatment of depression, insomnia, and diabetes in the older adult.
2. Outline the changes that you would make to the pharmacotherapeutic regimen for this patient if she had a history of each of the following comorbidities or characteristics:
   - Creatinine clearance <30 mL/min
   - Major depression
   - Moderate to severe Alzheimer's disease
3. What is Mrs Jones' CHADS-2 score for atrial fibrillation? What is her risk for venous thromboembolism? Should she receive warfarin or aspirin? Why or why not?
4. Assume that Mrs Jones exhibits further cognitive decline at her next neurological follow-up appointment. What would you consider the next step in treatment of her worsening Alzheimer's dementia?

## CLINICAL PEARL

Each year, an estimated one third of older adults fall, and the likelihood of falling increases substantially with advancing age. In 2005, a total of 15,802 persons aged ≥65 years died as a result of injuries from falls.[5]

## REFERENCES


1. Fick DM, Cooper JW, Wade WE, Waller JL, Maclean R, Beers MH. Updating the Beers criteria for potentially inappropriate medication use in older adults. Arch Intern Med 2003;163:2716–2724.
2. Centers for Medicare and Medicaid Services. Bridging the coverage gap. Available at: *www.medicare.gov/Publications/Pubs/pdf/11213.pdf*. Accessed February 21, 2010.
3. Tinetti ME, Kumar C. The patient who falls: "It's always a trade-off". JAMA 2010;303:258–266.
4. Inouye SK, Studenski S, Tinetti ME, Kuchel GA. Geriatric syndromes: clinical, research, and policy implications of a core geriatric concept. J Am Geriatr Soc 2007;55:780–791.
5. Centers for Disease Control and Prevention (CDC). Self-reported falls and fall-related injuries among persons aged 65 years—United States, 2006. MMWR Wkly Rep 2008;57(9):225–229.
6. National Osteoporosis Foundation. Clinician's Guide to Prevention and Treatment of Osteoporosis. Washington, DC, National Osteoporosis Foundation, 2010.
7. Gates BJ, Sonnett TE, DuVall CA, Dobbins EK. Review of osteoporosis pharmacotherapy for geriatric patients. Am J Geriatr Pharmacother 2009;7:293–323.
8. Garwood CL, Corbett TL. Use of anticoagulation in elderly patients with atrial fibrillation who are at risk for falls. Ann Pharmacother 2008;42:523–532.
9. Cummings JL, Frank JC, Cherry D, et al. Guidelines for managing Alzheimer's disease: part II. Treatment. Am Fam Physician 2002;65:2525–2534.
10. U.S. Preventive Services Task Force. Screening for depression in adults: U.S. Preventive Services Task Force recommendation statement. Ann Intern Med 2009;151:784–792.


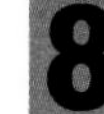

# 8

# PALLIATIVE CARE

Helpful Hospice . . . . . . . . . . . . . . . . . . . . . . . Level III

**Jennifer L. Swank, PharmD, BCOP**

## LEARNING OBJECTIVES

After completing this case study, students should be able to:

- Define the goals for pain management in a patient with chronic malignant pain with hospice services.
- Define a pharmacotherapeutic pain management plan.
- Differentiate between palliative care and hospice care.
- Select or recommend medication options for management of nausea in a hospice setting.
- Define the role of continuation of nutritional support and antibiotic therapy in a hospice setting.

## PATIENT PRESENTATION

### Chief Complaint

"I have been having fevers up to 102°F and chills for two days. I have also noticed that my skin is orange in color."

### HPI

Jamie Park is a 48-year-old woman with a history of metastatic gastric adenocarcinoma originally diagnosed 3 years ago. At that time, she had a subtotal gastrectomy with 16 out of 16 positive lymph nodes. She received adjuvant chemoradiation with 6 months of 5-fluorouracil. Two years ago, she developed gastric outlet obstruction and underwent laparotomy with extensive lysis of adhesions and revision of the gastrojejunostomy. She had no evidence of malignancy after this surgery. Three months later, she presented with symptoms of obstruction and underwent a sigmoid colectomy with pathology revealing metastatic gastric adenocarcinoma. She then was started on chemotherapy with epirubicin, cisplatin, and capecitabine × 6 cycles. Her chemotherapy course was complicated by neutropenia requiring significant dose reduction. After completing six cycles, she had worsening small bowel obstruction and underwent surgery where recurrent metastases to the small intestine were found. The metastases were resected, but several other malignant peritoneal nodules were seen during surgery. Four months after the surgery, she underwent colonoscopy due to further obstruction at the level of the colon. The procedure was complicated by cecal dilatation, requiring an urgent percutaneous cecostomy. A week later, she underwent a repeat exploratory laparotomy with jejunojejunal bypass and ileosigmoid bypass. After the last surgery, the patient did not recover any intestinal function and was started on chronic TPN therapy. Four months ago, the patient underwent elective external biliary drain placement for biliary obstruction due to tumor. She was recently enrolled in supportive hospice services but continues on TPN for treatment of chronic gastric outlet obstruction.

Mrs Park presents today with a 2-day history of fevers and chills, abdominal pain, and recurrent jaundice. She had been using Tylenol suppositories for the fevers at home without relief. Her abdominal pain has worsened over the past 2 days, and she currently rates the pain as 8 out of 10. This pain is not relieved by the use of as-needed oxycodone liquid.

## PMH

Cholangitis
Gastric outlet obstruction and small bowel obstruction
Subtotal gastrectomy 5 years ago
Sigmoid colectomy 2 years ago

## SH

Mrs Park is from Korea and has lived in the United States for 10 years. She is married and has two children. She denies the use of alcohol or tobacco.

## FH

Mother—cervical cancer
Maternal aunt—laryngeal cancer
Maternal uncle—liver cancer

## Meds

Total parental nutrition
Fentanyl 200-mcg patch, change every 72 hours
Oxycodone concentrated liquid 20 mg/mL, 1 mL po every 3 hours PRN pain
Ondansetron 8 mg ODT, one tablet po every 8 hours PRN nausea or vomiting
Acetaminophen suppository 650 mg, one every 6 hours PRN fever

## All

NKDA

## ROS

Ten organ systems were reviewed. Patient reports fever, chills, nausea, vomiting, headache, and abdominal pain rated as 8 out of 10. She denies chest pain, sore throat, cough, increased urinary frequency, rash, hematuria, hemoptysis, hematemesis, or black stool.

## Physical Examination

### *Gen*

Patient is a 48-year-old female in acute distress holding her abdomen.

### *VS*

BP 77/50, P 90, RR 16, T 100.9°F; Wt 45.8 kg, Ht 5′2″; pain 8/10 sharp, and stabbing in nature

### *Skin*

Warm; dry; jaundice is appreciated

### *HEENT*

PERRLA; EOMI; TMs intact; moist mucous membranes

### *Neck*

No JVD; full range of motion; no masses

### *Resp*

CTA; no crackles, rhonchi, or wheezes

### *CV*

Normal $S_1$, $S_2$; RRR; no murmurs

### *Abd*

Soft and distended; (+) BS; moderate RUQ pain with deep palpation and mild guarding; biliary drain is in place and noted to be draining appropriately but with foul-smelling, greenish liquid

### *Genit/Rect*

Deferred

### *MS/Ext*

Negative lower extremity edema; palpable pedal and radial pulsations

### *Neuro*

CN II–XII intact, A & O × 3; no sensory or focal deficits apparent

## Labs

| | | |
|---|---|---|
| Na 147 mEq/L | WBC 27.71 × $10^3$/mm$^3$ | T. Prot 8 g/dL |
| K 4.5 mEq/L | Neutros 65% | Alb 2.4 g/dL |
| Cl 115 mEq/L | Bands 12% | T. bili 13.5 mg/dL |
| CO2 19 mEq/L | Lymphs 22% | D. bili 11.2 mg/dL |
| BUN 50 mg/dL | Eos 0% | AST 402 IU/L |
| SCr 1.7 mg/dL | Monos 1% | ALT 400 IU/L |
| Glu 101 mg/dL | Hgb 10 g/dL | Alk phos 321 IU/L |
| Ca 8.8 mg/dL | Hct 31.1% | Cortisol 39.8 mcg/dL |
| Phos 3.9 mg/dL | Plt 158 × $10^3$/mm$^3$ | Lactic acid 0.7 mmol/L |
| Mg 3.0 mg/dL | | |

## Chest X-Ray

Mild increased interstitial lung markings; bilateral nonspecific changes that can be seen with pulmonary edema; no consolidation to suggest pneumonia

## RUQ Ultrasound

Sonographically abnormal appearance of the gallbladder, which is ill defined on this examination; no intrahepatic or extrahepatic biliary ductal dilatation; however, cholangitis cannot be excluded based on these findings.

## Blood Cultures × 2 Sets

Pending

## Urine Culture

Pending

## Biliary Drainage Culture

Pending

## Assessment

Acute-on-chronic abdominal pain due to peritoneal metastases from gastric cancer
Hypotension and probable cholangitis due to biliary obstruction
Chronic bowel obstruction requiring TPN for nutrition
Nausea due to pain medications and chronic gastric outlet and small bowel obstruction

# QUESTIONS

## Problem Identification

1.a. Create a list of the patient's drug therapy problems.

1.b. What clinical information indicates the presence of an acute-on-chronic pain syndrome?

1.c. What additional information is needed to satisfactorily assess this patient's pain?

1.d. What subjective and objective data support the diagnosis of cholangitis in this patient?

1.e. How does the role of hospice services affect the treatment plan for this patient's care?

## Desired Outcome

2. What are the goals of pharmacotherapy in this case?

## Therapeutic Alternatives

3.a. What nondrug therapies might be useful for this patient?

3.b. Compare the pharmacotherapeutic alternatives available for treatment of this patient's pain.

3.c. Compare the pharmacotherapeutic alternatives available for treatment of this patient's nausea and vomiting.

## Optimal Plan

4.a. What drug, dosage form, and schedule are best for treating this patient's pain?

4.b. What alternatives would be appropriate if the initial therapy fails or cannot be used?

4.c. Outline a drug regimen for the treatment of the patient's nausea.

## Outcome Evaluation

5. What clinical and laboratory parameters are necessary to evaluate the therapy for achievement of the desired therapeutic outcome and to detect or prevent adverse effects?

## Patient Education

6. What information should be provided to the patient to enhance compliance, ensure successful therapy, and minimize adverse effects?

# ■ CLINICAL COURSE

The patient was given IV fluids and started on empiric antibiotic therapy with meropenem 1g IV Q 8 h, vancomycin 750 mg IV daily, and fluconazole 100 mg IV daily. The patient's blood pressure normalized to 105/75 mm Hg, and SCr improved to 1.5 mg/dL with NS @ 150 mL/h. The blood and urine cultures were negative, but the biliary drainage cultures were positive for *Enterococcus faecalis* sensitive to vancomycin and *Pseudomonas stutzeri* sensitive to cefepime, ciprofloxacin, piperacillin/tazobactam, and tigecycline. The empiric antibiotic therapy was continued due to appropriate sensitivities to the antibiotics. Interventional radiology was consulted to evaluate the biliary drain for possible obstruction due to poor output. The internal/external catheter was exchanged with an external drain. The patient's bilirubin did not improve after the new external biliary drain was placed and remained in the range of 8–10 mg/dL. The patient was started on a fentanyl PCA pump at a basal rate of 30 mcg/h with on-demand dosing of 10 mcg every 8 minutes with an hourly lockout of 100 mcg/h, which resulted in adequate pain control rated 2 out of 10. The patient's overall prognosis is poor due to chronic jaundice from biliary obstruction, worsening renal function, and infection. She has metastatic gastric adenocarcinoma of the colon and small bowel and is not a candidate for further chemotherapy or surgery. The patient and her husband discussed her overall prognosis and made the choice to transition to full hospice services. The patient did choose to continue the 14-day course of IV antibiotic therapy. She was discharged home with home health services on IV meropenem 1 g IV Q 12 h, vancomycin 750 mg IV daily, and fluconazole 100 mg IV daily × 14 days, fentanyl PCA basal rate 30 mcg/h on demand 10 mcg Q 8 minutes, and TPN. After the patient completes the IV antibiotics, she will choose to stop the TPN and just continue with comfort measures only and enroll in full hospice services.

## Follow-Up Questions

1. Based on this new information of the patient discontinuing TPN and being discharged to hospice, are there any other supportive medications that may benefit the patient?
2. If the patient reports her pain to be 7 out of 10 at the time of discharge, how would you alter your treatment plan?

# ■ SELF-STUDY ASSIGNMENTS

1. Prepare a list of opioids and their corresponding equianalgesic dosing.
2. Prepare a set of guidelines for managing chronic malignant cancer pain.
3. Prepare a list of antiemetics and dosing regimens useful in palliative care.

# CLINICAL PEARL

Hospice is a specific type of palliative care team dedicated to managing patients with advanced illness who have a life expectancy of less than 6 months. Hospice has various levels of service and covers different therapies/services depending on the area in which the patient lives. Some hospice services will allow palliative therapy (i.e., chemotherapy), IV antibiotics, and IV nutrition, whereas other hospice agencies require the patient to stop all such therapies prior to enrolling in their services.

# REFERENCES


1. Cherny N. Cancer pain: principles of assessment and syndromes. In: Berger A, Shuster J, Roenn J, eds. Principles and Practice of Palliative Care & Supportive Oncology, 3rd ed. Philadelphia, PA, Lippincott Williams & Wilkins, 2007.
2. Williamson A, Hoggart B. Pain: a review of three commonly used pain rating scales. J Clin Nurs 2005;14:798–804.
3. Nersesyan H, Slavin KV. Current approach to cancer pain management: availability and implications of different treatment options. Ther Clin Risk Manage 2007;3:381–400.
4. World Heath Organization. WHO definition of palliative care. Available at: *http://www.who.int/cancer/palliative/definition/en/*. Accessed June 25, 2010.
5. Asch DA, Faber-Langendoen K, Shea JA, Christakis NA. The sequence of withdrawing life-sustaining treatment from patients. Am J Med 1999;107:153–156.
6. McCarberg BH, Barkin RL. Long-acting opioids for chronic pain: pharmacotherapeutic opportunities to enhance compliance, quality of life, and analgesia. Am J Ther 2001;8:181–186.

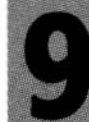



7. Davis M, Walsh D. Treatment of nausea and vomiting in advanced cancer. Support Care Cancer 2000;8:444–452.
8. Kress H, Von der Laage D, Hoerauf K, et al. A randomized, open, parallel group, multicenter trial to investigate analgesic efficacy and safety of a new transdermal fentanyl patch compared to standard opioid treatment in cancer pain. J Pain Symptom Manage 2008;36:268–279.

# 9

# CLINICAL TOXICOLOGY: ACETAMINOPHEN TOXICITY

To Sleep or Not to Sleep . . . . . . . . . . . . . . . . . Level II

**Elizabeth J. Scharman, PharmD, DABAT, BCPS, FAACT**

## LEARNING OBJECTIVES

After completing this case study, students should be able to:

- Determine when a potentially toxic acetaminophen exposure exists.
- Monitor a patient for signs and symptoms associated with acetaminophen toxicity.
- Recommend appropriate antidotal therapy for acetaminophen poisoning, and monitor its use for effectiveness and adverse effects.
- Describe the appropriate management of adverse drug reactions related to N-acetylcysteine.

## PATIENT PRESENTATION

### Chief Complaint

The patient is uncooperative and states he just wants to be left alone so that he can get some sleep.

### HPI

The poison center receives a telephone call at 1:40 AM from a physician in a local ED regarding a 54-year-old man named Steven Marks. Mr Marks was brought to the ED via ambulance accompanied by police because the patient had been belligerent and was refusing referral. According to his wife, he took a handful of pills following a heated argument she had with him that evening. She estimates the time of the fight was about 6:00 PM. She left the house and came back 2 hours later. When she returned, she found him lying on the bed and saw two empty bottles in the bathroom wastepaper basket that were not there before. The wife thinks he was trying to kill himself. He states that he took pills because he just wanted to sleep. The ambulance crew brings in the two empty bottles of medicine. The wife cannot remember how much, if any, was remaining in the bottles prior to today. According to the wife, all other medications in the house are accounted for. One of the bottles originally contained 60, 500-mg acetaminophen tablets, and the other bottle originally contained 30, 500-mg acetaminophen/25-mg diphenhydramine caplets. The physician reports that Mr Marks vomited twice in the ambulance and an additional four times since his arrival in the ED. He has not received any antiemetics.

### PMH

Patient states that he is healthy. He has not seen a physician "in years" according to his wife.

### FH

Father died of a heart attack when the patient was 12 years old. Mother is living. He has no sisters. He has one younger brother with "a bad heart."

### SH

Smokes two packs of cigarettes a day. Drinks "about as much as anybody else" according to his wife.

### Meds

No prescription medications
Often takes nonprescription sleeping pills because of insomnia

### All

None

### Physical Examination

*Gen*

The patient appears drowsy. There are no external signs of trauma. The patient has vomited a total of six times. The vomitus has not been bloody. His estimated height is 5′10″.

*VS*

BP 129/98, HR 72, RR 14, $O_2$ sat 96–98% on room air, T 37°C; Wt 98 kg

*Skin*

Mucous membranes are moist.

*HEENT*

Pupil size is normal; pupils are equal and reactive to light; retinal exam is unremarkable.

*Lungs/Thorax*

Occasional cough is noted.

*CV*

No murmurs or gallops heard

*Abd*

Bowel sounds are present. No guarding or tenderness.

*Neuro*

Patient is noticeably drowsy but is oriented to time and place; no tremors noted. Patient denies headache and is not in pain.

### Labs (Drawn at 01:00)

| | | |
|---|---|---|
| Na 142 mEq/L | Hgb 15.7 g/dL | Aspirin not detected |
| K 3.1 mEq/L | Hct 48.2% | Acetaminophen 124 mcg/mL |
| Cl 96 mEq/L | AST 38 U/L | Ethanol (EtOH) 278 mg/dL |
| $CO_2$ 23 mEq/L | ALT 27 U/L | |
| BUN 24 mg/dL | T. bili 0.8 mg/dL | |
| SCr 1.1 mg/dL | INR 1.2 | |
| Glucose 215 mg/dL | | |
| Urine: (+) THC, (+) PCP | | |

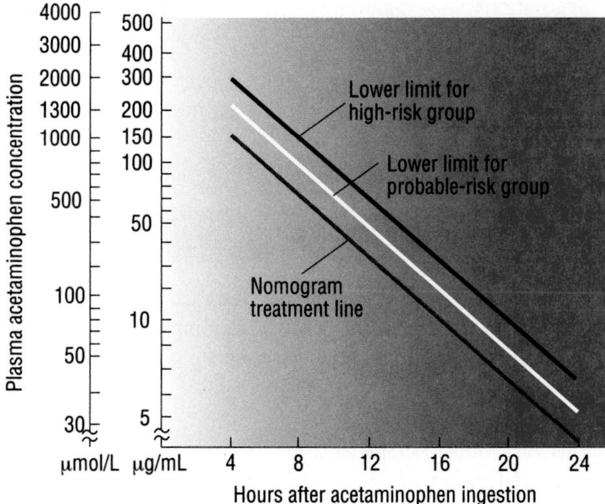


**FIGURE 9-1.** Nomogram for assessing hepatotoxic risk following acute ingestion of acetaminophen. *(Reprinted with permission from DiPiro JT, Posey LM, Talbert RL, et al., eds. Pharmacotherapy: A Pathophysiologic Approach, 7th ed. New York, McGraw-Hill, 2008.)*

#### ■ ECG

Normal sinus rhythm

#### ■ Assessment

The physician asks the poison center if acetaminophen toxicity is present (Fig. 9-1).

# QUESTIONS

## Problem Identification

1.a. Is determining the amount of acetaminophen the patient ingested an important factor in determining whether acetaminophen toxicity is present? Why or why not?

1.b. Which signs, symptoms, and laboratory values indicate that acetaminophen toxicity is present?

1.c. What are possible causes of vomiting in this patient?

1.d. Does toxicity from any other drug(s)/toxin(s) need to be considered in this patient? If so, which one(s) and why?

1.e. Develop a problem list for this patient. Identify the problem(s) that need to be addressed first. For the other problems, describe the rationale behind whether they need to be managed now or whether they just need to be addressed prior to discharge.

## Desired Outcome

2. What are the goals of pharmacotherapy for managing acetaminophen toxicity in this case?

## Therapeutic Alternatives

3. What feasible pharmacotherapeutic alternatives are available for treating acetaminophen toxicity in this patient?

## Optimal Plan

4.a. What antidote route, dose, schedule, and duration of therapy for acetaminophen toxicity are best for this patient, and when should therapy be initiated for optimal results?

4.b. If the physician asks the pharmacy to make an IV containing the exact dose of IV *N*-acetylcysteine (Acetadote) for this patient, instead of rounding to the nearest dose designated in the prescribing information dosing table, how many milliliters of *N*-acetylcysteine should this patient receive? Show all calculations, including how the total dose needed was obtained and how the amount of *N*-acetylcysteine in each milliliter of Acetadote was calculated.

4.c. Will administration of *N*-acetylcysteine have any influence on the pharmacologic management of the patient's other problems as identified in his problem list? Why or why not?

4.d. If this patient had been a female who was human chorionic gonadotropin (β-HCG) (+), would recommendations for *N*-acetylcysteine therapy change? Why or why not?

## Outcome Evaluation

5. What clinical and laboratory parameters are necessary to evaluate the therapy for achievement of the desired therapeutic outcome for acetaminophen toxicity and to detect adverse effects?

## Patient Education

6. What should the patient be told about the effectiveness of *N*-acetylcysteine therapy?

# ■ CLINICAL COURSE

At 02:20 the same day, the poison center gets a call from the patient's treating physician. He states that Mr Marks developed flushing and urticaria at the end of the loading dose; some faint wheezes were heard, and the baseline cough is unchanged. The physician thinks the patient may be having an anaphylactic reaction and has stopped the IV *N*-acetylcysteine. He wants poison center recommendations for an alternative antidote. The poison specialist determines that the correct mg/kg dosage was administered although the loading dose was administered over 15 minutes. Vital signs are BP 132/99, HR 65, and RR 14 and nonlabored. Blood chemistries are scheduled to be repeated at 08:00. Administration of ondansetron has controlled the vomiting.

## Follow-Up Questions

1. Do you agree that this is an anaphylactic reaction? If not, what type of reaction is this and how is it different from an anaphylactic reaction?
2. What are the appropriate management options for this reaction and for continued management of acetaminophen toxicity in this patient?
3. The prescribing information for IV *N*-acetylcysteine lists one contraindication. Do you agree with this contraindication? Why or why not?
4. If this patient is discharged from the hospital on medications to treat other medical problems, how will his history of an overdose affect the health care provider's decision on which medication(s) to select?

# ■ SELF-STUDY ASSIGNMENTS

1. Defend the argument that all patients with an intentional drug overdose, no matter what their stated history, should have an acetaminophen level drawn to rule out acetaminophen toxicity.
2. If this patient had been 104 kg instead of 98 kg, the dose given would have been the same as that of a person weighing 100 kg. Why do patients weighing over 100 kg not receive an IV *N*-acetylcysteine dose calculated on an mg/kg basis, and what is the rationale for this maximum dose being clinically effective?

## CLINICAL PEARL

The FDA Modernization Act of 1997 states that acceptable compounding practice excludes the extemporaneous compounding of commercially available products (e.g., Acetadote). Therefore, pharmacists should not prepare IV *N*-acetylcysteine extemporaneously using the oral formulation. Although compounding IV *N*-acetylcysteine in an emergency could be justified (as in this case), a pharmacy could not decide in advance to prepare IV *N*-acetylcysteine extemporaneously in lieu of purchasing the commercially available product. USP Chapter 797, which some state pharmacy boards have adopted, identifies the sterility conditions that would need to be met during the compounding process.

## REFERENCES


1. Dart RC, Erdman AR, Olson KR, et al. Acetaminophen poisoning: an evidence-based consensus guideline for out-of-hospital management. Clin Toxicol (Phila) 2006;44:1–18.
2. Payen C, Dachraoui A, Pulce C, et al. Prothrombin time prolongation in paracetamol poisoning: a relevant marker of hepatic failure? Hum Exp Toxicol 2003;22:617–621.
3. Rowden AK, Norvell J, Eldridge DL, et al. Acetaminophen poisoning. Clin Lab Med 2006;26:49–65.
4. Scharman EJ, Erdman AR, Wax PM, et al. Diphenhydramine and dimenhydrinate poisoning: an evidence-based consensus guideline for out-of-hospital management. Clin Toxicol (Phila) 2006;44:205–223.
5. Fontanella CA, Bridge JA, Campo JV. Psychotropic medication changes, polypharmacy, and the risk of early readmission in suicidal adolescent inpatients. Ann Pharmacother 2009;43:1939–1947.
6. Dribben WH, Porto SM, Jeffords BK. Stability and microbiology of inhalant N-acetylcysteine used as an intravenous solution for the treatment of acetaminophen poisoning. Ann Emerg Med 2003;42:9–13.
7. Acetadote Package Insert. Nashville, TN, Cumberland Pharmaceuticals Inc, 2006.
8. Wilkes JM, Clark LE, Herrera JL. Acetaminophen overdose in pregnancy. South Med J 2005;98:1118–1122.
9. Sandilands EA, Bateman DN. Adverse reactions associated with acetylcysteine. Clin Toxicol (Phila) 2009;47:81–88.


# 10

# CYANIDE EXPOSURE

Curtain Call . . . . . . . . . . . . . . . . . . . . . . . . . . . . Level II

**Colleen M. Terriff, PharmD**

## LEARNING OBJECTIVES

After completing this case study, students should be able to:

- Identify which signs, symptoms, and laboratory data indicate a possible cyanide exposure.
- Compare and contrast the two different antidotes for cyanide exposure.
- Recommend specific dosing regimens for antidotes and supportive care for children and adults.
- State monitoring parameters and management of antidote side effects.
- In a scenario with multiple patients, explain how providers will be able to obtain necessary antidotes from local or national stockpiles.

## PRESENTATION OF PATIENTS

Multiple patients present to your hospital's ED; some are seizing, some are comatose, and others present seemingly drunk, confused, and, when ambulating, stumbling around.

### HPI

Dozens of seriously ill patients arrive by ambulance at all area emergency departments. Many more turn up by car. They were attending a high school musical, and all emptied out into a foyer for intermission. Attendees then experienced nausea, dizziness, lightheadedness, and weakness. 911 was called when approximately six people passed out. The crowd estimate was 250, and most attendees ran out to the parking lot. Initial emergency medical technicians arriving on the scene recognized a mass incident. Medical Alert was activated for the town and surrounding communities. Fifty people are believed to still be in the auditorium. Decontamination areas are being set up in a high school parking lot and all local hospital emergency departments.

### PMH, PSH, FH, and SH

Most patients arriving via ambulance are unconscious; some are seizing. History for most of these patients is unobtainable. Patients able to communicate are providing information as needed.

### ROS

Patients are presenting with a variety of symptoms and severity. ED nurses and doctors do brief physical exams and start using triage tags. Some patients arrive with triage tags from the scene. Age, height, and weight are being estimated as needed.

### Physical Examination

*Gen*

Symptomatic patients appear weak and are breathing quickly. Some unconscious and seizing patients have required intubation. Some patients report headache, dizziness, vision changes, and feeling confused; some complain of abdominal pain and nausea, and a few experience emesis.

*VS*

BP: A few patients have mildly elevated BP, but many have hypotension.
HR: Most patients have bradycardia, but some have tachycardia.
RR: Most patients are tachypneic.
T: Most patients are normal.
Pain: Patients are anxious but do not have notable or consistent complaints of pain.
$O_2$ sat: Most patients are normal.

*Skin*

No notable contusions, abrasions, or obvious signs of trauma

*HEENT*

Mydriasis observed in some patients. Some nurses note "nutty" smelling breath in a few patients; nothing else is noted on quick exam.

*Neck/Lymph Nodes*

No lymphadenopathy

*Lungs/Thorax*

Rapid respiratory rate; lungs clear to auscultation

*CV*

Bradycardia for most patients, too noisy in ED to listen for heart sounds

*Abd*

Bowel sounds presents in most patients; normal exam

*Genital/Rect*

Digital rectal exam and guaiac not performed

*MS/Ext*

No abnormal movements noted

*Neuro*

Seizure activity noted in some patients; Glasgow coma scale on unconscious patients is 3.

### Labs

Example labs ordered for a symptomatic patient: Complete metabolic panel pending; CBC normal; toxicology screen pending; lactate 14 mmol/L

Serum cholinesterase and blood cyanide levels pending

### Other

Example blood gas ordered for an intubated patient: pH 7.1, $pCO_2$ 17, $pO_2$ 240, $HCO_3$6

Chest x-rays pending

### Physician's Assessment

Based on feedback from the scene and Regional Disaster Hospital, up to 250 people may have been affected by this unknown chemical release. Paramedic services are transporting patients to all area hospitals. Medical Alert has been issued for the city. The ED staff are also alerted to obtain information from victims and save patient belongings as evidence for the FBI. Incident Command at the scene has not officially received identification of a chemical agent and asks for clinical assistance from health care providers triaging victims. First responders on the scene relayed information to Incident Command that some of the crowd reported seeing vapor in bathrooms and in a few garbage cans, but no smoke or fire. The ED medical resident contacts the Regional Poison Control Center for guidance on identifying the agent based on patient symptoms. Cyanide exposure is suspected. The pharmacy department is also contacted for their assistance with antidote recommendations, including dosing and side-effect monitoring. The hospital administration announced that their Incident Command will be situated in the auditorium, and physicians are to report to floor nursing stations.

# QUESTIONS

## Problem Identification

1.a. List the abnormal signs and symptoms displayed in these patients presenting to area hospitals after exposure to the unknown chemical. Which of these findings are consistent with inhalation of cyanide?

1.b. List the laboratory tests that may be abnormal in patients exposed to cyanide. Explain the pathophysiology underlying these abnormalities.

1.c. What are the potential short- and long-term sequelae from this exposure?

## Desired Outcome

2. What are the goals of pharmacotherapy in these cases?

## Therapeutic Alternatives

3.a. What nonpharmacologic measures are available to treat cyanide poisoning?

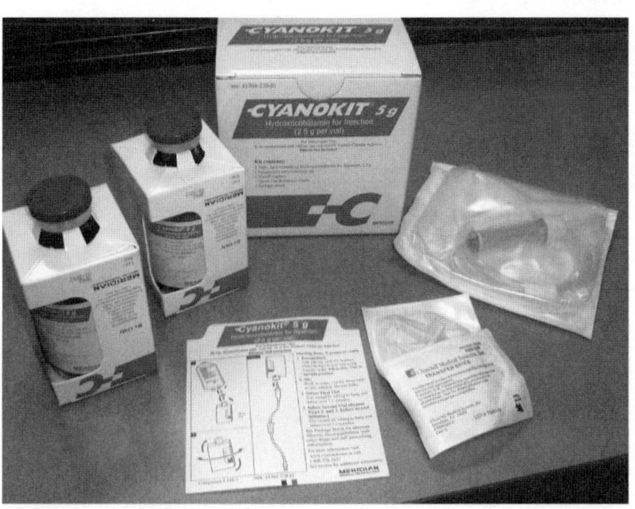


A

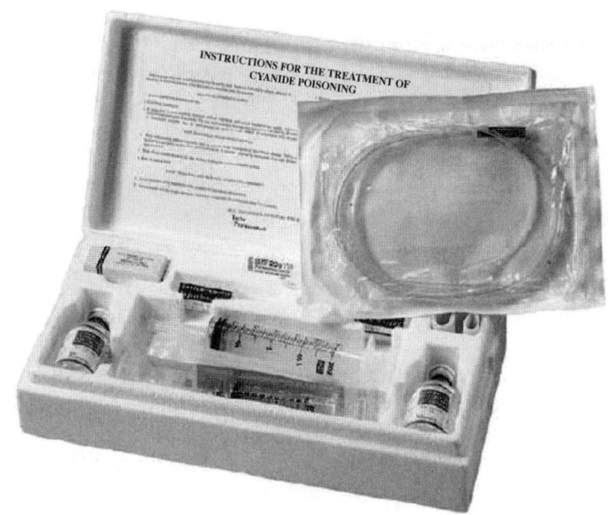


B

**FIGURE 10-1.** *A.* Cyanokit® (hydroxocobalamin for injection) for the treatment of known or suspected cyanide poisoning. Meridian Medical Technologies, Inc, Columbia, MD, September 2009. *B.* Cyanide antidote kit (sodium nitrite injection, sodium thiosulfate injection, amyl nitrite inhalants) for the treatment of cyanide poisoning. Taylor Pharmaceuticals, Decatur, IL, 2006.

3.b. What feasible pharmacotherapeutic alternatives are available for treating cyanide poisoning (see Fig. 10-1)?

### Optimal Plan

4.a. Outline your pharmacotherapeutic plan for treating cyanide poisoning in these patients. Include dose(s), route(s), and repeat dosing information (if any) for both adult and pediatric patients. Also describe use of administration devices or ancillary supplies.

4.b. What supportive care measures may be necessary for optimal management?

### Outcome Evaluation

5.a. Describe the clinical and laboratory parameters required to determine whether the treatment for these patients has been successful.

5.b. How often should the nursing staff attempt to assess and reassess the patients?

### Patient Education

6.a. For patients who are alert and oriented, what information would you share with them about the possible immediate side effects of each of the antidotes?

6.b. How long might it take for the patients to recover from potential long-term effects of acute cyanide exposure?

## CLINICAL COURSE

Throughout the next 24 hours, your ED treats 50 victims; 25 were treated and released, 20 were treated and admitted (10 to intensive care units), and 5 expired. Clinicians suspect that cyanide gas was released. This was later confirmed by HAZMAT units and federal response teams. During the next day, the FBI and local law enforcement discover that disgruntled former high school students obtained cyanide salt and a strong acid, quickly mixing and releasing a gas in bathrooms and garbage cans around the auditorium.

## FOLLOW-UP QUESTIONS

1. If your pharmacy department runs out of antidotes and more are needed emergently, where can you obtain additional antidote supplies: locally, regionally, and nationally?
2. Suppose there are 100 patients in your hospital's ED needing a cyanide antidote and you only have enough antidote to treat 25 patients. Who may be involved in making these ethical treatment decisions, and how would these decisions be made?

## CLINICAL PEARLS

The exhaled breath of cyanide exposure victims may smell like bitter almonds. Not everyone (only 40–60% of people) can detect this odor.

Hydroxocobalamin administration can interfere with co-oximetry and blood chemistry results. Draw pertinent labs quickly, prior to hydroxocobalamin administration, and refer to the package insert for more details about which tests can be affected.

## SELF-STUDY ASSIGNMENTS

1. Research information on the Strategic National Stockpile Program.
2. Describe the limitation of the cyanide antidote kit if concurrent carbon monoxide poisoning is suspected.

## REFERENCES


1. Leybell I, Borron SW, Roldan CJ. Emedicine [Internet]. New York, Web MD Inc, © 1996–2006 [updated December 14, 2009; cited February 28, 2010]. Toxicity, cyanide. Available at: *www.emedicine.com/emerg/topic118.htm.*
2. Emergency Preparedness and Response [Internet]. Atlanta, GA, Centers for Disease Control and Prevention [updated January 27, 2004; cited February 28, 2010]. Facts about cyanide. Available at: *www.bt.cdc.gov/agent/cyanide/basics/facts.asp.*
3. Mutlu GM, Keikin JB, Oh K, Factor P. An unresponsive biochemistry professor in the bathtub. Chest 2002;122:1073–1076.
4. Baud FJ. Cyanide: critical issues in diagnosis and treatment. Hum Exp Toxicol 2007;26:191–201.
5. Borron SW, Baud FJ, Barriot P, Imbert M, Bismuth C. Prospective study of hydroxocobalamin for acute cyanide poisoning in smoke inhalation. Ann Emerg Med 2007;49:794–801.
6. Gracia R, Shepherd G. Cyanide poisoning and its treatment. Pharmacotherapy 2004;24:1358–1365.
7. Cyanide Antidote Kit [package insert]. Decatur, IL, Taylor Pharmaceuticals, February 2006.
8. Cyanokit [package insert]. Columbia, MD, Meridian Technologies Inc, September, 2009.
9. Colley J, Baker DE. Hydroxocobalamin. In: Cada DJ, Baker DE, Levien TL, eds. Formulary Monograph Service. St. Louis, Wolters Kluwer Health Inc, January 2007.


# 11

# CHEMICAL EXPOSURE

Terrorism or Freak Accident? . . . . . . . . . . . . . . Level II

**Colleen M. Terriff, PharmD, BCPS**

## LEARNING OBJECTIVES

After completing this case study, students should be able to:

- Identify potential toxins or chemical agents that could be used in a terrorist attack.
- Determine the proper antidote or treatments, such as supportive care for seizures, and the dosing regimens for a potential chemical weapon, based on patient signs and symptoms.
- State the types and advantages of auto-injectors for treatment of chemical exposures.
- List ancillary supplies that will be needed to complement the drug stockpiles; compare and contrast what is needed for adults versus pediatric patients.

## PATIENT PRESENTATION

### Patient Scenario

Many patients present to your hospital's ED visibly teary, coughing, and having trouble breathing.

## HPI

Patients arrive at the ED via car, taxi, and ambulance. They were attending an all-day seminar at the downtown convention center when, after a loud explosion down the hall, they were exposed to smoke and "fumes." Paramedics also reported that patients complained of difficulty breathing and blurred vision. Patients were covering their eyes, coughing, crying, and even drooling.

Dozens of patients outside the ED are awaiting decontamination, and patients appear to be anxious and extremely concerned. Medical Alert has been activated for city and county, and the Regional Disaster Hospital has been notified of Alert. All local EDs are securing their perimeters and setting up decontamination units. Scene decontamination of patients is occurring before some are arriving via ambulance. Patients arriving by car or cab or by foot have not been decontaminated. Hospital administration activates the Incident Command System.

## PMH, PSH, FH, and SH

Not obtained

## ROS

Most patients can only nod to some questions, making individual interviews difficult. The ED lead physician instructs nurses to get patient vital signs and approximate age and weight. Medical residents are told to do brief triage physical exams on an estimated 25 patients each.

## Physical Examination

### *Gen*

Patients appear anxious, breathing quickly. Some have required intubation.

### *VS*

BP: A few patients have mildly elevated BP.
P: Most patients have tachycardia, but a few have bradycardia.
RR: Most patients are tachypneic.
T: Most patients are normal.
Pain: Most patients indicate that they do not have significant pain.
$O_2$ sat: Spot checks on most patients >94%.

### *Skin*

Some patients are sweating profusely; no cyanosis, clubbing, or edema present.

### *HEENT*

Bilateral pinpoint pupils, nonreactive to light, profuse rhinorrhea, and hypersalivation

### *Neck/Lymph Nodes*

Cursory exam reveals no swollen lymph nodes or other abnormalities.

### *Lungs/Thorax*

Rapid respiratory rate, rhonchi present throughout; a few patients exhibit bronchoconstriction and excessive respiratory secretions.

### *CV*

Tachycardia for most patients; too noisy to listen for heart sounds for most patients

### *Abd*

Some patients complain of nausea; a few experience emesis.

### *Genital/Rect*

DRE and stool guaiac not performed

### *MS/Ext*

Facial muscle twitching noticed in a few patients who also had substantial rhinorrhea and complaints of severe vision changes

### *Neuro*

Initially, five patients have flaccid paralysis and respiratory arrest requiring intubation; three of these five patients are actively seizing (tonic–clonic seizures).

## Labs

Complete metabolic panel: Hyperglycemia, hypokalemia, hypomagnesemia, and elevated amylase and liver function tests in some patients
CBC: Mild leukocytosis and elevated Hg/Hct suggestive of hemoconcentration
Pending: RBC and plasma cholinesterase levels, blood cyanide levels, and toxicology screen

## Other

Blood gases ordered on intubated patients reveal metabolic acidosis with or without a respiratory acidosis
Multiple chest x-rays: Pending

## Lead Physician's Assessment

Based on feedback from the scene and the Regional Disaster Hospital, 1,000 people may have been affected by this chemical release, going to four area hospitals. The ED staff is also alerted to get information from victims and save patient belongings as evidence for FBI. Scene fire chief acting as Incident Commander asks for assistance (request relayed from combined communications center to hospitals) from health care providers triaging victims in area hospitals to attempt to identify chemical agent based on symptomatology. An ED medical resident contacts the Regional Poison Control Center for guidance identifying the possible agent. The pharmacy department is also contacted for their assistance with antidote recommendations, including dosing and side-effect monitoring.

# QUESTIONS

## Problem Identification

1.a. Create a list of potential chemical agents that the patients may have been exposed to based on presenting signs and symptoms.

1.b. How serious is this exposure, and what could be some potential sequelae?

## Desired Outcome

2.a. What are the goals of pharmacotherapy in this case?

2.b. How do your goals change if there were 15 patients presenting with these symptoms and differing degrees of severity and exposure?

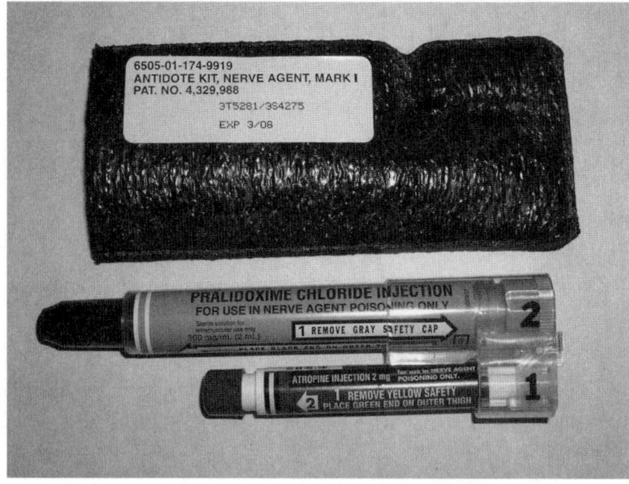


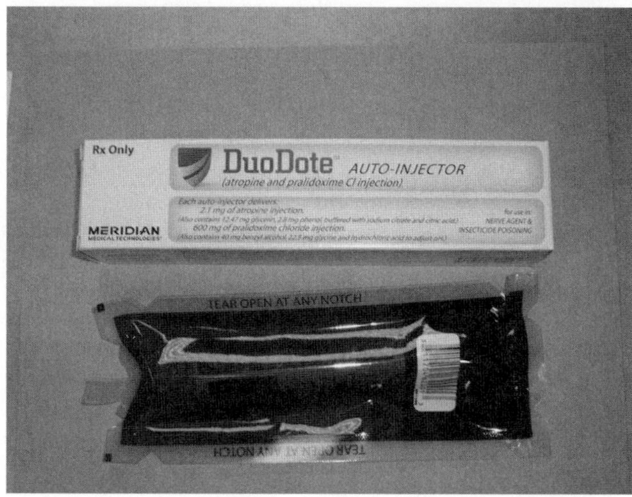


**FIGURE 11-1.** *A.* The Mark-I™ auto-injector, consisting of two antidotes to be used after exposures to a nerve or organophosphate agent in a disaster situation. The kit contains an atropine auto-injector (2 mg/0.7 mL) and a pralidoxime chloride (2-PAM) auto-injector (600 mg/2 mL). *B.* The Duodote™ auto-injector (replacing the Mark-I auto-injector) contains 2.1 mg atropine and 600 mg of pralidoxime chloride in one syringe.

## Therapeutic Alternatives

3.a. What nonpharmacologic measures are available to treat these patients?

3.b. What feasible pharmacotherapeutic alternatives are available for treating these patients?

3.c. Suppose there are 100 patients in your hospital's emergency department needing an antidote, and you only have enough antidote to treat 25 patients. How do you decide who gets life-saving treatment?

## Optimal Plan

4.a. What antidotes are required for this chemical exposure? Provide the adult doses, routes, and repeat dosing information for each antidote.

4.b. There are special dosing kits and administration devices available for these antidotes (see Figs. 11-1 and 11-2). Describe how these kits should be administered.

4.c. If a patient's condition worsens and seizure activity occurs, what class of medications should be used for this chemical-induced seizure?

FIGURE 11-2. Diazepam provided as a 10-mg dose in a military-designed auto-injector.

## Outcome Evaluation

5. Outline a monitoring plan to assess if the pharmacotherapy treatment for these patients is successful.

## Patient Education

6.a. What information would you share with the patients about immediate side effects of each of the antidotes?

6.b. How long might it take for patients to recover from the ocular effects of the chemical exposure? Incorporate this information into your educational efforts.

## CLINICAL COURSE

Students: Your instructor can provide you with the outcome of this incident.

## FOLLOW-UP QUESTION

1. If your pharmacy department runs out of antidotes and more are needed emergently, where can you obtain additional antidote supplies: locally, regionally, and nationally?

## CLINICAL PEARL

Most chemical agents that could be used for a terrorist attack would likely be exploded or released as a gas in order to increase respiratory exposure and allow for rapid systemic entry into victims. Therefore, clinicians need to quickly triage patients, classify symptoms for identification, and administer appropriate treatment if available.

## SELF-STUDY ASSIGNMENTS

1. Research information on the Strategic National Stockpile Program and the CHEMPACK program. Research the difference in response times and focus for both programs.
2. List ancillary supplies (i.e., syringes, needles, tubing) needed to complement the nerve agent stockpiles. Are there any differences for what is needed for adults versus pediatric patients?

## REFERENCES


1. North Carolina Statewide Program for Infection Control and Epidemiology (SPICE) [Internet]. Chemical terrorism agents and syndromes, 2002 [cited March 1, 2010]. Available at: *www.unc.edu/depts/spice/chemical-generic.pdf.*
2. US Army Medical Research Institute of Chemical Defense (USAMRICD). Field Management of Chemical Casualties Handbook, 2nd ed. [Intranet], July 2000 [cited April 2, 2010]. Available at: *https://www.rke.vaems.org/wvems/Libraryfiles/Dis/E_04.pdf.*
3. Department of Health and Human Services Agency for Toxic Substances and Disease Registry. Medical Management Guidelines for Nerve Agents: Tabun (GA); Sarin (GB); Soman (GD) and VX [Intranet]. Atlanta, GA [updated August 22, 2008; cited April 2, 2010]. Available at: *http://www.atsdr.cdc.gov/MHMI/mmg166.html.*
4. Ciottone GR, Arnold JL. CBRNE—chemical warfare agents. Emedicine [Internet]. New York, Web MD Inc, ©1994–2010 [updated July 11, 2008; cited April 2, 2010]. Available at: *http://emedicine.medscape.com/article/829454-overview.*
5. Bartlett JG, Sifton DW, Gwynned LK. PDR Guide to Biological and Chemical Warfare Response, 1st ed. Montvale, NJ, Thomson Healthcare, 2002:79–86, 101–102, 126–127.
6. National Center for Disaster Preparedness, Columbia University Mailman School of Public Health. Pediatric Preparedness for Disasters and Terrorism: A National Consensus Conference, 2003 [cited April 2, 2010]. Available at: *http://www.ncdp.mailman.columbia.edu/files/Executive%20Summary%20for%20Pediatric%20Preparedness%20National%20Consensus%20Conference.pdf.*
7. Cyanide Antidote Kit [package insert]. Decatur, IL, Taylor Pharmaceuticals, February 2006.
8. Cyanokit [package insert]. Columbia, MD, Meridian Technologies Inc, September 2009.
9. Atropen Auto-Injector [package insert]. Columbia, MD, Meridian Technologies Inc, November 2005.
10. Pralidoxime Chloride Injection Auto-Injector [package insert]. Columbia, MD, Meridian Technologies Inc, October 2003.
11. Duodote [package insert]. Columbia, MD, Meridian Technologies Inc, September 2006.

# SECTION 2 CARDIOVASCULAR DISORDERS

## 12

## CARDIAC ARREST

A Near-Death Experience . . . . . . . . . . . . . . . . Level II

**Tate N. Trujillo, PharmD, BCPS, FCCM**

**Christopher M. Scott, PharmD, BCPS, FCCM**

### LEARNING OBJECTIVES

After completing this case study, the reader should be able to:

- Discuss possible causes for cardiac arrest.
- Outline medications used to treat cardiac arrest.
- List the pharmacologic actions of medications used in cardioversion.
- Outline the Advanced Cardiac Life Support (ACLS) guidelines.
- Identify appropriate parameters to monitor a patient who has just been cardioverted.

### PATIENT PRESENTATION

#### Chief Complaint

"I don't know what happened. I don't remember a thing."

#### HPI

Megan Zolman is a 68-year-old female driver of a motor vehicle brought from an outside hospital by air ambulance who was involved in a crash. She was T-boned at high speed by a semitruck on the driver's side. There was no alcohol involved. The extrication time was 15 minutes. There was a loss of consciousness, and she does not remember the event.

#### PMH

Cervical dystonia
Endometriosis
Thyroid disease
HTN
Hyperlipidemia
Type 2 DM—diet controlled

#### PSH

Hysterectomy in 1985

#### FH

Mother had HTN and died of an AMI at age 69; no information available for father; one brother is alive with HTN and DM at age 73.

#### SH

Smoker; quit 8 years ago; previously 1.5 ppd

#### Meds PTA

Atorvastatin 20 mg po daily
Metoprolol 50 mg po twice daily

#### Meds

Metoclopramide 10 mg IV Q 6 H
Famotidine 20 mg IV Q 12 H
Labetalol 10 mg IV Q 10 minutes PRN for SBP >160 (three uses)
Enalaprilat 1.25 mg IV Q 6 H PRN SBP >120 (two uses)
Lorazepam 2 mg IV Q 4 H PRN (nine uses)
Morphine 2–4 mg IV Q 2 H PRN (two uses)
Fentanyl 150 mcg/h
Midazolam 3 mg/h
Nitroprusside 1.5 mcg/kg/min

#### All

Sulfa

#### ROS

Frequent chest pain and back pain with difficulty breathing

#### Physical Examination

*Gen*

Obese white woman

*VS*

BP 98/60, P 112, RR 24, T 37.9°C; dry Wt 120 kg; Ht 162.5 cm

*Skin*

Warm, dry

*HEENT*

PERRLA; EOMI; arteriolar narrowing on funduscopic exam; no hemorrhages, exudates, or papilledema; oral mucosa clear

*Neck/Lymph Nodes*

Supple with no JVD or bruits; no lymphadenopathy or thyromegaly

*Chest*

Mild bibasilar rales with decreased breath sounds on the left

*CV*

Tachycardic; $S_1$, $S_2$ normal; no $S_3$ or $S_4$; no murmurs or rubs

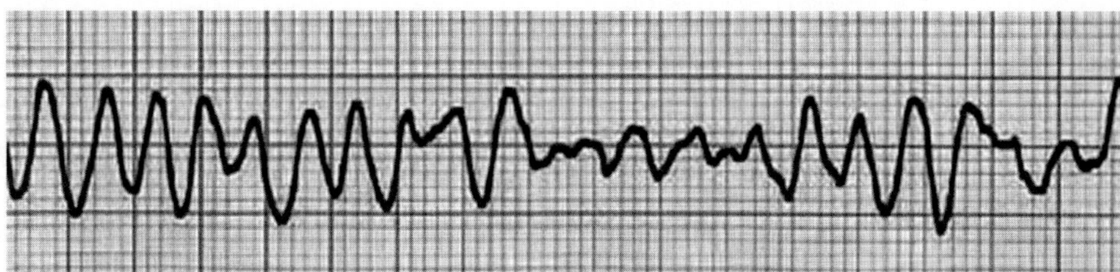

**FIGURE 12-1.** Electrocardiogram showing ventricular fibrillation.

*Abd*

Obese, soft, nontender; (+) BS; no HSM

*Genit/Rect*

Stool heme (−)

*MS/Ext*

Capillary refill <2 seconds; age-appropriate strength and ROM

*Neuro*

A & O × 3, GCS 15, CN II–XII intact

### Labs

| | | |
|---|---|---|
| Na 140 mEq/L | Mg 2.5 mg/dL | Hgb 9.3 g/dL |
| K 4.9 mEq/L | Phos 2.5 mg/dL | Hct 28% |
| Cl 106 mEq/L | Alb 2.5 g/dL | Plt 229 × $10^3$/mm$^3$ |
| $CO_2$ 20 mEq/L | | WBC 9.9 × $10^3$/mm$^3$ |
| BUN 35 mg/dL | | PMNs 79% |
| SCr 1.3 mg/dL | | Bands 1% |
| Glu 245 mg/dL | | Lymphs 17% |
| Ca 6.7 mg/dL | | Monos 3% |

### ECG

Sinus tachycardia at a rate of 112 bpm

### Clinical Course

The patient's clinical condition deteriorated, and she was subsequently intubated for respiratory failure and taken to CT scan for further work-up. The CT showed a normal head, bilateral acetabular fractures, bilateral inferior and superior pubic ramus fractures, a 50% left pneumothorax, and an aortic tear. She was emergently taken to the operating room for repair of the aortic tear by cardiovascular surgery. Postoperatively, she was taken to the intensive care unit. Approximately 36 hours S/P aortic repair, the patient developed multifocal PVCs that quickly changed to ventricular fibrillation (Fig. 12-1). A code was called.

### Assessment

68-Year-old multiple trauma patient S/P aortic repair currently in cardiac arrest 36 hours postoperatively

# QUESTIONS

## Problem Identification

1.a. What actual and potential drug-related problems does this patient have just prior to the development of ventricular fibrillation?

1.b. Discuss the possible causes for the development of ventricular fibrillation.

## Desired Outcome

2. What are the short-term goals of pharmacotherapy for this patient?

## Therapeutic Alternatives

3.a. What nonpharmacologic maneuvers should be taken immediately in a patient with ventricular fibrillation?

3.b. What pharmacotherapeutic agents are available for the acute therapy of this patient's condition?

## Optimal Plan

4.a. A pharmacist was not available to participate in this resuscitation effort. Assess the appropriateness of the treatment used to obtain a cardiac conversion in this patient (see the section "Clinical Course: Cardiopulmonary Resuscitation Record of Events and Orders").

4.b. On conversion to normal sinus rhythm, what is your pharmacotherapeutic plan to maintain the patient's stability?

## Clinical Course: Cardiopulmonary Resuscitation Record of Events and Orders

See the following table:

| Time | BP | Cardiac Rhythm | HR | Defib. (J) | Rhythm after Defib. | Drugs Given |
|---|---|---|---|---|---|---|
| 0220 | 56/? | VF (see Fig. 12-1) | 98 | 100 | Torsades (Fig. 12-2) | |
| 0221 | 46/? | Torsades | | 200 | Torsades | |
| 0222 | 116/? | Torsades | | 300 | Agonal | |
| 0225 | 88/? | Torsades | | 360 | Agonal to torsades | Epi 1 mg IVP<br>Atropine 1 mg IVP<br>Amio 150 mg IVP |
| 0232 | 302/133 | SVT | 160 | 360 | SVT | |
| 0238 | 160/84 | SVT | 180 | 360 | NSR | Amio 150 mg IVP |
| 0247 | 133/50 | NSR | 96 | | Torsades to NSR with PVC | |
| 0252 | | | | | NSR with PVC | |

Key: ?, not recorded; Amio, amiodarone; BP, blood pressure; HR, heart rate; Defib., defibrillation; Epi, epinephrine; IVP, intravenous push; NSR, normal sinus rhythm; PVC, premature ventricular contraction; SVT, supraventricular tachycardia; VF, ventricular fibrillation.

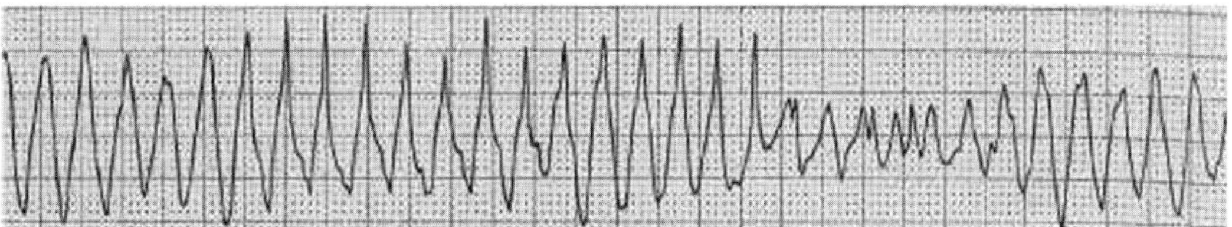

**FIGURE 12-2.** Electrocardiogram showing torsades de pointes.

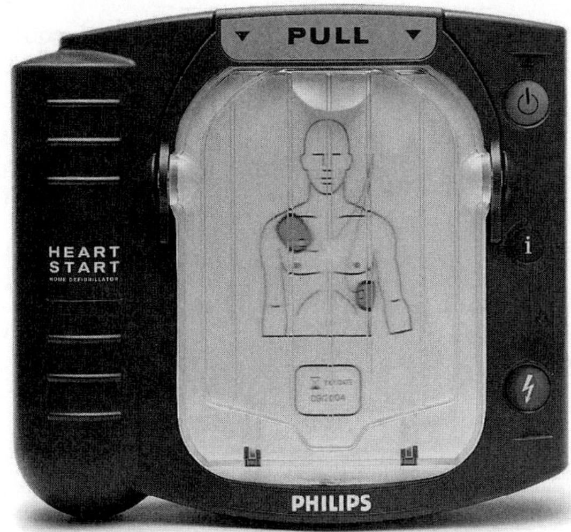


**FIGURE 12-3.** The Heartstart Home Defibrillator, an automated external defibrillator (AED) device approved by the FDA for home use. *(Photograph courtesy of Philips Medical Systems, Bothell, Washington.)*

## Outcome Evaluation

5. How should the patient be monitored to assess drug efficacy and to prevent or detect adverse effects? Describe how the therapy should be adjusted if adverse events occur.

## ■ SELF-STUDY ASSIGNMENTS

1. Search the Internet for commercially available automated external defibrillator (AED) devices (see Fig. 12-3 for one example). Explain how such a device would be used by a layperson during a cardiac arrest that occurred in the home or workplace.
2. Perform a literature search to determine the odds of surviving a cardiac arrest while hospitalized.
3. List medications that can be administered through an endotracheal tube in an emergent situation.
4. Investigate the effects of induced hypothermia following cardiac arrest on patient outcomes.

## CLINICAL PEARL

During a cardiac arrest, a patient's serum potassium will increase dramatically due to the presence of metabolic acidosis; this can worsen or complicate arrhythmia conversion.

## REFERENCES

1. Hazinski MF, Chameides L, Elling B, et al., eds. 2005 American Heart Association guidelines for cardiopulmonary resuscitation and emergency cardiovascular care. Circulation 2005;12: IV-1–IV-211.
2. Wenzel V, Krismer AC, Arntz HR, Sitter H, Stadlbauer KH, Lindner KH. A comparison of vasopressin and epinephrine for out-of-hospital cardiopulmonary resuscitation. N Engl J Med 2004;350: 105–113.
3. Zipes DP, Camm AJ, Borggrefe M, et al. ACC/AHA/ESC 2006 guidelines for management of patients with ventricular arrhythmias and the prevention of sudden cardiac death: a report of the American College of Cardiology/American Heart Association Task Force and the European Society of Cardiology Committee for Practice Guidelines (Writing Committee to Develop Guidelines for Management of Patients With Ventricular Arrhythmias and the Prevention of Sudden Cardiac Death). Circulation 2006;114:e385–e484.

# 13

# HYPERTENSION

Pass the Salt, Please .................... Level II

**Julia M. Koehler, PharmD, FCCP**

**James E. Tisdale, PharmD, BCPS, FCCP**

## LEARNING OBJECTIVES

After completing this case study, the reader should be able to:

- Classify blood pressure according to current hypertension guidelines, and discuss the correlation between blood pressure and risk for cardiovascular morbidity and mortality.
- Identify medications that may cause or worsen hypertension.
- Discuss complications (e.g., target organ damage, clinical vascular disease) that may occur as a result of uncontrolled and/or long-standing hypertension, and identify additional cardiovascular risk factors.
- Establish goals for the treatment of hypertension, and choose appropriate lifestyle modifications and antihypertensive regimens based on patient-specific characteristics and comorbid disease states.
- Provide appropriate patient counseling for antihypertensive drug regimens.

## PATIENT PRESENTATION

### ■ Chief Complaint

"I'm here to see my new doctor for a checkup. I'm just getting over a cold. Overall, I'm feeling fine, except for occasional headaches and some dizziness in the morning. My other doctor prescribed a low-salt diet for me, but I don't like it!"

## HPI

James Frank is a 64-year-old African-American man who presents to his new family medicine physician for evaluation and follow-up of his medical problems. He generally has no complaints, except for occasional mild headaches and some dizziness after he takes his morning medications. He states that he is dissatisfied with being placed on a low-sodium diet by his former primary care physician.

## PMH

Hypertension (HTN) × 14 years
Type 2 diabetes mellitus × 16 years
Chronic obstructive pulmonary disease (COPD), Stage 2 (moderate)
Benign prostatic hyperplasia
Chronic kidney disease
Gout

## FH

Father died of acute MI at age 73. Mother died of lung cancer at age 65. Father had HTN and dyslipidemia. Mother had HTN and diabetes mellitus.

## SH

Former smoker (quit 6 years ago; 35 pack-year history); reports moderate amount of alcohol intake. He admits he has been nonadherent to his low-sodium diet (states, "I eat whatever I want"). He does not exercise regularly and is limited somewhat functionally by his COPD. He is retired and lives alone.

## Meds

Triamterene/hydrochlorothiazide 37.5 mg/25 mg po Q AM
Insulin glargine 36 U subQ daily
Insulin lispro 12 U subQ TID with meals
Doxazosin 2 mg po Q AM
Carvedilol 12.5 mg po BID
Albuterol HFA MDI, two puffs Q 4–6 h PRN shortness of breath
Tiotropium DPI 18 mcg, one capsule inhaled daily
Fluticasone/salmeterol DPI 250/50, one inhaled BID
Mucinex D two tablets Q 12 h PRN cough/congestion
Naproxen 220 mg po Q 8 h PRN pain/HA
Allopurinol 200 mg po daily

## All

PCN—rash

## ROS

Patient states that overall he is doing well and recovering from a cold. He has noticed no major weight changes over the past few years. He complains of occasional headaches, which are usually relieved by naproxen, and he denies blurred vision and chest pain. He states that shortness of breath is "usual" for him, and that his albuterol helps. He denies experiencing any hemoptysis or epistaxis; he also denies nausea, vomiting, abdominal pain, cramping, diarrhea, constipation, or blood in stool. He denies urinary frequency, but states that he used to have difficulty urinating until his physician started him on doxazosin a few months ago. He has no prior history of arthritic symptoms and states that his occasional gout pain is also relieved with naproxen.

## Physical Examination

### *Gen*

WDWN, African-American male; moderately overweight; in no acute distress

### *VS*

BP 162/90 mm Hg (sitting; repeat 164/92 mm Hg), HR 76 bpm (regular), RR 16/min, T 37°C; Wt 95 kg, Ht 6′2″

### *HEENT*

TMs clear; mild sinus drainage; AV nicking noted; no hemorrhages, exudates, or papilledema

### *Neck*

Supple without masses or bruits, no thyroid enlargement or lymphadenopathy

### *Lungs*

Lung fields CTA bilaterally. Few basilar crackles, mild expiratory wheezing.

### *Heart*

RRR; normal $S_1$ and $S_2$. No $S_3$ or $S_4$.

### *Abd*

Soft, NTND; no masses, bruits, or organomegaly. Normal BS.

### *Genit/Rect*

Enlarged prostate

### *Ext*

No CCE; no apparent joint swelling or signs of tophi

### *Neuro*

No gross motor-sensory deficits present. CN II–XII intact. A & O × 3.

## Labs

| | | | |
|---|---|---|---|
| Na 138 mEq/L | Ca 9.7 mg/dL | *Fasting lipid panel* | *Spirometry (6 months ago)* |
| K 4.7 mEq/L | Mg 2.3 mEq/L | Total Chol 171 mg/dL | FVC 2.38 L (54% pred) |
| Cl 99 mEq/L | $HbA_{1C}$ 6.1% | LDL 99 mg/dL | $FEV_1$ 1.21 L (38% pred) |
| $CO_2$ 27 mEq/L | Alb 3.4 g/dL | HDL 40 mg/dL | $FEV_1$/FVC 51% |
| BUN 22 mg/dL | Hgb 13 g/dL | TG 158 mg/dL | |
| SCr 2.2 mg/dL | Hct 40% | | |
| Glucose 110 mg/dL | WBC 9.0 × $10^3$/mm$^3$ | | |
| Uric acid 6.7 mg/dL | Plts 189 × $10^3$/mm$^3$ | | |

## UA

Yellow, clear, SG 1.007, pH 5.5, (+) protein, (–) glucose, (–) ketones, (–) bilirubin, (–) blood, (–) nitrite, RBC 0/hpf, WBC 1–2/hpf, neg bacteria, 1–5 epithelial cells

## ECG

Normal sinus rhythm

## ECHO (6 Months Ago)

Mild LVH, estimated EF 45%

## Assessment

1. HTN, uncontrolled
2. Type 2 diabetes mellitus, controlled on current insulin regimen

3. Moderate COPD, stable on current regimen
4. BPH, symptoms improved on doxazosin
5. Gout, controlled on current regimen

## QUESTIONS

### Problem Identification

1.a. Create a list of this patient's drug-related problems, including any medications that may be contributing to his uncontrolled HTN.

1.b. How would you classify this patient's HTN, according to current HTN guidelines?

1.c. What are the patient's known cardiovascular risk factors, and what is his Framingham risk score?

1.d. What evidence of target organ damage or clinical cardiovascular disease does this patient have?

### Desired Outcome

2. List the goals of treatment for this patient (including his goal blood pressure).

### Therapeutic Alternatives

3.a. What lifestyle modifications should be encouraged for this patient to help achieve and maintain adequate blood pressure reduction?

3.b. What reasonable pharmacotherapeutic options are available for controlling this patient's blood pressure, and what comorbidities and individual patient considerations should be taken into account when selecting pharmacologic therapy for his HTN? How might Mr Frank's HTN medications potentially affect his other medical problems?

### Optimal Plan

4.a. Recommend specific lifestyle modifications for this patient.

4.b. Outline a specific and appropriate pharmacotherapeutic regimen for this patient's uncontrolled HTN, including drug(s), dose(s), dosage form(s), and schedule(s).

### Outcome Evaluation

5. Based on your recommendations, what parameters should be monitored after initiating this regimen and throughout the treatment course? At what time intervals should these parameters be monitored?

### Patient Education

6. Based on your recommendations, provide appropriate education to this patient.

## ■ SELF-STUDY ASSIGNMENTS

1. Review the American Heart Association Scientific Statement on the treatment of HTN in the prevention of and management of ischemic heart disease, and highlight the key differences in recommendations for managing a hypertensive patient with known CHD.

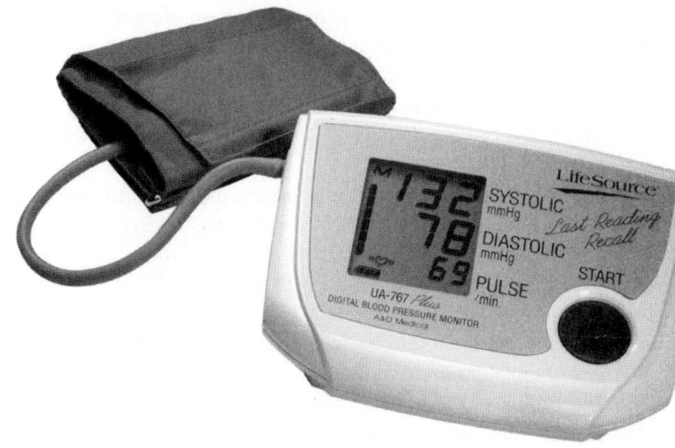


**FIGURE 13-1.** The LifeSource UA-767 Plus—One-Step Plus Memory digital home blood pressure monitor. *(Photo courtesy of A&D Medical, Milpitas, California.)*

2. Outline the changes, if any, that you would make to the pharmacotherapeutic regimen for this patient if he had a history of each of the following comorbidities or characteristics:
    - Severe persistent asthma
    - Major depression
    - Ischemic heart disease with a history of myocardial infarction
    - Cerebrovascular disease
    - Peripheral arterial disease
    - Isolated systolic HTN
    - Migraine headache disorder
    - Liver disease
    - Renovascular disease (bilateral or unilateral renal artery stenosis)
    - Heart failure due to left ventricular systolic dysfunction
3. Describe how you would explain to a patient how to use a digital home blood pressure monitor such as the one shown in Figure 13-1.

## CLINICAL PEARLS

1. The risk of hemorrhagic stroke may be increased by the use of aspirin therapy in patients with uncontrolled HTN.
2. The majority of hypertensive patients will require two or more blood pressuring lowering medications to achieve recommended blood pressure goals.

## REFERENCES

1. Salerno SM, Jackson JL, Berbano EP. Effect of oral pseudoephedrine on blood pressure and heart rate: a meta-analysis. Arch Intern Med 2005;165:1686–1694.
2. Chobanian AV, Bakris GL, Black HR, et al., the National High Blood Pressure Education Program Coordinating Committee. Seventh report of the Joint National Committee on Prevention, Detection, Evaluation, and Treatment of High Blood Pressure. Hypertension 2003;42:1206–1252.
3. Giles TD, Materson BJ, Cohn JN, Kostis JB. Definition and classification of hypertension: an update. J Clin Hypertens 2009;11:611–614.
4. Rosendorff C, Black HR, Cannon CP, et al. Treatment of hypertension in the prevention and management of ischemic heart disease: a scientific statement from the American Heart Association Council for

High Blood Pressure Research and the Councils on Clinical Cardiology and Epidemiology and Prevention. Circulation 2007;115:2761–2788.

5. Sacks FM, Svetkey LP, Vollmer WM, et al. Effects on blood pressure of reduced dietary sodium and the Dietary Approaches to Stop Hypertension (DASH) diet. DASH-Sodium Collaborative Research Group. N Engl J Med 2001;344:3–10.
6. Douglas JG, Bakris GL, Epstein M, et al. Management of high blood pressure in African Americans: consensus statement of the Hypertension in African Americans Working Group of the International Society on Hypertension in Blacks. Arch Intern Med 2003;163:525–541.
7. ALLHAT Officers and Coordinators for the ALLHAT Collaborative Research Group. Major outcomes in high-risk hypertensive patients randomized to angiotensin-converting enzyme inhibitor or calcium channel blocker vs diuretic: the Antihypertensive and Lipid-Lowering Treatment to Prevent Heart Attack Trial (ALLHAT). JAMA 2002;288:2981–2997.
8. UKPDS 39. Efficacy of atenolol and captopril in reducing risk of macrovascular and microvascular complications in type 2 diabetes: UKPDS 39. UK Prospective Diabetes Study Group. BMJ 1998;317:713–720.
9. Heart Outcomes Prevention Evaluation Study Investigators. Effects of an angiotensin-converting enzyme inhibitor, ramipril, on cardiovascular events in high-risk patients. N Engl J Med 2000;342:145–153.
10. Heart Outcomes Prevention Evaluation Study Investigators. Effects of ramipril on cardiovascular and microvascular outcomes in people with diabetes mellitus: results of the HOPE study and the MICRO-HOPE substudy. Lancet 2000;355:253–259.
11. American Diabetes Association. Treatment of hypertension in adults with diabetes. Diabetes Care 2002;25:S71–S73.
12. The ALLHAT Officers and Coordinators for the ALLHAT Collaborative Research Group. Major cardiovascular events in hypertensive patients randomized to doxazosin vs chlorthalidone: the Antihypertensive and Lipid-Lowering Treatment to Prevent Heart Attack Trial (ALLHAT). JAMA. 2000;283:1967–1975.
13. Hou FF, Zhang X, Xie D, et al. Efficacy and safety of benazepril for advanced chronic renal insufficiency. N Engl J Med 2006;354:131–140.
14. Hansson L, Zanchetti A, Carruthers SG, et al. Effects of intensive blood-pressure lowering and low-dose aspirin in patients with hypertension: principal results of the Hypertension Optimal Treatment (HOT) randomized trial. HOT Study Group. Lancet 1998;351:1755–1762.
15. Haymore BR, Yoon J, Mikita CP, Klote MM, DeZee KJ. Risk of angioedema with angiotensin receptor blockers in patients with prior angioedema associated with angiotensin-converting enzyme inhibitors: a meta-analysis. Ann Allergy Asthma Immunol 2008;101:495–499.

# 14

# HYPERTENSIVE CRISIS

Those Pills Made Me Sick . . . . . . . . . . . . . . . . . Level I

**James J. Nawarskas, PharmD, BCPS**

## LEARNING OBJECTIVES

After completing this case study, the reader should be able to:

- Distinguish a hypertensive urgency from a hypertensive emergency.
- Identify treatment goals for a patient with a hypertensive crisis.
- Develop an appropriate treatment plan for a patient with a hypertensive crisis.
- Describe how a pharmacist can educate a patient about hypertension and the importance of providing this education.

## PATIENT PRESENTATION

### Chief Complaint

"I'm having trouble seeing, and my legs are aching and tingling."

### HPI

Agnes Latham is a 61-year-old woman who is admitted to the emergency department with a chief complaint of difficulty seeing and severe tingling in her arms and legs. She describes "fuzzy vision" that started about 1 day ago. The aching and tingling in the extremities started about a week ago and was very mild at that time. It has gotten progressively worse since then and affects mainly her calves. The more she moves her legs, the worse the symptoms become, and she is having difficulty at work due to the discomfort. She takes ibuprofen, but that does not seem to help. Rest does help considerably. She has a past medical history significant for hypertension and hypothyroidism, and was diagnosed with diabetes about 3 months ago. She had been on chlorthalidone for several years with reasonable success and good tolerability, but was recently (3 months ago) switched to a combination product containing lisinopril and hydrochlorothiazide because her primary care provider wanted more aggressive blood pressure control for her hypertension in consideration of her newly diagnosed diabetes.

Ms Latham was convinced that these medications were making her feel worse, so she stopped taking them about 2 months ago. She did not inform her primary care provider of this and is not scheduled to see her provider again for another month. When asked, Ms Latham said that soon after starting these medications she developed a dry, hacking cough that was keeping her awake at night. She also claims that she got dizzy when rising from a seated position. She states that after stopping the medications, the cough went away, as did the dizziness, and she actually felt better. That is why she did not contact anyone until now.

### PMH

HTN × 7 years
Hypothyroidism × 10 years
Type 2 diabetes mellitus × 3 months

### FH

Both parents had HTN, and mother had diabetes. Father had a heart attack in his early 50s and died in his 70s of a second heart attack; mother died a few years later from a stroke. Two brothers, 57 and 60 years old, are both alive; the elder has HTN and hypercholesterolemia and underwent coronary artery bypass graft surgery 3 years ago, the younger has no chronic diseases. One sister who is 53 years old and in fairly good health, although there is suspicion that she may have impaired fasting glucose.

### SH

Married for 38 years with four children (two boys, two girls all over 25 years of age with no notable medical problems); she works part-time (2–3 days per week) as a cashier at a large department store. She smoked cigarettes rather heavily when she was younger, but cut back to 1–2 per day when she was raising her children. As her children got older, she gradually increased her cigarette use and is now smoking about 1.5 packs per day and has been doing so for about the past 10 years. She drinks alcohol infrequently (maybe once or twice a month), when she is at a social gathering. She denies ever using recreational drugs. She does not exercise and leads a rather sedentary lifestyle. In terms of diet, for breakfast she typically has a cup of coffee, toast with butter, and two eggs. For lunch, she usually eats a cold cut sandwich, although on days she works, she typically does not eat lunch at all and compensates by eating a large breakfast. She does munch on snack cakes and chips on breaks during her work shift, however. For dinner, she likes to eat baked chicken and prepares some canned vegetables as a side dish along with a dinner salad with Italian dressing. She admits to the liberal use of salt during breakfast and dinner. She has a high school education. Her husband is alive and well and works as an accountant. Her household income is average middle-class. She has good health insurance through her husband's employer.

## Meds

Lisinopril/HCTZ 20/25 mg po once daily (has not taken for approximately 2 months)
Levothyroxine 75 mcg po once daily
Metformin 500 mg po twice daily
Ibuprofen 400 mg po PRN headaches and leg pain; used to take infrequently, now takes 1–2 doses per day

## All

NKDA

## ROS

Ms Latham complains of vision trouble as mentioned above; no hearing problems. She does get headaches every couple of days, which she now admits is rather frequent for her; these are relieved with ibuprofen. She denies palpitations, chest pain, and dizziness. She does get short of breath more easily in the past few weeks and has felt a loss of energy over this same time period, although she never has been very active. She denies nausea, vomiting, and abdominal pain. She complains of leg discomfort as mentioned above. She denies mental status changes.

## Physical Examination

### *Gen*

The patient is a middle-aged African-American woman appearing to be in moderate distress.

### *VS*

BP 240/130 mm Hg right arm, 232/128 mm Hg left arm (manual readings performed in the emergency department). A repeat measurement in the right arm after several minutes yields a BP of 236/134 mm Hg.
P 58, RR 24, T 36.8°C; Wt 80 kg, Ht 5′5″

### *Skin*

Cool to touch, shiny, good turgor

### *HEENT*

PERRLA; EOMI; funduscopic exam revealed arterial tortuosity with A/V nicking and papilledema

### *Neck/Lymph Nodes*

Neck supple, no JVD, no bruits, no thyromegaly or lymphadenopathy

### *Chest*

CTA

### *CV*

PMI shifted laterally, RRR, no murmurs or rubs appreciated; +$S_4$ heard at apex

### *Abd*

Soft, NT/ND, no guarding, (+) BS, no abdominal bruits appreciated, liver span about 12 cm

### *Genit/Rect*

Normal female genitalia, heme-negative stool

### *MS/Ext*

Normal ROM, no CCE, pulses 2+ on upper extremities; 1+ femoral; absent pedal pulses

### *Neuro*

A & O × 3, CN II–XII intact, motor/sensory normal, DTRs 2+

## Labs

| | | |
|---|---|---|
| Na 140 mEq/L | Hgb 13.2 g/dL | AST 27 IU/L |
| K 4.9 mEq/L | Hct 43% | ALT 45 IU/L |
| Cl 100 mEq/L | WBC 6.6 × $10^3$/mm$^3$ | Cholesterol 196 mg/dL |
| $CO_2$ 28 mEq/L | Plt 222 × $10^3$/mm$^3$ | HDL 36 mg/dL |
| BUN 28 mg/dL | | Triglycerides 142 mg/dL |
| SCr 2.6 mg/dL | | LDL 132 mg/dL |
| Glu 122 mg/dL | | |

## UA

Specific gravity 1.010; pH 5.8; urine protein:creatinine ratio = 640; negative for blood; negative for recreational drugs

## Chest X-Ray

Enlarged heart, no infiltrates

## ECG

Normal sinus rhythm; LVH by voltage criteria. There are no ST-segment changes, although there does appear to be some T-wave flattening in the anterior leads.

## Assessment

A 61-year-old woman with a history of HTN, hypothyroidism, and newly diagnosed diabetes presents with an extremely elevated blood pressure and signs and symptoms of target organ damage. She admits to not taking any antihypertensive drug therapy for approximately 2 months due to unexpected medication-related side effects and a lack of understanding about her disease state.

# QUESTIONS

## Problem Identification

1.a. Did this patient's situation result from a drug-related problem? Why or why not?

1.b. What signs and symptoms are present that may be related to the severity of this patient's hypertension?

1.c. Is this a hypertensive urgency or an emergency? Explain your answer.

## Desired Outcome

2.a. What are the goals of pharmacotherapy for this patient's hypertension?

2.b. How would the treatment goals differ if this patient presented with the same blood pressure, but was asymptomatic with normal laboratory findings and no acute changes on physical examination?

## Therapeutic Alternatives

3.a. What nondrug therapies might be useful for this patient?

3.b. What feasible pharmacotherapeutic alternatives are available for the treatment of this patient's acute hypertension?

## Optimal Plan

4.a. What drug and dosage form are best for treating this patient's acute hypertension?

4.b. How would your treatment recommendations differ if this patient presented with the same blood pressure, but was asymptomatic with normal laboratory findings and no acute changes on physical examination?

## Outcome Evaluation

5. Which clinical and laboratory parameters are necessary to evaluate your therapy for reducing this patient's blood pressure and monitoring for adverse events?

## Patient Education

6. What information can you provide to Ms Latham to enhance adherence, ensure successful therapy, and minimize adverse effects?

## Clinical Course

Once Ms Latham's blood pressure is lowered to an acceptable level, her inpatient provider consults with you regarding chronic antihypertensive therapy for Ms Latham.

7.a. Do you recommend Ms Latham resume her lisinopril and HCTZ as prescribed or would you recommend alternative drug therapy? Rationalize your answer. If you would recommend alternative drug therapy, which drug(s) would you recommend and why?

7.b. What economic considerations are applicable to this patient regarding drug selection?

7.c. What nonpharmacologic measures can Ms Latham incorporate as part of an overall treatment plan for her chronic hypertension?

## ■ SELF-STUDY ASSIGNMENTS

1. Debate the need for aggressive blood pressure control (i.e., systolic blood pressure <140 mm Hg vs. <120 mm Hg) in a patient with diabetes.
2. Describe any ethnic and racial differences in response to antihypertensive medications and the impact these differences may have on drug selection.
3. Compare and contrast the safeties and antihypertensive efficacies of chlorthalidone and hydrochlorothiazide, and make a compelling argument for preferring one over the other.
4. List various measures that have historically been employed to treat ACE inhibitor–induced cough.

## CLINICAL PEARL

Of patients presenting to the emergency department with a hypertensive emergency, the vast majority of them have been diagnosed with hypertension and have been prescribed antihypertensive medication. Only 8% of hypertensive emergencies presenting to the emergency department involve patients unaware of having a diagnosis of hypertension.

## REFERENCES

1. Chobanian AV, Bakris GL, Black HR, et al. Seventh report of the Joint National Committee on Prevention, Detection, Evaluation, and Treatment of High Blood Pressure. Hypertension 2003;42:1206–1252.
2. Rodriguez MA, Kumar SK, De Caro M. Hypertensive crisis. Cardiol Rev 2010;18:102–107.
3. Hebert CJ, Vidt DG. Hypertensive crises. Prim Care Office Pract 2008;35:475–487.
4. Varon J, Marik PE. The diagnosis and management of hypertensive crises. Chest 2000;118:214–227.
5. Mansoor GA, Frishman WH. Comprehensive management of hypertensive emergencies and urgencies. Heart Dis 2002;4:358–371.
6. Varon J. Treatment of acute severe hypertension. Current and newer agents. Drugs 2008;68:283–297.
7. Aggarwal M, Khan I. Hypertensive crisis: hypertensive emergencies and urgencies. Cardiol Clin 2006;24:135–146.
8. Thach AM, Schultz PJ. Nonemergent hypertension. New perspectives for the emergency medicine physician. Emerg Med Clin North Am 1995;13:1009–1035.
9. Gales MA. Oral antihypertensives for hypertensive urgencies. Ann Pharmacother 1994;28:274–284.
10. Ross S, Walker A, MacLeod MJ. Patient compliance in hypertension: role of illness perceptions and treatment beliefs. J Hum Hypertens 2004;18:607–613.

# 15

# HEART FAILURE: SYSTOLIC DYSFUNCTION

Cross My Heart and Hope to Live . . . . . . . . . Level III

**Julia M. Koehler, PharmD, FCCP**

**Alison M. Walton, PharmD, BCPS**

## LEARNING OBJECTIVES

After completing this case study, the reader should be able to:

- Recognize the signs and symptoms of heart failure.
- Develop a pharmacotherapeutic plan for treatment of heart failure due to systolic dysfunction.
- Outline a monitoring plan for heart failure that includes both clinical and laboratory parameters.

## PATIENT PRESENTATION

### ■ Chief Complaint

"I've been more short of breath lately. I can't seem to walk as far as I used to, and either my feet are growing or my shoes are shrinking!"

### ■ HPI

Rosemary Quincy is a 68 yo African-American female who presents to her family medicine physician for evaluation of her shortness of breath and increased swelling in her lower extremities. She reports that her shortness of breath has been gradually increasing over the past 4 days. She has noticed that her shortness of breath is particularly worse when she is lying in bed at night, and she has to prop her head up with three pillows in order to sleep. She also reports exertional dyspnea that is usual for her, but especially worse over the last couple of days.

## PMH

Hypertension × 20 years
CHD with history of MI in 2005 (PCI performed and bare metal stents placed in LAD and RCA)
Heart failure (NYHA FC III)
Type 2 DM × 25 years
Atrial fibrillation
COPD (Stage 3)

## FH

Father died of lung cancer at age 71, mother died of MI at age 73

## SH

Reports occasional alcohol intake. States she has been trying to follow her low-cholesterol and low-sodium diet. Former smoker (35 pack-year history; quit approximately 10 years ago).

## Meds

Valsartan 160 mg po BID
Furosemide 40 mg po BID
Warfarin 2.5 mg po once daily
Carvedilol 3.125 mg po BID
Pioglitazone 30 mg po once daily
Glimepiride 2 mg po once daily
Potassium chloride 20 mEq po once daily
Atorvastatin 40 mg po once daily
Aspirin 81 mg po once daily
Albuterol MDI, 2 inhalations q 4–6 hours PRN shortness of breath
Tiotropium DPI 18 mcg, 1 inhalations daily
Fluticasone/salmeterol DPI 250 mcg/50 mcg, 1 inhalations BID

## All

Lisinopril (cough)

## ROS

Approximate 7-kg weight gain over the past week. No fever or chills. Denies any recent chest pain, palpitations, or dizziness. Reports worsening shortness of breath with exertion and three-pillow orthopnea. Describes a chronic, dry (nonproductive), hacking cough, which she describes as usual without recent worsening. No abdominal pain, nausea, constipation, or change in bowel habits. Denies joint pain or weakness.

## Physical Examination

*Gen*

African-American female in moderate respiratory distress

*VS*

BP 134/76 (sitting; repeat 138/80), HR 65 (irreg irreg), RR 24, T 37°C, $O_2$ sat 90% RA, Ht 5′5″, Wt 79 kg

*Skin*

Color pale and diaphoretic; no unusual lesions noted

*HEENT*

PERRLA; lips mildly cyanotic; dentures

*Neck*

(+) JVD at 30° (7 cm); no lymphadenopathy or thyromegaly

*Lungs/Thorax*

Crackles bilaterally, 2/3 of the way up; no expiratory wheezing

*Heart*

Irregularly irregular; (+) $S_3$; displaced PMI

*Abd*

Soft, mildly tender, nondistended; (+) HJR; no masses, mild hepatosplenomegaly; normal BS

*Genit/Rect*

Guaiac (–), genital examination not performed

*MS/Ext*

3+ pitting pedal edema bilaterally; radial and pedal pulses are of poor intensity bilaterally

*Neuro*

A & O × 3, CNs intact. No motor deficits.

## Labs

| | | | |
|---|---|---|---|
| Na 131 mEq/L | Hgb 13 g/dL | Mg 1.9 mEq/L | INR 2.3 |
| K 3.5 mEq/L | Hct 40% | Ca 9.3 mg/dL | $HbA_{1c}$ 6.1% |
| Cl 99 mEq/L | Plt 192 × $10^3$/mm$^3$ | Phos 4.3 mg/dL | |
| $CO_2$ 28 mEq/L | WBC 9.1 × $10^3$/mm$^3$ | AST 34 IU/L | |
| BUN 32 mg/dL | | ALT 27 IU/L | |
| SCr 2.3 mg/dL (baseline SCr 2.1 mg/dL) | | | |
| Glucose 124 mg/dL | | | |
| BNP 776 pg/mL (BNP drawn 2 months prior: 474 pg/mL) | | | |

## ECG

Atrial fibrillation, LVH

## Chest X-Ray

PA and lateral views (Fig. 15-1) show evidence of congestive failure with cardiomegaly, interstitial edema, and some early alveolar edema. There is a small right pleural effusion.
No evidence of infiltrates; evidence of pulmonary edema suggestive of congestive heart failure; enlarged cardiac silhouette

## Echocardiogram

LVH, reduced global left ventricular systolic function, estimated EF 20%; evidence of impaired ventricular relaxation, Stage 1 diastolic dysfunction

## Assessment

Acute exacerbation of heart failure with systolic dysfunction

# QUESTIONS

## Problem Identification

1.a. Create a list of this patient's drug-related problems.

1.b. What signs, symptoms, and other information indicate the presence and type of heart failure in this patient?

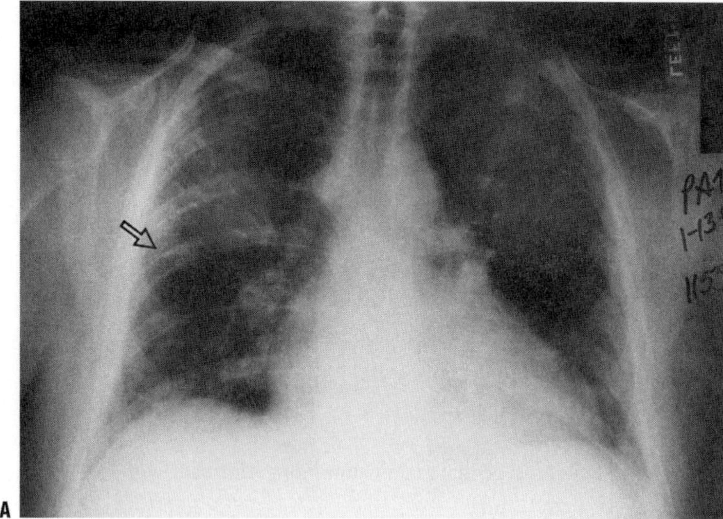


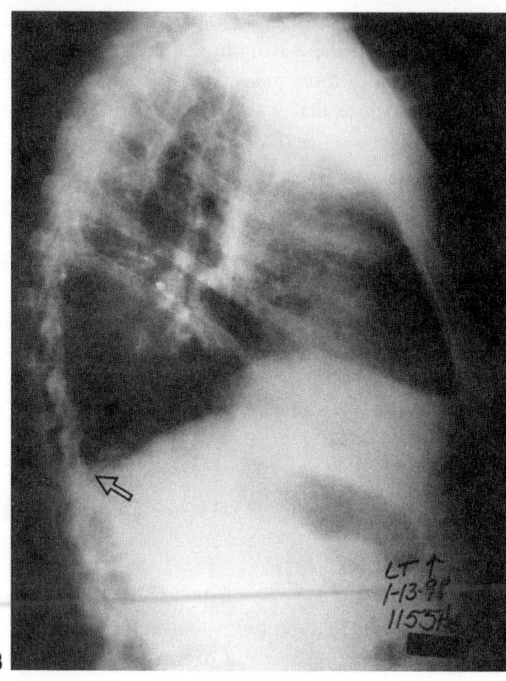


**FIGURE 15-1.** *A.* PA CXR demonstrates increased vascular markings representative of interstitial edema, with some early alveolar edema. The *arrow* points out fluid lying in the fissure of the right lung. Note the presence of cardiomegaly. *B.* Lateral view of CXR. *Arrow* points out the presence of pulmonary effusion.

1.c. What is the classification and staging of heart failure for this patient?

1.d. Could any of this patient's problems have been caused by drug therapy?

## Desired Outcome

2.a. What are the goals for the pharmacologic management of heart failure in this patient?

2.b. Considering her other medical problems, what other treatment goals should be established?

## Therapeutic Alternatives

3.a. What diuretic therapy should be recommended for this patient initially for acute treatment of her heart failure exacerbation?

3.b. How should this patient's pharmacotherapy be adjusted for chronic management of her systolic heart failure?

3.c. What nonpharmacologic therapy should be recommended for this patient with respect to her heart failure?

## Optimal Plan

4. What drugs, doses, schedules, and duration are best suited for the management of this patient?

## Outcome Evaluation

5. What clinical and laboratory parameters are needed to evaluate the therapy for achievement of the desired therapeutic outcome and to detect and prevent adverse events?

## Patient Education

6. What information should be provided to the patient about the medications used to treat her heart failure?

## ■ SELF-STUDY ASSIGNMENTS

1. Develop a table illustrating the recommended target doses for ACE inhibitors, angiotensin II receptor blockers, and beta-blockers in patients with heart failure due to systolic dysfunction.
2. Research the topic of diuretic resistance, and write a report describing the phenomenon and methods used to overcome it.
3. Review the guidelines and evidence describing the role of routine BNP monitoring in patients with heart failure.

## CLINICAL PEARL

The presence of pitting edema is associated with a substantial increase in body weight; it typically takes a weight gain of 10 lb to result in the development of pitting edema.

## REFERENCES

1. Nesto RW, Bell D, Bonow RO, et al. AHA/ADA consensus statement for thiazolidinedione use, fluid retention, and congestive heart failure. Circulation 2003;108:2941–2948.
2. Tang WH, Francis GS, Morrow DA, et al. National Academy of Clinical Biochemistry Laboratory Medicine practice guidelines: clinical utilization of cardiac biomarker testing in heart failure. Circulation 2007;116:99–109.
3. Hunt SA, Abraham WT, Chin MH, et al. 2009 focused update incorporated into the ACC/AHA 2005 guidelines for the diagnosis and management of heart failure in adults: a report of the American College of Cardiology Foundation/American Heart Association Task Force on Practice Guidelines. *Circulation* 2009;119:e391–e479.
4. Rosendorff C, Black HR, Cannon CP, et al. Treatment of hypertension in the prevention and management of ischemic heart disease: a scientific statement from the American Heart Association Council for High Blood Pressure Research and the Councils on Clinical Cardiology and Epidemiology and Prevention. Circulation 2007;115:2761–2788.

5. Pitt B, Poole-Wilson PA, Segal R, et al. Effect of losartan compared with captopril on mortality in patients with symptomatic heart failure: randomised trial—the Losartan Heart Failure Survival Study ELITE II. Lancet 2000;355:1582–1587.
6. Cohn JN, Tognoni G; Valsartan Heart Failure Trial Investigators. A randomized trial of the angiotensin-receptor blocker valsartan in chronic heart failure. N Engl J Med 2001;345:1667–1675.
7. Pfeffer MA, Swedberg K, Granger CB; for the CHARM Investigators and Committees. Effects of candesartan on morbidity and mortality in patients with chronic heart failure: the CHARM-Overall Programme. Lancet 2003;362:759–766.
8. CIBIS II Investigators. The Cardiac Insufficiency Bisoprolol Study II (CIBIS II): a randomized trial. Lancet 1999;353:9–13.
9. MERIT-HF Investigators. Effect of metoprolol CR/XL in chronic heart failure: Metoprolol CR/XL Randomised Intervention Trial in Congestive Heart Failure (MERIT-HF). Lancet 1999;353:2001–2007.
10. Colucci WS, Packer M, Bristow MR, et al.; for the US Carvedilol Heart Failure Study Group. Carvedilol inhibits clinical progression in patients with mild symptoms of heart failure. Circulation 1996;94:2800–2806.
11. Pitt B, Zannad F, Remme WJ. The effect of spironolactone on morbidity and mortality in patients with severe heart failure. Randomized Aldactone Evaluation Study Investigators. N Engl J Med 1999;341:709–717.
12. Pitt B, Remme W, Zannad F, et al. Eplerenone, a selective aldosterone blocker, in patients with left ventricular dysfunction after myocardial infarction. N Engl J Med 2003;348:1309–1321.
13. The Digitalis Investigation Group. The effect of digoxin on mortality and morbidity in patients with heart failure. N Engl J Med 1997;336:525–533.
14. Lindenfeld J, Albert NM, Boehmer JP, et al. Executive summary: HFSA 2010 comprehensive heart failure practice guideline. J Card Fail 2010;16:475–539.
15. Taylor AL, Ziesche S, Yancy C, et al.; for the African-American Heart Failure Trial Investigators. Combination of isosorbide dinitrate and hydralazine in blacks with heart failure. N Engl J Med 2004;351:2049–2057.
16. Tang WH, Girod JP, Lee MJ, et al. Plasma B-type natriuretic peptide levels in ambulatory patients with established chronic symptomatic systolic heart failure. Circulation 2003;108:2964–2966.


# 16

# HEART FAILURE: DIASTOLIC DYSFUNCTION

A Balancing Act . . . . . . . . . . . . . . . . . . . . . . . . Level II

**Joel C. Marrs, PharmD, BCPS (AQ Cardiology), CLS**

**Joseph P. Vande Griend, PharmD, BCPS**

## LEARNING OBJECTIVES

After completing this case study, the reader should be able to:

- Recognize the signs and symptoms of diastolic heart failure.
- Develop a pharmacotherapeutic plan for treatment of diastolic heart failure.
- Outline a monitoring plan for heart failure that includes both clinical and laboratory parameters.
- Initiate, titrate, and monitor β-adrenergic blocker, calcium channel blocker, angiotensin-converting enzyme inhibitor, angiotensin receptor blocker, and diuretic therapy in diastolic heart failure when indicated.

## PATIENT PRESENTATION

### Chief Complaint

"Why do I keep gaining all this weight?"

### HPI

Lawrence Smith is a 62-year-old man who presents to the ED with shortness of breath and lower extremity edema. He reports his symptoms started approximately 1–1.5 weeks ago. He noted that he was gaining about 2 lb daily and gained approximately 20 lb of weight over the week prior to admission. He attempted to use his albuterol/ipratropium MDI for relief of symptoms at home without improvement. As his symptoms worsened, he called his primary care doctor, who increased his furosemide dose over the phone to 80 mg twice daily. In the ED he was noted to be hypoxic with an increased oxygen need from 2 to 4 L by nasal cannula. He was given one dose of IV furosemide with improvement and then admitted to the medicine service for further evaluation and management.

### PMH

CAD (s/p STEMI 6 years ago)
COPD × 3 years
Diastolic heart failure × 2 years
Dyslipidemia × 10 years
HTN × 20 years
Type 2 DM × 3 years

### FH

Father is alive at age 78 with type 2 DM; mother is alive at age 76 and has HTN and dyslipidemia; two brothers (age 48 and 54) alive and both have type 2 DM and HTN.

### SH

History of tobacco use (30 pack-year history), but quit 3 years ago. Denies any alcohol or substance abuse. Lives alone.

### Meds

Albuterol/ipratropium MDI, two puffs inhaled Q 6 H PRN
Aspirin 325 mg po daily
Amlodipine 5 mg po daily
Carvedilol 6.25 mg po BID
Furosemide 80 mg po BID (previously 40 mg po BID)
Isosorbide mononitrate ER 30 mg po QAM
Metformin 500 mg po BID
Nitroglycerin 0.4 mg po q 5 minutes PRN chest pain
Potassium chloride 20 mEq po BID
Rosuvastatin 10 mg po daily

### All

NKDA

### ROS

*Gen*

Patient reports a recent 20-lb weight gain over the past week.

*CV*

No complaints of chest pain but reports dyspnea on exertion

*Resp*

Reports an increase in shortness of breath from baseline.

*GI*

No recent changes noted in bowel habits

*GU*

No complaints

*MS*

No complaints of MS pain or weakness

*Neuro*

No complaints

## Physical Examination

*Gen*

Patient with 20-lb weight gain over past week with increased shortness of breath

*VS*

BP 165/94, P 81 (regular), RR 20, T 36.9°C; Wt 100 kg (usual weight 90 kg), Ht 5′6″, oxygen saturation of 95% on 4-L nasal cannula

*Skin*

Chronic venous stasis changes on bilateral lower extremities and 2+ edema to the knees

*HEENT*

PERRLA, EOMI, fundi were not examined. Normocephalic, atraumatic. Nasal cannula in place.

*Neck*

(+) JVD at 30° (4 cm). Carotid bruit is not appreciated. No lymphadenopathy or thyromegaly.

*Lungs/Thorax*

Respirations are even. Crackles noted in the right lung base.

*Heart*

RRR. No murmurs, rubs, or gallops.

*Abd*

Obese with a nontender, nondistended abdomen; hypoactive bowel sounds

*Genit/Rect*

Guaiac (–), genital examination not performed

*MS/Ext*

2+ pitting pedal edema bilaterally; radial and pedal pulses are of poor intensity bilaterally; grip strength even.

*Neuro*

A & O × 3; CNs intact; DTR intact

## Labs

| | | | |
|---|---|---|---|
| Na 140 mEq/L | Hgb 15.3 g/dL | Mg 1.7 mEq/L | CK 20 IU/L |
| K 4.2 mEq/L | Hct 47.2% | Ca 9.1 mg/dL | CK-MB 0.8 IU/L |
| Cl 103 mEq/L | Plt 298 × $10^3$/mm$^3$ | AST 50 IU/L | PT 12.6 s |
| $CO_2$ 26 mEq/L | WBC 6.4 × $10^3$/mm$^3$ | ALT 43 IU/L | INR 1.1 |
| BUN 20 mg/dL | Troponin I | Alk phos 80 IU/L | TSH 2.01 mIU/L |
| SCr 0.9 mg/dL | 0.5 ng/mL | GGT 24 IU/L | $HbA_{1c}$ 7.2% |
| Glucose 108 mg/dL | | T. bili 0.2 mg/dL | |
| BNP 900 pg/mL | | | |

## ECG

Sinus rate of 70; QRS 0.08; no ST–T wave changes; low voltage

## CXR

PA and lateral views show evidence of interstitial edema and some early alveolar edema.

## Assessment

Decompensated heart failure with pulmonary and lower extremity edema

# CLINICAL COURSE

The patient was admitted to a telemetry unit. The patient has a known history of diastolic dysfunction but preserved systolic function (EF 60%) per an echocardiogram from 2 years ago. A 2D echocardiogram was obtained today to evaluate the patient's current LV and valvular function. Results revealed evidence of impaired ventricular relaxation and elevated left atrial filling pressures consistent with grade II diastolic dysfunction. EF was estimated at 55%; there was no evidence of mitral stenosis or pericardial disease. A dilated inferior vena cava suggests increased right atrial pressure. Moderate pulmonary hypertension is evident.

# QUESTIONS

## Problem Identification

1.a. Create a list of this patient's drug-related problems.

1.b. What signs, symptoms, and other information indicate the presence and severity of the patient's heart failure?

1.c. What are the classification and staging of this patient's heart failure on presentation?

1.d. Could any of this patient's problems have been caused by drug therapy or lack of optimal drug therapy?

## Desired Outcome

2.a. What are the goals for the pharmacologic management of heart failure in this patient?

2.b. Considering this patient's other medical problems, what other treatment goals should be established?

## Therapeutic Alternatives

3. What medications are indicated in the long-term management of this patient's diastolic heart failure based on his stage of heart failure?

## Optimal Plan

4. What drugs, doses, schedules, and duration are best suited for the management of this patient?

## Outcome Evaluation

5. What clinical and laboratory parameters are needed to evaluate the therapy for achievement of the desired therapeutic outcome and to detect and prevent adverse events?

## ■ CLINICAL COURSE

Over the next 3 days, the patient received maximal drug therapy, and his condition improved. He was discharged on lisinopril 10 mg po daily, carvedilol 12.5 mg po BID, furosemide 40 mg po twice daily, metformin 500 mg po twice daily, rosuvastatin 10 mg po daily, albuterol/ipratropium MDI two puffs po four times a day, and aspirin 325 mg po daily. On the day of discharge his serum potassium was 3.8 mEq/L, creatinine 1.1 mg/dL, BUN 18 mg/dL, and he had a blood pressure of 140/92 mm Hg with a heart rate of 75 beats/min.

## Patient Education

6. What information should be provided to the patient about the medications used to treat his heart failure?

## ■ CLINICAL COURSE

On follow-up with his primary care doctor, the patient is noted to have sustained a 5-lb weight gain from baseline dry weight at discharge. He feels much better than prior to coming to the hospital and is back to most of his daily living activities.

## ■ FOLLOW-UP QUESTIONS

1. Outline a plan for maximizing the patient's current medication regimen for diastolic heart failure.
2. Outline a therapeutic plan for titration of the lisinopril for this patient.
3. Would you consider titrating up his carvedilol to a higher dose? If so, why? Is switching the patient to a long-acting, once-daily carvedilol product indicated?

## ■ SELF-STUDY ASSIGNMENTS

1. Describe the common causes of heart failure in patients with a preserved LVEF.
2. Describe how you would evaluate and monitor this patient's quality of life.
3. Evaluate whether evidence exists to support the role of aldosterone antagonists in the chronic management of diastolic heart failure.

## CLINICAL PEARL

Patients with heart failure who require chronic diuretic therapy with furosemide and still struggle to maintain fluid balance (e.g., multiple hospitalizations for fluid overload despite maximized furosemide as an outpatient) may need their diuretic therapy optimized by switching to another loop diuretic with better oral bioavailability (i.e., torsemide, bumetanide).

## REFERENCES


1. Tang WH, Francis GS, Morrow DA, et al. National Academy of Clinical Biochemistry Laboratory Medicine Practice Guidelines: clinical utilization of cardiac biomarker testing in heart failure. Circulation 2007;116:e99–e109.
2. Hunt SA, Abraham WT, Chin MH, et al. 2009 focused update incorporated into the ACC/AHA 2005 guidelines for the diagnosis and management of heart failure in adults: a report of the American College of Cardiology Foundation/American Heart Association Task Force on Practice Guidelines. J Am Coll Cardiol 2009;53:e1–e90.
3. Lindenfeld J, Albert NM, Boehmer JP, et al. Executive summary: HFSA 2010 comprehensive heart failure practice guideline. J Card Fail 2010;16:475–539.
4. Rosendorff C, Black HR, Cannon CP, et al. Treatment of hypertension in the prevention and management of ischemic heart disease: a scientific statement from the American Heart Association Council for High Blood Pressure Research and the Councils on Clinical Cardiology and Epidemiology and Prevention. Circulation 2007;115:2761–2788.
5. The Digitalis Investigation Group. The effect of digoxin on mortality and morbidity in patients with heart failure. N Engl J Med 1997;336:525–533.
6. Aronow WS, Kronzon I. Effect of enalapril on congestive heart failure treated with diuretics in elderly patients with prior myocardial infarction and normal left ventricular ejection fraction. Am J Cardiol 1993;71:602–604.
7. Philbin EF, Rocco TA Jr, Lindenmuth NW, Ulrich K, Jenkins PL. Systolic versus diastolic heart failure in community practice: clinical features, outcomes, and the use of angiotensin-converting enzyme inhibitors. Am J Med 2000;109:605–613.
8. Warner JG Jr, Metzger DC, Kitzman DW, Wesley DJ, Little WC. Losartan improves exercise tolerance in patients with diastolic dysfunction and a hypertensive response to exercise. J Am Coll Cardiol 1999;33:1567–1572.
9. Yusuf S, Pfeffer MA, Swedberg K, et al. Effects of candesartan in patients with chronic heart failure and preserved left-ventricular ejection fraction: the CHARM-Preserved Trial. Lancet 2003;362:777–781.
10. Massie BM, Carson PE, McMurrary JJ, et al. Irbesartan in patients with heart failure and preserved ejection fraction. N Engl J Med 2008;359:2456–2467.
11. Hernandez AF, Hammill BG, O'Connor CM, Schulman KA, Curtis LH, Fonarow GC. Clinical effectiveness of beta-blockers in heart failure: findings from the OPTIMIZE-HF (organized program to initiate lifesaving treatment in hospitalized patients with heart failure) registry. J Am Coll Cardiol 2009;53:184–192.
12. Aronow WS, Ahn C, Kronzon I. Effect of propranolol versus no propranolol on total mortality plus nonfatal myocardial infarction in older patients with prior myocardial infarction, congestive heart failure, and left ventricular ejection fraction > or = 40% treated with diuretics plus angiotensin-converting enzyme inhibitors. Am J Cardiol 1997;80:207–209.
13. Chen HH, Lainchbury JB, Redfield MM. Factors influencing survival of patients with diastolic heart failure in Olmsted County, MN in 1996–97. Circulation 2000;102:II-412–II-413.
14. Setaro JF, Zaret BL, Schulman DS, Black HR, Soufer R. Usefulness of verapamil for congestive heart failure associated with abnormal left ventricular diastolic filling and normal left ventricular systolic performance. Am J Cardiol 1990;66:981–986.
15. Aldosterone antagonist therapy in adults with heart failure and preserved systolic function (TOPCAT). Available at: *http://www.clinicaltrials.gov/ct/gui/show/NCT00094302*. Accessed February 1, 2010.

# 17

# ISCHEMIC HEART DISEASE: CHRONIC STABLE ANGINA

An Uphill Battle . . . . . . . . . . . . . . . . . . . . . . . . Level III

**Shawn R. Hansen, PharmD**

**Megan Ose, PharmD**

## LEARNING OBJECTIVES

After completing this case study, the reader should be able to:

- Identify modifiable risk factors for IHD, and discuss the potential benefit to be gained by their modification in an individual patient.
- Optimize medical therapy in a patient with persistent angina considering response to current therapy and the presence of comorbidities.
- Assess clinical response to antianginal therapy by identifying relevant monitoring parameters for efficacy and adverse effects.

## PATIENT PRESENTATION

### Chief Complaint

"Doc, the drugs aren't working for my chest pain!"

### HPI

Jack Palmer is a 72-year-old man with coronary artery disease. He is an avid golfer and prefers to walk the course, but this is becoming progressively more difficult for him due to frequent angina. He has had two coronary artery bypass operations in the past. A coronary angiogram performed 1 month ago revealed significant disease in the RCA proximal to his graft but this was considered high risk for angioplasty. His dose of isosorbide mononitrate was increased at that time from 60 to 120 mg once daily. This had no effect on his angina. He is still using about 30 nitroglycerin tablets a week, and these do relieve his chest pain. He reports that most often the chest discomfort comes on with activity, such as walking up slight inclines on the golf course. The discomfort is located in the center of his chest and rated as a 3–4/10 on average. He reports that the chest discomfort slowly fades as he slows his activity. He also complains of occasional lightheadedness with a pulse around 50 bpm and SBP near 100 mm Hg.

### PMH

1. Acute anterior wall MI with CABG in 1976
2. Posterior lateral MI in 1990 and PTCA to the circumflex at that time
3. Redo CABG in 1998
4. Ischemic cardiomyopathy
5. Heart failure with an ejection fraction of 40%
6. Dyslipidemia
7. COPD (mild)
8. Chronic low back pain
9. Depression

### FH

Noncontributory for premature coronary artery disease

### SH

Retired dairy farmer, lives with wife, drinks occasionally, previous smoker—quit in 1998

### Meds

Carvedilol 6.25 mg twice daily
Digoxin 0.25 mg once daily
Lisinopril 5 mg once daily
Furosemide 40 mg once daily
Aspirin 325 mg once daily
Isosorbide mononitrate, extended release 120 mg once daily
Diltiazem, extended-release 240 mg once daily
St. John's wort 300 mg three times daily
Celecoxib 200 mg once daily
Simvastatin 40 mg once daily
Nitroglycerin 0.4 mg SL PRN

### All

NKDA

### ROS

No fever, chills, or night sweats. No recent viral illnesses. No shortness of breath; occasional cough with cold weather. No nausea, vomiting, diarrhea, constipation, melena, or hematochezia. No dysuria or hematuria. No myalgias or arthralgias.

### Physical Examination

*Gen*

Pleasant, cooperative man in no acute distress

*VS*

BP 105/68, P 50, RR 22, T 36.4°C, Ht 5′11″, Wt 93 kg, waist circumference 43 in

*Skin*

Intact, no rashes or ulcers

*HEENT*

PERRL; EOMI; oropharynx is clear

*Neck*

Supple, no masses; no JVD, lymphadenopathy, or thyromegaly

*Lungs*

Bilateral air entry is clear. No wheezes.

*CV*

RRR, $S_1$, $S_2$ normal; no murmurs or gallops; PMI palpated at left fifth ICS, MCL

*Abd*

Soft, NT/ND; bowel sounds normoactive

*Genit/Rect*

Heme (−) stool

*Ext*

No CCE; pulses 2+ throughout

*Neuro*

A & O × 3, CN II–XII intact; speech is fluent; no motor or sensory deficit; no facial asymmetry; tongue midline

### Labs

| | | |
|---|---|---|
| Na 137 mEq/L | Hgb 11.8 g/dL | Fasting lipid profile |
| K 4.8 mEq/L | Hct 35.1% | Chol 202 mg/dL |
| Cl 103 mEq/L | Plt 187 × $10^3$/mm$^3$ | LDL 125 mg/dL |
| $CO_2$ 21 mEq/L | WBC 7.9 × $10^3$/mm$^3$ | HDL 38 mg/dL |
| BUN 24 mg/dL | MCV 77 μm$^3$ | Trig 215 mg/dL |
| SCr 1.2 mg/dL | MCHC 29 g/dL | |
| Glu 98 mg/dL | | |

Digoxin serum concentration: 1.8 ng/mL

### ECG

Sinus rhythm, first-degree AVB, 50 bpm, old AWMI, no ST–T wave changes noted, QT/QTc 406/431

### Assessment

A 72-year-old man with poorly controlled angina on multiple medications who is a poor candidate for angioplasty

# QUESTIONS

## Problem Identification

1.a. What drug-related problems appear to be present in this patient?

1.b. Could any of these problems potentially be caused or exacerbated by his current therapy?

## Desired Outcome

2. What are the goals of pharmacotherapy for IHD in this case?

## Therapeutic Alternatives

3.a. Does this patient possess any modifiable risk factors for IHD?

3.b. What pharmacotherapeutic options are available for treating this patient's IHD? Discuss the agents in each class with respect to their relative utility in his care.

## Optimal Plan

4. Given the patient information provided, construct a complete pharmacotherapeutic plan for optimizing management of his IHD.

## Outcome Evaluation

5. When the patient returns to the clinic in 2 weeks for a follow-up visit, how will you evaluate the response to his new antianginal regimen for efficacy and adverse effects?

## CLINICAL COURSE

Mr Palmer improved hemodynamically following a switch from diltiazem to amlodipine. However, due to continued frequent episodes of angina, his amlodipine was titrated to 10 mg once daily. He returned to cardiology clinic today stating that his angina frequency has improved somewhat on the maximum dose of amlodipine but is still bothersome to him. His cardiologist decided to add ranolazine 500 mg twice daily to his regimen in an attempt to further decrease his angina frequency.

## Patient Education

6. What information will you communicate to the patient about his antianginal regimen to help him experience the greatest benefit and fewest adverse effects?

## FOLLOW-UP QUESTION

1. What drug therapy changes would you recommend to avoid or minimize drug interactions with ranolazine?

## SELF-STUDY ASSIGNMENTS

1. Summarize the potential role of L-arginine in the treatment of chronic angina.
2. Describe the potential role of allopurinol in the treatment of chronic angina.

## CLINICAL PEARL

The COURAGE trial made major headlines in 2007 by showing that coronary stenting with optimal medical therapy is no better at preventing future coronary events than optimal medical therapy alone in patients with stable coronary disease, potentially saving the US health care system $5 billion a year.[14]

## REFERENCES


1. Jessup M, Abraham WT, Casey DE, et al. 2009 focused update: ACCF/AHA guidelines for the diagnosis and management of chronic heart failure in adults: a report of the American College of Cardiology Foundation/American Heart Association Task Force on Practice Guidelines developed in collaboration with the International Society for Heart and Lung Transplantation. J Am Coll Cardiol 2009;53:1343–1382.
2. Lindenfeld J, Albert NM, Boehmer JP, et al. Executive summary: HFSA 2010 comprehensive heart failure practice guideline. J Card Fail. 2010;16:475–539.
3. Fraker TD, Fihn SD, on behalf of the 2002 Chronic Stable Angina Writing Committee. 2007 chronic angina focused update of the ACC/AHA 2002 guidelines for the management of patients with chronic stable angina. J Am Coll Cardiol 2007;50:2264–2274.
4. The CAPRICORN Investigators. Effect of carvedilol on outcome after myocardial infarction in patients with left-ventricular dysfunction: the CAPRICORN randomized trial. Lancet 2001;357:1385–1390.
5. Chaitman BR. Ranolazine for the treatment of chronic angina and potential use in other cardiovascular conditions. Circulation 2006;113:2462–2472.
6. Morrow DA, Scirica BM, Karwatowska-Prokopczuk E, et al. Effects of ranolazine on recurrent cardiovascular events in patients with non-ST-elevation acute coronary syndromes. The MERLIN-TIMI 36 randomized trial. JAMA 2007;297:1775–1783.
7. Antithrombotic Trialists' Collaboration. Collaborative meta-analysis of randomised trials of antiplatelet therapy for prevention of death, myocardial infarction, and stroke in high risk patients. BMJ 2002;324:71–86.
8. Smith SC, Allen J, Blair SN, et al. AHA/ACC Guidelines for Secondary Prevention for Patients With Coronary and Other Atherosclerotic Vascular Disease: 2006 update. J Am Coll Cardiol 2006;47:2130–2139.
9. CAPRIE Steering Committee. A randomised, blinded, trial of clopidogrel versus aspirin in patients at risk of ischaemic events (CAPRIE). Lancet 1996;348:1329–1339.

# 18

# ACUTE CORONARY SYNDROME: ST-ELEVATION MYOCARDIAL INFARCTION

I can't handle the pressure . . . . . . . . . . . . . . . Level III

**Kelly C. Rogers, PharmD**

**Robert B. Parker, PharmD, FCCP**

## LEARNING OBJECTIVES

After completing this case study, the reader should be able to:

- Determine the goals of pharmacotherapy for patients with ST-segment elevation myocardial infarction (STEMI).
- Discuss interventional strategies for patients with STEMI, and understand the pharmacotherapeutic agents used with interventions.
- Design an optimal therapeutic plan for management of STEMI, and describe how the selected drug therapy achieves the therapeutic goals.
- Identify appropriate parameters to assess the recommended drug therapy for both efficacy and adverse effects.
- Provide appropriate education to a patient who has suffered an STEMI.

## PATIENT PRESENTATION

### Chief Complaint

"This is the worst pain I have ever felt in my life."

### HPI

Gary Roberts is a 68-year-old man admitted to the ED complaining of chest pressure/pain lasting 20–30 minutes occurring at rest. He describes the pain as substernal, crushing, and pressurelike that radiates to his jaw and is accompanied by nausea and diaphoresis. The pain first started approximately 6 hours ago after he ate breakfast and was unrelieved by antacids or SL NTG × 3. He also states he has been experiencing intermittent chest pain over the past 3–4 weeks with minimal exertion.

### PMH

HTN
Type 2 DM
Dyslipidemia
CAD with PCI with a bare metal stent 10 years ago

### FH

Father died from heart failure at age 75 and mother is alive at age 88 with HTN and type 2 DM.

### SH

(+) Tobacco × 20 years but quit when he received his BMS 10 years ago; drinks beer usually on weekends; denies illicit drug use.

### Meds

Aspirin 81 mg po daily
Metoprolol tartrate 25 mg po BID
Simvastatin 40 mg po QHS
Metformin 500 mg po BID
SL NTG PRN CP

### All

NKDA

### ROS

Positive for some baseline CP on exertion for the past 3–4 weeks, now with CP at rest

### Physical Examination

*Gen*

WDWN man, A & O × 3, still with ongoing chest pain, somewhat anxious

*VS*

BP 145/92, P 89, RR 18, T 37.1°C; Wt 95 kg, Ht 5′10″

*HEENT*

PERRLA, EOMI, fundi benign; TMs intact

*Neck*

No bruits; mild JVD; no thyromegaly

*Lungs*

Few dependent inspiratory crackles; bibasilar rales; no wheezes

*CV*

Normal $S_1$ and $S_2$, no MRG

*Abd*

Soft, nontender; liver span 10–12 cm; no bruits

*Genit/Rect*

Deferred

*MS/Ext*

Normal ROM; muscle strength on right 5/5 UE/LE; on left 4/5 UE/LE; pulses 2+; no femoral bruits or peripheral edema

*Neuro*

CNs II–XII intact; DTRs decreased on left; negative Babinski's sign

### Labs

| | | | |
|---|---|---|---|
| Na 134 mEq/L | Ca 9.8 mg/dL | Hgb 14.0 g/dL | *Fasting lipid profile* |
| K 4.4 mEq/L | Mg 2.0 mg/dL | Hct 44% | T. chol 159 mg/dL |
| Cl 102 mEq/L | $PO_4$ 2.4 mg/dL | WBC 5.0 × $10^3$/$mm^3$ | Trig 92 mg/dL |
| $CO_2$ 23 mEq/L | AST 22 U/L | Plt 268 × $10^3$/$mm^3$ | LDL 105 mg/dL |
| BUN 15 mg/dL | ALT 30 U/L | PT 12.5 sec | HDL 36 mg/dL |
| SCr 1.0 mg/dL | Alk Phos 75 U/L | aPTT 32.4 sec | $HbA_{1c}$ 7.6% |
| Glu 140 mg/dL | Troponin I 8.6 ng/mL | INR 1.0 | |

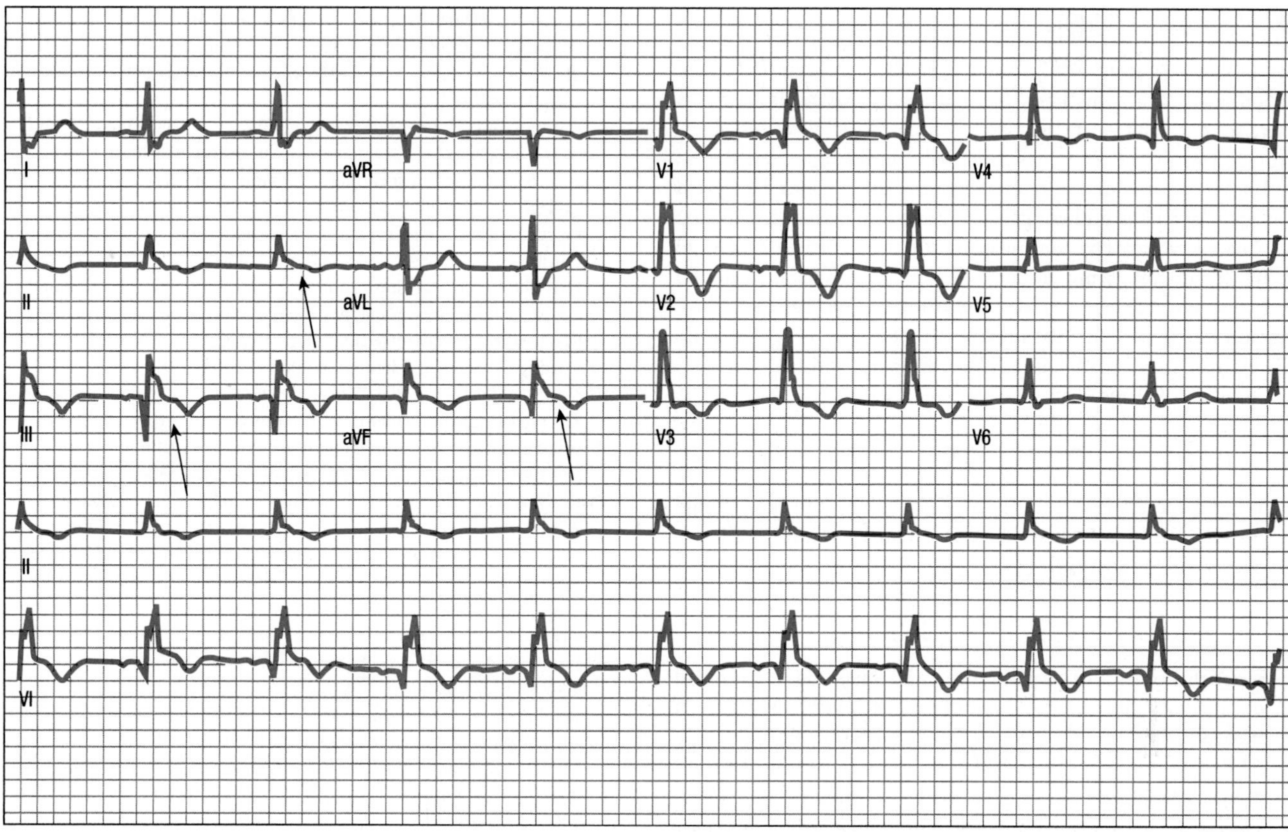


**FIGURE 18-1.** ECG taken on arrival in the emergency department showing ST-segment elevation *(arrows)* in leads II, III, and aVF, consistent with acute inferior myocardial infarction. Right bundle branch block is also present in leads $V_1$–$V_3$.

■ ECG

2- to 3-mm ST-segment elevation in leads II, III, and aVF (Fig. 18-1)

■ Assessment

Acute inferior STEMI

## QUESTIONS

### Problem Identification

1.a. Which findings in this patient's case history are consistent with acute STEMI?

1.b. What risk factors for the development of coronary artery disease are present in this patient?

### Desired Outcome

2.a. What is the immediate goal of therapy in this patient?

2.b. How can this goal be achieved using pharmacotherapy?

### Therapeutic Alternatives

3.a. What nonpharmacologic therapeutic alternative can also achieve the immediate goal in this patient?

3.b. What is the role of adjunctive anticoagulant therapy during PCI, and how should these therapies be monitored?

3.c. What is the role of adjunctive antiplatelet therapy before, during, and after PCI, and how should these therapies be monitored?

### Optimal Plan

4.a. What are other important goals of therapy in this patient?

4.b. Based on the history and presentation, what initial drug therapy is indicated in this patient?

### Outcome Evaluation

5. How should the recommended therapy be monitored for efficacy and adverse effects?

## ■ CLINICAL COURSE

The patient received aspirin, morphine, oxygen, IV unfractionated heparin (UFH), IV nitroglycerin, and oral metoprolol. An interventional cardiologist was consulted and discussed with the patient the need for primary PCI to restore blood flow to the heart. Within 1 hour of his arrival to the ED, the patient was transported to the cardiac catheterization lab. The catheterization revealed a 60–70% proximal stenosis in the RCA with thrombus. Additionally, there was a 40% mid-LAD obstruction and 20–30% distal circumflex disease, neither of which was amenable to PCI. In the catheterization lab, the patient was loaded with oral clopidogrel 600 mg and an eptifibatide infusion was started. The left ventricular ejection fraction (LVEF) by echocardiogram was 35%. The remainder of the patient's hospital stay was uncomplicated, and he was discharged 4 days post-MI.

### Patient Education

6.a. Based on his hospital course, which discharge medications would be most appropriate for this patient?

6.b. What education should you provide to this patient?

## CLINICAL COURSE

Mr Roberts presents to his cardiologist for a routine follow-up appointment 6 months later. He states that he is really trying to exercise more and eat better. He has been taking all of his medications. He states that he has some pain in his calves and thighs, and he thinks it is due to his walking exercise regimen he started 4 months ago. It is bothering him enough that he has had to stop walking every day. His current medications are aspirin 81 mg po daily, clopidogrel 75 mg po daily, metoprolol succinate 50 mg po daily, lisinopril 20 mg po daily, metformin 1 g po BID, and simvastatin 80 mg po daily. Labs reveal the following: TC 135 mg/dL, TG 89 mg/dL, HDL 39 mg/dL, LDL 78 mg/dL, and CK 450 IU/L. Vitals: BP 130/80 and P 65.

## FOLLOW-UP QUESTION

1. What is the cause of this patient's myopathy, and how should his regimen be modified taking into consideration his adverse effects and his goal LDL?

## SELF-STUDY ASSIGNMENTS

1. A patient comes into your pharmacy and states that he has heard on the news that you should not take clopidogrel and stomach medicine together. He tells you that he takes omeprazole for his GERD and recently started taking clopidogrel because of a stent in his heart. Review the potential drug–drug interaction between clopidogrel and PPIs. How should you respond to him?
2. A 54 yo man is admitted to the hospital for an acute MI. He states that he heard on the news that taking antioxidant vitamins might help his heart. Review the available literature on the cardiovascular impact of antioxidant vitamins. How would you respond to him?
3. Perform a literature search and evaluate the use of thiazolidinediones in diabetic patients and the possible increased risk of ischemic cardiovascular events.

## CLINICAL PEARLS

1. The administration of oral β-blockers in the first 24 hours of presentation with an AMI is a class I recommendation from the ACC/AHA guidelines for patients who do not have any contraindications such as (1) signs of heart failure, (2) evidence of low output state, (3) increased risk for cardiogenic shock, or (4) other relative contraindications such as heart block, active asthma, or reactive airway disease. Routine early use of intravenous β-blockers is associated with increased risk of cardiogenic shock. It is reasonable to administer intravenous β-blockers to patients with hypertension who do not have any contraindications.
2. The appropriate recommendation for use of SL NTG is to use **one** sublingual tablet if a patient experiences chest pain or discomfort. If symptoms are unimproved or worsening 5 minutes after **one** dose, it is recommended that the patient should call 9-1-1 immediately to access EMS. This is to avoid a delay in patients with STEMI in seeking rapid medical attention in order to receive life-saving reperfusion therapy. This recommendation was modified in the 2004 ACC/AHA STEMI guidelines.

## REFERENCES


1. Antman EM, Anbe DT, Armstrong PW, et al. ACC/AHA guidelines for the management of patients with ST-elevation myocardial infarction: a report of the American College of Cardiology/American Heart Association Task Force on Practice Guidelines (Committee to Revise the 1999 Guidelines for the Management of Patients with Acute Myocardial Infarction). Circulation 2004;110:e82–e292.
2. Antman EM, Hand M, Armstrong PW, et al. 2007 focused update of the ACC/AHA 2004 guidelines for the management of patients with ST-elevation myocardial infarction: a report of the American College of Cardiology/American Heart Association Task Force on Practice Guidelines: developed in collaboration with the Canadian Cardiovascular Society endorsed by the American Academy of Family Physicians: 2007 writing group to review new evidence and update the ACC/AHA 2004 guidelines for the management of patients with ST-elevation myocardial infarction, writing on behalf of the 2004 Writing Committee. Circulation 2008;117:296–329.
3. Smith SC Jr, Allen J, Blair SN, et al. AHA/ACC guidelines for secondary prevention for patients with coronary and other atherosclerotic vascular disease: 2006 update endorsed by the National Heart, Lung, and Blood Institute. J Am Coll Cardiol 2006;47:2130–2139.
4. Kushner FG, Hand M, Smith SC Jr, et al. 2009 focused updates: ACC/AHA guidelines for the management of patients with ST-elevation myocardial infarction (updating the 2004 guideline and 2007 focused update) and ACC/AHA/SCAI guidelines on percutaneous coronary intervention (updating the 2005 guideline and 2007 focused update): a report of the American College of Cardiology Foundation/American Heart Association Task Force on Practice Guidelines. Circulation 2009;120:2271–2306.
5. Reinhart KM, White CM, Baker WL. Prasugrel: a critical comparison with clopidogrel. Pharmacotherapy 2009;29:1441–1451.
6. Wiviott SD, Braunwald E, McCabe CH, et al. Prasugrel versus clopidogrel in patients with acute coronary syndromes. N Engl J Med 2007;357:2001–2015.
7. Cannon CP, Braunwald E, McCabe CH, et al. Intensive versus moderate lipid lowering with statins after acute coronary syndromes. N Engl J Med 2004;350:1495–1504.
8. Skyler JS, Bergenstal R, Bonow RO, et al. Intensive glycemic control and the prevention of cardiovascular events: implications of the ACCORD, ADVANCE, and VA diabetes trials: a position statement of the American Diabetes Association and a scientific statement of the American College of Cardiology Foundation and the American Heart Association. Circulation 2009;119:351–357.
9. FDA Drug Safety Communication: Ongoing safety review of high-dose Zocor (simvastatin) and increased risk of muscle injury, 2010. Available at: *http://www.fda.gov/Drugs/DrugSafety/SafetyInformationforPatientsandProviders/ucm204882.htm*. Accessed March 6, 2010.
10. Joy TR, Hegele RA. Narrative review: statin-related myopathy. Ann Intern Med 2009;150:858–868.


# 19

# VENTRICULAR ARRHYTHMIA

Julia's Parking Lot Accident . . . . . . . . . . . . . . . Level III

**Kwadwo Amankwa, PharmD**

## LEARNING OBJECTIVES

After completing this case study, the reader should be able to:

- Understand the risk factors for development of drug-induced torsades de pointes (TdP).

- Differentiate TdP from other cardiac arrhythmias.
- Select appropriate first-line therapy for acute treatment of TdP.
- Identify appropriate dosing, common adverse effects, and monitoring parameters for pharmacologic agents used to treat TdP.
- Discuss long-term approaches to prevention of drug-induced TdP.

## PATIENT PRESENTATION

### Chief Complaint

"I was not feeling well, and I think I passed out."

### HPI

Julia Doellefeld is a 55-year-old woman who experiences syncope while parking her car in the parking lot of the neighborhood grocery store. There were no injuries from the accident, and she was brought to the ED for evaluation. She reports being in her usual state of relatively good health until she developed a "cold" approximately 4 days before admission. She called her primary care physician complaining of her upper respiratory tract symptoms, and the physician called in a prescription for erythromycin 500 mg QID (for 10 days) to her pharmacy. She took the first dose on the morning of admission. She started feeling something was wrong on her way to the grocery store approximately 1 hour after taking the second dose of erythromycin. She reports symptoms of lightheadedness, shortness of breath, as well as palpitations while driving. She passed out while parking, and her car collided with another car with minimal impact, damage, or injury. On medic arrival, she was awake and alert but looked shaken. She was transported to the ED without further events.

While being evaluated in the ED, she had another syncopal episode. ACLS protocol was initiated, and a rhythm strip showed TdP.

### PMH

CAD S/P PTCA
Heart failure (EF 30%)
Dyslipidemia
Paroxysmal atrial fibrillation

### SH

She lives with her husband and does not smoke or drink alcohol.

### Meds

Carvedilol 3.125 mg po BID
Pravastatin 40 mg po once daily
Furosemide 40 mg po BID (recently increased from 40 mg po once a day due to increased edema)
Warfarin 4 mg po once daily as directed
Amiodarone 200 mg po BID
Centrum Silver po once daily
Ranitidine 150 mg po once daily
Candesartan 8 mg po once daily
Aspirin 325 mg po once daily
Erythromycin 500 mg po QID (started day of admission)

### All

NKDA

### ROS

The patient has no complaints other than those mentioned in the HPI.

### Physical Examination

*Gen*

The patient is awake on an ED bed in moderate distress.

*VS*

BP 104/50, P 98 (200 during syncope), RR 30, T 36.3°C; Ht 5′7″, Wt 90 kg

*Skin*

Warm and dry; no rashes seen

*HEENT*

Normocephalic, atraumatic. PERRLA. EOMI. Oropharynx is clear.

*Neck/Lymph Nodes*

Supple; no JVD or bruits; no lymph nodes palpated

*Lungs/Thorax*

CTA bilaterally

*Breasts*

Deferred

*CV*

RRR with no murmurs or gallops

*Abd*

NTND; no rebound or guarding; (+) bowel sounds

*Genit/Rect*

Deferred

*MS/Ext*

Trace edema in the lower extremities; pulses intact

*Neuro*

A & O × 3

### Labs

| | | |
|---|---|---|
| Na 140 mEq/L | Hgb 12.1 g/dL | WBC 12 × $10^3$/mm$^3$ |
| K 2.8 mEq/L | Hct 35% | |
| Cl 100 mEq/L | RBC 3.88 × $10^6$/mm$^3$ | |
| $CO_2$ 29 mEq/L | Plt 200 × $10^3$/mm$^3$ | |
| BUN 36 mg/dL | MCV 90.5 μm$^3$ | |
| SCr 1.4 mg/dL | MCHC 34.4 g/dL | |
| Glu 110 mg/dL | INR 2.3 | |
| Mg 1.2 mg/dL | | |

### ECG

NSR, QTc 605 milliseconds; rhythm strip from oscilloscope during syncope: TdP (Fig. 19-1)

### Assessment

A 55-year-old white woman S/P syncopal episodes from drug-induced TdP; upper respiratory tract symptoms; drug-induced electrolyte imbalance

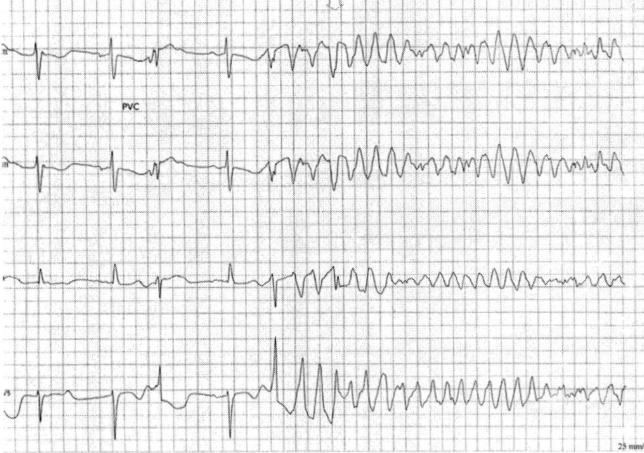

**FIGURE 19-1.** Electrocardiogram showing torsades de pointes.

# QUESTIONS

## Problem Identification

1.a. What risk factors predisposed the patient to drug-induced arrhythmia?

1.b. What features of the patient's ECG are characteristic of TdP?

1.c. Discuss pharmacologic and nonpharmacologic factors that may have contributed to drug-induced TdP in this patient.

## Desired Outcome

2. What are the short-term goals of pharmacotherapy for this patient?

## Therapeutic Alternatives

3.a. What nonpharmacologic therapies may be useful for this patient?

3.b. What pharmacotherapy options are available for acute treatment of TdP?

## Optimal Plan

4. Design a pharmacotherapeutic plan for the treatment of acute drug-induced TdP for this patient.

## Outcome Evaluation

5. What monitoring parameters should be used to assess efficacy and toxicity of treatment?

## Patient Education

6. What medication counseling should be provided for the patient to prevent recurrence?

## ■ CLINICAL COURSE

The patient was treated with a magnesium infusion, and she converted to normal sinus rhythm. The erythromycin was stopped. Potassium and magnesium were replaced, and the patient was admitted for further electrophysiology workup.

## ■ SELF-STUDY ASSIGNMENTS

1. List the most common drug classes associated with TdP.
2. List 10 commonly used medications that have a potential to cause TdP.

# CLINICAL PEARL

There is a need for increased pharmacovigilance regarding drug-induced arrhythmias in the outpatient setting because a large number of pharmacologic agents and/or conditions that cause QT prolongation and TdP are present in the outpatient population.

# REFERENCES

1. Gowda RM, Khan IA, Wilbur SL, Vasavada BC, Sacchi TJ. Torsades de pointes: the clinical considerations. Int J Cardiol 2004;95:219–222.
2. Arizona CERT—Center for Education and Research on Therapeutics. Available at: *http://www.azcert.org/*. Accessed February 1, 2010.
3. Yee GY, Camm AJ. Drug induced QT prolongation and torsades de pointes. Heart 2003:89;1363–1372.
4. Owens RC, Nolin TD. Antimicrobial-associated QT interval prolongation: pointes of interest. Clin Infect Dis 2006;43:1603–1611.
5. Tisdale JT. Torsades de pointes. In: Tisdale JE, Miller DA, eds. Drug-Induced Diseases: Prevention, Detection and Management. Bethesda, MD, American Society of Health-Systems Pharmacists, 2010:485–515.
6. ACC/AHA/ESC 2006 guidelines for management of patients with ventricular arrhythmias and the prevention of sudden cardiac death: a report of the American College of Cardiology/American Heart Association Task Force and the European Society of Cardiology Committee for Practice Guidelines (Writing Committee to Develop Guidelines for Management of Patients With Ventricular Arrhythmias and the Prevention of Sudden Cardiac Death): developed in collaboration with the European Heart Rhythm Association and the Heart Rhythm Society. J Am Coll Cardiol 2006;48:247–346.
7. Berul CI, Seslar SP, Zimetbaum PJ, et al. Acquired QT syndrome. In: Triedman J, Levy S, eds. UpToDate, Waltham, MA. Available at: *http://www.uptodateonline.com*. Accessed February 4, 2010.

# 20

# ATRIAL FIBRILLATION

Go Easy on My Beating Heart. . . . . . . . . . . . . Level III

**Virginia H. Fleming, PharmD**

**Bradley G. Phillips, PharmD, BCPS, FCCP**

## LEARNING OBJECTIVES

After completing this case study, the reader should be able to:

- Describe the cornerstones of atrial fibrillation (AF) treatment.
- Determine therapeutic goals for managing AF in patients with heart failure (HF).
- Recommend an optimal agent for anticoagulation in AF patients with HF.

## PATIENT PRESENTATION

### ■ Chief Complaint

"Lately, I feel like my heart has been racing a bit. It really doesn't bother me that much, but I wanted to have it checked out to be sure."

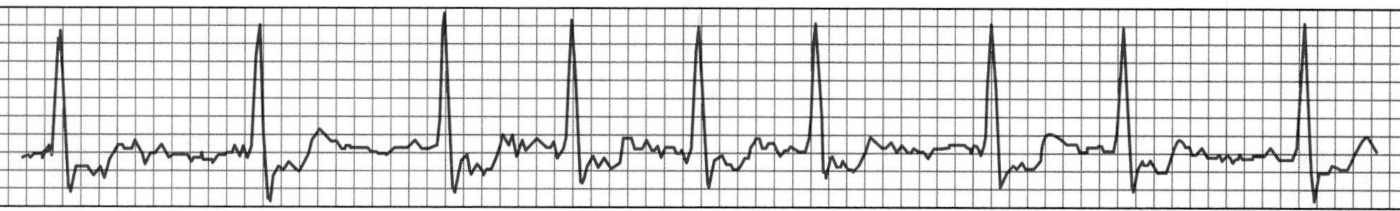

**FIGURE 20-1.** Rhythm recorded in Mr Riley's physician's office that depicts atrial fibrillation with a ventricular response rate of 110 bpm. Atrial fibrillation is characterized by the absence of atrial "p" waves with varying distances between QRS complexes. Atrial fibrillation is sometimes referred to as an irregularly irregular rhythm: irregular because it is not normal sinus rhythm; irregular because it produces an irregular ventricular response rate or peripheral pulse.

## HPI

Cooper Riley is a 64-year-old man with HF and a history of persistent AF who presents to his primary care physician complaining of palpitations that he first noticed 7 days ago. He reports that he is aware of the palpitations but that he has remained relatively asymptomatic. There has not been a noticeable change in his level of fatigue or exercise capacity during his normal daily activities. Mr Riley has had congestive HF for 6 years. For the past few years, his baseline exercise capacity would be described as slight limitation of physical activity with some symptoms during normal daily activities but asymptomatic at rest. He has a history of AF that was cardioverted to NSR, and he has been on amiodarone to maintain normal sinus rhythm for the past 8 months. In the office today, Mr Riley's ECG shows that he is in AF (see Fig. 20-1).

## PMH

Hypertension
Persistent AF (previously in NSR with amiodarone therapy)
Systolic HF (LVEF 34%)
Obstructive sleep apnea (AHI 28 events/h), alleviated with CPAP therapy

## FH

Both parents are deceased. Father died from AMI at age 64. Mother died of breast cancer at age 70 years.

## SH

Mr Riley works as an accountant. He is married with two healthy children. He does not smoke but occasionally "drinks a few beers on the weekend."

## Medications

Carvedilol 6.25 mg po BID
Digoxin 0.0625 mcg po once daily
Amiodarone 400 mg po once daily
Furosemide 40 mg po once daily
KCl 20 mEq po once daily
Lisinopril 10 mg po once daily
Warfarin 5 mg po once daily
CPAP therapy (8 cm $H_2O$) at night

## Allergies

NKDA

## ROS

Reports no change in level of fatigue, some exercise intolerance; no headache, lightheadedness, chest pain, angina, or fainting spells; 2+ pitting edema

## Physical Examination

*Gen*

Cooperative overweight man in no apparent distress

*VS*

BP 138/90, P 110 (irregular), RR 20, T 36.3°C, Wt 108.3 kg, Ht 5′11″

*Skin*

Cool to touch, normal turgor and color

*HEENT*

PEERLA, EOMI, funduscopic exam reveals mild arteriolar narrowing but no hemorrhages, exudates, or papilledema

*Neck*

Large and supple, no carotid bruits; no lymphadenopathy or thyromegaly, (−) JVD

*Lungs/Thorax*

Inspiratory and expiratory rales bilaterally, no rhonchi

*CV*

Pulse 110 bpm and irregular; normal $S_1$, $S_2$, (+) $S_3$, no $S_4$

*Abd*

NT/ND, (+) BS; no organomegaly, (−) HJR

*Genit/Rect*

Normal male anatomy; stool heme (−)

*MS/Ext*

Pulses 1+ weak, full ROM, no clubbing or cyanosis; mild edema (2+)

*Neuro*

A & O X 3; CN II–XII intact; DTR 2+, negative Babinski

## Labs

| | | |
|---|---|---|
| Na 140 mEq/L | Hgb 12.0 g/dL | Ca 8.5 mg/dL |
| K 4.0 mEq/L | Hct 35.8 | Mg 2.1 mEq/L |
| Cl 105 mEq/L | Plt 212 × $10^3/mm^3$ | Dig 0.08 ng/mL |
| $CO_2$ 24 mEq/L | WBC 9.5 × $10^3/mm^3$ | |
| BUN 22 mg/dL | Polys 65% | |
| SCr 1.1 mg/dL | Bands 2% | |
| Glu 109 mg/dL | Lymphs 30% | |
| INR 2.3 | Mono 3% | |

## ECG

Persistent AF, ventricular rate 110 bpm (see Fig. 20-1)

## Echo

Evidence of systolic dysfunction (LVEF 34%) and moderate left atrial enlargement (5.2 cm). No thrombus seen.

■ Chest X-Ray

Enlarged cardiac silhouette; no evidence of acute pulmonary infection or edema

■ Assessment

Persistent AF, previously in NSR on amiodarone therapy: mildly symptomatic, appropriately anticoagulated with warfarin therapy. Ventricular response rate not controlled.
HF: mildly symptomatic, standard meds not at target doses
HTN: not controlled, optimize therapy for blood pressure control
OSA: controlled on CPAP therapy

## QUESTIONS

### Problem Identification

1.a. List and prioritize the patient's drug therapy problems.

1.b. How effective is amiodarone therapy in maintaining normal sinus rhythm long-term in patients with AF?

1.c. What factors may hinder preservation of normal sinus rhythm in Mr Riley?

1.d. Mr Riley has persistent AF. How is this different from permanent AF?

### Desired Outcomes

2.a. What are the goals for pharmacotherapy in patients with AF?

2.b. What are the goals for pharmacotherapy for this patient's comorbid disease states or conditions?

### Therapeutic Alternatives

3.a. What therapeutic rhythm control alternatives exist for patients with AF and HF?

3.b. What are therapeutic options for rate control?

3.c. What nondrug therapies might be options for Mr Riley's AF?

### Optimal Plan

4. How would you manage Mr Riley's AF at this time?

### Outcome Evaluation

5. How would you monitor and adjust Mr Riley's drug therapies for AF?

### Patient Education

6. What patient education would you provide Mr Riley about his AF and HF at this time to explain choice of management strategy, ensure adherence, and minimize risk of side effects?

## ■ SELF-STUDY ASSIGNMENTS

1. Recommend a management strategy/plan for Mr Riley if he returned in 2 weeks with a therapeutic INR, a heart rate of 95 bpm, and no symptoms of tachycardia but with 2+ pitting edema and a 1.2-kg gain in body weight.
2. List the drugs that have been demonstrated to improve mortality in the setting of HF and AF.
3. Based on recent clinical trials, update the ACC/AHA/ESC 2006 guidelines for the management of patients with AF, specifically the section on recommendations for the pharmacologic management of AF in patients with HF.

## CLINICAL PEARL

In treating AF with concomitant systolic HF, lenient ventricular rate control (<110 bpm) plus anticoagulation is a viable treatment option over maintaining normal sinus rhythm with antiarrhythmic therapy.

## REFERENCES


1. Hunt SA, Abraham WT, Chin MH, et al. 2009 focused update incorporated into the ACC/AHA 2005 guidelines for the diagnosis and management of heart failure in adults: a report of the American College of Cardiology Foundation/American Heart Association Task Force on Practice Guidelines developed in collaboration with the International Society for Heart and Lung Transplantation. J Am Coll Cardiol 2009;53:e1–e90.
2. Fuster V, Ryden LE, Cannom DS, et al. ACC/AHA/ESC 2006 guidelines for the management of patients with atrial fibrillation: a report of the American College of Cardiology/American Heart Association Task Force on Practice Guidelines and the European Society of Cardiology Committee for Practice Guidelines (Writing Committee to Revise the 2001 Guidelines for the Management of Patients With Atrial Fibrillation): developed in collaboration with the European Heart Rhythm Association and the Heart Rhythm Society. Circulation 2006;114:e257–e354.
3. Shelton RJ, Clark AL, Goode K, et al. A randomized, controlled study of rate versus rhythm control in patients with chronic atrial fibrillation and heart failure: (CAFE-II Study). Heart 2009;95(11):924–930.
4. Roy D, Talajic M, Nattel S, et al. Rhythm control versus rate control for atrial fibrillation and heart failure. N Engl J Med 2008;358:2667–2677.
5. Van Gelder IC, Groenveld HF, Crijns HJ, et al. Lenient versus strict rate control in patients with atrial fibrillation. N Engl J Med 2010;362(15):1363–1373.


# 21

# DEEP VEIN THROMBOSIS

Trouble from Deep Within . . . . . . . . . . . . . . . . Level II


**James D. Coyle, PharmD**

**Patrick J. Fahey, MD**


## LEARNING OBJECTIVES

After completing this case study, the reader should be able to:

- Define acute deep vein thrombosis (DVT), and discuss its pathophysiology.
- Discuss the clinical presentation of patients with a DVT.
- Develop a pharmacotherapeutic care plan for the management of a patient with a DVT.
- Educate a patient receiving anticoagulation therapy for the treatment of a DVT.

## PATIENT PRESENTATION

### Chief Complaint

"I'm having pain in my leg."

### HPI

Rodney Cross is a 48-year-old man who presents to his primary care physician because of pain in his right leg. He states that he awoke with the pain 3 days ago and that it has been continuous, although it hurts more when he walks. The pain is located behind his right knee and extends down into his calf. He rates the pain intensity as 3/10 at this time. The patient denies CP and SOB. He denies recent travel, immobility, and leg injury. The patient did start pravastatin 40 mg daily for treatment of dyslipidemia approximately 3 months prior to this visit. He stopped the pravastatin 3 days ago because he thought it might be causing his leg pain, but the pain has continued.

### PMH

Hypertension
Dyslipidemia
Graves' disease with thyroid ablation
Gout
Left ankle fracture 9 years ago that required a cast but no surgery
Remote history of depression

### PSH

Left herniorrhaphy about 10 years ago. Pilonidal cyst excision in remote past.

### FH

Father died at age 81 of liver failure. Mother, one brother, and son all alive and well. No family history of venous thromboembolism or clotting disorders.

### SH

Married, one adult child. Drinks one to two alcoholic beverages daily. Smokes one cigar per month, no cigarettes. Denies illicit drug use.

### Meds

Allopurinol 300 mg po once daily
Hydrochlorothiazide 12.5 mg once daily
Lisinopril 10 mg once daily
Levothyroxine 150 mcg po once daily
Pravastatin 40 mg po once daily (discontinued 3 days ago)

### All

NKDA

### ROS

Constitutional: No chills, no fatigue.
Eyes: No eye pain or changes in vision.
ENT: No sore throat.
Skin: No pigmentation changes, no nail changes.
Cardiovascular: No CP, palpitations, or syncope.
Respiratory: No cough, SOB, wheezing, or stridor.
GI: No abdominal pain, nausea, diarrhea, or vomiting.
Musculoskeletal: No neck pain, back pain, or injury.
Neurologic: No dizziness, headache, or focal weakness.
Psychiatric/behavioral: Remote history of depression. Not a current problem.

### Physical Examination

*Gen*

Somewhat overweight, Caucasian man who appears comfortable. Cooperative, A & O × 3, normal affect.

*VS*

BP 132/76, P 75 regular, R 16, T 98.3°F, $O_2$ sat 97/ra; Wt 194 lb, Ht 6′0″

*Skin*

Warm, dry, normal color. No rash or induration.

*HEENT*

Pupils equal and reactive to light. EOM intact. Mucous membranes moist and pink.

*Neck*

Normal range of motion with no meningeal signs

*Lungs/Thorax*

Breath sounds normal, no respiratory distress

*CV*

RRR, no rubs, murmurs, or gallops

*Abd*

Nontender, no masses, no distension, no peritoneal signs

*MS/Ext*

Upper extremities: Normal by inspection, no CCE, normal ROM.

Lower extremities: Right calf tight, warm to touch, and tender with 1+ pretibial pitting edema. LLE without redness, warmth, and swelling. Lower extremity pulses and sensation are normal bilaterally. Normal ROM.

*Neuro*

Glasgow coma scale of 15, no focal motor deficits, no focal sensory deficits

### Labs

| | |
|---|---|
| Na 140 mEq/L | WBC 5.9 × $10^3$/μL |
| K 3.9 mEq/L | RBC 4.28 × $10^6$/μL |
| Cl 103 mEq/L | Hgb 13.5 g/dL |
| $CO_2$ 27 mEq/L | Hct 39.3% |
| BUN 10 mg/dL | MCV 92.0 fL |
| SCr 0.84 mg/dL | MCHC 34.4 g/dL |
| Glucose 88 mg/dL | RBC dist 14.3 |
| Uric acid 5.0 mg/dL | Platelets 175 × $10^3$/μL |
| CK 117 IU/L | Mean platelet volume 7.2 fL |
| | Granulocytes, electronic 51.0% |
| | Lymphocytes, electronic 38.2% |
| | Monocytes, electronic 8.4% |
| | Eosinophils, electronic 1.9% |
| | Basophils, electronic 0.5% |
| | INR 1.0 |

Lower extremity venous duplex ultrasonography: "Acute DVT of right distal superficial femoral, popliteal, and peroneal veins. No compression or flow in these vessels."

(**Note to reader:** *The "superficial femoral vein" is actually a deep vein, in spite of its name. Use of the name "femoral vein" is preferred because it is less confusing. However, the name "superficial femoral vein" is still encountered, as it is in this patient's venous duplex report.*)

■ Assessment

Acute DVT in right distal femoral, popliteal, and peroneal veins

# QUESTIONS

## Problem Identification

1.a. Create a list of this patient's medication-related problems.

1.b. What subjective and objective findings support the diagnosis of a lower extremity DVT?

## Desired Outcome

2. What are the short- and long-term goals of pharmacotherapy for this patient's DVT?

## Therapeutic Alternatives

3. What therapeutic alternatives are available for the pharmacologic management of this patient's DVT?

## Optimal Plan

4. Design a treatment plan for the initial management of this patient's DVT. Be sure to include dosage form, dose, schedule, and duration of therapy for each drug that is part of the plan.

## Outcome Evaluation

5. Design a monitoring plan for this patient's DVT therapy. Be sure to include monitoring for both safety and efficacy.

## Patient Education

6. What education should be provided for this patient to optimize the probability of therapeutic success while minimizing the risk of adverse events?

## ■ CLINICAL COURSE

Mr Cross presents to his primary care physician 3 days after his first visit. He has been administering his injections and taking warfarin 5 mg daily, as instructed. He continues to experience RLE pain and swelling, but these symptoms are somewhat improved. He denies new CP or SOB. He reports no missed warfarin doses, no changes in his other medications, a diet with consistent vitamin K intake, no change in his alcohol intake, and no acute health problems. He denies bruising and bleeding, other than minor bruising related to his injections. His INR is 1.7.

## Follow-Up Question

1.a. Identify the patient's anticoagulation therapy–related drug therapy problem(s), and design treatment and monitoring plans for managing each problem you identify.

## ■ CLINICAL COURSE

Mr Cross presents to his primary care physician's office approximately 2 months after his acute DVT episode. He reports that he experienced an episode of very dark brown, "cola"-colored urine 2 days before this visit. He has had no recurrences. The patient denies dysuria, back or groin pain, and blood in his bowel movements. His current dose of warfarin is 2.5 mg on Monday, Wednesday, Friday, and Saturday and 5 mg on Tuesday, Thursday, and Sunday. Physical examination reveals no CVA tenderness. His INR is 2.3.

## Follow-Up Question

1.b. Identify the patient's anticoagulation therapy–related drug therapy problem(s), and design treatment and monitoring plans for managing each problem you identify.

## ■ CLINICAL COURSE

Three months after his initial presentation, you see Mr Cross in the new anticoagulation clinic at his primary care physician's office. He is currently taking warfarin 2.5 mg on Monday, Wednesday, Friday, and Saturday and 5 mg on Tuesday, Thursday, and Sunday. His INR is 4.3. The patient's INR 4 weeks ago was 2.3 on the same warfarin dose. Mr Cross has not experienced any symptoms suggesting DVT recurrence or PE occurrence. He states that he has not had any problem with bleeding, has not missed doses or taken extra doses of warfarin in the past month, and has not changed his diet or alcohol intake. His medications have been unchanged, except for a switch from pravastatin 40 mg daily to simvastatin 40 mg daily for the treatment of his dyslipidemia approximately 2–3 weeks ago. You note that the following thrombophilia tests were completed prior to the initiation of anticoagulation therapy:

| Test | Result | Reference Interval |
|---|---|---|
| Antithrombin III (% activity) | 101 | 85–118 |
| Protein C (% activity) | 122 | 72–220 |
| Protein S (% activity) | 111 | 50–168 |
| Factor V Leiden mutation | Negative | Normal: negative |
| Prothrombin G-20210-A mutation | Negative | Normal: negative |
| Anticardiolipin antibodies IgG (GPL units) | 5.0 | 0.0–15.0 |
| Anticardiolipin antibodies IgM (MPL units) | <4.7 | 0.0–12.5 |
| Thrombin time (s) | 15.5 | 13.0–20.0 |
| DRVVT (s) | 63.2 | 35.0–47.0 |
| DRVVT confirm (s) | 36.3 | – |
| DRVVT ratio | 1.74 | 1.10–1.41 |
| StaClot LA | Positive | Normal: negative |
| Homocysteine, plasma (μmol/L) | 10.0 | 3.7–13.9 |

The laboratory summarizes the above results as consistent with the presence of lupus anticoagulants.

## Follow-Up Question

1.c. Identify this patient's anticoagulation therapy–related drug problem(s), and design a treatment and monitoring plan for each problem that you identify. Be sure to specify the anticipated duration of his anticoagulation therapy.

## ■ SELF-STUDY ASSIGNMENTS

1. Create a summary of antiphospholipid syndrome, including its definition, clinical presentation, and management.
2. Summarize the existing literature regarding the effects of various statins on response to warfarin. Does warfarin alter the effect of statins?

## CLINICAL PEARL

Current evidence does not clearly establish the appropriate duration of anticoagulation therapy for many patients with DVTs. A decision must therefore be based on a careful comparison of the benefits of continuing anticoagulation (primarily a decreased risk of DVT recurrence and potential sequelae) versus the risk of adverse events (primarily bleeding) in each patient.

## REFERENCES


1. Clive K, Kahn SR, Giancarlo A, et al. Antithrombotic therapy for venous thromboembolic disease: American College of Chest Physicians evidence-based clinical practice guidelines (8th edition). Chest 2008;133:454S–545S.
2. Kearon C, Ginsberg JS, Julian JA, et al. Comparison of fixed-dose weight-adjusted unfractionated heparin and low-molecular-weight heparin for acute treatment of venous thromboembolism. JAMA 2006;296:935–942.
3. Nutescu EA, Wittkowsky AK, Dobesh PP, Hawkins DW, Dager WE. Choosing the appropriate antithrombotic agent for the prevention and treatment of VTE: a case-based approach. Ann Pharmacother 2006;40:1558–1571.
4. Schulman S, Kearon C, Kakkar AK, et al. Dabigatran versus warfarin in the treatment of acute venous thromboembolism. N Engl J Med 2009;361:2342–2352.
5. Baetz BE, Spinler SA. Dabigatran etexilate: an oral direct thrombin inhibitor for prophylaxis and treatment of thromboembolic diseases. Pharmacotherapy 2008;28:1354–1373.
6. Van Dongen CJ, MacGillavry MR, Prins MH. Once versus twice daily LMWH for the initial treatment of venous thromboembolism. Cochrane Database Syst Rev 2005;(3):CD003074.
7. Westergren T, Johansson P, Molden E. Probable warfarin–simvastatin interaction. Ann Pharmacother 2007;41:1292–1295.
8. Sconce EA, Khan TI, Daly AK, Wynne HA, Kamali F. The impact of simvastatin on warfarin disposition and dose requirements. J Thromb Haemost 2006;4:1422–1424.
9. Schellerman H, Bilker WB, Brensinger CM, Wan F, Yang YX, Hennessy S. Fibrate/statin initiation in warfarin users and gastrointestinal bleeding risk. Am J Med 2010;123:151–157.
10. Miyakis S, Lockshin MD, Atsumi T, et al. International consensus statement on an update of the classification criteria for definite antiphospholipid syndrome (APA). J Thromb Haemost 2006;4:295–306.
11. Ansell J, Hirsh J, Hylek E, et al. Pharmacology and management of the vitamin K antagonists: American College of Chest Physicians evidence-based clinical practice guidelines (8th edition). Chest 2008;133:160S–198S.


# 22

# PULMONARY EMBOLISM

HIT Can Happen . . . . . . . . . . . . . . . . . . . . . . . Level II

**Kristen L. Longstreth, PharmD, BCPS**

## LEARNING OBJECTIVES

After completing this case study, the reader should be able to:

- Identify the signs, symptoms, and risk factors associated with pulmonary embolism.
- Evaluate a patient for heparin-induced thrombocytopenia (HIT).
- Select an appropriate anticoagulant for the treatment of pulmonary embolism complicated by HIT.
- Recommend a pharmacotherapeutic plan to initiate and monitor anticoagulation for the treatment of pulmonary embolism complicated by HIT.
- Provide patient education on anticoagulation therapy.

## PATIENT PRESENTATION

### Chief Complaint

"I'm having chest pain and I can't catch my breath."

### HPI

Mary Anton is a 70-year-old woman who arrives at the hospital's emergency department by ambulance transfer from her home. The patient is S/P right TKR (postoperative day #10) for severe osteoarthritis. She was discharged from the hospital's orthopedic nursing unit 4 days ago with a prescription for enoxaparin for DVT prophylaxis. The patient was scheduled to receive physical therapy at a local rehabilitation center; however, she canceled therapy due to pain. She has been inactive at home with the exception of completing her activities of daily living with the assistance of her husband. This morning, the patient developed sharp chest pain and shortness of breath while watching television. She denies nausea, vomiting, and diaphoresis. The patient has a nonproductive cough. She is anxious and also complains of pain in her right knee and right lower extremity.

### PMH

HTN × 30 years
Dyslipidemia × 25 years
Chronic stable angina × 2 years (negative adenosine stress test 2 months ago)
CKD secondary to previously uncontrolled HTN, stage 4 (baseline creatinine 1.8–2.0 mg/dL)
Osteoarthritis
Obesity
S/P TKR right leg (postoperative day #10)

### FH

Father died at age 74 (lung CA)
Mother died at age 89 (MI)
No siblings

### SH

The patient is retired. She lives at home with her husband. Prior to surgery, she avoided most physical activity due to severe osteoarthritis. Negative for tobacco abuse. Denies alcohol use.

### Meds

Home medications:
- Aspirin 81 mg po once daily
- Metoprolol 50 mg po BID
- Amlodipine 10 mg po once daily
- Hydralazine 25 mg po TID
- Atorvastatin 20 mg po once daily
- Nitroglycerin 0.4 mg sublingually PRN chest pain
- Calcium acetate 667 mg po TID with meals
- Enoxaparin 30 mg SC Q 24 hours
- Oxycodone sustained release 20 mg po Q 12 hours
- Oxycodone immediate release 5 mg po Q 6 hours PRN pain
- Docusate 100 mg po QHS

### All

Lisinopril (angioedema)

### ROS

Positive for shortness of breath and nonproductive cough. Positive for sharp chest pain at rest. The pain does not radiate and is not reproducible by touch. No palpitations, diaphoresis, nausea, vomiting, or diarrhea. The patient denies headache, fever, and chills. Pain rated by patient as 7/10 in right knee and lower extremity.

### PE

*Gen*

The patient is alert and oriented × 3; moderate respiratory distress.

*VS*

BP 128/68, P 101, RR 21, T 36.9°C; Wt 85 kg, Ht 5′4″, $O_2$ sat 88% in room air

*Skin*

Warm and dry; no rashes

*HEENT*

Head: atraumatic; PERRLA; EOMI

*Neck/Lymph Nodes*

No carotid bruits; no lymphadenopathy; no thyromegaly

*Lungs/Thorax*

CTA; no wheezing or crackles

*CV*

Tachycardia with regular rhythm; normal heart sounds; no MRG

*Abd*

Obese, soft; NT/ND; +BS; no organomegaly

*Genit/Rect*

WNL

*MS/Ext*

S/P TKR right leg; right lower extremity ROM limited with slight redness, warmth, and edema; pain in right knee and lower extremity

*Neuro*

No focal deficits noted; cranial nerves intact

### Labs (Nonfasting)

| | | | |
|---|---|---|---|
| Na 144 mEq/L | Magnesium 1.9 mEq/L | Cholesterol 171 mg/dL | D-dimer 975 ng/mL |
| K 4.5 mEq/L | Phosphate 4.4 mg/dL | LDL 103 mg/dL | CK 67 IU/L (time: 1245) |
| Cl 108 mEq/L | Calcium 8.9 mg/dL | HDL 42 mg/dL | CK-MB 1.1 IU/L (time: 1245) |
| $CO_2$ 26 mEq/L | Albumin 3.5 g/dL | Triglycerides 130 mg/dL | Troponin I 0.03 ng/mL (time: 1245) |
| BUN 35 mg/dL | AST 21 IU/L | Hgb 11.5 g/dL | |
| SCr 1.8 mg/dL | ALT 15 IU/L | Hct 34.7% | |
| Glu 106 mg/dL | Alk Phos 57 IU/L | Plt 86 × $10^3$/mm$^3$ | |
| $HbA_{1c}$ 6.0% | | WBC 6 × $10^3$/mm$^3$ | |

### ECG

Sinus tachycardia. No T wave or ST changes present.

### Venous Doppler Ultrasound of Right Lower Extremity

Occlusive deep venous thrombosis from the right popliteal vein to the right common femoral vein

### CXR

No evidence of acute cardiopulmonary disease

### Assessment

1. Chest pain, SOB—history of chronic stable angina; R/O ACS, R/O PE
2. Right lower extremity DVT
3. Thrombocytopenia—R/O HIT
4. S/P TKR right leg (postoperative day #10)— no signs of infection, pain not controlled
5. CKD—stage 4, creatinine at patient's baseline
6. HTN—stable on current regimen
7. Dyslipidemia—stable on current regimen

## CLINICAL COURSE

The patient is admitted to a telemetry nursing unit within the hospital for treatment of the DVT and further workup for chest pain and shortness of breath. A V/Q scan is ordered. The patient's medical chart from the previous admission is reviewed to obtain a more complete medication and laboratory history.

An internal medicine resident physician discontinues enoxaparin and restarts all of the patient's other home medications. The resident physician also orders the following: consult clinical pharmacist to dose and monitor fondaparinux and warfarin; morphine 2–4 mg IV or IM Q 4 hours PRN pain; propoxyphene napsylate and acetaminophen 100/325 mg po Q 4 hours PRN pain.

### V/Q Scan

Multiple segmental perfusion defects, indicating a ventilation–perfusion mismatch and high probability of pulmonary embolism (Fig. 22-1).

Cardiac enzymes (second set; time: 1905):

CK 45 IU/L
CK-MB 0.7 IU/L
Troponin I 0.02 ng/mL

Pertinent medication and laboratory history from the previous admission:

| | | | |
|---|---|---|---|
| TKR | Plt 239 × $10^3$/mm$^3$ | Hgb 11.8 g/dL | |
| Postoperative day #1 | Plt 233 × $10^3$/mm$^3$ | Hgb 11.5 g/dL | Enoxaparin 30 mg SC Q 24 hours started |
| Postoperative day #2 | Plt 227 × $10^3$/mm$^3$ | Hgb 11.7 g/dL | |
| Postoperative day #3 | Plt 229 × $10^3$/mm$^3$ | | |
| Postoperative day #4 | Plt 221 × $10^3$/mm$^3$ | | |
| Postoperative day #5 | Plt 234 × $10^3$/mm$^3$ | | |
| Postoperative day #6 | Plt 141 × $10^3$/mm$^3$ | Hgb 11.6 g/dL | Discharged from hospital on enoxaparin 30 mg SC Q 24 hours |

## QUESTIONS

### Problem Identification

1.a. What subjective and objective information is consistent with a diagnosis of PE for this patient?

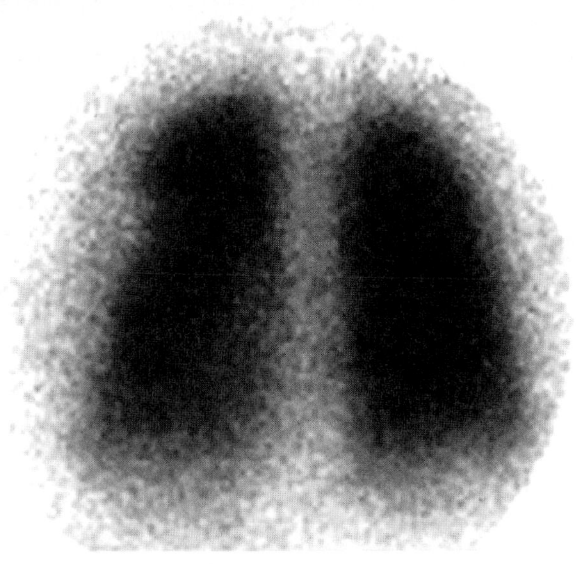


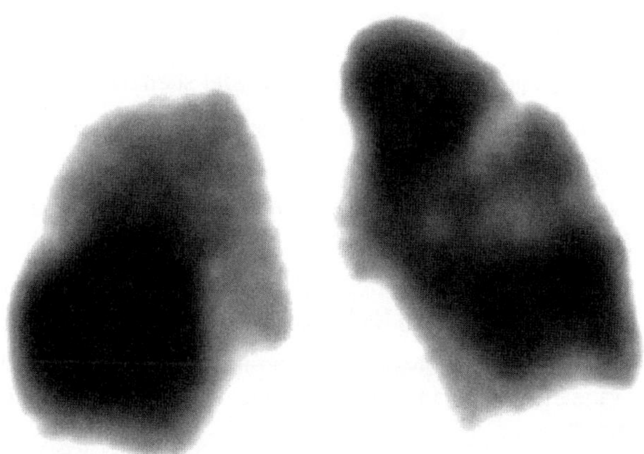


**FIGURE 22-1.** Ventilation–perfusion lung scan. *(A)* Normal ventilation; *(B)* multiple segmental perfusion defects, indicating a ventilation–perfusion mismatch and high probability of pulmonary embolism. *(Reproduced with permission from Rao RK. Pulmonary embolic disease. In: Crawford MH, ed. Current Diagnosis and Treatment in Cardiology, 3rd ed. New York, NY, The McGraw-Hill Companies Inc, 2009:369.)*

1.b. What risk factors for PE are present for this patient?

1.c. Discuss the process to confirm or rule out a suspected diagnosis of HIT for this patient (see Table 22-1).[2,3]

1.d. Develop a list of the potential drug therapy problems for this patient.

## Desired Outcome

2.a. What are the goals of therapy for the treatment of PE?

2.b. What additional goals of therapy exist for this patient with HIT?

# ■ CLINICAL COURSE

A heparin-induced platelet antibody ELISA is drawn and sent to an outside laboratory. An order is written to avoid all heparin (including heparin catheter flushes). Prior to initiating anticoagulation, a baseline aPTT (29.5 seconds), PT (10.8 seconds), and INR (1.0) are obtained to assist with anticoagulation dosing. The nursing unit notifies the clinical pharmacist of the consultation order to dose and monitor fondaparinux and warfarin.

## Therapeutic Alternatives

3.a. Which agents are available to initiate anticoagulation for the treatment of PE in this patient?

3.b. What nonanticoagulant alternatives (pharmacologic and nonpharmacologic) are available? Is this patient an appropriate candidate for any of these therapeutic alternatives?

## Optimal Plan

4.a. Select an appropriate parenteral anticoagulant to begin therapy and calculate the initial dose for this patient.

4.b. Design a pharmacotherapeutic plan to transition the patient to warfarin therapy and discontinue the parenteral anticoagulant.

4.c. Determine the appropriate length of warfarin therapy for this patient.

## Outcome Evaluation

5.a. Choose an appropriate therapeutic monitoring parameter and calculate a therapeutic range for the anticoagulant selected for this patient.

5.b. In addition to the therapeutic monitoring parameter selected above, what clinical and laboratory parameters will you use to monitor the efficacy and safety of anticoagulation in this patient?

**TABLE 22-1** Estimating the Pretest Probability of HIT: The "Four T's"

| | **Points (0, 1, or 2 for each of four categories: maximum possible score = 8)** | | |
|---|---|---|---|
| | **2** | **1** | **0** |
| Thrombocytopenia | >50% platelet fall to nadir ≥20 | 30–50% platelet fall, or nadir 10–19 | <30% platelet fall, or nadir <10 |
| Timing[a] of onset of platelet fall (or other sequelae of HIT) | Days 5–10, or ≤day 1 with recent heparin (past 30 days) | >Day 10 or timing unclear; or <day 1 with recent heparin (past 31–100 days) | <Day 4 (no recent heparin) |
| Thrombosis or other sequelae | Proven new thrombosis, skin necrosis, or acute systemic reaction after intravenous UFH bolus | Progressive or recurrent thrombosis, erythematous skin lesions, suspected thrombosis (not proven) | None |
| Other cause(s) of platelet fall | None evident | Possible | Definite |

[a]First day of immunizing heparin exposure considered day 0.

Pretest probability score: 6–8, high; 4–5, intermediate; and 0–3, low.

*Reproduced with permission from Warkentin TE. Heparin-induced thrombocytopenia: diagnosis and management. Circulation 2004;110:e454–e458.*

## CLINICAL COURSE

The results of the heparin-induced platelet antibody ELISA were reported as positive with an optical density (OD) of 0.58 (laboratory reports OD values greater than 0.41 as positive for heparin-induced antibodies). The parenteral anticoagulant was discontinued, and the patient's INR has been therapeutic for 72 hours. The patient will be discharged home today.

### Patient Education

6.a. Prior to discharge, what information should be provided to this patient about warfarin therapy to enhance adherence and ensure efficacy and safety?

6.b. Discuss the information that you will provide to this patient concerning the future use of heparin and low-molecular-weight heparin therapy.

## SELF-STUDY ASSIGNMENTS

1. Determine the appropriate frequency of platelet count monitoring when therapeutic or prophylactic unfractionated heparin, low-molecular-weight heparin, or fondaparinux is used in medical or postoperative patients.
2. Investigate the sensitivity and specificity of the various activation and antigen assays available to confirm the diagnosis of HIT.
3. Compare the effects of lepirudin, bivalirudin, and argatroban on INR measurement and warfarin monitoring.
4. Review the literature for available options to reverse the effects of the direct thrombin inhibitors if excessive anticoagulation occurs.

## CLINICAL PEARL

The optimal duration of anticoagulation in a patient with HIT who does not have evidence of thrombosis (isolated HIT) is unknown. Anticoagulation with a direct thrombin inhibitor or fondaparinux should be continued until the platelet count has recovered (to at least $150 \times 10^3/mm^3$) and stabilized; however, some clinicians may also initiate warfarin therapy for several months to prevent HIT-related thrombosis.

## REFERENCES


1. Tapson VF. Acute pulmonary embolism. N Engl J Med 2008;358:1037–1052.
2. Warkentin TE. Heparin-induced thrombocytopenia: diagnosis and management. Circulation 2004;110:e454–e458.
3. Warkentin TE, Greinacher A, Koster A, Lincoff AM. Treatment and prevention of heparin-induced thrombocytopenia: the American College of Chest Physicians evidence-based clinical practice guidelines (8th edition). Chest 2008;133(6 Suppl):340S–380S.
4. Lo GK, Juhl D, Warkentin TE, Sigouin CS, Eichler P, Greinacher A. Evaluation of pretest clinical score (4 T's) for the diagnosis of heparin-induced thrombocytopenia in two clinical settings. J Thromb Haemost 2006;4:759–765.
5. Blackmer AB, Oertel MD, Valgus JM. Fondaparinux and the management of heparin-induced thrombocytopenia: the journey continues. Ann Pharmacother 2009;43:1636–1646.
6. Bartholomew JR. Transition to an oral anticoagulant in patients with heparin-induced thrombocytopenia. Chest 2005;127(2 Suppl):27S–34S.
7. Kearon C, Kahn SR, Giancarlo A, Goldhaber S, Raskob GE, Comerota AJ. Antithrombotic therapy for venous thromboembolic disease: American College of Chest Physicians evidence-based clinical practice guidelines (8th edition). Chest 2008;133(6 Suppl):454S–545S.
8. Lexi-Comp Online, Lexi-Drugs Online, Hudson, OH, Lexi-Comp Inc, 2010. Accessed March 14, 2010.


# 23

# CHRONIC ANTICOAGULATION

To Bridge or Not to Bridge, That is the Question. . . . . . . . . . . . . . . . . . . . Level III


**Mikayla L. Spangler, PharmD, BCPS**

**Beth Bryles Phillips, PharmD, FCCP, BCPS**


## LEARNING OBJECTIVES

After completing this case study, the reader should be able to:

- List the goals of anticoagulant therapy for periprocedural management of anticoagulation.
- Appropriately assess a patient's response to chronic warfarin therapy.
- Determine thromboembolic risk for patients receiving warfarin therapy and the need for bridging therapy.
- Develop a patient-specific pharmacotherapeutic plan for warfarin therapy and periprocedural management of anticoagulation.
- Educate patients appropriately about administration of low-molecular-weight heparins (LMWH) and chronic warfarin therapy.

## PATIENT PRESENTATION

### Chief Complaint

"I am scheduled to have a colonoscopy and my physician said to talk to you about what to do with my warfarin."

### HPI

Elizabeth Heartly is a 53-year-old woman with a past medical history of a DVT × 2 and APL antibodies. After the first DVT, she was treated for 1 year and then tested for thrombophilias. A diagnosis of APL was made at that time. She recently experienced another DVT 4 months ago when her INR was subtherapeutic for an extended period of time. Today, she presents to the anticoagulation clinic for a follow-up appointment. She also reports that she is scheduled for a colonoscopy 2 weeks from today. She states her physician has been recommending the colonoscopy for routine screening since she turned 50. However, she has been reluctant to schedule it. She realized the need for the procedure after a friend was diagnosed with colon cancer. Although no biopsy is planned, her physician explained that she should be off warfarin in case a biopsy is needed. Ms Heartly states she uses a medication box and has not missed any of her warfarin doses during the last month. She denies any bleeding, excessive bruising, severe headaches, abdominal pain, chest pain, shortness of breath, or pain or swelling in the lower extremities. She states that her arthritis has been really flaring up and therefore has been taking ibuprofen 800 mg three times daily for the last 2.5 weeks. She has one glass of red wine with dinner each evening. She has had no medication changes over the last month.

### PMH

Recurrent DVT × 2, 5 years ago and 4 months ago
APL antibodies
Hypothyroidism
Osteoarthritis of the knee

### FH

Father—colon polyps removed when he was in his 50s but is currently alive and well in his 80s.
Mother—hypertension and is 79 years of age.
Brother—healthy.
She has two children who are alive and well.

### SH

(+) ETOH—one glass of red wine each evening with supper; (–) smoking

### Meds

Ibuprofen 200 mg one to two tablets po TID PRN for osteoarthritis pain
Calcium carbonate 600 mg po BID with meals
Levothyroxine 125 mcg po once daily
Warfarin 2.5 mg po Tue, Sat; 5 mg 5 days per week

### All

Penicillin—bumps, rash/hives

### ROS

(–) For CP, SOB, severe headaches, abdominal pain, leg pain, bruises, or change in color of stool or urine

### Physical Examination

*Gen*

Pleasant obese woman in NAD

*VS*

BP 116/78, HR 76, RR 14, T 36.5°C; Wt 96.3 kg, Ht 5′6″

*Skin*

Normal turgor and color; warm

*HEENT*

PERRLA, EOMI; disks flat; fundi with no hemorrhages or exudates

*Neck/Lymph Nodes*

No lymphadenopathy, thyromegaly, or carotid bruits

*Lungs*

CTA bilaterally

*CV*

RRR; normal $S_1$ and $S_2$; no $S_3$ or $S_4$; no M/R/G

*Abd*

Obese, soft, nontender, nondistended, (+) BS

*Genit/Rect*

Deferred

*Ext*

Warm with no clubbing, cyanosis, or edema

*Neuro*

A & O × 3; CN II–XII intact; DTR 2+; Babinski negative

### Labs

| Date | INR | Warfarin Dose |
|---|---|---|
| Today | 2.8 | 2.5 mg Tue, Sat; 5 mg 5 days per week |
| 1 month ago | 2.7 | 2.5 mg Tue, Sat; 5 mg 5 days per week |
| 2 months ago | 2.8 | 2.5 mg Tue, Sat; 5 mg 5 days per week |
| 3 months ago | 2.4 | 2.5 mg Tue, Sat; 5 mg 5 days per week |

1 month ago TSH 1.93 mIU/L

### Assessment

History of recurrent DVT and APL requiring chronic anticoagulation with target INR 2.5 (range 2.0–3.0)
Therapeutic INR (target 2.5; range, 2.0–3.0)
Periprocedural management of anticoagulation needed
Euthyroid with current dose of levothyroxine
High-dose ibuprofen use for recent osteoarthritis flare

## QUESTIONS

### Problem Identification

1.a. Create a list of this patient's drug-related problems.

1.b. What questions would you ask this patient to assess her current warfarin therapy?

1.c. What signs or symptoms might she experience if she developed a venous thromboembolism?

1.d. What is her risk of thromboembolism during interruption of warfarin therapy?

1.e. What are the risks of using nonsteroidal anti-inflammatory drugs (NSAIDs) in combination with warfarin?

### Desired Outcome

2. What are the goals of anticoagulation therapy in this patient?

### Therapeutic Alternatives

3. What are the options for periprocedural management of anticoagulation?

### Optimal Plan

4.a. Based on today's laboratory result, what is your recommendation for this patient's warfarin therapy?

4.b. How should the plan for periprocedural management of anticoagulation be implemented?

### Outcome Evaluation

5. How will you monitor this patient's warfarin therapy?

## Patient Education

6.a. What information should this patient know regarding her upcoming bridging therapy for her colonoscopy procedure?

6.b. What information should this patient know about her warfarin therapy, especially to minimize subtherapeutic or supratherapeutic INRs and potential hemorrhagic and thromboembolic complications?

## ■ CLINICAL COURSE

On return to clinic 1 week after the colonoscopy, Ms Heartly reports that the procedure went well and she has taken her usual weekly dose of warfarin therapy and continues on her bridging therapy. Her INR is 2.0, and she is in need of further instructions regarding her warfarin and bridging therapy.

## Follow-Up Question

1. Based on this information, what are your recommendations for her warfarin and LMWH therapy?

## ■ ADDITIONAL CASE QUESTION

1. Ms Heartly has been diagnosed with hypothyroidism. Although her TSH is within normal range at this time, how would untreated hypothyroidism affect the INR?

## ■ SELF-STUDY ASSIGNMENTS

1. Research the options for bridging in patients with a history of heparin-induced thrombocytopenia, and create a table highlighting the various management options.
2. Research the data on LMWH dosing in morbidly obese patients, and write a one-page paper summarizing how LMWH should be dosed in such patients?

## CLINICAL PEARL

Dosing LMWH in obese patients can present challenges due to product availability of dosage strengths. Doses may need to be rounded up or down to the nearest available syringe. The availability of dosage forms may also determine whether enoxaparin may be administered once or twice daily.

## REFERENCES


1. Ansell J, Hirsh J, Hylek E, Jacobson A, Crowther M, Palareti G. Pharmacology and management of the vitamin K antagonists. Chest 2008;133:160S–198S.
2. Douketis JD, Berger PB, Dunn AS, et al. The perioperative management of antithrombotic therapy. Chest 2008;133:299S–339S.
3. Haines ST, Witt DM, Nutescu E. Venous thromboembolism. In: DiPiro JT, Talbert RL, Yee GC, Matzke GR, Wells BG, Posey LM, eds. Pharmacotherapy: A Pathophysiologic Approach, 7th ed. New York, NY, McGraw-Hill 2008:331–371.
4. Choudari CP, Rajgopal C, Palmer KR. Acute gastrointestinal haemorrhage in anticoagulated patients: diagnoses and response to endoscopic treatment. Gut 1994;35:464–466.
5. ASGE Standards of Practice Committee, Anderson MA, Ben-Menachem T, et al. Management of antithrombotic agents for endoscopic procedures. Gastrointest Endosc 2009;70:1060–1070.
6. Warkentin TE, Greinacher A, Koster A, Lincoff AM. Treatment and prevention of heparin-induced thrombocytopenia. Chest 2008;133;340S–380S.
7. Hirsh J, Bauer KA, Donati MB, Gould M, Samama MM, Weitz JI. Parenteral anticoagulants. Chest 2008;133;141S–159S.
8. Lovenox SC Injection Technique. Available at: *http://www.lovenox.com/hcp/dosing/lovenox-administration.aspx*. Accessed March 1, 2010.


# 24

# ISCHEMIC STROKE

One Stroke Off Par. . . . . . . . . . . . . . . . . . . . . . Level II

**Alexander J. Ansara, PharmD, BCPS**

**Michael R. Holowatyj, PharmD, BCPS**

## LEARNING OBJECTIVES

After completing this case study, the reader should be able to:

- Identify risk factors for ischemic stroke.
- Discuss the role of thrombolytics in the management of acute ischemic stroke.
- Formulate an appropriate patient-specific drug regimen for the treatment of an acute ischemic stroke.
- Discuss the approach to multidisease state management for the secondary prevention of ischemic stroke, including the management of hypertension, hyperlipidemia, and the use of antiplatelet agents.
- Educate a patient regarding secondary stroke prevention strategies.

## PATIENT PRESENTATION

### ■ Chief Complaint

"My dad is having trouble talking and seems to be losing feeling in his left arm and leg."

### ■ HPI

Marvin Palmer is a 57-year-old man who was brought to the EO by his son at 10 am after experiencing left arm numbness, slurred speech, and dizziness. His son states that the two of them were enjoying their typical Saturday morning golf outing at the country club when Mr Palmer, on teeing off on hole 6 at 9:30 am, dropped his golf club and went down on one knee. Mr Palmer's words were "slow and disjointed" according to his son who immediately called 9-1-1. While in the ER, Mr Palmer began to have a left-sided facial droop. He admitted noticing minor dizziness and slight tingling in his left hand at 8 am that both resolved soon thereafter. He assumed these were symptoms due to low blood pressure and therefore opted not to take his blood pressure medications this morning.

### ■ PMH

HTN, diagnosed 10 years ago
Dyslipidemia

■ FH

Both parents alive and relatively healthy. Sister, age 62, also has HTN. Son, age 31, has type 1 DM.

■ SH

Married, lives with wife and three children. Occasional recreational beer or wine consumption. Denies tobacco use.

■ Meds

Amlodipine 2.5 mg po daily
Simvastatin 10 mg po daily
Chlorthalidone 25 mg po daily

■ All

Shellfish (hives)

■ ROS

Mild blurry vision, but no double vision, loss of vision, or oscillopsia

■ Physical Examination

*Gen*

Slender Caucasian man lying in bed in no acute distress, responsive with occasionally slurred speech

*VS*

BP 192/98, P 70, RR 19, T 98.6°F, $O_2$ sat 97% in room air; Wt 80 kg, Ht 6′0″

*Skin*

Warm, dry

*HEENT*

PERRLA, EOMI; no nystagmus, exudates, hemorrhages, or papilledema; mild left-sided facial droop. Normal hearing acuity bilaterally.

*Neck*

(–) Carotid bruits, (–) lymphadenopathy

*Chest*

Lungs clear to auscultation bilaterally

*CV*

RRR, $S_1$ and $S_2$ normal, no $S_3$ or $S_4$

*Abd*

Soft, nontender, nondistended, (+) BS

*GU*

Deferred

*MS/Ext*

RUE: 5/5; RLE 4/5; LUE: 2/5; LLE: 3/5. No abnormal or involuntary movements. Strong peripheral pulses and brisk capillary refill; no CCE; DTR: 2+ throughout, normal Babinski reflex.

*Neuro*

Awake, A & O × 3. No aphasia, agnosia, or apraxia. Attention, concentration, and vocabulary are all excellent. No impairment of facial sensation noted with light touch bilaterally. Moderate left facial weakness, as noted by the presence of left-sided facial droop. Mild dysarthria. Shoulder shrug is symmetrical, and tongue is midline on protrusion. Can easily touch chin to chest, and there are no other signs of meningismus.

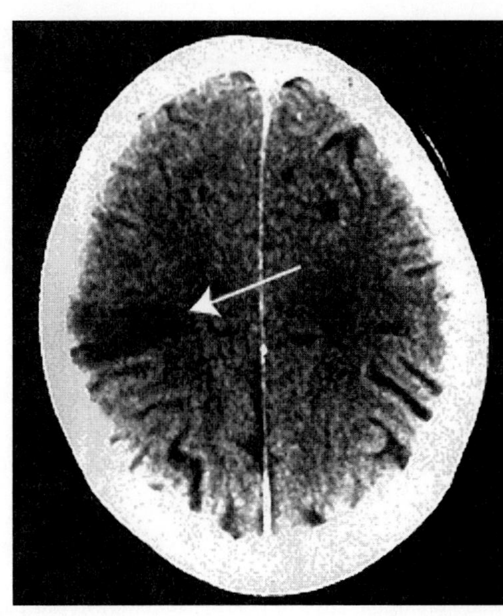

**FIGURE 24-1.** Head CT scan without contrast negative for hemorrhage and showing right-sided middle cerebral artery infarct.

■ Labs

| | | |
|---|---|---|
| Na 140 mEq/L | WBC 5.9 × $10^3$/mm$^3$ | **Fasting lipid profile** |
| K 4.2 mEq/L | Hgb 16.4 g/dL | Total cholesterol 200 mg/dL |
| Cl 103 mEq/L | Hct 49.6% | LDL-C 118 mg/dL |
| $CO_2$ 28 mEq/L | Plt 310 × $10^3$/mm$^3$ | Triglycerides 160 mg/dL |
| BUN 10 mg/dL | aPTT 25.3 sec | HDL-C 50 mg/dL |
| SCr 0.6 mg/dL | | |
| Glu 98 mg/dL | | |

Head CT scan: right-sided middle cerebral artery infarct; no evidence of hemorrhage (Fig. 24-1)
Carotid Dopplers: normal blood flow bilaterally, no appreciable ischemia or stenosis
Angiogram: not performed.
Echocardiogram: no evidence of LV thrombus, ejection fraction 55–60%; overall unremarkable
EKG: normal sinus rhythm (Fig. 24-2)

■ Assessment

Acute ischemic stroke secondary to atherosclerosis and ischemic disease in a patient with hypertension, dyslipidemia, and no prior history or stroke or transient ischemic attack

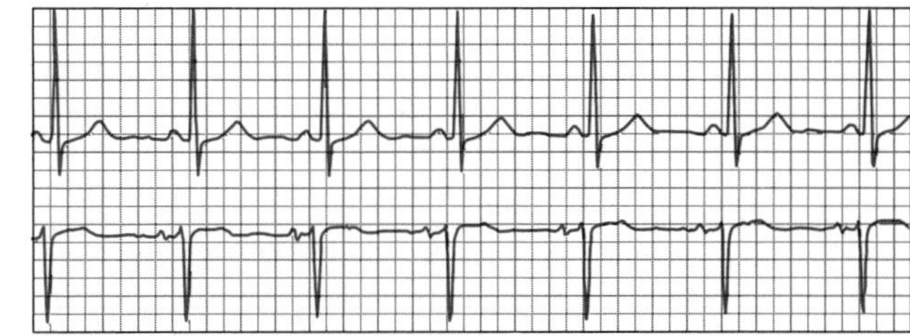

**FIGURE 24-2.** EKG showing normal sinus rhythm.

## CLINICAL COURSE

It is now 11:00 am, and you are seeing the patient with the rest of the neurology team.

## QUESTIONS

### Problem Identification

1.a. Create a list of the patient's drug therapy problems.

1.b. Identify the nonmodifiable, modifiable, and Framingham risk factors for CHD present in this patient.

1.c. Which signs, symptoms, and other tests indicate the presence of an acute ischemic stroke?

### Desired Outcome

2.a. What are the initial goals of pharmacotherapy in this patient?

2.b. What are the long-term goals of pharmacotherapy in this patient?

### Therapeutic Alternatives

3.a. What nondrug therapies might be useful for this patient?

3.b. What feasible pharmacotherapeutic alternatives are available for the treatment of acute ischemic stroke?

### Optimal Plan

4.a. What is your recommendation for the acute use of antihypertensives in this patient?

4.b. What pharmacotherapeutic regimen would you recommend for the acute treatment of stroke in this patient (include drug, dose, route, frequency, and duration)?

### Outcome Evaluation

5. What clinical and laboratory parameters are necessary to evaluate the therapy for achievement of the desired therapeutic outcome(s) and to detect or prevent adverse effects?

### Patient Education

6. What information should be provided to Mr Palmer to enhance adherence, ensure successful therapy, and minimize adverse effects?

## ■ CLINICAL COURSE

Mr Palmer is currently 4 days poststroke and will be discharged home today. He has regained motor coordination and strength in his extremities, and his speech has improved significantly. A mild facial droop is still noted to be present when he is prompted to smile and show his teeth.

### Follow-Up Questions

1. What antiplatelet regimen would you recommend for the secondary prevention of acute ischemic stroke in Mr Palmer (include drugs, dose and dosage form, schedule, and duration)?
2. Which parameters related to Mr Palmer's treatment should be monitored to ensure optimal secondary prevention?
3. What recommendations would you make to Mr Palmer's home drug regimen to optimally manage his hypertension and dyslipidemia?

## ■ SELF-STUDY ASSIGNMENTS

1. Explain which patients are candidates to receive aspirin instead of warfarin for the prevention of stroke in the setting of atrial fibrillation.
2. Summarize the role of HMG Co-A reductase inhibitors in the primary and secondary prevention of ischemic stroke.
3. Read the CURE and MATCH trials, and explain when and why patients should be treated with the combination of aspirin and clopidogrel. Explain what the MATCH results tell us about the use of combination antiplatelet therapy for the prevention of ischemic stroke.
4. Write a one-page report summarizing the findings of the NINDS and ECASS III trials pertaining to the use of thrombolytics for the treatment of acute ischemic stroke.
5. Read the PRoFESS trial, and explain the clinical implications of this trial pertaining to the use of clopidogrel and extended-release aspirin and dipyridamole for secondary stroke prevention.

## CLINICAL PEARLS

1. Hypoglycemia results in a clinical presentation similar to ischemic stroke and therefore should be ruled out as a diagnosis before treatment for an acute stroke is initiated.
2. Initially elevated blood pressures often decrease, without the use of antihypertensive therapy, within the first few days after an ischemic stroke. When initiating antihypertensive therapy after an acute ischemic stroke, caution should be used to not reduce blood pressures too aggressively unless clinically indicated.

## REFERENCES


1. Chaturvedi S, Bruno A, Feasby T, et al. Carotid endarterectomy—an evidence-based review. Report of the American Academy of Neurology. Neurology 2005;65:794–801.
2. National Institute of Neurological Disorders and Stroke rt-PA Stroke Study Group. Tissue plasminogen activator for acute ischemic stroke. N Engl J Med 1995;333:1581–1587.
3. Hacke W, Kaste M, Bluhmki E, et al., ECASS III Investigators. Thrombolysis with alteplase 3 to 4.5 hours after acute ischemic stroke. N Engl J Med 2008;359:1317–1329.
4. del Zoppo GJ, Saver JL, Jauch EC, et al. Expansion of the time window for treatment of acute ischemic stroke with intravenous tissue plasminogen activator. Stroke 2009;40:2945–2948.
5. Chinese Acute Stroke Trial Collaborative Group (CAST). Randomized placebo-controlled trial of early aspirin use in 20,000 patients with acute ischemic stroke. Lancet 1997;349:1641–1649.
6. International Stroke Trial Collaborative Group (IST). A randomized trial of aspirin, subcutaneous heparin, both, or neither among 19435 patients with acute ischaemic stroke. Lancet 1997;349:1569–1581.
7. Adams HP Jr, del Zoppo G, Alberts MJ, et al. Guidelines for the early management of adults with ischemic stroke: a guideline from the American Heart Association/American Stroke Association Stroke Council, Clinical Cardiology Council, Cardiovascular Radiology and Intervention Council, and the Atherosclerotic Peripheral Vascular Disease and Quality of Care Outcomes in Research Interdisciplinary Working Groups: the American Academy of Neurology affirms the value of this guideline as an educational tool for neurologists. Circulation 2007;115:e478–e534.
8. Kennedy J, Hill MD, Ryckborst BA, et al. FASTER Investigators. Fast assessment of stroke and transient ischaemic attack to prevent early

recurrence (FASTER): a randomised controlled pilot trial. Lancet Neurol 2007;6:961–969.

9. Bath PM, Iddenden R, Bath FJ. Low-molecular-weight heparins and heparinoids in acute ischemic stroke: a meta-analysis of randomized controlled trials. Stroke 2000;31:1770–1778.
10. CAPRIE Steering Committee. A randomized, blinded, trial of clopidogrel versus aspirin in patients at risk of ischemic events (CAPRIE): CAPRIE Steering Committee. Lancet 1996;348:1329–1339.
11. Yusuf S, Zhao F, Mehta SR, et al., for the Clopidogrel in Unstable Angina to Prevent Recurrent Events Trial Investigators. Effects of clopidogrel in addition to aspirin in patients with acute coronary syndromes without ST-segment elevation. N Engl J Med 2001;345:494–502.
12. Diener HC, Cunha L, Forbes C, et al. European Stroke Prevention Study 2: dipyridamole and acetylsalicylic acid in the secondary prevention of stroke. J Neurol Sci 1996;143:1–13.
13. Sacco RL, Diener HC, Yusuf S, et al. Aspirin and extended-release dipyridamole versus clopidogrel for recurrent stroke. N Engl J Med 2008;359:1238–1251.
14. Chobanian AV, Bakris GL, Black HR, et al., for the National Heart, Lung, and Blood Institute Joint National Committee on Prevention, Detection, Evaluation, and Treatment of High Blood Pressure, National High Blood Pressure Education Program Coordinating Committee. The seventh report of the Joint National Committee on Prevention, Detection, Evaluation, and Treatment of High Blood Pressure: the JNC 7 report. JAMA 2003;289:2560–2571.

# 25

# DYSLIPIDEMIA

I Need Refills . . . . . . . . . . . . . . . . . . . . . . . . . . Level II

**Laurajo Ryan, PharmD, MSc, BCPS, CDE**

## LEARNING OBJECTIVES

After completing this case study, the reader should be able to:

- Identify patients who require treatment for dyslipidemia.
- Stratify individual patients for risk of coronary heart disease (CHD) and stroke.
- Determine appropriate LDL, HDL, triglyceride, total cholesterol, and non-HDL goals based on individual risk factors.
- Recommend a cholesterol management strategy that includes therapeutic lifestyle changes (TLC), drug therapy, patient education, and monitoring parameters.

## PATIENT PRESENTATION

### Chief Complaint

"I need refills."

### HPI

Felecia A. Thorngrass is a 56-year-old woman who presents to pharmacotherapy clinic for intake. She has recently moved to your area, and states she has not seen her primary care provider for the last 11 months. Her prescriptions have expired, and she is coming to you for "refills."

### PMH

Obesity (BMI 31.5 kg/m$^2$)
Dyslipidemia × 4 years
HTN × 15 years
Postmenopausal—has not had GYN screening since onset of menopause (14 years ago)

### FH

Father; age 74 with extensive cardiovascular history, most notably first MI at age 42.
Mother; died at age 61 from MVA, medical history unknown.
Patient has one older sister with hypertension and history of "mini-strokes" and one younger sister with hypertension only.
Her children's medical conditions are noncontributory.

### SH

Patient is married with three children, all of whom live out of state.
College graduate, works as librarian.
Denies current alcohol and tobacco use, but does admit to occasional marijuana use when she is visiting her children.
Began sporadic exercise regimen when diagnosed with dyslipidemia.

### Meds (Per Patient History; She Did Not Bring Records)

Metoprolol tartrate 50 mg po BID
Ezetimibe 10 mg po once daily
Aspirin 81 mg po once daily
Ibuprofen 200 mg, four tablets po PRN leg cramps
Naproxen 220 mg, two tablets po PRN leg cramps
Garlic capsules

### All

"Statin" drugs—states she had occasional leg cramps after starting atorvastatin

### ROS

Patient states that she just needs refills. She is argumentative about getting labs done and cannot understand why you would not just refill her medications. She denies any acute changes in health. She denies unilateral weakness, numbness/tingling, or changes in vision. She denies CP, and only has SOB when she walks in the park. With further questioning you find that she rarely exercises, but when she does go for a walk she typically overdoes it. She denies changes in bowel or urinary habits and states she does not need to have GYN follow-ups anymore, because she has gone through "the change." She denies any lower extremity edema.

### Physical Examination

*Gen*

Obese, somewhat agitated Caucasian woman

*VS*

BP 162/92, P 89, RR 18, T 37.2°C; Wt 94 kg, Ht 5′8″

*Skin*

Warm and dry to touch, normal turgor, (−) for acanthosis nigricans

*HEENT*

PERRLA; EOMI; funduscopic exam deferred; TMs intact; oral mucosa clear

*Neck/Lymph Nodes*

Neck supple, no lymphadenopathy, thyroid smooth and firm without nodules

*Chest*

CTA bilaterally, no wheezes, crackles, or rhonchi

*Breasts*

Normal, slightly fibrotic, no lumps or discharge

*CV*

RRR, no MRG, normal $S_1$ and $S_2$; no $S_3$ or $S_4$

*Abd*

(+) BS, no hepatosplenomegaly

*Genit/Rect*

Deferred

*Ext*

No pedal edema, pulses 2+ throughout

*Neuro*

No gross motor–sensory deficits present

### Labs (Fasting)

| | | *Fasting Lipid profile:* |
|---|---|---|
| Na 142 mEq/L | Ca 8.2 mg/dL | TC 240 mg/dL |
| K 4.9 mEq/L | Mg 2.0 mEq/L | HDL 41 mg/dL |
| Cl 103 mEq/L | AST 28 U/L | LDL 163 mg/dL |
| $CO_2$ 23 mEq/L | ALT 31 U/L | TG 183 mg/dL |
| BUN 16 mg/dL | T. bili 0.5 mg/dL | hsCRP 4.6 mg/L |
| SCr 0.9 mg/dL | T. prot 7.1 g/dL | |
| Glucose 105 mg/dL | | |
| Hgb 11.6mg/dL | | |
| Hct 34% | | |

### Assessment

Mrs Thorngrass is an obese Caucasian woman who presents to pharmacotherapy clinic for intake. She has a significant family history of cardiovascular disease. She has uncontrolled hypertension, treated with metoprolol tartrate, and dyslipidemia, treated only with ezetimibe and garlic. She reports an allergy to atorvastatin, but admits that her leg cramps have not improved since discontinuing the drug and coincide with her rare bouts of exercise. She reports liberal use of ibuprofen and naproxen to relieve the cramps. She also has previously undiagnosed anemia.

# QUESTIONS

## Problem Identification

1.a. What drug-related problems does this patient have?

1.b. What laboratory values indicate the presence and severity of dyslipidemia in this patient?

1.c. What are the patient's risk factors (both modifiable and non-modifiable) for cardiovascular disease?

1.d. What is this patient's risk classification for cardiovascular disease, and how does this relate to her individual lipid goals?

## Desired Outcome

2. What are the pharmacologic and nonpharmacologic goals of treatment in this patient?

## Therapeutic Alternatives

3.a. What nonpharmacologic therapies are necessary for this patient to achieve and maintain target cholesterol values?

3.b. What pharmacotherapeutic options are available for controlling this patient's dyslipidemia and preventing future CVD events?

## Optimal Plan

4.a. Design a plan that details specific lifestyle modifications for this patient.

4.b. Develop a specific pharmacotherapeutic regimen for this patient's dyslipidemia and uncontrolled HTN. This regimen should include drugs, dosages, and duration of therapy.

4.c. What options are available if the pharmacotherapy regimen you chose fails, or if she develops an adverse drug reaction?

## Outcome Evaluation

5. Based on your treatment regimen, what are the monitoring parameters for each pharmacologic agent selected?

## Patient Education

6.a. Based on your recommendations, provide appropriate education to this patient regarding pharmacologic and nonpharmacologic treatments.

6.b. What steps can you take to ensure that patient is successful in implementing nonpharmacologic measures?

# CLINICAL COURSE: ALTERNATIVE THERAPY

Mrs Thorngrass is already taking garlic capsules, but she is not sure about the type or dose. Because you are making changes to her current prescription regimen, you need to investigate the advisability of continuing the garlic. If Mrs Thorngrass does begin a statin drug as indicated, she would not be able to take red yeast rice (duplicative therapy because of mevacolin K content, a lovastatin analog). Would fish oil be a possible option for her? See Section 19 in this casebook for questions about the use of garlic and fish oil (omega-3 fatty acids) for treatment of dyslipidemia.

# SELF-STUDY ASSIGNMENTS

1. Describe how this patient's other drug/disease interactions issues that are unrelated to dyslipidemia should be managed.
2. What changes, if any, you would make to the pharmacotherapy regimen for this patient if she had presented at the initial visit with each of the following characteristics:
   - Childbearing age
   - Cirrhosis of the liver
   - Renal disease
   - Significant alcohol use

## CLINICAL PEARL

Rosuvastatin has been FDA-approved to decrease risk of stroke, MI, and need for revascularization procedures in men and women without evidence of CHD and normal LDL, if they are considered to be at increased risk based on age, elevated hsCRP, and one or more additional risk factors.

## REFERENCES


1. Ridker PM, Danielson E, Fonseca FA, et al. Rosuvastatin to prevent vascular events in men and women with elevated C-reactive protein. N Engl J Med 2008;359:2195–2207.
2. Third report of the National Cholesterol Education Program (NCEP) Expert Panel on Detection, Evaluation, and Treatment of High Blood Cholesterol in Adults (Adult Treatment Panel III) final report. Circulation 2002;106:3143–3421.
3. Grundy SM, Cleeman JI, Merz CNB, et al. Implications of recent clinical trials for the National Cholesterol Education Program Adult Treatment Panel III guidelines. Circulation 2004;110:227–239.
4. Lichtenstein AH, Appel LJ, Brands M, et al. Diet and lifestyle recommendations revision 2006: a scientific statement from the American Heart Association Nutrition Committee. Circulation 2006;114: 82–96.
5. Kastelein JJ, Akdim F, Stroes ES, et al. Simvastatin with or without ezetimibe in familial hypercholesterolemia. N Engl J Med 2008; 358:1431–1443.
6. Mosca L, Banka CL, Benjamin EJ, et al. Evidence-based guidelines for cardiovascular disease prevention in women: 2007 update. Circulation 2007;115:1481–1501.
7. Ridker PM, Cook NR, Lee IM, et al. A randomized trial of low-dose aspirin in the primary prevention of cardiovascular disease in women. *N Engl J Med* 2005;352:1293–1304.


# 26

# PERIPHERAL ARTERIAL DISEASE

Cold Feet? . . . . . . . . . . . . . . . . . . . . . . . . . . . . . Level II

**Tracy L. Sprunger, PharmD, BCPS**

## LEARNING OBJECTIVES

After completing this case study, the reader should be able to:

- Identify risk factors for peripheral arterial disease (PAD).
- Describe the symptoms and diagnosis of PAD.
- Recommend appropriate nonpharmacologic strategies for PAD, including risk factor modification, exercise, and revascularization.
- Design an appropriate pharmacologic treatment plan for a patient with PAD.
- Provide appropriate education to a patient with PAD.

## PATIENT PRESENTATION

### Chief Complaint

"I am having pain in both legs and in my left foot."

### HPI

Angie Belden is a 47-year-old woman with a history of hypertension, diabetes, stroke, hypothyroidism, dyslipidemia, and a history of bilateral leg weakness for the previous year. She reports to her primary care provider today with increased numbness and weakness when she walks. She reports that it is painful to walk even for 4–5 minutes and that her legs are often weak and "give out." She is concerned because she lives alone and is responsible for walking her beloved Labrador retriever, Jules. Her symptoms tend to get better when she is able to rest and prop her feet up. She would also like a "check-up" on her other chronic conditions as well.

### PMH

HTN
Diabetes
Stroke
Hypothyroidism
Dyslipidemia

### FH

Mother died of a stroke at age 67, father died of pneumonia at the age of 62.

### SH

Works as a biller in a dentist's office; has one child; lives alone; smokes 1 ppd × 25 years; denies ETOH and illicit drug use; has one dog in home

### Meds

Atenolol 50 mg po daily
Clopidogrel 75 mg po daily
Gabapentin 600 mg po TID
Hydrocodone/acetaminophen 7.5/500 mg q 6 hours PRN pain
Levothyroxine 75 mcg po daily
Metformin 1,000 mg po BID
Simvastatin 40 mg po daily

### All

NKDA

### ROS

Complains of dyspnea on exertion, lower extremity muscle aches, and muscle weakness. Denies chest pains, palpitations, syncope, and orthopnea. Denies nausea, vomiting, diarrhea, constipation, change in bowel habits, abdominal pain, or melena. Denies transient paralysis, seizures, syncope, and tremors.

### Physical Examination

*Gen*

The patient is a pleasant woman in NAD. She appears older than her stated age.

*VS*

BP 149/87, P 73, RR 17, T 98.2°F; Wt 85 kg, Ht 5′4″

*Skin*

Distal to mid shin with shiny-appearing skin, skin atrophy, and lack of hair growth. No evidence of skin breakdown or ulceration.

*HEENT*

PERRLA; conjunctivae and lids normal; TM intact; normal dentition, no gingival inflammation, no labial lesions; tongue normal, posterior pharynx without erythema or exudate

*Neck/Lymph Nodes*

Supple, no masses, trachea midline; no carotid bruit; no lymphadenopathy or thyromegaly

*Lungs/Thorax*

No rales, rhonchi, or wheezes; no intercostal retractions or use of accessory muscles

*CV*

RRR, $S_1$, $S_2$ normal; no murmurs, rubs, or gallops; no thrill or palpable murmurs, no displacement of PMI

*Abd*

Soft, nontender, no masses, bowel sounds normal; no enlargement or nodularity of liver or spleen

*Genit/Rect*

Deferred

*MS/Ext*

Normal gait; no clubbing, cyanosis, petechiae, or nodes; normal ROM and strength, good stability, and no joint enlargement or tenderness; pedal pulses 1+, symmetric

*Neuro*

CN II–XII grossly intact; DTRs 2+, no pathologic reflexes; sensory and motor levels intact

### Labs

| | | |
|---|---|---|
| Na 137 mEq/L | Hgb 12.7 g/dL | WBC $6.3 \times 10^3$/mm$^3$ |
| K 3.9 mEq/L | Hct 34.4% | CPK 71 IU/L |
| Cl 97 mEq/L | Plt $313 \times 10^3$/mm$^3$ | AST 22 U/L |
| $CO_2$ 24 mEq/L | TSH 1.12 mIU/L | ALT 30 U/L |
| BUN 12 mg/dL | TC 224 mg/dL | |
| SCr 1.0 mg/dL | TG 220 mg/dL | |
| Glu 99 mg/dL | LDL 140 mg/dL | |
| A1C 6.3% | HDL 40 mg/dL | |

Lower extremity arterial Doppler; ankle–brachial index (ABI)—right: 0.53; left: 0.62

### Assessment

A 47-year-old woman with a significant smoking history presents with uncontrolled hypertension, dyslipidemia, and new symptoms of intermittent claudication (IC).

## QUESTIONS

### Problem Identification

1.a. Create a list of this patient's drug-related problems.

1.b. What information presented in this case supports the diagnosis of IC?

1.c. Identify this patient's risk factors for PAD.

### Desired Outcome

2. What are the goals of therapy for IC in this case?

### Therapeutic Alternatives

3.a. Does this patient have any modifiable risk factors for PAD? If so, what are your recommendations for these conditions?

3.b. What pharmacologic options are available for the treatment of this patient's PAD?

3.c. What treatment options are available to patients who have severe disease or fail pharmacologic therapy?

### Optimal Plan

4. What drug, dose, and schedule would be most appropriate for treating this patient's IC and concomitant disease states?

### Outcome Evaluation

5. Based on your recommendations, what clinical and laboratory parameters are necessary to evaluate the therapy for achievement of the desired therapeutic outcome and to detect or prevent adverse effects?

### Patient Education

6. What information should be provided to the patient to enhance adherence, ensure successful therapy, and minimize adverse effects?

## SELF-STUDY ASSIGNMENTS

1. Review the recommendations for dual antiplatelet therapy for the treatment of PAD. Would a patient benefit from aspirin plus clopidogrel or an aspirin/dipyridamole combination?
2. Review the literature on the use of herbal medications in the treatment of PAD. What are your recommendations to a patient inquiring about their use?
3. Perform a literature search to determine the role of warfarin for the management of PAD.

## CLINICAL PEARL

Although cilostazol has antiplatelet effects, it is currently not recommended for the prevention of atherosclerotic events or the treatment of atherosclerotic disease.

## REFERENCES


1. Chobanian AV, Bakris GL, Black HR, et al. The seventh report of the Joint National Committee on Prevention, Detection, Evaluation, and Treatment of High Blood Pressure: the JNC 7 report. JAMA 2003;289:2560–2572.
2. Rosendorff C, Black HR, Cannon CP, et al. Treatment of hypertension in the prevention and management of ischemic heart disease: a scientific statement from the American Heart Association Council for High Blood Pressure Research and the Councils on Clinical Cardiology and Epidemiology and Prevention. Circulation 2007:115; 2761–2788.
3. Hirsch AT, Haskal ZJ, Hertzer NR, et al. ACC/AHA guidelines for the management of patients with peripheral arterial disease (lower extremity, renal, mesenteric, and abdominal aortic): executive summary a collaborative report from the American Association for Vascular Surgery, Society for Cardiovascular Angiography and Interventions, Society of Interventional Radiology, Society for Vascular Medicine and Biology, and the ACC/AHA Task Force on Practice Guidelines. J Am Coll Cardiol 2006;47:1239–1312.
4. White C. Intermittent claudication. N Engl J Med 2007;356:1241–1250.
5. Gornick HL, Creager MA. Contemporary management of peripheral arterial disease: cardiovascular risk-factor modification. Cleve Clin J Med 2006;73:S30–S37.
6. CAPRIE Steering Committee. A randomized, blinded, trial of clopidogrel vs. aspirin in patients at risk of ischaemic events (CAPRIE). Lancet 1996;348:1329–1339.
7. Dawson DL, Cutler BS, Meissner MH, Strandness DE. Cilostazol has beneficial effects in treatment of intermittent claudication: results from a multicenter, randomized, prospective, double-blind trial. Circulation 1998;98:678–686.

# 27

# HYPOVOLEMIC SHOCK

A Glass Half Full . . . . . . . . . . . . . . . . . . . . . . . Level II

Brian L. Erstad, PharmD, FCCP, FCCM, FASHP

## LEARNING OBJECTIVES

After completing this case study, the reader should be able to:

- Develop a plan for implementing fluid or medication therapies for treating a patient in the initial stages of shock.
- Outline the major parameters used to monitor hypovolemic shock and its treatment.
- List the major disadvantage of using isolated hemodynamic recordings, such as blood pressure measurements, for monitoring the progression of shock.
- Compare and contrast fluids and medications used for treating hypovolemic shock.

## PATIENT PRESENTATION

### Chief Complaint

"I'm beat. I have vomited four times in the last 24 hours and had diarrhea last evening. Now is not a great time to get sick since I'm in college and have finals next week."

### HPI

Four days PTA, Mr Hobbs had abdominal pain that he attributed to a flare-up in his Crohn's disease due to the stress of final examinations. He has an infliximab infusion scheduled for next week; he has them every 8 weeks and does not miss these infusions. However, he admits that he forgets to take his oral medications now that he lives away from his family. When he has Crohn's pain, he does not feel like eating since eating causes more stomach pain. Furthermore, he has vomiting and diarrhea, which is aggravated by food intake. Per the recommendation of his community pharmacist, Mr Hobbs purchased a commercially available rehydration solution and attempted to drink the small but frequent volumes recommended by his pharmacist, but he could not keep up with fluid losses. His primary care physician referred this 20-year-old college student to the local hospital for rehydration and further evaluation.

### PMH

Crohn's disease, diagnosed 4 years ago
Ankylosing spondylitis, diagnosed 3 years ago
Pulmonary coccidiodomycosis (small ill-defined mass in lungs with positive cocci titers), diagnosed 1 year ago

### FH

Noncontributory

### SH

Does not smoke or use illicit drugs; admits to occasional ETOH use at parties

### Meds

Infliximab 300 mg by IV infusion over 3 hours every 8 weeks
Azathioprine 100 mg po daily
Fluconazole 200 mg po BID
Fish oil (unknown strength) one capsule po BID
Multivitamin one tablet po daily
Whey shakes for protein supplementation, one shake po daily

### All

NKDA

### ROS

Patient has had a recent increase in weight over the past month (6 kg), although this has decreased by 2 kg in the past few days. Hearing is intact with no vertigo. No dizziness or fainting episodes. Colorless sputum. No chest pain or dyspnea, but heart has been "racing." Has had one episode of diarrhea and four episodes of vomiting with abdominal pain in the past 24 hours. No musculoskeletal pain or cramping.

### Physical Examination

*Gen*

Thin, somewhat anxious man in mild distress

*VS*

BP 84/58 (baseline 122/78), but possible orthostatic changes not determined, HR 132 (baseline 80), RR 16, T 38.2°C; admission Wt 60 kg, Ht 5′10″

*Skin*

Pale color (including nail beds) and dry, but not cyanotic; no lesions

*HEENT*

Normal scalp/skull; conjunctivae pale and dry with clear sclerae; PERRLA, dry oral mucosa; remainder of ophthalmologic exam not performed

*Neck/Lymph Nodes*

Supple, no lymphadenopathy or thyromegaly

*Lungs/Thorax*

Clear by palpation and auscultation

*CV*

RRR; $S_1$ and $S_2$ normal; apical pulse difficult to palpate; no MRG

*Abd*

Perigastric pain on light palpation, no hepatosplenomegaly or masses; bowel sounds present

*Genit/Rect*

Normal male genitalia; prostate smooth, not enlarged; no hemorrhoids noted; stool heme (–)

*MS/Ext*

No deformities with normal ROM of joints except for hips and knees (somewhat limited ROM); no edema, ulcers, or tenderness

*Neuro*

Mild muscular atrophy with weak grip strength; CN II–XII intact; 2+ reflexes throughout; Babinski downgoing

### Labs

| | | |
|---|---|---|
| Na 149 mEq/L | Hgb 11.9 g/dL | Phos 2.9 mg/dL |
| K 3.3 mEq/L | Hct 34.3% | AST 35 IU/L |
| Cl 112 mEq/L | Plt 151 × $10^3$/mm$^3$ | ALT 23 IU/L |
| $CO_2$ 30 mEq/L | WBC 13 × $10^3$/mm$^3$ | T. bili 1.1 mg/dL |
| BUN 32 mg/dL | PT 12.1 sec | Alk phos 83 IU/L |
| SCr 1.4 mg/dL[a] | PTT 33 sec | CRP 16 mg/dL |
| Glu 105 mg/dL | Albumin 3.3 g/dL | ESR 48 mm/h |
| [a]Baseline SCr 1.1 mg/dL | Prealbumin 12 mg/dL | |

### Other Test Results

CXR negative. I/O 1,200/75 (urinary catheter) for first 3 hours of hospitalization. Results pending for blood and urine cultures, gastroenteric pathogens on stool culture, O & P, and *Clostridium difficile* titer. ABGs and synthetic ACTH adrenal stimulation testing pending.

### Assessment

Volume depletion, possible infectious process, malnutrition

# QUESTIONS

## Problem Identification

1.a. Create a list of the patient's drug-related problems.

1.b. What information (signs, symptoms, laboratory values) indicates the presence or severity of hypovolemic shock?

## Desired Outcome

2. What are the goals of pharmacotherapy in this case?

## Therapeutic Alternatives

3.a. What nondrug therapies might be useful for this patient?

3.b. What feasible pharmacotherapeutic alternatives are available for treatment of shock and the associated laboratory alterations?

## Optimal Plan

4. What drug, dosage form, dose, schedule, and duration of therapy are best for this patient?

## Outcome Evaluation

5. What clinical and laboratory parameters are necessary to evaluate the therapy for achievement of the desired therapeutic outcome and to detect or prevent adverse events?

## Patient Education

6. What information should be provided to the patient to enhance adherence, ensure successful therapy, and minimize adverse effects?

## CLINICAL COURSE

No evidence of infection was found, including a negative titer for *C. difficile*. All cultures were negative, and the elevated temperature abated within 12 hours of admission. However, the patient had a complicated clinical course since inadequate nonisotonic fluids were given early in his hospital course. After approximately 10 days, the patient had to be admitted to the ICU for renal failure precipitated by inadequate vascular expansion.

## FOLLOW-UP QUESTION

1. Explain why hypotonic IV fluids such as 5% dextrose are not indicated in a patient with overt hypovolemia who is going into shock.

## SELF-STUDY ASSIGNMENTS

1. Search the literature and be able to discuss the results of comparative trials involving crystalloids and colloids for plasma expansion.
2. Write a two-page report that compares the advantages and limitations of each type of fluid for the plasma expansion indication.

## CLINICAL PEARL

Isotonic or near-isotonic IV crystalloid solutions are indicated in patients with extracellular fluid depletion who cannot receive oral rehydration solutions due to the severity of presentation or inability to absorb adequate volumes. Isotonic solutions replenish the extracellular space and have minimal intracellular distribution.

## REFERENCES

1. Brunkhorst FM, Engel C, Bloos F, et al. Intensive insulin therapy and pentastarch resuscitation in severe sepsis. N Engl J Med 2008;358: 125–139.
2. Choi PT, Yip G, Quinonez LG, Cook DJ. Crystalloids vs. colloids in fluid resuscitation: a systematic review. Crit Care Med 1999;27: 200–210.
3. Finfer S, Bellomo R, Boyce N, French J, Myburgh J, Norton R. SAFE Study Investigators. A comparison of albumin and saline for fluid resuscitation in the intensive care unit. N Engl J Med 2004;350: 2247–2256.

SECTION 3
# RESPIRATORY DISORDERS

# 28

## ACUTE ASTHMA

A Little Influenza, a Big Asthma Attack . . . . . . Level I

**Jennifer A. Donaldson, PharmD**

### LEARNING OBJECTIVES

After completing this case study, the reader should be able to:

- Recognize the signs and symptoms of an acute asthma exacerbation.
- Formulate therapeutic endpoints based on the initiation of a pharmacotherapy plan used to treat the acute asthma symptoms.
- Identify appropriate dosage form selection based on the patient's age, ability to take medication, or adherence to technique.
- Determine an appropriate home pharmacotherapy plan, including discharge counseling, as the patient nears discharge from a hospital setting.

### PATIENT PRESENTATION

#### Chief Complaint

"My daughter has had a bad fever, and now she is having trouble breathing and albuterol doesn't help."

#### HPI

Terri Collins is an 8-year-old African-American girl who presents to the emergency department with a 2-day history of fevers, malaise, and nonproductive cough. The mother gave acetaminophen and ibuprofen to help control the fever. Mother stated that "a lot of other kids in her class have been sick this fall, too." Terri started having trouble breathing the morning of admission, and the mother gave her albuterol, 2.5 mg via nebulization twice within an hour. Terri still sounded wheezy to the mother after the albuterol, and Terri stated it was "hard to breath." Terri was previously well controlled regarding asthma symptoms. Previous clinic notes reported symptoms during the day only with active play at school or at home and rare nighttime symptoms. She uses prn albuterol to help with symptoms after playing. Her assessment in the emergency department revealed Terri to have labored breathing, such that she could only complete four- to five-word sentences. She had subcostal retractions, tracheal tugging with tachypnea at 54 breaths/min. Her other vital signs were a heart rate of 160 beats/min, blood pressure of 115/59, temperature of 38.8°C, and a weight of 22.7 kg. The initial oxygen saturation was 88%, and she was started on oxygen at 3 L/min via nasal cannula. Bilateral expiratory and inspiratory wheezes were noted on examination. A chest x-ray revealed a right lower lobe consolidation consistent with pneumonia and possible effusion. After receiving three albuterol/ipratropium nebulizations, her breath sounds and oxygenation did not improve, so she was started on hourly albuterol nebulizations at 5 mg. She was also given a dose of 25 mg IV methylprednisolone and a dose of 600 mg IV magnesium sulfate. Terri was then transferred to the Pediatric Intensive Care Unit for further treatment and monitoring.

#### PMH

Asthma, last hospitalization 4 years ago, and last course of oral corticosteroids over a year ago

#### FH

Asthma on dad's side of the family

#### SH

Lives with mother, father, and two siblings, both of whom have asthma. There are two cats and a dog in the home. Father is a smoker, but states that he tries to smoke outside and not around the kids. She is in the second grade and is very active on the playground.

#### Meds

Albuterol 2.5 mg nebulized Q 4–6 h PRN wheezing
Fluticasone 44 mcg MDI two puffs BID
Acetaminophen 160 mg/5 mL—10 mL PRN fever
Ibuprofen 100 mg/5mL—10 mL PRN fever

#### All

NKA

#### ROS

(+) Fever, cough, increased work of breathing

#### Physical Examination

*Gen*

Alert and oriented but in mild distress with difficulty breathing

*VS*

BP 125/69, P 120, T 37.9°C, R 40, $O_2$ sat 94% on 3 L/min nasal cannula

*Skin*

No rashes, no bruises

*HEENT*

NC/AT, PERRLA

*Neck/LN*

Soft, supple, no cervical lymphadenopathy

*Chest*

Wheezes throughout all lung fields, still with subcostal retractions

*CV*

RRR, no m/r/g

*Abd*

Soft, NT/ND

*Ext*

No clubbing or cyanosis

*Neuro*

A & O, no focal deficits

### Labs

| | |
|---|---|
| Na 141 mEq/L | WBC 34.2 × $10^3$/mm$^3$ |
| K 3.1 mEq/L | Neut 91% |
| Cl 104 mEq/L | Lymph 5% |
| $CO_2$ 29 mEq/L | Mono 4% |
| BUN 16 mg/dL | RBC 5.07 × $10^6$/mm$^3$ |
| SCr 0.52 mg/dL | Hgb 13 g/dL |
| Glu 154 mg/dL | Hct 41% |
| | Plt 310 × $10^3$/mm$^3$ |

Respiratory viral panel nasal swab: positive for influenza A (probably H1N1 strain)

### Chest X-Ray

RLL consolidation

### Assessment

Asthma exacerbation with viral pneumonia

## QUESTIONS

### Problem Identification

1.a. Create a list of the patient's drug-related problems.

1.b. What information (signs, symptoms, laboratory values) indicates the severity of the acute asthma attack?

### Desired Outcome

2. What are the acute goals of pharmacotherapy in this case?

### Therapeutic Alternatives

3.a. What nondrug therapies might be useful for this patient?

3.b. What feasible pharmacotherapeutic alternatives are available for the treatment of acute asthma?

### Optimal Plan

4.a. What drug, dosage form, dose, schedule, and duration of therapy are best for this patient's acute asthma exacerbation?

4.b. What other pharmacotherapy would you recommend in the acute treatment of this patient?

## CLINICAL COURSE

Within 48 hours of initiation of the treatment plan for management of the acute exacerbation, Terri was stable enough to transfer to the general pediatric floor. Her vital signs were BP 103/70, P 82, R 35, T 37.2°C, and $O_2$ sat 99% on 1 L/min nasal cannula. Mother states that she is able to speak in full sentences now and no longer seems to have trouble breathing.

4.c. What drug, dosage form, dose, schedule, and duration of therapy are best for this patient's discharge plan?

### Outcome Evaluation

5.a. Once the patient has transferred to the general medical floor and her vitals have improved (see the section "Clinical Course"), what clinical and laboratory parameters are necessary to evaluate the therapy for achievement of the desired therapeutic outcome and to detect or prevent adverse effects at that point in the patient's care?

5.b. What clinical parameters are necessary to evaluate the efficacy of the patient's asthma therapy after hospital discharge?

### Patient Education

6.a. What should the family monitor for regarding the potential adverse effects from the drug therapy, and how should they be counseled on the use of the asthma medications, especially regarding the differences between quick-relief and controller medications?

6.b. Describe the information that should be provided to the family regarding medication delivery technique and possible asthma triggers.

## FOLLOW-UP QUESTIONS

1. Should any cough and cold products be used for asthma symptoms? Why or why not?
2. What information should be given to patients/families regarding influenza?
3. What information can be given to families who are concerned about giving their child "steroids" for asthma treatment (either in an acute asthma exacerbation or for controller therapy)?

## SELF-STUDY ASSIGNMENTS

1. Research the efficacy of systemic corticosteroids for treatment of acute asthma exacerbation when given intravenously versus orally (enterally).
2. Discuss the differences in acute asthma exacerbation symptoms in an adult patient versus a pediatric patient, and describe when you would refer a patient (or family) to the physician or emergency department based on an individualized asthma action plan.
3. Discuss the appropriate use of intravenous magnesium in an acute asthma exacerbation.

## CLINICAL PEARL

For proper treatment of an acute asthma exacerbation, the patient (or family) needs to be aware of the first symptoms of an exacerbation and possible triggers. At this point, the patient (family) should initiate their asthma action plan to minimize the symptoms, duration of drug therapy, and severity of the exacerbation. This, in turn, should decrease the number of severe exacerbations and hospital admissions.

## REFERENCES


1. National Asthma Education and Prevention Program Expert Panel report 3: guidelines for the diagnosis and management of asthma. Bethesda, MD, National Institutes of Health, 2007. Available at: *http://www.nhlbi.nih.gov/guidelines/asthma/asthgdln.htm*. Accessed March 16, 2010.
2. Aldington S, Beasley R. Asthma exacerbations 5: assessment and management of severe asthma in adults in hospital. Thorax 2007;62:447–458.
3. Andrew T, McGintee E, Mittal MK, et al. High-dose continuous nebulized levalbuterol for pediatric status asthmaticus: a randomized trial. J Pediatr 2009;155:205–210.
4. Rodrigo GJ, Castro-Rodriguez JA. Anticholinergics in the treatment of children and adults with acute asthma: a systematic review with meta-analysis. Thorax 2005;60:740–746.
5. Rowe BH, Camargo CA. The role of magnesium sulfate in the acute and chronic management of asthma. Curr Opin Pulm Med 2008;15:70–76.
6. Cheuk DKL, Chau TCH, Lee SL. A meta-analysis on intravenous magnesium sulphate for treating acute asthma. Arch Dis Child 2005;90:74–77.
7. Hendeles L. Selecting a systemic corticosteroid for acute asthma in young children. J Pediatr 2003;142:S40–S44.
8. Rank MA, Li JT. Clinical pearls for preventing, diagnosing, and treating seasonal and 2009 H1N1 influenza infections in patients with asthma. J Allergy Clin Immunol 2009;124:1123–1126.


# 29

# CHRONIC ASTHMA

## Cat Got Your Tongue? . . . . . . . . . . . . . . . . . . Level II

**Julia M. Koehler, PharmD, FCCP**

**Carrie Maffeo, PharmD, BCPS, CDE**

## LEARNING OBJECTIVES

After completing this case study, the reader should be able to:

- Recognize signs and symptoms of uncontrolled asthma.
- Identify potential causes of uncontrolled asthma.
- Formulate a patient-specific therapeutic plan (including drugs, route of administration, and appropriate monitoring parameters) for management of a patient with chronic asthma.
- Develop a self-management action plan for improving control of asthma.

## PATIENT PRESENTATION

### Chief Complaint

"Please don't tell me we have to get rid of the cats!"

### HPI

Shiloh Eddingfield is a 17-year-old girl who presents to her primary care physician for follow-up and evaluation regarding her asthma. During her visit, she reports having had to use her albuterol MDI approximately three to four times per week over the past 2 months, but over the past week she admits to using albuterol once daily. She reports being awakened by a cough three times over the past month. She states she especially becomes short of breath when she exercises, although she admits that her shortness of breath is not always brought on by exercise and sometimes occurs when she is not actively exercising. In addition to her albuterol MDI, which she uses PRN, she also has a fluticasone MDI, which she uses "most days of the week." She indicates that her morning peak flows have been running around 300 L/min (personal best = 400 L/min) over the past several weeks.

### PMH

Asthma (previously documented as "mild persistent") diagnosed at age 7; no prior history of intubations; hospitalized twice in the past year for poorly controlled asthma; three visits to the ED in the past 6 months; treated with oral systemic corticosteroids during both hospitalizations and at each ED visit

Migraine headache disorder (diagnosed at age 15); currently taking prophylactic medication; has had only one migraine attack in the past year

### FH

Mother 47-years old with HTN, migraine HA disorder; father 48-years old (smoker) with HTN and type 2 DM; brother, age 21 (smoker); twin sister, age 17 (nonsmoker)

### SH

No alcohol or tobacco use. Single, sexually active. Lives at home with parents (father is a cabinet maker), twin sister, and two cats. Brother is currently away at college.

### Meds

Fluticasone HFA 44 mcg, two puffs BID
Albuterol HFA two puffs Q 4–6 h PRN shortness of breath
Yaz one po daily
Propranolol 80 mg po BID
Maxalt-MLT 5 mg po PRN acute migraine

### All

PCN (rash)

### Physical Examination

*Gen*

Normal-appearing Caucasian female in NAD complaining of symptoms of shortness of breath throughout the week requiring increased need for albuterol

*VS*

BP 110/68, HR 72, RR 16, T 37°C; Wt 58 kg, Ht 5′5″

*HEENT*

PERRLA; mild oral thrush; TMs intact

*Neck/Lymph Nodes*

Supple; no lymphadenopathy or thyromegaly

*Lungs/Thorax*

Mild expiratory wheezes bilaterally

*Breasts*

Nontender without masses

*CV*

RRR; no MRG

*Abd*

Soft, NTND; (+) BS

*Genit/Rect*

Deferred

*Ext*

Normal ROM; peripheral pulses 3+; no CCE

*Neuro*

No motor deficits; CN II–XII grossly intact; A & O × 3

### Labs

| | | |
|---|---|---|
| Na 136 mEq/L | Hgb 12 g/dL | WBC 6.0 × $10^3$/$mm^3$ |
| K 3.8 mEq/L | Hct 36% | PMNs 56% |
| Cl 99 mEq/L | RBC 5.0 × $10^6$/$mm^3$ | Bands 1% |
| $CO_2$ 27 mEq/L | MCH 28 pg | Eosinophils 3% |
| BUN 18 mg/dL | MCHC 34 g/dL | Basophils 2% |
| SCr 0.6 mg/dL | MCV 90 $\mu m^3$ | Lymphocytes 33% |
| Glu 98 mg/dL | Plts 192 × $10^3$/$mm^3$ | Monocytes 5% |
| Ca 9.3 mg/dL | | |

### Assessment

17 yo girl with uncontrolled chronic asthma and mild oral thrush

# QUESTIONS

## Problem Identification

1.a. Create a list of the patient's drug therapy problems.

1.b. What information indicates the presence of uncontrolled chronic asthma?

1.c. What factors may have contributed to this patient's uncontrolled asthma?

1.d. How would you classify this patient's level of asthma control (well controlled, not well controlled, or very poorly controlled), according to NIH guidelines?

## Desired Outcome

2. What are the goals of pharmacotherapy in this case?

## Therapeutic Alternatives

3.a. What nonpharmacologic therapies might be useful for this patient?

3.b. What feasible pharmacotherapeutic alternatives are available for treatment of this patient's chronic asthma?

## Optimal Plan

4.a. Outline an optimal plan of treatment for this patient's chronic asthma.

4.b. What alternatives would be appropriate if the initial therapy fails?

## Outcome Evaluation

5. What clinical parameters are necessary to evaluate the therapy for achievement of the desired therapeutic effect and to detect or prevent adverse effects?

## Patient Education

6. What information should be provided to the patient regarding the use of her asthma medications, and how can she use her peak flow readings to better manage her disease?

# SELF-STUDY ASSIGNMENTS

1. Review the NIH guidelines on the management of asthma during pregnancy, and develop a pharmacotherapeutic treatment plan for this patient's asthma if she were to become pregnant.
2. Review the literature on the impact of chronic inhaled corticosteroid use on the risk for development of osteoporosis, and write a two-page paper summarizing the available published literature on this topic.

# CLINICAL PEARL

Patients with asthma who report that taking aspirin makes their asthma symptoms worse may respond well to leukotriene modifiers. Aspirin inhibits prostaglandin synthesis from arachidonic acid through inhibition of cyclooxygenase. The leukotriene pathway may play a role in the development of asthma symptoms in such patients, as inhibition of cyclooxygenase by aspirin may shunt the arachidonic acid pathway away from prostaglandin synthesis and toward leukotriene production. Although inhaled corticosteroids are still the preferred anti-inflammatory medications for patients with asthma and known aspirin sensitivity, leukotriene modifiers may also be useful in such patients based on this theoretical mechanism.

# REFERENCES

1. National Asthma Education and Prevention Program. Executive summary of the NAEPP expert panel report 3: guidelines for the diagnosis and management of asthma. Bethesda, MD, U.S. Department of Health and Human Services, Public Health Service, National Institutes of Health, National Heart, Lung, and Blood Institute, 2007. Full report. Available at: *http://www.nhlbi.nih.gov/guidelines/asthma/index.htm*. Accessed July 26, 2010.
2. Global Initiative for Asthma (GINA). Global strategy for asthma management and prevention (updated December 2009), 2009. Available at: *http://www.ginasthma.com*. Accessed July 26, 2010.
3. Lemanske RF, Mauger DT, Sorkness CA, et al. Step-up therapy for children with uncontrolled asthma while receiving inhaled corticosteroids. N Engl J Med 2010; 362: 975–985.
4. Busse W, Raphael GD, Galant S, et al. Fluticasone Propionate Clinical Research Study Group. Low-dose fluticasone propionate compared with montelukast for first-line treatment of persistent asthma: a randomized clinical trial. J Allergy Clin Immunol 2001;107:461–468.
5. Busse W, Nelson H, Wolfe J, Kalberg C, Yancey SW, Rickard KA. Comparison of inhaled salmeterol and oral zafirlukast in patients with asthma. J Allergy Clin Immunol 1999;103:1075–1080.
6. Humbert M, Beasley R, Ayres J, et al. Benefits of omalizumab as addon therapy in patients with severe persistent asthma who are inadequately controlled despite best available therapy (GINA 2002 step 4 treatment): INNOVATE. Allergy 2005;60:309–316.

7. Food and Drug Administration (FDA) 2007. FDA alert: omalizumab (marketed as Xolair) information, February 2007. Available at: *http://www.fda.gov/Drugs/DrugSafety/PostmarketDrugSafetyInformationforPatientsandProviders/ucm103291.htm*. Accessed July 28, 2010.

# 30

# CHRONIC OBSTRUCTIVE PULMONARY DISEASE

## Treading on Thin Air . . . . . . . . . . . . . . . . . . . Level II

**Joseph P. Vande Griend, PharmD, BCPS, CGP**

**Joel C. Marrs, PharmD, BCPS (AQ Cardiology), CLS**

## LEARNING OBJECTIVES

After completing this case study, the reader should be able to:

- Recognize modifiable risk factors for the development of COPD.
- Interpret spirometry readings to evaluate and appropriately stage the severity of COPD for an individual patient.
- Identify the importance of nonpharmacologic therapy in patients with COPD.
- Develop an appropriate medication regimen for a patient with COPD based on disease severity.
- Educate patients on the proper use of inhaled medications, and determine which patients may benefit from spacers and/or holding chambers.

## PATIENT PRESENTATION

### Chief Complaint

"My wife says I need to get my lungs checked. Ever since we moved, I'm having a hard time breathing."

### HPI

Dwayne Morrison is a 59-year-old man who is presenting to a new provider at the family medicine clinic today with complaints of increasing shortness of breath. He points out that he first noticed some difficulty catching his breath at his job 3 years ago. He had been able to carry heavy loads up and down a flight of stairs daily for the last 35 years without any problem. However, his shortness of breath began to make this very difficult. Coincidently at that time, he accepted a managerial position at his company that significantly reduced his activity level. After taking this position, he no longer noticed any problems, but admits that he avoids activities that cause him to physically exert himself. He noticed significant shortness of breath again after he moved to Colorado from a lower elevation 2 months ago to be closer to his grandchildren. His shortness of breath is worst when he is outside playing with his grandchildren. His previous physician had placed him on salmeterol/fluticasone (Advair) one inhalation twice daily 2 years ago. He thinks his physician initiated the medication for the shortness of breath, but he is not entirely sure. He is hoping to get a good medication that will help relieve his shortness of breath because the gardening season is right around the corner and he enjoys this hobby.

### PMH

CAD (MI 7 years ago, resulting in stent placement at that time; additional stent placed 2 years ago; normal ECHO and stress test 3 months ago)
Chronic bronchitis × 8 years (has received antibiotic treatment on multiple occasions over last 3 years)
Cervical radiculopathy

### FH

Father with COPD (smoked a pipe for 40 years). Mother with coronary artery disease and cerebrovascular disease.

### SH

He lives with his wife, who is a nurse. He has a 40 pack-year history of smoking. When he had an MI at age 52, he quit smoking temporarily. At present, he continues to smoke five to six cigarettes per day. He drinks two to three beers most nights of the workweek.

### Meds

Aspirin 81 mg po once daily
Bupropion SR 150 mg twice daily
Clopidogrel 75 mg po once daily
Fluticasone/salmeterol 100/50, one inhalation BID
OTC ibuprofen 200 mg po four to six times daily PRN neck pain
Rosuvastatin 20 mg po once daily

### All

NKDA

### ROS

(+) Chronic cough with sputum production; (+) exercise intolerance

### Physical Examination

*Gen*

WDWN man in NAD

*VS*

BP 110/68, P 60, RR 16, T 37°C; Wt 82 kg, Ht 5′9″

*Skin*

Warm, dry; no rashes

*HEENT*

Normocephalic; PERRLA, EOMI; normal sclerae; mucous membranes are moist; TMs intact; oropharynx clear

*Neck/Lymph Nodes*

Supple without lymphadenopathy

*Lungs*

Decreased breath sounds; no rales, rhonchi, or crackles

*CV*

RRR without murmur; normal $S_1$ and $S_2$

*Abd*

Soft, NT/ND; (+) bowel sounds; no organomegaly

*Genit/Rect*

No back or flank tenderness; normal male genitalia

*MS/Ext*

No clubbing, cyanosis, or edema; pulses 2+ throughout

*Neuro*

A & O × 3; CN II–XII intact; DTRs 2+; normal mood and affect

### Labs

| | | | |
|---|---|---|---|
| Na 135 mEq/L | Hgb 13.5 g/dL | AST 40 IU/L | Ca 9.6 mg/L |
| K 4.2 mEq/L | Hct 41.2% | ALT 19 IU/L | Mg 3.6 mg/L |
| Cl 108 mEq/L | Plt 195 × $10^3$/mm$^3$ | T. bili 1.1 mg/dL | Phos 2.9 mg/dL |
| $CO_2$ 26 mEq/L | WBC 5.4 × $10^3$/mm$^3$ | Alb 3.8 g/dL | |
| BUN 19 mg/dL | Pulse Ox 93% (RA) | | |
| SCr 1.1 mg/dL | | | |
| Glu 89 mg/dL | | | |

### Pulmonary Function Tests (During Clinic Visit Today)

Prebronchodilator $FEV_1$ = 2.98 L (predicted is 4.02 L)
FVC = 4.5 L
Postbronchodilator $FEV_1$ = 2.75 L

### Assessment

This is a normal-appearing 59 yo man presenting to the clinic with complaints of shortness of breath that is limiting his activity and affecting his quality of life. Given the results of spirometry and patient history, patient has COPD in addition to a history of CAD, daily pain from cervical radiculopathy, and chronic cough. Cardiac pathology as a cause of current symptoms is unlikely, given lack of chest pain and recent normal cardiovascular stress test. The patient states that he is adherent to his medication regimen.

## QUESTIONS

### Problem Identification

1.a. Create a list of this patient's drug-related problems.

1.b. What objective information indicates the presence and severity of COPD?

1.c. What subjective information (e.g., patient history) suggests the diagnosis of COPD in this patient?

1.d. How would you stage this patient's COPD?

### Desired Outcome

2. What are the desired goals of pharmacotherapy for the treatment of COPD in this patient?

### Therapeutic Alternatives

3.a. What nonpharmacologic therapies would be useful to improve this patient's COPD symptoms?

3.b. What pharmacotherapeutic alternatives are available for the treatment of COPD based on the most recent GOLD guideline recommendations?

3.c. Should home oxygen therapy be considered for the patient at this time? Why or why not?

### Optimal Plan

4. Evaluate the patient's current COPD regimen, and develop recommendations to continue or change the current COPD medications at his clinic visit today. Make sure to include specific doses, route, frequency, and duration of therapy.

### Outcome Evaluation

5.a. What clinical parameters will you monitor to assess the COPD pharmacotherapy regimen in this patient?

5.b. What laboratory tests can be performed and how often should they be performed to assess the efficacy of the current COPD regimen as well as progression of the patient's lung disease?

### Patient Education

6. What information should be provided to the patient to enhance adherence, ensure successful therapy, and minimize adverse effects?

## SELF-STUDY ASSIGNMENTS

1. Describe and compare the expectations for deterioration in pulmonary function in patients with COPD who have quit smoking with those who continue smoking. In particular, emphasis should be placed on expected patterns of change in $FEV_1$, FVC, and general health over time in years.
2. Research and describe the appropriate use of inhaled corticosteroids for the management of stable chronic obstructive pulmonary disease. Be able to compare and contrast the benefits and risks of this therapy.

## CLINICAL PEARL

COPD can lead to exercise reconditioning, mood disorders such as depression, progressive muscle loss, and weight loss. A pulmonary rehabilitation program including mandatory exercise training of the muscles used in respiration is recommended for patients with COPD because of the established benefit related to improvements seen in dyspnea symptoms, health-related quality of life, and reduced number of hospital days secondary to exacerbations.

## REFERENCES

1. Global Initiative for Chronic Obstructive Lung Disease. Global strategy for the diagnosis, management, and prevention of chronic obstructive pulmonary disease: executive summary. Updated 2009. Available at: *http://www.goldcopd.com*. Accessed March 10, 2010.
2. American Thoracic Society/European Respiratory Society Task Force. Standards for the diagnosis and management of patients with COPD [Internet]. Version 1.2. New York, American Thoracic Society, 2004. Updated September 8, 2005. Available at: *http://www.thoracic.org/go/copd*. Accessed March 10, 2010.
3. Mahler DA, Wire P, Horstman D, et al. Effectiveness of fluticasone propionate and salmeterol combination delivered via the diskus device in the treatment of chronic obstructive pulmonary disease. Am J Respir Crit Care Med 2002;166:1084–1091.
4. Szafranski W, Cukier A, Ramirez A, et al. Efficacy and safety of budesonide/formoterol in the management of chronic obstructive pulmonary disease. Eur Respir J 2003;21:74–81.
5. Jones PW, Willits LR, Burge PS, Calverley P. Disease severity and the effect of fluticasone propionate on chronic obstructive pulmonary disease exacerbations. Eur Respir J 2003;21:68–73.

6. Calverley P, Pauwels R, Vestbo J, et al. Combined salmeterol and fluticasone in the treatment of chronic obstructive pulmonary disease: a randomized controlled trial. Lancet 2003;361:449–456.
7. Nichols J. Combination inhaled bronchodilator therapy in the management of chronic obstructive pulmonary disease. Pharmacotherapy 2007;27:447–454.
8. Chen AM, Bollmeier SG, Finnegan PM. Long-acting bronchodilator therapy for the treatment of chronic obstructive pulmonary disease. Ann Pharmacother 2008;42:1832–1842.
9. Toogood JH. Helping your patients make better use of MDIs and spacers. J Respir Dis 1994;15:151–166.
10. Package Insert. Spiriva (tiotropium bromide). New York, Boehringer Ingelheim Pharmaceuticals Inc, December 2009.
11. Package Insert. Serevent Diskus (salmeterol xinafoate). North Carolina, GlaxoSmithKline, March 2008.
12. Package Insert. Foradil Aerolizer (formoterol fumarate). New Jersey, Novartis Pharmaceuticals Corporation, June 2006.


# 31

# PULMONARY ARTERIAL HYPERTENSION

Windy Cindy . . . . . . . . . . . . . . . . . . . . . . . . Level II

**Brian C. Sedam, PharmD, BCPS**

## LEARNING OBJECTIVES

After completing this case study, the reader should be able to:

- Determine risk factors for developing pulmonary arterial hypertension.
- Discuss common signs and symptoms associated with pulmonary arterial hypertension.
- List the pharmacologic agents used to treat pulmonary arterial hypertension.
- List the nonpharmacologic agents used to treat pulmonary arterial hypertension.
- Recommend appropriate pharmacologic and nonpharmacologic education for a patient with pulmonary arterial hypertension.

## PATIENT PRESENTATION

### Chief Complaint

"I felt really dizzy and short of breath, and I suddenly passed out on the bathroom floor."

### HPI

Cindy Price is a 32-year-old woman who presents to the ED complaining of episodes of dyspnea and dizziness. While stepping out of the shower this morning, she became very weak and experienced a syncopal episode. She remembers falling to the floor and hitting her head but remembers nothing after that. She was brought to the ED this morning by her sister.

### PMH

Hypertension × 4 years
Diabetes mellitus × 2 years
Asthma (intermittent)

### FH

Father died of heart failure at age of 62. Mother is 57 and was diagnosed with pulmonary hypertension 4 years ago. Cindy is single and lives with her sister (her only sibling).

### SH

Denies tobacco or alcohol use. Admits to heavy cocaine use in her late 20s. Has tried various fad diets (including prescription amphetamines) since she was in college.

### Meds

Hydrochlorothiazide 12.5 mg po Q AM
Glyburide 5 mg po daily with breakfast
Albuterol MDI one to two puffs Q 6 h PRN SOB

### All

NKDA

### ROS

Today, Cindy says she is comfortable at rest but complains of having experienced increased dyspnea, fatigue, and dizziness with her everyday activities for the past 6 months. She says that these symptoms only mildly limit her physical activity and denies experiencing these symptoms at rest. Over the past 2–3 months, she has developed palpitations and noticeable swelling in her ankles. She denies episodes of syncope before this acute incident. Approximately 9 months ago, Cindy was seen by her family doctor for increasing shortness of breath. Her physician believed that her increasing dyspnea was attributed to asthma, so he prescribed an albuterol inhaler for her to use. The patient says that the albuterol inhaler did not improve her shortness of breath.

### Physical Examination

*Gen*

Patient is lying in ED bed and appears to be in moderate distress.

*VS*

BP 128/78, P 120, RR 26, T 37°C; Wt 128 kg, Ht 5′6″, $O_2$ sat 88% on room air

*Skin*

Cool to touch; no diaphoresis

*HEENT*

PERRLA; EOMI; dry mucous membranes; TMs intact

*Neck/Lymph Nodes*

(+) JVD; no lymphadenopathy; no thyromegaly; no bruits

*Lungs/Thorax*

Clear without wheezes, rhonchi, or rales

*Breasts*

Deferred

*CV*

Split $S_2$, loud $P_2$, $S_3$ gallop

*Abd*

Soft; (+) HJR; liver slightly enlarged; normal bowel sounds; no guarding

*Genit/Rect*

Deferred

*MS/Ext*

Full range of motion; 2+ edema to both lower extremities; no clubbing or cyanosis; pulses palpable

*Neuro*

A & O × 3; normal DTRs bilaterally

### Labs

| | | | |
|---|---|---|---|
| Na 138 mEq/L | Hgb 14 g/dL | WBC 8.8 × $10^3$/mm$^3$ | Mg 2.1 mg/dL |
| K 3.8 mEq/L | Hct 40% | Neutros 62% | Ca 8.4 mg/dL |
| Cl 98 mEq/L | RBC 5.1 × $10^6$/mm$^3$ | Bands 2% | BNP 60 pg/mL |
| $CO_2$ 28 mEq/L | Plt 311 × $10^3$/mm$^3$ | Eos 1% | |
| BUN 12 mg/dL | MCV 84 μm$^3$ | Lymphs 32% | |
| SCr 0.9 mg/dL | MCHC 34 g/dL | Monos 3% | |
| Glu 88 mg/dL | | | |

### ECG

Sinus tachycardia (rate 120 bpm); right-axis deviation; ST-segment depression in right precordial leads; tall P waves in leads 2, 3, and aVF

### Chest X-Ray

Cardiomegaly; prominent main pulmonary artery; no apparent pulmonary edema

### Two-Dimensional Echocardiography

Right ventricular and atrial hypertrophy; tricuspid regurgitation; estimated mean pulmonary arterial pressure (mPAP) 55 mm Hg

### Ventilation/Perfusion Scan

Negative for pulmonary embolism

### Pulmonary Function Tests

$FEV_1$ = 1.87 L (61% of predicted)

FVC = 2.10 L (57% of predicted)

$FEV_1$/FVC = 0.89

### Assessment

A 32 yo woman presents with signs/symptoms of pulmonary arterial hypertension (likely familial).

## QUESTIONS

### Problem Identification

1.a. What potential risk factors does this patient have for developing pulmonary arterial hypertension?

1.b. What subjective and objective clinical evidence is suggestive of pulmonary arterial hypertension?

### Desired Outcome

2. What are the initial and long-term goals of therapy in this case?

### Therapeutic Alternatives

3.a. What pharmacologic alternatives are available for the treatment of pulmonary arterial hypertension? Include each medication's role in disease state management/indication, mechanism of action, dose, potential adverse effects, contraindications, significant drug interactions, and monitoring parameters.

3.b. What nonpharmacologic alternatives are available for the treatment of pulmonary arterial hypertension?

## CLINICAL COURSE

After admission into the ED, the patient underwent a right heart catheterization for vasoreactivity testing. The results indicated that after receiving the short-acting vasodilator epoprostenol, the patient did not have significant reductions in mPAP and therefore was deemed a nonresponder. The patient's pulmonologist wants to start the patient on bosentan and asks for your recommendation.

### Optimal Plan

4.a. Design a treatment plan for the initial management of this patient's pulmonary arterial hypertension with bosentan. Include patient-specific information, including dosage form, dose, and schedule. Be sure to evaluate the patient's entire medication regimen.

4.b. After 3 months of bosentan therapy the patient's liver function tests (LFTs) are elevated, so the patient's pulmonologist tells the patient to stop the bosentan for 1 month. It has now been 1 month and the patient returns with normal LFTs. The pulmonologist asks you to recommend an appropriate alternative agent(s), including dosage form, dose, and schedule.

### Outcome Evaluation

5. How should the recommended therapy be monitored for efficacy and adverse effects?

### Patient Education

6. What information should be provided to the patient to enhance compliance, ensure successful therapy, and minimize adverse effects?

## SELF-STUDY ASSIGNMENTS

1. Perform a literature search to determine which medications used for the treatment of PAH have been shown to be safe in pregnancy. Identify the risks associated with pregnancy in female patients with PAH.
2. Use primary and tertiary literature to identify the potential visual side effects associated with oral phosphodiesterase inhibitors. Identify the visual side effect that is a medical emergency.
3. Review primary and tertiary literature to compare the advantages and disadvantages of using the vasodilators epoprostenol, treprostinil, and iloprost for PAH.

## CHAPTER 32

4. Use two different drug information sources to develop a recommendation for transitioning a patient from intravenous epoprostenol to subcutaneous treprostinil.

## CLINICAL PEARL

Calcium channel blockers should only be used in patients with PAH who respond favorably to short-acting vasodilators during right heart catheterization.

## REFERENCES


1. Badesch DB, Abman SH, Simonneau G, et al. Medical therapy for pulmonary hypertension: ACCP evidence-based clinical practice guidelines. Chest 2007;131:1917–1928.
2. Raiesdana A, Loscalzo J. Pulmonary arterial hypertension. Ann Med 2006;38:95–110.
3. McGoon MD, Kane GC. Pulmonary hypertension: diagnosis and management. Mayo Clin Proc 2009;84(2):191–207.
4. McLaughlin VV, McGoon M. Pulmonary arterial hypertension. Circulation 2006;114:1417–1431.
5. Nagaya N. Drug therapy of primary pulmonary hypertension. Am J Cardiovasc Drugs 2004;4:75–85.
6. Archer SL, Michelakis ED. Phosphodiesterase type 5 inhibitors for pulmonary hypertension. N Engl J Med 2009;361:1864–1871.
7. McLaughlin VV, Archer SL, Badesch DB, et al. ACCF/AHA 2009 expert consensus document on pulmonary hypertension: a report of the American College of Cardiology Foundation Task Force on Expert Consensus Documents and the American Heart Association developed in collaboration with the American College of Chest Physicians; American Thoracic Society, Inc.; and the Pulmonary Hypertension Association. J Am Coll Cardiol 2009;53(17):1573–1619.
8. Humbert M, Sitbon O, Simonneau G. Treatment of pulmonary arterial hypertension. N Engl J Med 2004;351:1425–1436.


# 32

# CYSTIC FIBROSIS

Blood, Sweat, Lungs, and Gut . . . . . . . . . . . . Level II

**Kimberly J. Novak, PharmD, BCPS**

## LEARNING OBJECTIVES

After completing this case study, the reader should be able to:

- Identify signs and symptoms of common problems in patients with cystic fibrosis (CF).
- Develop an antimicrobial therapy plan and appropriate monitoring strategy for treatment of an acute pulmonary exacerbation in CF.
- Devise treatment strategies for common complications of drug therapy in patients with CF.
- Provide education on aerosolized medications to patients with CF, including appropriate instructions for dornase alfa and inhaled tobramycin.

## PATIENT PRESENTATION

### Chief Complaint

As reported by patient's father: "My daughter's experiencing shortness of breath, fast breathing, increasing cough and sputum production, and decreased energy, and she has a poor appetite."

### HPI

Jenna O'Mally is a 7-year-old girl with a lifetime history of CF; she was diagnosed with CF at birth after presenting with meconium ileus. She had been doing well until 4 weeks ago, when she developed coldlike symptoms, with a runny nose, dry cough, sore throat, and subjective fever. She was seen at her local pediatrician's office and prescribed a 5-day course of azithromycin suspension 200 mg/5 mL 160 mg (10 mg/kg) po on Day 1 and 80 mg (5 mg/kg) po daily on Days 2–5 for possible pneumonia. After completing the antibiotic course, Jenna was not feeling any better. Father called the pulmonary clinic regarding her symptoms, and Jenna's pulmonologist called in a prescription to a local pharmacy for ciprofloxacin suspension 250 mg/5 mL, 325 mg po BID (~40 mg/kg per day), and prednisolone syrup 15 mg/5 mL, one teaspoonful po twice daily. Father was also instructed to perform three chest physiotherapy sessions (vest treatments) per day and increase her hypertonic saline schedule from once per day to twice daily with her vest treatments. The patient now presents to the pulmonary clinic for a follow-up to her outpatient treatment course. She describes worsening shortness of breath and chest pain, lung and sinus congestion, poor appetite, and severe fatigue. Father reports increasing cough productive of very dark green sputum but no fever. The patient has lost 2 lb since her last clinic visit and has missed 7 days of school. Her oxygen saturation is 88% in clinic in room air, and she was immediately placed on 1 L of $O_2$ by nasal cannula.

### PMH

Significant for seven hospitalizations for acute pulmonary exacerbations of CF and two hospitalizations for distal intestinal obstruction syndrome (DIOS) since her initial neonatal intensive care unit (NICU) stay at birth; last hospitalization was 4 months ago

Sinus surgery × 2, last 1 year ago

Pancreatic insufficiency

Poor nutritional status

Recurrent constipation/DIOS

Pulmonary changes c/w long-standing CF with mild bronchiectasis

Seasonal allergies

Asthma

Broken clavicle previous summer after falling from a tree

ADHD

### FH

Both parents are alive and generally well (father has hypercholesterolemia). Jenna has an older half-brother (age 15) without CF who had a recent bout of gastroenteritis and a younger sister (age 2) with CF who was recently diagnosed with RSV bronchiolitis. Two maternal uncles died at ages 13 and 17 from CF.

### SH

Jenna is in first grade and is enrolled in the gifted program at her school. Family is considering home schooling due to frequent absences in the past school year. Lives with her mother, father, and younger sister approximately 100 miles from the nearest CF center. Her older half-brother visits every other weekend. They have well water and a small mixed-breed family dog; father smokes but only outside of the home. Family is experiencing financial difficulties due to a job layoff and recently lost health insurance. Family is in the process of applying for state Medicaid assistance.

### Meds

Ciprofloxacin suspension 250 mg/5 mL, 325 mg po BID
Prednisolone syrup 15 mg/5 mL, one teaspoonful po BID
Aerosolized tobramycin (TOBI) 300 mg BID via nebulizer (every other month, currently "on")
Albuterol 0.083% 3 mL (one vial) BID via nebulizer with vest therapy (currently using TID)
Dornase alfa (Pulmozyme) 2.5 mg via nebulizer once daily with morning vest therapy
Sodium chloride 7% aerosol (Hyper-Sal) 4 mL via nebulizer once daily with evening vest therapy (currently using BID)
Fluticasone (Flovent HFA) 44 mcg, one puff once daily
Budesonide (Rhinocort AQ) one spray each nostril once daily
Saline nasal rinse (neti pot) daily
Loratadine 5 mg po once daily
Creon 12,000 two caps with meals (1,500 U of lipase/kg/meal) and one cap with snacks and supplement shakes (750 U of lipase/kg/snack)
Omeprazole 20 mg po once daily
Ferrous sulfate 324 mg po BID
ADEK one tablet po once daily
Children's multivitamin with iron one tablet po once daily
Polyethylene glycol 17 g po once daily
Atomoxetine 25 mg po once daily
Ibuprofen 200 mg po three to four times daily as needed for chest pain
Pediasure two cans per day

### All

Codeine (itching), bacitracin cream (rash), strawberries (anaphylaxis)

### ROS

Patient complains of chest pain when coughing and large amounts of expectorated green sputum. Reduced ability to perform usual daily activities and play because of SOB. No current hemoptysis, constipation, vomiting, or abdominal pain. Reports having three to four loose or partially formed stools each day. Patient usually has a large appetite but has not been able to finish a meal for the past week.

### Physical Examination

#### *Gen*

A shy, thin, cooperative, 7 yo girl who has shortness of breath with her oxygen cannula removed during the examination

#### *VS*

BP 100/65, P 144, RR 45, T 37.8°C; Wt 16 kg, Ht 3′10″; oxygen saturation 95% on 1 L of oxygen; 88% in room air

#### *Skin*

Normal tone and color, some eczematous lesions at the elbows

#### *HEENT*

EOMI, PERRLA; nares with dried mucus in both nostrils; sinuses tender to palpation; no oral lesions, but secretions noted in the posterior pharynx

#### *Neck/Lymph Nodes*

Supple; no lymphadenopathy or thyromegaly

#### *Lungs*

Crackles heard bilaterally in the upper lobes greater than in the lower lobes; mild scattered wheezes; chest pain not reproducible with palpation

#### *Breasts*

Tanner Stage I

#### *CV*

Tachycardic, regular rate without murmurs

#### *Abd*

Ticklish during examination; (+) bowel sounds; abdomen soft and supple; mild bloating noted, with palpable stool

#### *Genit/Rect*

Tanner Stage I, deferred internal exam

#### *MS/Ext*

Clubbing noted, with no cyanosis; capillary refill <2 seconds

#### *Neuro*

Jenna is alert and awake though reserved; CNs intact; somewhat uncooperative with the full neurologic examination

### Labs

| | | | |
|---|---|---|---|
| Na 149 mEq/L | Hgb 15.4 g/dL | WBC 16.5 ×μ10³/mm³ | AST 30 IU/L |
| K 4.5 mEq/L | Hct 45.2% | Segs 72% | ALT 20 IU/L |
| Cl 108 mEq/L | MCV 78 μm³ | Bands 10% | LDH 330 IU/L |
| $CO_2$ 34 mEq/L | MCH 31.1 pg | Lymphs 10% | GGT 75 IU/L |
| BUN 18 mg/dL | MCHC 34 g/dL | Monos 2% | T. Prot 7.3 g/dL |
| SCr 0.45 mg/dL | $Ca_i$ 4.6 mEq/L[a] | Eos 6% | Alb 3.1 g/dL |
| Glu 195 mg/dL | Phos 4.6 mEq/L | Mg 2.1 mg/dL | IgE 85 IU/mL |

[a]$Ca_i$, ionized calcium.

### Virology/Serology Results

Respiratory viral antigen panel: negative
Influenza A/B PCRs: negative
*B. pertussis* PCR: negative

### Sputum Culture Results

Organism A: *Pseudomonas aeruginosa*
Sensitive: piperacillin/tazobactam, ticarcillin/clavulanate, cefepime, ceftazidime, meropenem, aztreonam, tobramycin, amikacin
Intermediate: ciprofloxacin
Resistant: gentamicin
Organism B: *Stenotrophomonas maltophilia*
Sensitive: ticarcillin/clavulanate, trimethoprim-sulfamethoxazole, minocycline, moxifloxacin
Resistant: ceftazidime, meropenem, all aminoglycosides
Organism C: *P. aeruginosa*, mucoid strain
Sensitive: piperacillin/tazobactam, ticarcillin/clavulanate, cefepime, ceftazidime, meropenem, aztreonam, tobramycin
Resistant: ciprofloxacin, gentamicin, amikacin
Organism D: *Staphylococcus aureus*
Sensitive: vancomycin, linezolid, trimethoprim-sulfamethoxazole, minocycline
Resistant: nafcillin, cefazolin, clindamycin, erythromycin

Organism E: *Achromobacter xylosoxidans*

Sensitive: piperacillin/tazobactam, ticarcillin/clavulanate, ceftazidime, trimethoprim-sulfamethoxazole, minocycline

Resistant: meropenem, ciprofloxacin, all aminoglycosides

#### PFTs

$FEV_1$ 65% of predicted (baseline 90%); FVC 82% of predicted (baseline 95%)

#### Chest X-Ray

Bronchiectatic and interstitial fibrotic changes consistent with CF

#### High-Resolution Chest CT (HRCT)

Interval worsening of bronchiectasis in all lobes; increased mucus plugging in left lower lobe

#### Sinus CT

Panopacification of ethmoid and maxillary sinuses, possible polyp extending into right nasal passage

#### Assessment

A 7 yo CF patient with failed outpatient management of acute pulmonary exacerbation and sinusitis, also with nutritional failure

## QUESTIONS

### Problem Identification

1.a. Identify this patient's drug-related problems. Include those relating to both her acute medical issue and her chronic CF management.

1.b. What information indicates the disease severity and the need to treat Jenna's acute pulmonary exacerbation pharmacologically?

1.c. Could any of her problems be caused by drug therapy?

### Desired Outcome

2. What are the goals of pharmacotherapy in this case?

### Therapeutic Alternatives

3.a. What nonpharmacologic therapies might be useful for this patient?

3.b. What pharmacotherapeutic alternatives are available for treatment of this patient's acute pulmonary exacerbation?

3.c. What economic and psychosocial considerations are important in this patient's acute and chronic CF management?

### Optimal Plan

4.a. What drugs, dosage forms, doses, schedules, and durations of therapy are best for this patient?

4.b. During the clinical course, serum tobramycin concentrations were drawn around the fourth dose of tobramycin 80 mg (5 mg/kg/dose) IV Q 12 h. Levels are reported as follows:

- Peak: 11.2 mcg/mL collected 1 hour after the end of the 30-minute infusion
- Trough: 0.4 mcg/mL collected 30 minutes before the next scheduled dose

Based on this new information, evaluate her drug therapy. Calculate the true peak (30 minutes after the end of infusion), true trough, elimination rate, half-life, volume of distribution, and clearance (standardized for BSA) of her tobramycin therapy. If necessary, suggest modifications. Assume that the previous doses were administered on time.

4.c. What pharmacologic therapies should be considered for Jenna's chronic CF management?

### Outcome Evaluation

5. What clinical and laboratory parameters are necessary to evaluate the efficacy and safety of therapy for CF exacerbations?

### Patient Education

6. What information should you provide the patient regarding the administration of aerosolized drug therapy? The patient will be going home on aerosolized dornase alfa, hypertonic saline, tobramycin, and albuterol.

7. Where can you obtain information about the patient assistance programs that are available for children, adolescents, and adults with CF on a national and state/local level?

## SELF-STUDY ASSIGNMENTS

1. Investigate the new CF drug therapy aztreonam lysine for inhalation (Cayston) and the unique drug delivery device required for administration (Altera Nebulizer System). How are these products prescribed and dispensed to patients?
2. Research the potential problems associated with the use of very-high-dose pancreatic enzymes in patients with CF. What dosage guidelines should be followed to minimize potential risk? Why did the FDA mandate that these previously unapproved products seek FDA approval?
3. Analyze the role of azithromycin in the chronic medical management of CF. What is/are the proposed mechanism(s) of action of azithromycin in CF management?
4. Review the recommendations for the administration of high-dose ibuprofen in patients with CF. When would you suggest that serum concentrations be drawn, and what levels are thought to be necessary to optimize therapy in a patient with CF?
5. Review the recommendations for use of fluoroquinolones in children. What data support these recommendations?
6. Perform a literature search to determine the progress of gene therapy in CF.

## CLINICAL PEARL

Chronic gastric acid suppression (proton pump inhibitor or histamine-2 receptor antagonist) is often used in CF patients to improve efficacy of pancreatic enzyme replacement therapy regardless of presence of gastroesophageal reflux symptoms. Due to defective bicarbonate transport in the small intestine and subnormal pH, enteric coating may not dissolve consistently in CF patients. Suppression of gastric acid can subsequently raise small intestine pH through mixing of gastrointestinal fluids.

## REFERENCES

1. Konstan MW, Butler SM, Wohl ME, et al. Growth and nutritional indexes in early life predict pulmonary function in cystic fibrosis. J Pediatr 2003;142:624–630.

2. Elkins MR, Robinson M, Rose BR, et al. A controlled trial of long-term inhaled hypertonic saline in patients with cystic fibrosis. N Engl J Med 2006;54:229–240.
3. Yee CL, Duffy C, Gerbino PG, Stryker S, Noel GJ. Tendon or joint disorders in children after treatment with fluoroquinolones or azithromycin. Pediatr Infect Dis J 2002;21:525–529.
4. Moss RB. Long-term benefits of inhaled tobramycin in adolescent patients with cystic fibrosis. Chest 2002;121:55–63.
5. Stevens DA, Moss RB, Kurup VP, et al. Allergic bronchopulmonary aspergillosis in cystic fibrosis—state of the art: cystic fibrosis foundation consensus conference. Clin Infect Dis 2003;37(Suppl 3):S225–S264.
6. Saiman L, Marshall BC, Mayer-Hamblett N, et al. Azithromycin in patients with cystic fibrosis chronically infected with *Pseudomonas aeruginosa*: a randomized controlled trial. JAMA 2003;20:1749–1756.
7. Konstan MW, Byard PJ, Hoppel CL, Davis PB. Effect of high-dose ibuprofen in patients with cystic fibrosis. N Engl J Med 1995;332:848–854.
8. McCoy KS, Quittner AL, Oermann CM, Gibson RL, Retsch-Bogart GZ, Montgomery AB. Inhaled aztreonam lysine for chronic airway *Pseudomonas aeruginosa* in cystic fibrosis. Am J Respir Crit Care Med 2008:178(9):921–928.

# SECTION 4 GASTROINTESTINAL DISORDERS

## 33

## GASTROESOPHAGEAL REFLUX DISEASE

A Burning Question . . . . . . . . . . . . . . . . . . . . . Level II

**Brian A. Hemstreet, PharmD, BCPS**

### LEARNING OBJECTIVES

After completing this case study, students should be able to:

- Describe the clinical presentation of gastroesophageal reflux disease (GERD), including typical, atypical, and alarm symptoms.
- Discuss appropriate diagnostic approaches for GERD, including when patients should be referred for further diagnostic evaluation.
- Recommend appropriate nonpharmacologic and pharmacologic measures for treating GERD.
- Develop a treatment plan for a patient with GERD, including both nonpharmacologic and pharmacologic measures and monitoring for efficacy and toxicity of selected drug regimens.
- Effectively counsel patients with GERD on the proper use of their drug therapy.

### PATIENT PRESENTATION

#### Chief Complaint

"I'm having a lot of heartburn. These pills I have been using have helped a little but it's still keeping me up at night."

#### HPI

Janet Swigel is a 68-year-old woman who presents to the GI clinic with complaints of heartburn four to five times a week over the last 5 months. She also reports some regurgitation after meals. She states that her symptoms are much worse at night, particularly when she goes to bed. She finds that her heartburn worsens and she coughs a lot at night, which keeps her awake. She has had difficulty sleeping over this time period and feels fatigued during the day. She reports no difficulty swallowing food or liquids. She has tried OTC Prevacid 24HR once daily for the last 3 weeks. This has reduced the frequency of her symptoms to 3–4 days per week, but they are still bothering her, and she needs help.

#### PMH

Atrial fibrillation × 12 years
Asthma × 10 years
Type 2 DM × 5 years
HTN × 10 years

#### SH

Patient is married with three children. She is a retired school bus driver. She drinks one to two glasses of wine 4–5 days per week. She does not use tobacco. She has Blue Cross prescription drug coverage.

#### FH

Father died of pneumonia at age 75, mother died at age 68 of gastric cancer.

#### Meds

Diltiazem CD 240 mg po once daily
Metformin 500 mg po twice daily
Aspirin 81 mg po daily
Fluticasone/salmeterol DPI 100/50 one puff twice daily

#### All

Peanuts (hives)

#### ROS

Reports being tired all the time, (–) SOB or hoarseness; (+) cough at night, (+) frequent episodes of heartburn, sometimes after meals, but is worse at night; (–) N/V; (–) BRBPR or dark/tarry stools; (–) dysuria, nocturia, or frequency

#### Physical Examination

*Gen*

Well-developed African-American woman in NAD

*VS*

BP 139/82, P 90, RR 17, T 36°C; Wt 100 kg, Ht 5′7″

*Skin*

No lesions or rashes

*HEENT*

PERRLA; EOMI; moist mucous membranes; intact dentition; oropharynx clear

*Neck/Lymph Nodes*

Trachea midline; (–) thyromegaly; (–) lymphadenopathy; (–) JVD

*Lungs/Thorax*

Mostly CTA bilaterally, some intermittent wheezes

*CV*

Tachycardia with irregularly irregular rhythm; no MRG

*Abd*

Obese; NT/ND; (+) BS; (–) HSM

*Genit/Rect*

Gyn exam deferred; heme (–) brown stool

*MS/Ext*

No CVA tenderness

*Neuro*

A & O × 3, CN II–XII intact, 5/5 upper- and lower-extremity strength bilaterally

### Labs

| | | |
|---|---|---|
| Na 138 mEq/L | Hgb 13 g/dL | AST 21 IU/L |
| K 3.8 mEq/L | Hct 39% | ALT 24 IU/L |
| Cl 108 mEq/L | RBC 4.6 × $10^6$/mm$^3$ | Alk Phos 55 IU/L |
| $CO_2$ 21 mEq/L | Plt 400 × $10^3$/mm$^3$ | *Fasting lipid panel:* |
| BUN 18 mg/dL | WBC 8.7 × $10^3$/mm$^3$ | TC 230 mg/dL |
| SCr 1.3 mg/dL | Neutros 60% | LDL 130 mg/dL |
| FBG 220 mg/dL | Bands 1% | TG 170 mg/dL |
| Ca 8.9 mg/dL | Eos 2% | HDL 42 mg/dL |
| Phos 4.1 mg/dL | Lymphs 32% | |
| | Monos 5% | |
| | A1C 9.0% | |

### EGD

Grade B esophagitis; normal gastric and duodenal mucosa; small hiatal hernia. Biopsy results of esophagus and stomach are negative for atypical cells and *H. pylori*.

### Assessment

A 68-year-old woman presenting with uncontrolled GERD symptoms despite self-treatment with OTC PPI therapy. EGD show erosive esophagitis and a hiatal hernia.

## QUESTIONS

### Problem Identification

1.a. Develop a list of this patient's drug therapy problems.

1.b. Classify the GERD symptoms this patient is experiencing. Are they typical or atypical in nature? Are any alarm symptoms or features present?

1.c. What factors could be contributing to the development of GERD symptoms in this patient?

1.d. If you saw this patient in the community pharmacy setting, what factors would cause you to refer her for further diagnostic evaluation versus recommending empiric drug therapy?

1.e. What are other potential complications of long-standing untreated GERD?

### Desired Outcome

2. Develop a list of pharmacotherapeutic goals for this patient.

### Therapeutic Alternatives

3.a. What lifestyle modifications or nonpharmacologic therapies may improve this patient's GERD symptoms?

3.b. What drug therapies could be used to treat this patient's GERD symptoms?

### Optimal Plan

4. Develop a complete treatment plan for managing this patient's GERD symptoms.

### Outcome Evaluation

5. What parameters should be monitored to assess both the efficacy and toxicity of your selected drug regimen?

### Patient Education

6. How will you educate the patient about her GERD therapy to enhance compliance, minimize adverse effects, and promote successful therapeutic outcomes?

## CLINICAL COURSE

Four weeks later, Mrs Swigel returns to the clinic for follow-up. Her symptoms have greatly improved, but she is considering stopping therapy because she heard that "all sorts of bad side effects" can happen to her. She saw on television that she could get osteoporosis and that she should be taking calcium. Someone told her that she may also develop some "nasty infections." She does not think it is worth staying on the medication. She also states that she sometimes has brief episodes of heartburn after meals and wishes to know if she should take more of her medication to manage these symptoms.

## FOLLOW-UP QUESTIONS

1. Should the patient be placed on calcium and vitamin D supplementation because of her acid-suppressive therapy?
2. How would you address her concerns regarding the potential for developing infections due to acid-suppressive therapy?
3. What recommendations could you give her regarding management of the breakthrough symptoms after meals?

## SELF-STUDY ASSIGNMENTS

1. Surgical intervention is a well-accepted option for treating GERD in certain patients. Conduct a primary literature search and identify two articles that compare surgery with drug therapy for treatment of GERD. What conclusions can you draw from the results of these articles? When is surgery indicated in patients with GERD?
2. Pharmacy practice involves providing care to diverse patient populations. Identify and review tertiary drug references and Internet Web sites that provide educational materials about GERD or its treatment in languages other than English.

## CLINICAL PEARL

PPIs may cause false-negative results in patients undergoing urease-based *H. pylori* testing, such as with the urea breath test or rapid urease test, or stool antigen tests. Ideally, these drugs should be discontinued 2 weeks before performing these diagnostic tests.

## REFERENCES


1. American Gastroenterological Association Institute. Medical position statement on the management of gastroesophageal reflux disease. Gastroenterology 2008;135:1383–1391.

2. American Gastroenterological Association Institute. Technical review on the management of gastroesophageal reflux disease. Gastroenterology 2008;135:1392–1413.
3. Haag S, Andrews JM, Katelaris PH, et al. Management of reflux symptoms with over-the-counter proton pump inhibitors: issues and proposed guidelines. Digestion 2009;80:226–234.
4. Chey WD, Wong BC, Practice Parameters Committee of the American College of Gastroenterology. American College of Gastroenterology guideline on the management of *Helicobacter pylori* infection. Am J Gastroenterol 2007;102:1808–1825.
5. Fennerty MB. The continuum of GERD complications. Cleve Clin J Med 2003;70(Suppl 5):S33–S50.
6. Becher A, El-Serag HB. Mortality associated with gastroesophageal reflux disease and its non-malignant complications: a systematic review. Scand J Gastroenterol 2008;43:645–653.
7. Fass R. Erosive esophagitis and nonerosive reflux disease (NERD): comparison of epidemiologic, physiologic, and therapeutic characteristics. J Clin Gastroenterol 2007;41:131–137.
8. Vakil N. Review article: new pharmacological agents for the treatment of gastroesophageal reflux disease. Aliment Pharmacol Ther 2004;19:1041–1049.
9. Ali T, Roberts DN, Tierney WM. Long-term safety concerns with proton pump inhibitors. Am J Med 2009;122:896–903.

# 34

# PEPTIC ULCER DISEASE

Feel the Burn . . . . . . . . . . . . . . . . . . . . . . . . . . Level II

**Ashley H. Vincent, PharmD, BCPS**

## LEARNING OBJECTIVES

After completing this case study, the reader should be able to:

- List the options for the evaluation and treatment of a patient with symptoms suggestive of peptic ulcer disease (PUD).
- Identify the desired therapeutic outcomes for patients with PUD.
- Identify the factors that guide selection of a *Helicobacter pylori* eradication regimen and improve adherence with the regimen.
- Compare the efficacy of two-, three-, and four-drug *H. pylori* treatment regimens and regimens lasting 7 and 14 days.
- Create a treatment and monitoring plan for a patient diagnosed with PUD, given patient-specific information.

## PATIENT PRESENTATION

### Chief Complaint

"My stomach has been hurting really badly for the past month or so. It seems to get worse at night."

### HPI

Justine Ward is a 67-year-old woman who presents to her primary care physician with complaints of episodic epigastric pain for the past 6 weeks. Her pain is nonradiating. It is sometimes worse with meals, but sometimes eating helps improve the pain. She has been experiencing occasional nausea, bloating, and heartburn. She denies any change in color or frequency of bowel movements. She does not have a history of PUD or GI bleeding. She mentions that she has been having frequent headaches for the past month and has been taking naproxen sodium one to two times daily.

### PMH

CAD × 1 year (s/p Taxus stents × 2)
Hypothyroidism × 22 years
Hyperlipidemia × 10 years
Lactose intolerance × 47 years
Postmenopausal; LMP ~13 years ago

### FH

Her mother died at the age of 75 from lymphoma. Her father is alive and has a history of glaucoma, prostate cancer, and AMI at age 70. She has five siblings who are alive. All siblings have a history of hypertension and hyperlipidemia.

### SH

She is married and has raised three children; she is not employed outside the home. She has never smoked and drinks one to two glasses of wine most days of the week.

### Meds

Plavix 75 mg po daily
Lisinopril 5 mg po daily
Aspirin 325 mg po daily
Synthroid 125 mcg po daily
Simvastatin 40 mg po daily
MVI tablet po daily
Tums 500 mg po PRN stomach pain
Naproxen sodium 220 mg po PRN headache
Lactaid one tablet po PRN dairy product consumption

### All

NKDA

### ROS

Unremarkable except for complaints noted above

### Physical Examination

*Gen*

Slightly overweight woman in moderate distress

*VS*

BP 110/72 left arm (seated), P 99, RR 16 reg, T 37.2°C, Wt 68 kg, Ht 5′3″

*Skin*

Warm and dry

*HEENT*

Normocephalic; PERRLA; EOMI

*Chest*

CTA

*CV*

RRR; $S_1$ and $S_2$ normal; no MRG

*Abd*

Soft; mild epigastric tenderness; (+) BS; no splenomegaly or masses; liver size normal

*Rect*

Nontender; stool heme (+)

*Ext*

Normal ROM; no cyanosis, clubbing, or edema

*Neuro*

CN II–XII intact; A & O × 3

## Labs

| | | |
|---|---|---|
| Na 142 mEq/L | Hgb 10.1 g/dL | Ca 9.5 mg/dL |
| K 4.7 mEq/L | Hct 30% | Mg 2.2 mEq/L |
| Cl 98 mEq/L | Plt 320 × $10^3$/$mm^3$ | Phos 3.8 mg/dL |
| $CO_2$ 30 mEq/L | WBC 7.6 × $10^3$/$mm^3$ | Albumin 5.0 g/dL |
| BUN 8 mg/dL | MCV 72 $\mu m^3$ | |
| SCr 0.7 mg/dL | Retic 0.4% | |
| FBG 92 mg/dL | Fe 48 mcg/dL | |

## Assessment

Suspected PUD

# QUESTIONS

## Problem Identification

1.a. Identify this patient's drug therapy problems.

1.b. What information (signs, symptoms, diagnostic tests, and laboratory values) indicates the presence of PUD?

## CLINICAL COURSE (PART 1)

Justine's PCP referred her for a nonemergent EGD, which revealed a 5.5-mm superficial ulcer in the superior duodenum (Fig. 34-1). The ulcer base was clear and without evidence of active bleeding. In addition, inflammation of the duodenum was detected and biopsied. Refer to Table 34-1 for the characteristics of common causes of PUD.

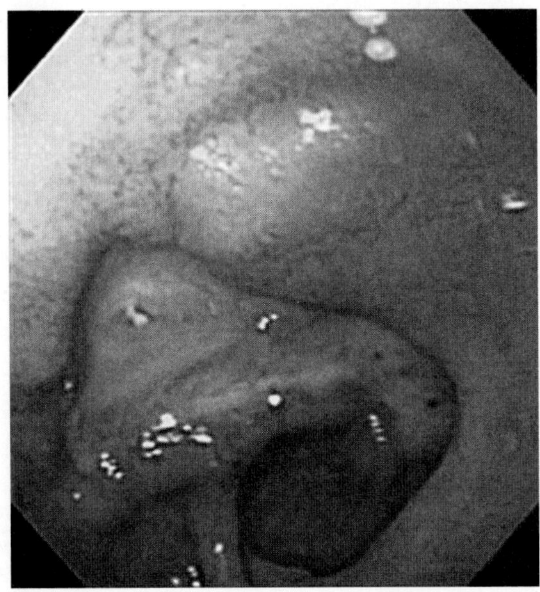

**FIGURE 34-1.** A duodenal ulcer with a clean base. *Reprinted with permission from Fauci AS, Kasper DL, Braunwald E, et al. Harrison's Principles of Internal Medicine, 17th ed. New York, McGraw-Hill, 2008.*

## Desired Outcome

2. What are your treatment goals for treating this patient's PUD?

## Therapeutic Alternatives

3.a. Considering the patient's presentation, what nonpharmacologic alternatives are available to treat her PUD?

3.b. In the absence of information about the presence of *H. pylori*, what pharmacologic alternatives are available to treat duodenal ulcers?

## Optimal Plan

4. Based on the patient's presentation and the current medical assessment, design a pharmacotherapeutic regimen to treat her duodenal ulcer, anemia, and frequent headaches.

## Outcome Evaluation

5. What clinical and laboratory parameters are necessary to evaluate therapy for achievement of the desired therapeutic outcomes and to detect or prevent adverse effects?

## Patient Education

6. What information should be provided to the patient to ensure successful therapy, enhance compliance, and minimize adverse effects?

## CLINICAL COURSE (PART 2)

At the time of the EGD, a biopsy of the duodenal mucosa was taken and indicated the presence of inflammation and abundant *H. pylori*–like organisms.

## FOLLOW-UP QUESTIONS

1. What is the significance of finding *H. pylori* in the duodenal biopsy?
2. Based on this new information, how would you modify your goals for treating this patient's PUD?
3. What pharmacotherapeutic alternatives are available to achieve the new goals?
4. Design a pharmacotherapeutic regimen for this patient's ulcer that will accomplish the new treatment goals.
5. How should the PUD therapy you recommended be monitored for efficacy and adverse effects?
6. What information should be provided to the patient about her therapy?
7. How should her frequent headaches now be treated?

## SELF-STUDY ASSIGNMENTS

1. Describe the advantages and limitations of both endoscopic and nonendoscopic diagnostic tests to detect *H. pylori*.
2. After performing a literature search on *H. pylori* eradication therapy, compare the efficacy of two-, three-, and four-drug regimens.

**TABLE 34-1 Characteristics of Common Causes of Peptic Ulcer Disease**

| | *H. pylori* | NSAID | SRMD |
|---|---|---|---|
| Onset | Chronic | Chronic | Acute |
| Primary location of damage | Duodenum | Stomach | Stomach |
| Presence of symptoms | Frequent | Rare | Rare |
| Primary mechanism for ulceration | Infection resulting in inflammatory state | Loss of defense mechanisms | Loss of defense mechanisms |
| Depth of ulcers | Superficial | Deep | Superficial |
| Dependence on acid for mucosal damage | Greater | Lesser | Lesser |
| Characterization of GI bleeding | Minor | Major | Major |
| Responsiveness to acid-suppressive therapy | No | Yes | Yes |

GI, gastrointestinal; *H. pylori, Helicobacter pylori;* NSAID, nonsteroidal anti-inflammatory drug; SRMD, stress-related mucosal damage.
*Reprinted with permission from Fong JJ, Devlin JW. Peptic ulcer disease. In: Chisholm MA, Well BG, Schwinghammer TL, et al., eds. Pharmacotherapy Principles & Practice. New York, McGraw-Hill, 2007.*

3. Based on the literature search on *H. pylori* eradication therapy, determine whether therapy should be continued for 7–14 days.
4. Describe the role of pharmacists and nurse practitioners in treating patients with PUD.

## CLINICAL PEARL

Rapid urease breath tests for diagnosis of *H. pylori* should not be used for patients who have received bismuth-containing medications, proton pump inhibitors, or antimicrobials within the previous 4 weeks due to the increased risk of a false-negative result.

## REFERENCES


1. Suerbaum S, Micchetti P. *Helicobacter pylori* infection. N Engl J Med 2002;347:1175–1186.
2. Howden CW, Hunt RH. Guidelines for the management of *Helicobacter pylori* infection. Ad hoc Committee on Practice Parameters of the American College of Gastroenterology. Am J Gastroenterol 1998;93:2330–2338.
3. Laheij RJ, Rossum LG, Jansen JB, et al. Evaluation of treatment regimens to cure *Helicobacter pylori* infection: a meta analysis. Aliment Pharmacol Ther 1999;13:857–864.
4. ASHP Commission on Therapeutics. ASHP therapeutic position statement on the identification and treatment of *Helicobacter pylori*-associated peptic ulcer disease in adults. Am J Health Syst Pharm 2001;58:331–337.
5. Soll AH. Consensus conference. Medical treatment of peptic ulcer disease. Practice guidelines. JAMA 1996;275:622–629.
6. Gilard M, Arnaud B, Cornily JC, et al. Influence of omeprazole on the antiplatelet action of clopidogrel associated with aspirin: the randomized, double-blind OCLA (Omeprazole CLopidogrel Aspirin) study. J Am Coll Cardiol 2008;51:256–260.
7. Sibbing D, Morath T, Stegherr J, et al. Impact of proton pump inhibitors on the antiplatelet effects of clopidogrel. Thromb Haemost 2009;101:714–719.
8. Siller-Matula JM, Spiel AO, Lang IM, et al. Effects of pantoprazole and esomeprazole on platelet inhibition by clopidogrel. Am Heart J 2009;157:148.e1–148.e5.
9. Juurlink DN, Gomes T, Ko DT, et al. A population-based study of the drug interaction between proton pump inhibitors and clopidogrel. CMAJ 2009;180:713–718.


# 35

# NSAID-INDUCED ULCER DISEASE

To Protect and Serve .................... Level II

**Craig Williams, PharmD**

## LEARNING OBJECTIVES

After completing this case study, the student should be able to:

- Debate the role of aspirin therapy in development of peptic ulcer disease (PUD).
- Determine whether this patient with diabetes should remain on aspirin and at what dose.
- Identify the hallmark signs and symptoms of NSAID-induced PUD.
- Recommend appropriate therapy for the treatment of NSAID-induced PUD while taking into account *Helicobacter pylori* infection and its appropriate diagnosis and follow-up.
- Recommend alternative therapies besides traditional NSAIDs for treatment of pain and inflammation in patients with PUD.
- Educate patients effectively on treatment options for NSAID-induced PUD.

## PATIENT PRESENTATION

### Chief Complaint

"I have had some stomach pain in the past 2 weeks and am worried that my ulcers have come back."

### HPI

Tom Jackson is a 55-year-old man who presents to his PCP with complaints of epigastric pain for 2 weeks. He stated that he started taking OTC Zantac for the pain with partial relief but the symptoms persisted. They are consistent with those he experienced 1 year ago when he was diagnosed empirically with bleeding gastric ulcers. When questioned, he cannot recall what diagnostic tests were done but he does recall having a prescription for several medications that he did not finish because he felt better after about a week and the medications gave him an odd taste in his mouth. He also says that acetaminophen has failed to provide much symptom relief from his osteoarthritis, so he currently uses a variety of OTC NSAID products. Additional review of his pharmacy records shows that he was prescribed a 10-day course of amoxicillin, clarithromycin, and omeprazole 1 year ago.

## PMH

Osteopenia (presumed to be secondary to intermittent prednisone use for OA) diagnosed with bone densitometry of left ankle 2 years ago
H/O PUD with *H. pylori* eradication
GERD with hiatal hernia
OA primarily in right wrist and hand but also left hip
HTN
Type 2 DM
S/P appendectomy after appendicitis in the 1970s

## FH

Father died of MI at age 55; mother died of cervical CA in her eighties.

## SH

Police officer; smokes one to two packs per week down from two packs per day 6 years ago; drinks one alcoholic drink per day but admits to occasionally having more; plays basketball one to two nights per week as he can tolerate with OA symptoms

## Meds

ASA 325 mg po once daily
Lisinopril 20 mg po once daily
Alendronate 5 mg po once daily
Gemfibrozil 600 mg po twice daily
Pioglitazone 20 mg po daily
OTC naproxen 200 mg, one to two tablets po one to three times daily for OA pain
OTC ranitidine 75 mg, one tablet two to three times daily for stomach pain

## All

Codeine; bee pollen; tetracycline → rash/hives

## ROS

Denies headache or chest pain. Occasional SOB. No heartburn, weakness, polyphagia, polydipsia, or polyuria. Gait slow but steady. Complains of some chronic pain in left hip, which he has been told is from OA.

## Physical Examination

*Gen*

The patient is a pleasant man in mild distress.

*VS*

BP 130/60, P 80, RR 12, T 36.3°C; Wt 74.8 kg, Ht 5′8″

*HEENT*

PERRLA; funduscopic exam without hemorrhages, exudates, or papilledema; mild cataracts bilaterally

*Neck/Lymph Nodes*

Supple; no JVD or thyromegaly; no carotid bruits

*Lungs*

CTA

*Cor*

RRR, normal $S_1$, $S_2$

*Abd*

Normal BS, moderate epigastric pain on palpation

*Genit/Rect*

FOBT positive × 3

*MS/Ext*

No CCE; no skin breakdown or ulcers; mild weakness of RUE; mild deformity of right first finger at MCP joint and swelling of DIP joints on first and second finger

*Neuro*

A & O × 3; CN II–XII intact; negative Babinski. Normal sensation in hands bilaterally, decreased pain and vibratory sensation in right foot, normal in left.

## Labs

| | | |
|---|---|---|
| Na 141 mEq/L | Hgb 8.9 g/dL | *Fasting lipid profile:* |
| K 4.6 mEq/L | Hct 27% | T. Chol 195 mg/dL |
| Cl 107 mEq/L | Plt 390 × $10^3$/mm$^3$ | LDL-C 115 mg/dL |
| $CO_2$ 27 mEq/L | WBC 7.0 × $10^3$/mm$^3$ | HDL-C 39 mg/dL |
| BUN 21 mEq/L | Retic 1.8% | TG 205 mg/dL |
| SCr 1.3 mg/dL | A1C 6.9% | TSH 2.93 μIU/mL |
| Glu 119 mg/dL | | |

## *H. pylori* Testing

Serology positive but rapid urease test of gastric biopsy negative. Urea breath test not performed.

## UA

SG 1.005; straw-colored; pH 4.9; trace protein; glucose negative; ketones negative

## EGD

Two small gastric ulcers approximately 6 mm in diameter, trace blood seen but no obvious active bleeding

# QUESTIONS

## Problem Identification

1.a. Create a list of the patient's drug therapy problems.

1.b. What signs, symptoms, and laboratory values indicate the presence of PUD in this patient?

1.c. What other diagnostic test could be ordered to assess the patient's current *H. pylori* status?

1.d. What are the strengths and weaknesses of the different methods available for *H. pylori* diagnosis?

## Desired Outcome

2. What are the goals of pharmacotherapy in this case?

## CHAPTER 36

## Therapeutic Alternatives

3.a What pharmacologic alternatives are available for treating the gastric ulcers in this patient?

3.b. What feasible pharmacotherapeutic options are available for preventing future gastric ulcers in this patient?

3.c. Should this patient remain on aspirin with his documented recurrent gastric ulcers?

## Optimal Plan

4.a. What is the optimal pharmacotherapeutic regimen for treating this patient's gastric ulcers?

4.b. What pharmacotherapeutic regimen is best for treating this patient's osteoarthritis?

4.c. Is this patient a candidate for prophylaxis of future NSAID-induced ulcers? If so, what drug and regimen would you recommend?

## Outcome Evaluation

5. What measures would you implement for monitoring the efficacy and toxicity of the treatment regimen for gastric ulcers in this patient?

## Patient Education

6. What information should be shared with this patient about management of his gastric ulcers to enhance adherence, ensure successful therapy, and minimize adverse effects?

## ■ SELF-STUDY ASSIGNMENTS

1. Perform a literature search and assess current information on the efficacy of various agents for secondary prevention of NSAID-induced ulcers. Review recent expert opinion on the data specific to prevention of aspirin-induced PUD in the ACCF/ACG/AHA 2008 consensus document on antiplatelet therapy and PUD.
2. Review the recent Antithrombotic Trialists' (ATT) Collaboration study examining the cardiac benefits of low-dose aspirin and describe the risk of gastric bleeding in patients with and without coronary disease.
3. Perform a literature search and assess the cost effectiveness of *H. pylori* screening in patients on chronic NSAID therapy.

## CLINICAL PEARL

Documented or undocumented use of NSAIDs plays a role in 60% of peptic ulcers that occur in patients who are *H. pylori* negative.

Due to documented risk of COX-2 agents, celecoxib is contraindicated for the acute management of pain after cardiac surgery.

Risk factors for developing NSAID-induced ulcer disease include: (1) prior history of PUD; (2) age >60 years; (3) higher NSAID doses; and (4) concomitant use of anticoagulants, antiplatelet agents, and corticosteroids or other immunosuppressants.

## REFERENCES


1. Suerbaum S, Michetti P. *Helicobacter pylori* infection. N Engl J Med 2002;347:1175–1186.
2. Chey WD, Wong BCY, Committee of the American College of Gastroenterology. American College of Gastroenterology guideline on the management of *Helicobacter pylori infection*. Am J Gastroenterol 2007;102:1808–1825.
3. Bannwarth B, Dorval E, Caekert A, et al. Influence of *Helicobacter pylori* eradication therapy on the occurrence of gastrointestinal events in patients treated with conventional nonsteroidal anti-inflammatory drugs combined with omeprazole. J Rheumatol 2002;29;1975–1980.
4. Hawkey CJ, Karrasch JA, Szczepanski L, et al. Omeprazole compared with misoprostol for ulcers associated with nonsteroidal anti-inflammatory drugs. N Engl J Med 1998;338:727–734.
5. Graham DY, Agrawal NM, Campbell DR, et al. NSAID-Associated Gastric Ulcer Prevention Study Group. Ulcer prevention in long-term users of nonsteroidal anti-inflammatory drugs: results of a double-blind, randomized, multicenter, active- and placebo-controlled study of misoprostol vs. lansoprazole. Arch Intern Med 2002;162:169–175.
6. Silverstein FE, Faich G, Goldstein JL, et al. Gastrointestinal toxicity with celecoxib vs nonsteroidal anti-inflammatory drugs for osteoarthritis and rheumatoid arthritis: the CLASS study. JAMA 2000;284:1247–1255.
7. American Diabetes Association. Standards of medical care in diabetes—2010. Diabetes Care 2010;33:S11–S61.
8. Antithrombotic Trialists' (ATT) Collaboration. Aspirin in the primary and secondary prevention of vascular disease: collaborative meta-analysis of individual participant data from randomized trials. Lancet 2009;373:1849–1860.
9. Bhatt DL, Scheiman J, Abraham N, et al. ACCF/ACG/AHA 2008 expert consensus document on reducing the gastrointestinal risks of antiplatelet therapy and NSAID use. Circulation 2008;118:1894–1909.


# 36

# STRESS ULCER PROPHYLAXIS/ UPPER GI HEMORRHAGE

A Bloody Bad Time . . . . . . . . . . . . . . . . . . . . . . Level I

**Jay L. Martello, PharmD**

**Lena M. Maynor, PharmD, BCPS**

## LEARNING OBJECTIVES

After completing this case study, students should be able to:

- Identify risk factors associated with stress gastritis/ulceration and determine which critically ill patients should receive pharmacologic prophylaxis.
- Recommend appropriate pharmacologic alternatives including agent, route of administration, and dose for the prevention of stress-induced gastritis/ulceration.
- Identify and implement monitoring parameters for the recommended stress gastritis/ulceration prophylactic regimens.
- Discuss the pharmacologic approaches to the management of stress ulcer–induced bleeding.

## PATIENT PRESENTATION

### ■ Chief Complaint

No complaint—patient is unresponsive.

## HPI

Penny Robinson is a 26-year-old woman who presents to the ED after a motor vehicle accident. She was the restrained driver of a car who was hit on the driver's side by a tractor-trailer that ran a red light. When EMS arrived in the field, the patient was unresponsive, and her breathing was labored. She was given fentanyl 50 mcg and midazolam 5 mg, and was intubated prior to transfer to the hospital. The EMS report indicates that the intubation was very difficult. The extraction time from the vehicle to the ED was 25 minutes.

## PMH (Provided by Patient's Mother)

PE × 1 about 3 months ago
IBS-C × 10 years
S/P cholecystectomy about 6 months ago

## FH

Both mother and father are still alive and in "good health."

## SH

Patient is a graduate student at a local university. She smoked cigarettes 1 ppd × 6 years until she was hospitalized for PE and has since quit. She does not drink alcohol or use illicit drugs.

## ROS

Patient is unresponsive after an MVA.

## Meds

Ortho Tri-Cyclen Lo po daily
Lubiprostone 24 mcg po Q 12 h
Warfarin 5 mg po at bedtime Mon–Wed–Fri
Warfarin 2.5 mg po at bedtime Thu–Sat–Sun

## Allergies

Sulfamethoxazole/trimethoprim (shortness of breath)
Clindamycin (hives)
Cimetidine (shortness of breath and thrombocytopenia)

## Physical Examination

*Gen*

Young unresponsive woman; no obvious bleeding on exam

*VS*

BP 108/68, P 106, RR 24, T 37.3°C; Wt 51 kg, Ht 5′11″

*Skin*

Warm, dry; small lacerations across forehead and chest; ecchymoses present on both legs and arms

*Neck/Lymph Nodes*

Supple, no palpable areas of deformity or masses

*HEENT*

No blood visible in the nose or ears; no obvious damage to the ears, eyes, or nose

*Lungs*

Patient is intubated.

*CV*

$S_1$, $S_2$ normal; sinus tachycardia with no $S_3$, $S_4$

*Abd*

Firm; no bowel sounds appreciated

*Genit/Rect*

No obvious damage to the genital area

*Neuro*

Glasgow Coma Score = 7; negative Babinski; 2+ deep tendon reflexes

*Labs*

| | | |
|---|---|---|
| Na 135 mEq/L | Hgb 9.0 g/dL | $PO_4$ 3.0 mg/dL |
| K 3.6 mEq/L | Hct 27.3% | Ca 10.2 mg/dL |
| Cl 101 mEq/L | WBC 8.0 × $10^3$/mm$^3$ | AST 29 IU/L |
| $CO_2$ 22 mEq/L | Plt 151 × $10^3$/mm$^3$ | ALT 22 IU/L |
| BUN 20 mg/dL | | Alk Phos 66 IU/L |
| SCr 0.8 mg/dL | | T. bili 0.4 mg/dL |
| Glu 91 mg/dL | | Alb 3.8 g/dL |
| | | INR 3.2 |

## ABG

pH 7.43, $PaCO_2$ 40 mm Hg, $PaO_2$ 74 mm Hg, pulse ox 92%

## AP Chest X-Ray

Multiple left and right rib fractures. There is evidence of a right hemopneumothorax with protrusion to the right lung.

## Focused Assessment with Sonography in Trauma (FAST) Exam

No evidence of fluid in the perihepatic, hepatorenal, perisplenic, pericardial, or pelvic spaces

## CT Abdomen/Pelvis with IV Contrast

There is no evidence for bowel obstruction. The common bile duct does not appear to be dilated. No free fluid present in the abdominal cavity.

## Urinalysis

Yellow color, specific gravity 1.026, pH 4.6, ketones negative, protein negative, nitrite negative, bilirubin negative, glucose negative, bacteria 0, WBC 0, RBC 3+, hCG negative

## Clinical Course

The patient is given 1 L NS, correcting her BP to 122/76. She is also given a six-pack of platelets and IV phytonadione 10 mg. She is transferred to the OR for repair of her rib fractures and hemopneumothorax. A central line is placed intraoperatively. She is given cefazolin 1 g as antimicrobial prophylaxis, which will continue for 24 hours after repair. Her fractures are repaired without significant incident and a chest tube is placed to drain fluid. During the surgery, the patient was given 2 L of LR and 2 units of PRBC to correct for blood and fluid loss. The patient's vitals on exiting surgery and arriving in the surgical/trauma ICU are BP 106/62, P 92. She is currently on assist/control mechanical ventilation. The patient's urine output has been 40 mL/h for the last 2 hours. The Hgb is 9.6 g/dL, K 3.2 mEq/L, INR 2.0, and pulse ox 94%. She is started on NS at 100 mL/h, enoxaparin 30 mg SQ Q 12 h, fentanyl drip, and midazolam drip. An NG tube is also placed.

# QUESTIONS

## Problem Identification

1.a. Prior to patient rounds, you review the medications the patient was taking prior to admission. Which of these chronic medications should be maintained during the hospitalization? Provide your rationale for continuing, discontinuing, or changing each drug regimen.

1.b. Identify all of the patient's drug therapy problems at this point in her hospital course (include both potential and actual drug therapy problems).

## Clinical Course

Two days later, the patient is still in the surgical/trauma ICU. She is hemodynamically stable and is still mechanically ventilated. She has bowel sounds and is currently receiving tube feeds through her NG tube. Labs include: Na 138 mEq/L, K 3.5 mEq/L, Cl 103 mEq/L, $CO_2$ 21 mEq/L, BUN 16 mg/dL, SCr 0.7 mg/dL, Hgb 8.6 g/dL, WBC 8.1 × $10^3$/mm$^3$, platelets 122 × $10^3$/mm$^3$, and INR 2.4. She has not had a bowel movement since admission and is given a glycerin suppository. The surgical resident realizes that no GI prophylaxis was provided initially but is not sure if it is needed at this point.

## Follow-Up Questions

1.c. What are the risk factors for developing stress gastritis/ulceration in critically ill patients, and which risk factors does this patient have?

1.d. Do this patient's risk factors warrant prophylactic therapy to prevent stress ulceration? Provide the rationale for your answer.

## Desired Outcome

2. What are the goals of pharmacotherapy for preventing stress gastritis and ulceration?

## Therapeutic Alternatives

3. What pharmacologic options are available for prophylaxis of stress ulceration in this critically ill patient?

## Optimal Plan

4. Create a pharmacotherapeutic plan for stress ulcer prophylaxis (SUP) in this patient.

## Outcome Evaluation

5. What clinical and laboratory parameters should be monitored to assess the effectiveness and potential adverse effects of the regimen you selected?

# ■ CLINICAL COURSE

Early the next morning, the patient is extubated and begun on a clear liquid diet. Later that day, the patient has a large, dark red/black bowel movement that tests heme positive. The nurse checks the patient's vitals, which show BP 92/58 and P 100. A stat Hgb comes back 7.8 g/dL, with a repeat value of 7.9 g/dL. The patient is given 1 L of LR to correct the blood pressure to 112/68 and pulse to 88, which is considered sufficiently stable for endoscopic evaluation. Multiple small gastric lesions oozing blood are visualized by EGD. The patient is diagnosed with an upper GI bleed.

## Follow-Up Questions

1. What are the differences in clinical presentation between an upper GI bleed and a lower GI bleed?
2. What are the pharmacotherapeutic goals for treating an upper GI bleed?
3. Discuss the pharmacologic options for treating an upper GI bleed.
4. Outline a pharmacotherapeutic plan for treating this patient's upper GI bleed.
5. What clinical and laboratory parameters should be monitored to assess the effectiveness and potential adverse effects of the regimen you recommended?

# ■ SELF-STUDY ASSIGNMENTS

1. Describe how to mix and store omeprazole and lansoprazole suspensions.
2. Identify commercially available GI protective products that may be administered via nasogastric or orogastric tube.
3. List the agents that are FDA-approved for preventing stress-related mucosal damage (SRMD; also known as SUP).
4. Discuss how to mix, store, and administer IV pantoprazole, lansoprazole, and esomeprazole.
5. Discuss the administration of sucralfate to renally compromised patients who may be at risk for aluminum accumulation.
6. Identify potential drug interactions and adverse effects with antacids, sucralfate, $H_2$-receptor antagonists, and proton pump inhibitors.
7. Discuss whether or not sucralfate use for SUP decreases the incidence of nosocomial pneumonia in comparison to the use of $H_2$-receptor antagonists.
8. Describe the impact of *Helicobacter pylori* infection on SUP and GI bleeding.

# CLINICAL PEARL

When performing medication reconciliation, always be on the lookout for antiulcer agents on the patient's profile. They are often relics from a previous problem that has resolved and are no longer indicated. Patients on antiulcer agents without an indication incur increased health care costs and are at increased risk for drug interactions and side effects, including a greater risk of pneumonia and *Clostridium difficile* infection.

# REFERENCES


1. American Society of Health-System Pharmacists. ASHP therapeutic guidelines on stress ulcer prophylaxis. Am J Health Syst Pharm 1999;56:347–379.
2. Cook D, Heyland D, Griffith L, et al. Risk factors for clinically important upper gastrointestinal bleeding in patients requiring mechanical ventilation. Crit Care Med 1999;27:2812–2817.
3. Herzig SJ, Howell MD, Ngo LH, Marcantonio ER. Acid-suppressive medication use and the risk for hospital-acquired pneumonia. JAMA 2009;301:2120–2128.
4. Wade EE, Rebuck JA, Healey MA, Rogers FB. H(2) antagonist-induced thrombocytopenia: is this a real phenomenon? Intensive Care Med 2002;28:459–462.
5. Kim YI, Park CK, Park DJ, Wi JO, Han ER, Koh YI. A case of famotidine-induced anaphylaxis. J Investig Allergol Clin Immunol 2010;20:166–169.
6. Gralnek IM, Barkun AN, Bardou M. Management of acute bleeding from a peptic ulcer. N Engl J Med 2008;359:928–937.
7. Rupp T, Singh S, Waggenspack W. Gastrointestinal hemorrhage: the prehospital recognition, assessment & management of patients with a GI bleed. JEMS 2004;29:80–81, 83–95.
8. Barkun A, Bardou M, Marshall JK. Consensus recommendations for managing patients with nonvariceal upper gastrointestinal bleeding. Ann Intern Med 2003;139:843–857.

# 37

# CROHN'S DISEASE

## A Sense of Urgency .................... Level II

Brian A. Hemstreet, PharmD, BCPS

## LEARNING OBJECTIVES

After completing this case study, students should be able to:

- Describe the typical clinical presentation of active Crohn's disease, including signs, symptoms, and disease distribution and severity.
- Identify exacerbating factors and potential complications of Crohn's disease.
- Recommend appropriate pharmacologic treatment for active Crohn's disease.
- Review major toxicities of drugs commonly used for managing Crohn's disease.
- Educate a patient on the proper use of medications used to treat Crohn's disease.

## PATIENT PRESENTATION

### Chief Complaint

"I'm having occasional diarrhea, sometimes with blood. I occasionally have mild abdominal pain and feel run down lately."

### HPI

John Jensen is a 28-year-old man who presents to the clinic with a 3-month history of intermittent episodes of watery diarrhea. He states that he has been having one to two loose bowel movements a day over this time. This is different from his typical bowel pattern. Over the last 4 weeks, he has also noticed blood in some of his stools. The episodes of diarrhea are infrequently accompanied by brief periods of mild abdominal pain. These symptoms have caused problems with his job, as he is a sales representative for a pharmaceutical company and spends a lot of time driving. He has tried OTC naproxen for the abdominal pain and Pepto-Bismol for the diarrhea, both of which have provided little relief. He does not recall any exposure to sick contacts. He reports no recent international travel. His PCP referred him to a gastroenterologist. A colonoscopy revealed a patchy "cobblestone" pattern of inflammation in the terminal ileum. The inflammatory process extends below the intestinal mucosa, and there is evidence of mucosal friability and recent bleeding. A biopsy of the intestinal mucosa revealed leukocyte infiltration and submucosal granulomas consistent with active Crohn's disease.

### PMH

GERD
Sinusitis (last treated with antibiotics 8 months ago)
Seasonal allergic rhinitis
Exercise-induced bronchoconstriction
ACL repair of the right knee 2 years ago

### FH

Father with DM, mother with HTN. Older sister with Crohn's disease.

### SH

Single. Works as a sales representative for a pharmaceutical company. Occasional alcohol use on the weekends. Smokes 0.5 ppd × 10 years.

### Meds

Loratidine10 mg po once daily
Fluticasone two sprays each nostril as needed
Naproxen sodium 220 mg po Q 8–12 h PRN pain
Albuterol MDI PRN prior to exercise

### All

Hydrocodone (GI upset)
Sulfa drugs (severe rash)

### ROS

No recent weight loss or sick contacts. Heartburn one to two times a week and rhinorrhea one to two times a week. No cough, SOB, HA, or mental status changes. No knee or joint pain. No jaundice or rashes. No mouth sores.

### Physical Examination

*Gen*

Well-developed Caucasian male in no apparent distress

*VS*

Sitting: BP 139/89, P 82; standing: BP 136/70, P 85; RR 17, T 37.9°C; Wt 175 lb, Ht 5′9″

*Skin*

No lesions or rashes

*HEENT*

PERRLA, EOMI, pale conjunctivae, moist mucous membranes, intact dentition, oropharynx clear

*Neck/Lymph Nodes*

Trachea midline, (–) thyromegaly, (–) lymphadenopathy, (–) JVD

*Lungs/Thorax*

CTA bilaterally

*CV*

Regular rate and rhythm, no MRG

*Abd*

Nontender, nondistended, no rebound; (+) BS, (–) HSM

*Genit/Rect*

Prostate size WNL, (–) tenderness, heme (+) stool, no evidence of hemorrhoids

*MS/Ext*

No CVA tenderness

*Neuro*

A & O × 3, CN II–XII intact, 5/5 upper and lower extremity strength bilaterally

### Labs

| | | |
|---|---|---|
| Na 139 mEq/L | Hgb 13 g/dL | AST 25 IU/L |
| K 3.0 mEq/L | Hct 39% | ALT 28 IU/L |
| Cl 100 mEq/L | RBC 2.86 × $10^6$/mm$^3$ | Alk phos 50 IU/L |
| $CO_2$ 26 mEq/L | Plt 400 × $10^3$/mm$^3$ | Total bili 1.2 mg/dL |
| BUN 15 mg/dL | MCV 80 $\mu$m$^3$ | Direct bili 0.6 mg/dL |
| SCr 1.1 mg/dL | WBC 12.7 × $10^3$/mm$^3$ | Albumin 4.1 g/L |
| Glu 104 mg/dL | Neutros 67% | CRP 13 mg/dL |
| Ca 8.7 mg/dL | Bands 1% | Lipase 15 U/L |
| Phos 3.9 mg/dL | Eos 2% | ESR 65 mm/h |
| | Lymphs 26% | Stool O & P (–) |
| | Monos 4% | Stool *C. diff* toxin (–) |

### Radiology

An abdominal x-ray reveals no evidence of obstruction, dilation, or free air.

### Assessment

A 28-year-old man presenting with new-onset Crohn's disease involving the terminal ileum requiring treatment

# QUESTIONS

## Problem Identification

1.a. Create a list of this patient's drug therapy problems.

1.b. What signs, symptoms, and laboratory alterations in this patient are consistent with Crohn's disease?

1.c. How would you classify the severity of this patient's Crohn's disease? Provide the rationale for your answer.

1.d. What factors could lead to the development or exacerbation of Crohn's disease in this patient?

1.e. What extraintestinal manifestations can develop in patients with Crohn's disease?

## Desired Outcome

2. Develop a list of pharmacotherapeutic goals for this patient.

## Therapeutic Alternatives

3. What drug therapies could be used to treat this patient's Crohn's disease?

## Optimal Plan

4.a. Develop a complete treatment plan for managing this patient's Crohn's disease.

4.b. How would your drug management differ if the disease involved the entire ileum and the colon?

## Outcome Evaluation

5. What parameters should be monitored to assess both the efficacy and toxicity of your selected drug regimen?

## Patient Education

6. How will you educate the patient about his Crohn's disease therapy in order to enhance compliance, minimize adverse effects, and promote successful therapeutic outcomes?

## CLINICAL COURSE

It is now 12 months after treatment was started. Mr Jensen achieved remission after 3 months of initial treatment. He then continued therapy for an additional 12-week period, after which he was withdrawn from drug treatment. He has had only a few intermittent episodes of diarrhea and abdominal pain over the next 6 months. However, over the last week he has had an increase in the frequency of bowel movement to three to four times per day with intermittent blood. He has developed significant abdominal pain, malaise, fever, and dehydration requiring hospitalization. He is admitted to the general medicine floor of the hospital with a recurrence of active Crohn's disease.

## FOLLOW-UP QUESTIONS

1. Given this new information, how would you modify the patient's drug therapy?
2. What baseline testing would be required if infliximab, adalimumab, or certolizumab were to be used in this instance?

## SELF-STUDY ASSIGNMENTS

1. Search for Web sites containing information about local support groups in your area to which you may refer patients with Crohn's disease for help and support.
2. Construct a table outlining the major differences between Crohn's disease and ulcerative colitis.
3. Review the FDA pregnancy categories for the major drug classes used for treatment of both active Crohn's disease and maintenance of remission.

## CLINICAL PEARL

Hospitalized patients with active Crohn's disease are at high risk for blood clots due to their inflammatory state and should be placed on prophylactic therapy for deep vein thrombosis.

## REFERENCES


1. Lichtenstein GR, Hanauer SB, Sandborn WJ, Practice Parameters Committee of the American College of Gastroenterology. Management of Crohn's disease in adults. Am J Gastroenterol 2009;104:465–483.
2. Podolsky DK. Inflammatory bowel disease. N Engl J Med 2002;347: 417–429.
3. Kethu SR. Extraintestinal manifestations of inflammatory bowel diseases. J Clin Gastroenterol 2006;40:467–475.
4. Cummings JRF, Keshav S, Travis SPL. Medical management of Crohn's disease. BMJ 2008;336;1062–1066.
5. Kozuch PL, Hanauer SB. Treatment of inflammatory bowel disease: a review of medical therapy. World J Gastroenterol 2008;14: 354–377.
6. Lichtenstein GR, Abreu MT, Cohen R, et al. American Gastroenterological Association Institute technical review on corticosteroids, immunomodulators, and infliximab in inflammatory bowel disease. Gastroenterology 2006;130:940–987.
7. Guslandi M. Antibiotics for inflammatory bowel disease: do they work? Eur J Gastroenterol Hepatol 2005;17:145–147.

# 38

# ULCERATIVE COLITIS

Seriously? Four times a day? . . . . . . . . . . . . . . Level I

Nancy S. Yunker, PharmD, BCPS

William R. Garnett, PharmD, FCCP, FAPhA

## LEARNING OBJECTIVES

After completing this case study, students should be able to:

- Identify the common signs and symptoms of ulcerative colitis.
- Evaluate treatment options for an acute episode of ulcerative colitis and recommend a specific treatment plan that includes the medication, dosing regimen, potential side effects, and monitoring parameters.
- Develop a pharmacotherapeutic plan for an ulcerative colitis patient whose disease is in remission.
- Discuss recent advances in the pharmacotherapy of ulcerative colitis.

## PATIENT PRESENTATION

### Chief Complaint

"I can't take the pain and diarrhea anymore. I thought I could make it until I got home to see my doctor but today I realized I needed to see someone."

### HPI

Bonnie Smith is a 32-year-old woman who presents to the ED with the chief complaint of a 1.5-week history of abdominal pain associated with cramping bloody diarrhea and mucus that she states is typical of her ulcerative colitis flares. She states that she has been having about four to five bloody bowel movements a day for most of the time that she has been in our city on vacation, but today she was dizzy when she stood up; she did not have any symptoms while sitting or lying down. She has been here on vacation for almost 2 weeks and is scheduled to return home in 3 days. She has not traveled outside the country, been hospitalized, or received antibiotics recently. She was diagnosed with UC approximately 3 years ago and has had approximately one exacerbation a year that her physician has treated with Pentasa capsules four times a day during each exacerbation. Each time her symptoms have resolved with 4–6 weeks of therapy. She has refused maintenance therapy because she does not want to take a medication four times a day; it is not conducive to her work and social life and she has refused rectal medications for the same reason. Her last exacerbation was approximately 10 months ago.

### PMH

Ulcerative colitis, diagnosed 3 years ago
Type 1 DM on insulin

### FH

Mother has a history of CAD and lung CA; father has a history of ulcerative colitis, S/P colectomy 18 years ago.

### SH

Works as an office manager; lives with her fiancée; no children; denies tobacco use; drinks one to two glasses of wine every few weeks; acknowledges marijuana use in the 1990s but states none in the past 10 years.

### ROS

Negative for chest pain, SOB, dysuria, fever, chills, N/V, myalgias, arthralgias, polyuria, or recent allergic reaction. Positive for mild abdominal soreness.

### Meds

NPH insulin 22 U in the morning and evening; insulin aspart 6 U for blood glucose >300 mg/dL.
Vaccination history is unavailable.

### All

NKDA

### Physical Examination

*Gen*

A & O, pleasant, healthy-appearing Caucasian woman in NAD

*VS*

At 8 AM:
BP (lying down) 100/58 mm Hg, P 60 bpm
BP (standing) 80/40 mm Hg, P 75 bpm
RR 18/min, T 37.0°C
Wt 66 kg (usual weight 68 kg), Ht 5′7″, BMI 23.5 kg/m$^2$

*Skin*

No lesions; warm, adequate turgor

*HEENT*

PERRLA; EOMI; mucous membranes without lesions or exudates; TMs intact

*Lungs*

CTA, no rales or rhonchi

*CV*

RRR, normal $S_1$ and $S_2$; no $S_3$, $S_4$

*Abd*

Normal active BS, soft, nondistended; tender to deep palpation but no palpable mass; no liver or spleen enlargement; no rebound tenderness or guarding

*Rect*

Somewhat tender; no hemorrhoids, fissures, or lesions by anoscopy; heme (+) stool

*MS/Ext*

No CCE; pulses 2+; normal ROM; strength 5/5 bilaterally

*Neuro*

A & O × 3; CN II–XII intact; DTRs 2+

### Labs

At 10:00 AM:

| | | | |
|---|---|---|---|
| Na 137 mEq/L | Hgb 13 g/dL | WBC $4.5 \times 10^3$/mm$^3$ | AST 22 IU/L |
| K 3.4 mEq/L | Hct 38% | PMNs 52% | ALT 20 IU/L |
| Cl 105 mEq/L | Plt $242 \times 10^3$/mm$^3$ | Bands 5% | Alk phos 36 IU/L |
| $CO_2$ 27 mEq/L | MCV 85.3 $\mu m^3$ | Lymphs 36% | T. Bili 0.5 mg/dL |
| BUN 26 mg/dL | MCH 29.1 pg | Basos 1% | PT 12.0 sec |
| SCr 1. 0mg/dL | MCHC 34.1 g/dL | Monos 6% | INR 1.0 |
| Glu 113 mg/dL | | | Ca 8.9 mg/dL |
| | | | Mg 1.9 mEq/L |
| | | | $PO_4$ 4.2 mg/dL |
| | | | Alb 3.9 g/dL |
| | | | A1c 6.2% |

### Urinalysis

Color yellow; transparency clear; negative for protein, leukocyte esterase, nitrite, blood, ketones, RBCs, WBCs, and bilirubin; pH 7.0; specific gravity 1.019

### Clinical Course

The patient received 1 L of 0.9% saline with KCl 40 mEq over 4 hours starting at 11:00 AM. Vital signs at 3:00 PM were as follows: BP (lying down) 110/74 mm Hg, P 62 bpm; BP (standing) 112/74 mm Hg, P 64 bpm. Repeat laboratory tests were as follows:

| | |
|---|---|
| Na 139 mEq/L | Hgb 12.5g/dL |
| K 3.9 mEq/L | Hct 36.3% |
| Cl 107 mEq/L | Plt $240 \times 10^3$/mm$^3$ |
| $CO_2$ 27 mEq/L | MCV 85.2 $\mu m^3$ |
| BUN 14 mg/dL | MCH 25.8 pg |
| SCr 0.89 mg/dL | MCHC 31.4 g/dL |
| Glu 119 mg/dL | WBC $4.4 \times 10^3$/mm$^3$ |

### ED Assessment

1. Lower GI bleeding with a history of ulcerative colitis; patient is stable after volume repletion.
2. D/C with instructions to return to ED if symptoms worsen and to contact PCP on return home.

## QUESTIONS

### Problem Identification

1.a. List all of the patient's drug therapy problems, including those existing at her initial presentation to the ED.

1.b. List the signs, symptoms, and laboratory values that indicate the presence and severity of ulcerative colitis; also include pertinent negative findings.

1.c. Could the manifestations of the patient's ulcerative colitis have been precipitated by an event?

### Desired Outcome

2. What are the short- and long-term pharmacotherapeutic goals for this patient?

### Therapeutic Alternatives

3.a. What nondrug therapies might be useful for this patient?

3.b. What feasible pharmacotherapeutic alternatives should be considered for the treatment of ulcerative colitis?

3.c. What other general health maintenance issues and therapies should be considered in patients with ulcerative colitis?

### Optimal Plan

4.a. What drug, dosage form, schedule, and duration of therapy are best for this patient based on your assessment of the patient's disease severity?

4.b. What alternatives should be considered if the patient fails to respond to initial therapy?

### Outcome Evaluation

5. What clinical and laboratory parameters are necessary to evaluate the therapy for achievement of the desired therapeutic outcome and to detect or prevent adverse effects?

### Patient Education

6. What information should be provided to the patient to enhance adherence, ensure successful therapy, and minimize adverse effects?

## CLINICAL COURSE

The patient presents to her local PCP for follow-up 1 month after her initial presentation to the ED. She states that her bowel movements are "completely normal" and she no longer has pain. She states that the symptoms started to resolve about 2 weeks after she started treatment. She has had no further complaints of weakness or dizziness. The repeat Hgb today is 12.9 g/dL.

## FOLLOW-UP QUESTIONS

1. Considering this new information, what therapeutic intervention(s) do you recommend at this time?
2. What additional information should be provided to the patient?

## SELF-STUDY ASSIGNMENTS

1. Review the literature comparing mesalamine, olsalazine, balsalazide, and sulfasalazine preparations regarding efficacy, adverse effects, and cost; include all currently available mesalamine dosage forms.
2. Perform a literature search to determine what new therapies are being evaluated for ulcerative colitis, including biologics other than infliximab.
3. Review the literature supporting use of cyclosporine, tacrolimus, and infliximab in patients with severe, extensive disease poorly responsive to initial corticosteroid treatment.
4. Conduct a literature search to determine how pharmacogenomics is affecting therapy of ulcerative colitis patients.

## CLINICAL PEARL

Patients may require both mesalamine and a thiopurine analog (azathioprine or 6-mercaptopurine) for maintenance of remission. However, concurrent therapy can lead to increased levels of thiopurine metabolites and has been associated with thiopurine toxicity. Withdrawal of mesalamine in a stable patient leads to a decrease in the active metabolites (6-thioguanine nucleotides [6-TGN]). Theoretically, this could reduce the efficacy but the clinical significance of this pharmacokinetic interaction is not well documented.

## REFERENCES


1. Travis SPL, Stange EF, Lemann M, et al., for the European Crohn's and Colitis Organisation (ECCO). European evidence-based consensus on the management of ulcerative colitis: current management. J Crohn's Colitis 2008;2:24–62.
2. Kornbluth A, Sachar DB, Practice Parameters Committee of the American College of Gastroenterology. Ulcerative colitis practice guidelines in adults: American College of Gastroenterology, Practice Parameters Committee. Am J Gastroenterol 2010;105:501–523.
3. Ng SC, Kamm MA. Therapeutic strategies for the management of ulcerative colitis. Inflamm Bowel Dis 2009;15:935–950.
4. Velayos FS, Terdiman JP, Walsh JM. Effect of 5-aminosalicylate use on colorectal cancer and dysplasia risk: a systematic review and metaanalysis of observational studies. Am J Gastroenterol 2005;100:1345–1353.
5. Hoentjen F, van Bodegraven AA. Safety of anti-tumor necrosis factor therapy in inflammatory bowel disease. World J Gastroenterol 2009;15:2067–2073.
6. AGA Institute. American Gastroenterological Association consensus development conference on the use of biologics in the treatment of inflammatory bowel disease, June-21–23, 2006. Gastroenterology 2007;133:312–339.
7. Pham CQ, Efros CB, Berardi RR. Cyclosporine for severe ulcerative colitis. Ann Pharmacother 2006;40:96–101.
8. Lichtenstein GR, Abreu MT, Cohen R, Tremaine W, American Gastroenterological Association. American Gastroenterological Association Institute medical position statement on corticosteroids, immunomodulators, and infliximab in inflammatory bowel disease. Gastroenterology 2006;130:935–939.
9. Mallon P, McKay D, Kirk S, Gardiner K. Probiotics for induction of remission in ulcerative colitis. Cochrane Database Syst Rev 2007;(4):CD005573.
10. Moscandrew M, Mahadevan U, Kane S. General health maintenance in IBD. Inflamm Bowel Dis 2009;15:1399–1409.


# 39

# NAUSEA AND VOMITING

In for a Tune-Up . . . . . . . . . . . . . . . . . . . . . . . Level II

**Kelly K. Nystrom, PharmD, BCOP**

**Amy M. Pick, PharmD, BCOP**

## LEARNING OBJECTIVES

After completing this case study, students should be able to:

- Develop a regimen of prophylactic antiemetics based on the emetogenic risk associated with cancer chemotherapeutic agents to optimize the management of nausea and vomiting.
- Design an appropriate treatment regimen for anticipatory, breakthrough, acute, and delayed nausea and vomiting.
- Design a monitoring plan to assess the effectiveness of an antiemetic regimen.
- Discuss with patients and caregivers the reason for antiemetics, their appropriate use, and the management of side effects.
- Recommend appropriate alternative antiemetic strategies based on patient-specific conditions, such as previous response to chemotherapy and side effects.

## PATIENT PRESENTATION

### Chief Complaint

"I have stomach pain and back pain."

### HPI

Mr Jones is a 57-year-old man who presents to the ED with complaints of lower back and abdominal pain, decreased appetite, and constipation since previous discharge from the hospital 3 days ago. He was recently hospitalized for prolonged abdominal pain, fatigue, a persistent cough, and a 14-lb weight loss over the previous 2 months. An ultrasound revealed marked cholelithiasis with changes of chronic cholecystitis for which he was started on Augmentin. He was found to have a 1.4-cm pulmonary mass in the lower left lung associated with endobronchial obstruction, a 4-mm noncalcified left pulmonary nodule, slightly enlarged left hilar lymph nodes, and an enlarged liver with evidence of metastasis. A diagnosis of small cell lung cancer was made with the plan to begin treatment in the outpatient setting. He currently reports that he does not have trouble swallowing but does have a productive cough. The sputum is sometimes clear but is usually brownish with one episode of blood (two small spots).

### PMH

BPH (untreated)
Cholelithiasis with chronic cholecystitis
Metastatic small cell lung cancer
GERD

### FH

Father died at age 82 of CHF and renal failure; mother died at age 68 with emphysema, obesity, MI, hypertension; two sisters, one with diabetes; three adult children, alive and healthy.

### SH

Single and works as a salesman at a car dealership. He has smoked 1–1.5 packs of cigarettes a day starting at the age of 14. He still smokes but is on a nicotine patch because his hospital has a campus-wide no smoking policy. History of alcohol and substance abuse, but he has not had alcohol for 14 years.

### ROS

Complaints include hoarseness for 1 week and fatigue. Lower extremity weakness, productive cough with brownish sputum, abdominal pain and bloating, nausea and constipation.

### Home Meds

Ibuprofen 400 mg po TID with food
Esomeprazole 40 mg po daily
Nicotine patch 21 mg topically daily
Oxycontin 10 mg po Q 12 h
Augmentin 875 mg po BID × 6 more days
Oxycodone 5 mg po Q 3 h PRN

### All

NKA

### Physical Examination

*Gen*

This is a pleasant thin Caucasian man who appears to be in acute distress due to back pain.

*VS*

BP 160/82, P 91, RR 20, T 36.6°C; Wt 68 kg, Ht 6′0″

*Skin*

Warm and dry

*HEENT*

No discharge noted in the external ear canals. Oral mucosa is intact. Mouth is pink and dry.

*Neck/Lymph Nodes*

Nontender, supple. No JVD, lymphadenopathy, or thyromegaly noted.

*Lungs/Thorax*

Good air movement. No wheezes or rhonchi noted. No spinal abnormalities appreciated.

*CV*

RRR. No rubs, murmurs, or gallops.

*Abd*

Abdomen is firm and slightly distended; hypoactive bowel sounds; tender across his midsection with hepatomegaly.

*Genit/Rect*

Deferred

*MS/Ext*

Normal range of motion and equal strength in upper and lower extremities. Positive for 2+ pitting edema in the feet and ankles.

*Neuro*

Patient is awake, alert, and oriented. Cranial nerves intact. Gait was not assessed. Patient is very anxious about his diagnosis and chemotherapy.

### Labs

| | | |
|---|---|---|
| Na 141 mEq/L | Hgb 12.4 g/dL | T. bili 2.8 mg/dL |
| K 4.3 mEq/L | Hct 36.3% | Albumin 2.4 g/dL |
| Cl 106 mEq/L | Plt 148 × $10^3$/mm$^3$ | AST 154 IU/L |
| $CO_2$ 21 mEq/L | WBC 18.4 × $10^3$/mm$^3$ | ALT 131 IU/L |
| BUN 21 mg/dL | Neutros 72% | Alk Phos 321 IU/L |
| SCr 0.7 mg/dL | Bands 8% | GGT 102 IU/L |
| Glu 97 mg/dL | Lymphs 11% | |
| | Monos 4% | |
| | Eos 1% | |
| | Basos 1% | |
| | Promyelo 1% | |
| | Meta 2% | |

### Clinical Course

Mr Jones is admitted to the hospital for severe abdominal and back pain. Although afebrile on admission, he is started on levofloxacin and metronidazole because of concerns of increased WBC count and possible abdominal infection. His Oxycontin is increased to 20 mg po Q 12 h for severe pain. He will receive his first chemotherapy cycle as an inpatient to try and improve his abdominal and back pain. He is very anxious about his diagnosis and the chemotherapy he is about to receive. Orders include:

Ondansetron 8 mg IV 30 minutes prior to chemotherapy × 3 days
Dexamethasone 20 mg IV 30 minutes prior to chemotherapy × 3 days
Aprepitant 125 mg po 1 hour prior to chemotherapy on day 1, and then 80 mg po daily on days 2 and 3
Cisplatin 75 mg/m$^2$ IV on day 1
Etoposide 100 mg/m$^2$ IV on days 1–3
Radiation therapy 250 cGy/fraction for a total dose of 3,500 cGy to the spine
Ondansetron 4–8 mg IV Q 8 H PRN nausea and vomiting

## QUESTIONS

### Problem Identification

1.a. Create a list of this patient's drug therapy problems.

1.b. What are this patient's risk factors for chemotherapy-induced nausea and vomiting?

1.c. What factors may be contributing to his nausea and vomiting?

### Desired Outcome

2. What are the goals of therapy in this case?

### Therapeutic Alternatives

3.a. Assess the patient's antiemetic regimen for prophylaxis of acute and delayed nausea and vomiting and for the treatment of breakthrough nausea and vomiting. Make any changes as necessary.

3.b. What nondrug therapies may be useful to prevent nausea and vomiting?

### Patient Education

4. How would you educate this patient on his antiemetic regimen?

## CLINICAL COURSE

You review Mr Jones' antiemetics, and the physician makes changes based on your recommendations. Mr Jones does well for the first 24 hours, but around hour 30, he develops nausea and vomiting. The nurse gives him a dose of ondansetron and is surprised when it does not work. Mr Jones is also given two other antiemetics ordered by the physician over the next 2 days with little relief.

### Follow-Up Questions

1. How might you educate the nurse about using ondansetron for breakthrough nausea and vomiting?
2. What pharmacologic alternatives may be helpful for the initial treatment of this patient?

## CLINICAL COURSE

After implementation of your recommendations, Mr Jones' nausea and vomiting have resolved and he is ready to be discharged. He will return to the clinic in about 2 weeks to receive cycle 2 of his chemotherapy.

### Follow-Up Questions (Continued)

3. Design a plan for preventing delayed nausea and vomiting in this patient for subsequent chemotherapy cycles.

4. Design a plan to prevent anticipatory nausea and vomiting in this patient for subsequent cycles.

## Outcome Evaluation

5.a. Describe how you will determine whether the antiemetic regimen he received was effective for preventing acute and delayed nausea and vomiting.

5.b. Describe the information you will need to assess the efficacy and adverse effects of the prophylactic antiemetic regimen prior to each future course of chemotherapy.

## SELF-STUDY ASSIGNMENTS

1. Compare the indications, doses, and costs of the 5-$HT_3$ antagonists dolasetron, ondansetron, granisetron, and palonosetron.
2. Discern in which patients it would be appropriate to use palonosetron or aprepitant, and the advantages and limitations of each drug.
3. Perform a literature search for antiemetic options for refractory nausea and vomiting.

## CLINICAL PEARL

Appropriate use of antiemetics is essential. The 5-$HT_3$ antagonists continue to be the drugs of choice for preventing acute nausea and vomiting, and the newer agents aprepitant and palonosetron are useful for preventing delayed nausea and vomiting. Antiemetic therapy decisions should be based on efficacy, patient-specific factors, and cost.

## REFERENCES


1. The NCCN Clinical Practice Guidelines in Oncology™ Antiemesis (Version 1.2010). © 2010 National Comprehensive Cancer Network Inc. Available at: *NCCN.org*. Accessed February 19, 2010. To view the most recent and complete version of the NCCN guidelines, go online to *NCCN.org*.
2. Hesketh PJ. Chemotherapy-induced nausea and vomiting. N Engl J Med 2008;358:2482–2494.
3. Lohr L. Chemotherapy-induced nausea and vomiting. Cancer J 2008;14:85–93.
4. Baribeault D, Erb CH. New directions in the treatment of chemotherapy-induced nausea and vomiting. Oncol Pharm 2009;2(Suppl):1–12.
5. Navari RM. Pharmacological management of chemotherapy-induced nausea and vomiting. Drugs 2009;69:515–533.
6. Herrstedt J. Antiemetics: an update and the MASCC guidelines applied in clinical practice. Nature 2008:5:32–43.
7. Grunberg SM, Osoba D, Hesketh PJ, et al. Evaluation of new antiemetic agents and definition of antineoplastic agent emetogenicity—an update. Support Care Cancer 2005;13:80–84.
8. Grunberg SM. Antiemetic activity of corticosteroids in patients receiving cancer chemotherapy: dosing, efficacy and tolerability analysis. Ann Oncol 2007;18:233–240.
9. Srivastava M, Brito-Dellan N, Davis MP, et al. Olanzapine as an antiemetic in refractory nausea and vomiting in advanced cancer. J Pain Symptom Manage 2003;25:578–582.
10. Musso M, Scalone R, Bonanno V, et al. Palonosetron (Aloxi®) and dexamethasone for the prevention of acute and delayed nausea and vomiting in patients receiving multiple-day chemotherapy. Support Care Cancer 2009;17:205–209.


# 40

# DIARRHEA

Diner's Diarrhea . . . . . . . . . . . . . . . . . . . . . . . . Level I


**Marie A. Abate, BS, PharmD**

**Charles D. Ponte, BS, PharmD, BC-ADM, BCPS, CDE, CPE, FAPhA, FASHP, FCCP**


## LEARNING OBJECTIVES

After completing this case study, students should be able to:

- Identify the common causes of acute diarrhea.
- Establish primary goals for the treatment of acute diarrhea.
- Recommend appropriate nonpharmacologic therapy for patients experiencing acute diarrhea.
- Explain the place of drug therapy in the treatment of acute diarrhea and recommend appropriate products.

## PATIENT PRESENTATION

### Chief Complaint

"I've had the runs for a couple of days, along with vomiting. I haven't been able keep anything down and I feel awful."

### HPI

Mindy Colonada is a 25-year-old woman who comes to the Family Medicine Clinic with a complaint of nausea, vomiting, and diarrhea. She had been well until yesterday, when she began to experience severe nausea that occurred about 6 hours after eating out at a local sushi restaurant. She had eaten a plate of sushi along with two glasses of iced tea. She had a few sips of her boyfriend's beer but did not have any milk or other dairy products. She woke up from sleep with severe nausea. She took two tablespoonfuls of Maalox Plus at that time. The nausea persisted, and she began to vomit "several times" with some relief. As the night progressed, she still felt "queezy" and took two Prilosec OTC tablets to settle her stomach. She began to feel dizzy, achy, and warm, and her temperature at the time was 38.2°C. These complaints continued to persist and she vomited a few more times. She has not tolerated any solid foods but she has been able to keep down small amounts of fluid. Since yesterday, she has had four to six liquid stools along with crampy abdominal pain. She has not noticed any blood or mucus in the bowel movements. Her boyfriend brought her to the clinic because she was becoming weak and lightheaded when she tried to stand up. She denies antibiotic use, laxative use, or excessive caffeine intake. She usually drinks bottled water and has not been traveling outside the country. She often experiences stress-related constipation and occasionally (once every 2 months) has loose stools alternating with constipation. These are usually accompanied by abdominal discomfort that is relieved by a bowel movement. She states that this episode is different.

### PMH

IBS × 2 years
Migraine headaches × 10 years

GERD × 5 years
Depression × 3 years
UTI—6 months ago (treated successfully with ciprofloxacin ×10 days)

## FH

Noncontributory

## SH

No current tobacco use, uses marijuana occasionally; drinks wine or a mixed drink socially, usually not more than one glass per week; has about two cups of caffeinated coffee daily. She works as an administrative associate for a local bank. Single, sexually active (one partner, monogamous relationship).

## ROS

Dizzy on standing but no complaints of vertigo; denies headache, sore throat, ear pain, or nasal discharge. Denies coughing or congestion. Frequent bouts of nausea. Frequent loose stools associated with significant cramping. Decreased urination; no dysuria or frequency. Complains of generalized lassitude, mild aching, feels like her heart is skipping beats.

## Meds

Valproic acid 500 mg po BID × 6 years
Triphasil oral contraceptive one po at bedtime × 3 years
Omeprazole 20–40 mg po daily as needed
Women's Health Formula Multivitamin one po daily
Metamucil one tablespoonful daily
St. John's wort two 900-mg tablets daily

## All

Penicillin → itching, rash on legs, 10 years ago; dust → nasal congestion, watery eyes

## Physical Examination

*Gen*

White female, appears ill, in moderate distress

*VS*

BP 125/82, P 80 (supine), BP 90/60, P 90 (standing), RR 16, T 38°C; Wt 75 kg, Ht 5′4″

*Skin*

Slightly warm to touch, fair skin turgor (mild tenting noted)

*HEENT*

Dry mucous membranes, nonerythematous TMs, PERRLA, fundi benign, slight erythema in throat

*Neck/Lymph Nodes*

Without masses, lymphadenopathy, or thyromegaly

*Chest*

Clear to A & P

*CV*

RRR without MRG

*Abd*

Diffuse tenderness, no guarding or rebound, without organomegaly, nondistended, hyperactive bowel sounds

*Genit/Rect*

Heme (–) stool in the rectal vault; no gross blood

*MS/Ext*

Normal muscle strength, no CCE

*Neuro*

A & O × 3; CN II–XII intact; normal reflexes, normal sensory and motor function

## Labs

| | | |
|---|---|---|
| Na 135 mEq/L | Hgb 12.0 g/dL | AST 35 IU/L |
| K 3.2 mEq/L | Hct 35% | ALT 30 IU/L |
| Cl 97 mEq/L | Plt 350 × $10^3$/mm$^3$ | T. bili 1.5 mg/dL |
| $CO_2$ 25 mEq/L | WBC 12.0 × $10^3$/mm$^3$ | |
| BUN 20 mg/dL | PMNs 62% | |
| SCr 1.2 mg/dL | Lymphs 36% | |
| Glu 90 mg/dL | Monos 2% | |

Serum pregnancy test—negative

## UA

Clear, dark amber; SG 1.030; pH 6.0; protein (–); glucose (–); acetone (–), bilirubin (–), blood (–); microscopic: 0–2 WBC/hpf, 0–2 RBC/hpf, several hyaline casts

## Assessment

Probable acute gastroenteritis; R/O other causes
Depression
Migraine headaches
GERD
Irritable bowel syndrome

## Plan

Admit to observation unit for acute therapy

# QUESTIONS

## Problem Identification

1.a. Create a list of the patient's drug therapy problems.

1.b. What signs and symptoms indicate the presence and severity of the diarrhea?

1.c. What questions should you ask the patient or members of the medical team to obtain the additional information needed for a complete assessment of this patient?

1.d. Could any of this patient's problems have been caused by her drug therapy?

1.e. What are other possible causes of this patient's diarrhea?

## Desired Outcome

2. What are the goals of therapy for this patient?

## Therapeutic Alternatives

3.a. What nonpharmacologic therapies should be considered for this patient?

3.b. What feasible pharmacotherapeutic alternatives are available for treatment of diarrhea in this patient?

## Optimal Plan

4. What nonpharmacologic interventions and specific pharmacotherapeutic regimens would you recommend for treating this patient's diarrhea?

## Outcome Evaluation

5. What clinical and laboratory parameters are necessary to evaluate the diarrhea therapy for achievement of the desired outcome and to detect or prevent adverse effects?

## Patient Education

6. What information should be provided to this patient to enhance adherence, ensure successful therapy, and minimize adverse effects?

## FOLLOW-UP QUESTIONS

1. How should this patient's contraception be managed after she is rehydrated and returns home?
2. Does the patient need any changes in her prophylactic migraine headache therapy?
3. How should her IBS be managed?
4. Is there a relationship between the development of IBS and bacterial gastroenteritis?

## CLINICAL COURSE

The treatment and monitoring plan you recommended was initiated on admission. The patient's diarrhea slowed by the evening of day 1. The patient had no further episodes of diarrhea or vomiting after midnight. On the morning of day 2, her orthostasis had resolved, her temperature was normal, the IV fluids were stopped, and she received clear liquids by mouth for breakfast and lunch. The patient was discharged during the late afternoon.

## SELF-STUDY ASSIGNMENTS

1. Identify the infectious causes of diarrhea. Design an effective pharmacotherapy treatment regimen for each cause.
2. Provide recommendations for the prevention of traveler's diarrhea.
3. Describe whether or not antidiarrheal drug products can be safely recommended for use in very young children (<3 years old) or in patients with bloody diarrhea and, if so, the specific products that could be used.
4. Describe when oral rehydration products should be used, and recommend a specific product and dosage for young or older patients who present with mild to moderate diarrhea and minimal dehydration.

## CLINICAL PEARL

Broad-spectrum antibiotics (especially fluoroquinolones) are a common cause of *Clostridium difficile* colitis. Diarrhea is a common sign of the disease and may begin 3 days after initiating an antibiotic or up to 3 months after a course of antibiotics (the Rule of 3s).

## REFERENCES


1. DuPont HL. Bacterial diarrhea. N Engl J Med 2009;361:1560–1569.
2. Guerrant RL, Van Gilder T, Steiner TS, et al. Practice guidelines for the management of infectious diarrhea. Clin Infect Dis 2001;32:331–350.
3. St. John's Wort. Natural Medicines Comprehensive Database. Stockton, CA, 2010. Available at: *www.naturalmedicinesdatabase.com*. Accessed March 22, 2010.
4. DuPont HL. New insights and directions in travelers' diarrhea. Gastroenterol Clin North Am 2006;35:337–353.
5. Pawlowski SW, Warren CA, Guerrant R. Diagnosis and treatment of acute or persistent diarrhea. Gastroenterology 2009;136:1874–1886.
6. Steffen R, Gyr K. Diet in the treatment of diarrhea: from tradition to evidence. Clin Infect Dis 2004;39:472–473 [editorial].
7. Wingate D, Phillips SF, Lewis SJ, et al. Guidelines for adults on self-medication for the treatment of acute diarrhoea. Aliment Pharmacol Ther 2001;15:773–782.
8. Guarino A, Lo Vecchio A, Canani RB. Probiotics as prevention and treatment for diarrhea. Curr Opin Gastroenterol 2009;25:18–23.
9. Videlock EJ, Chang L. Irritable bowel syndrome: current approach to symptoms, evaluation, and treatment. Gastroenterol Clin North Am 2007;36:665–685.
10. Jung IS, Kim HS, Park H, Lee SI. The clinical course of postinfectious irritable bowel syndrome. J Clin Gastroenterol 2009;43:534–540.


# 41

# IRRITABLE BOWEL SYNDROME

Life in the Slow Lane. . . . . . . . . . . . . . . . . . . . Level II

**Nancy S. Yunker, PharmD, BCPS**

**William R. Garnett, PharmD, FCCP, FAPhA**

## LEARNING OBJECTIVES

After completing this case study, students should be able to:

- Identify the signs and symptoms of irritable bowel syndrome associated with constipation (IBS-C).
- Devise patient management strategies for patients with IBS, including pharmacologic and nonpharmacologic options.
- Outline parameters for monitoring the safety and efficacy of therapy used in patients with IBS-C.
- Identify treatment options for IBS with diarrhea (IBS-D).
- Evaluate the efficacy of treatment options for patients with IBS.

## PATIENT PRESENTATION

### Chief Complaint

"My IBS is acting up again. I feel all bloated and I really have to strain to have a bowel movement. I have been really uncomfortable for the past 4 weeks. Most recently, I added FiberCon tablets to the docusate I was already taking because someone in the past told me that I would probably be able to tolerate FiberCon better than Metamucil. I haven't seen much improvement in the 8 weeks that I have been using them, plus it is hard to remember to take them four times a day. I have tried to live with this but I really think I need to try something else. Is there anything you can give me?"

## HPI

Jane Hoffman is a 28-year-old woman who presents to her PCP with the chief complaint of a 5-month history of hard pelletlike stools and difficulty passing stools. She was diagnosed with IBS her freshman year in college. She has been able to tolerate the minimal symptoms until about 6 months ago when she began to notice some bloating and a decrease in the number of bowel movements per week. She states that she now constantly feels bloated and has taken to wearing loose-fitting clothing because she cannot tolerate anything tight around her abdomen. She attributes the worsening symptoms to the stress associated with trying to complete classes for a graduate degree and serving as a teaching assistant (TA) for two courses. In addition to the 20 hours a week that she serves as a TA, she also works at least two weekends a month in a department store as a sales assistant. She also states the symptoms have gotten worse since she went back to school. In the past 2 years, they have been worse when she has midterms or finals or when she needs to complete a major college writing assignment. Other than stress, she cannot think of anything else that has changed in her life. She does not remember having any gastroenteritis symptoms in the past year, and she dislikes eating yogurt.

Prior to 6 months ago, she states that she averaged about six stools a week. She estimates that she has had one or two bowel movements a week for the past 6 weeks. She complains of straining to pass her stools and states that she is getting up 60 minutes early in the morning to allow for an attempt to pass a stool and uses the additional time exercising in order to "stimulate her bowels." She also tried eating more bran products but felt like that made the pain and bloating worse, so she stopped. She states that the abdominal pain is not limited to when she passes a stool. She complains of abdominal pain and bloating almost continuously throughout the day for the past 2 months, although her symptoms are somewhat alleviated by passing a "good stool." She resumed taking docusate 6 months ago. She briefly took senna in addition to the docusate but found that she sometimes had to go to the bathroom at inopportune times and felt that it caused additional cramping. She tried psyllium several years ago but hated the taste and felt it made her more bloated; she does not want to try that again. She thought about MiraLAX but her mother took that prior to a GI procedure and said that it caused diarrhea, so the patient is hesitant to try it with all her responsibilities.

## PMH

Seasonal allergies
Anxiety
UTIs

## PSH

Cholecystectomy 2 years ago

## FH

Lives alone. She separated from her boyfriend 2 months ago due to school and other job commitments. She became solely responsible for the apartment rent when he left. He has been "hassling" her recently, and there is a question of verbal and physical abuse. Her mother is alive with HTN and recently had an MI, and her father is alive with hypercholesterolemia. No siblings.

## SH

No alcohol use or smoking. No history of military service.

## ROS

Occasional headaches, usually associated with stress or allergy symptoms; occasional nausea, no vomiting; (–) blood in the stool or tarry stools; (+) flatulence and bloating. States that the abdominal symptoms may improve at night before bedtime especially if she uses a heating pad; she is not awakened at night with abdominal pain.

## Meds

Diphenydramine 25 mg po Q 6 h allergy symptoms
Ibuprofen 200 mg, two tablets po Q 4–6 h PRN headaches, menstrual cramps
FiberCon two tablets po three to four times daily
Docusate 100 mg po twice daily
Mircette (discontinued 2 months ago)

## All

NKDA

## Physical Examination

*Gen*

A & O, WDWN pleasant Caucasian female appearing slightly anxious

*VS*

BP 116/78, P 68, RR 18, T 37.0°C; Wt 61 kg, Ht 5′6″

*Skin*

Dry skin on lower extremities, no rashes noted

*HEENT*

PERRLA, EOMI, moist mucus membranes, TMs intact

*Neck/Lymph Nodes*

No thyromegaly, lymphadenopathy, or JVD

*Lungs*

CTA; no rales or rhonchi

*Breasts*

Symmetric; no lumps or masses detected; nipples without discharge

*CV*

RRR, normal S1 and S2; no S3 or S4

*Abd*

(+) BS, slightly tender in LLQ, no HSM

*Genit/Rect*

Vulva normal; no palpable rectal masses; brown stool with no occult blood; no hemorrhoids

*MS/Ext*

No CCE, pulses 2+, normal ROM, normal strength bilaterally

### Labs

| | |
|---|---|
| Na 142 mEq/L | WBC 5.2 × $10^3$/mm$^3$ |
| K 4.0 mEq/L | Hgb 14.1 g/dL |
| Cl 106 mEq/L | Hct 42.4% |
| $CO_2$ 27 mEq/L | |
| BUN 9 mg/dL | |
| SCr 0.8 mg/dL | |
| Glu 88 mg/dL | |

Lactulose $H_2$ breath test: Negative
Serum pregnancy test: Negative

### Assessment

IBS associated with abdominal discomfort, bloating, and constipation

## QUESTIONS

### Problem Identification

1.a. Create a list of the patient's drug therapy problems.

1.b. What information (signs, symptoms, and laboratory values) indicates the presence and severity of IBS-C? What are the pertinent negative findings in this patient?

1.c. Could any of the patient's problems have been caused by drug therapy?

1.d. What additional information is needed to satisfactorily assess this patient?

### Desired Outcome

2. Differentiate the patient's goals of therapy from those of her health care providers.

### Therapeutic Alternatives

3.a. What nondrug therapies might be useful for this patient?

3.b. What feasible pharmacotherapeutic alternatives are available for the treatment of IBS-C?

3.c. What pharmacotherapeutic alternatives are available for the treatment of IBS-D?

### Optimal Plan

4.a. What drug, dosage form, dose, schedule, and duration of therapy are best for this patient?

4.b. What alternatives would be appropriate if the initial therapy fails or cannot be used?

### Outcome Evaluation

5. What clinical and laboratory parameters are necessary to evaluate the therapy for achievement of the desired therapeutic outcome and to detect or prevent adverse effects?

### Patient Education

6. What information should be provided to the patient to enhance compliance, ensure successful therapy, and minimize adverse effects?

## CLINICAL COURSE

The patient returns to the physician 6 weeks later and reports that her symptoms are much improved and that the abdominal pain has resolved. She is happy with her medication regimen, but her friends have suggested that herbal medications may be just as effective. She would like more information about the use of these products for IBS.

## FOLLOW-UP QUESTIONS

1. What therapeutic regimen would you recommend for the patient at this time?
2. What information would you provide regarding the addition or substitution of alternative medications (e.g., herbal medications) to this patient's regimen?

## SELF-STUDY ASSIGNMENTS

1. Conduct a literature search to determine what types of alternative therapies, including probiotics, have been evaluated in IBS. Include a discussion of the scientific rigor of these studies.
2. Conduct a search of IBS drug treatment studies on www.clinicaltrials.gov for potential patient referral.
3. Conduct a literature search to identify clinical trials of antibiotics in IBS and evaluate the scientific rigor of these studies.
4. Conduct an informal survey among friends, family members, coworkers, and fellow students about the incidence of IBS and what therapeutic options they would recommend to a person suffering from IBS.
5. Conduct a literature search to identify new and emerging therapies for IBS and determine their commercial availability.
6. Search the Medicare.gov prescription drug plans database via Medicare prescription drug plan finder. Select five plans in your county and state and view their formulary to compare the affordability of specific IBS treatment options.

## CLINICAL PEARL

Linaclotide, an investigational agent for the treatment of IBS-C, is a guanylate cyclase C receptor activator that stimulates chloride and bicarbonate secretion and indirectly increases motility and gastrointestinal transit. In initial clinical trials, it resulted in an acceleration of time to the first bowel movement, improvement in stool frequency and consistency, and decreased straining in female patients with IBS-C.

## REFERENCES


1. American College of Gastroenterology IBS Task Force. An evidence-based systematic review on the management of irritable bowel syndrome. Am J Gastroenterol 2009;104(Suppl 1):S8–S35.
2. Videlock EJ, Chang L. Irritable bowel syndrome: current approach to symptoms, evaluation, and treatment. Gastroenterol Clin North Am 2007;36:665–685.
3. Longstreth GF, Thompson WG, Chey WD, Houghton LA, Mearin F, Spiller RC. Functional bowel disorders. Gastroenterology 2006;130:1480–1491.
4. Miller S, Heck A. Irritable bowel syndrome. US Pharm 2000;25 (Suppl 11):03–13.
5. Lacy BE, Weiser K, De Lee R. The treatment of irritable bowel syndrome. Ther Adv Gastroenterol 2009;2:221–238.
6. Ford AC, Talley NJ, Spiegel BM, et al. Effect of fibre, antispasmodics, and peppermint oil in the treatment of irritable bowel syndrome: systematic review and meta-analysis. BMJ 2008:337:a2313 [doi:10:1136/bmj.a2313].

7. Ford AC, Brandt LJ, Young C, Chey WD, Foxx-Orenstein AE, Moayyedi F. Efficacy of 5-HT3 antagonists and 5-HT4 agonists in irritable bowel syndrome: systematic review and met-analysis. Am J Gastroenterol 2009:104:1831–1843.
8. Drossman DA, Chey WD, Johanson JF, et al. Clinical trial: lubiprostone in patients with constipation-associated irritable bowel syndrome: results of two randomized placebo-controlled studies. Aliment Pharmacol Ther 2009;29:329–341.
9. Ford AC, Talley NJ, Schoenfeld PS, Quigley EMM, Moayyedi P. Efficacy of antidepressants and psychological therapies in irritable bowel syndrome: systematic review and meta-analysis. Gut 2009:58: 367–378.
10. Brenner DM, Moeller MJ, Chey WD, Schoenfeld PS. The utility of probiotics in the treatment of irritable bowel syndrome: a systematic review. Am J Gastroenterol 2009;104:1033–1049.
11. Liu J, Yang M, Liu Y, Wei M, Grimsgaard S. Herbal medicines for treatment of irritable bowel syndrome. Cochrane Database Syst Rev 2006;(1):CD004116.

# 42

# PEDIATRIC GASTROENTERITIS

One Thing You *Should* Try at Home. . . . . . . . Level II

**William McGhee, PharmD**

**Laura Panko, MD, FAAP**

## LEARNING OBJECTIVES

After completing this case study, students should be able to:

- Recognize the signs and symptoms of diarrhea with dehydration and be able to assess the severity of the problem.
- Describe the two available rotavirus vaccines, compare their dosage and availability, understand their safety and efficacy compared to the previously available vaccine, and explain their potential impact on rotavirus-induced diarrhea.
- Recommend appropriate oral rehydration therapy (ORT) products and treatment regimens for varying degrees of dehydration severity.
- Properly assess the effectiveness of ORT using both clinical and laboratory parameters.
- Be able to educate parents about the limited role of all antidiarrheal and antiemetic products and the limitations and concerns about probiotics that prevent their routine use for treatment of acute diarrhea in children.
- Identify the signs and symptoms of severe dehydration that require referral to an ED for immediate IV volume replacement.

## PATIENT PRESENTATION

### Chief Complaint

Lydia Mason is a 9-month-old female who presented to the ED with a 3-day history of fever, vomiting, and diarrhea.

### HPI

The child was in her baseline state of health, having just been seen by her pediatrician for her 9-month well-child check earlier in the week. Three days before presentation, she was noted to have a tactile fever, confirmed at 100.4°F (38.0°C) axillary, as well as diminished energy. Two days before presentation, she awoke from sleep, experiencing nonbilious, nonbloody emesis. Throughout that day, she had five similar episodes of vomiting, typically after attempts at oral intake. She continued to have low-grade fevers.

One day before presentation to the ED, she had only two episodes of emesis, but she developed diarrhea. The stools, totaling five that day, were initially described as slightly formed. As the day progressed, the stools became watery, voluminous, and contained small specks of blood. The patient's appetite continued to be poor, with very limited solid intake. On the pediatrician's recommendation, the family offered the patient liquids including formula, water, and Pedialyte, but she refused, preferring cola and diluted apple juice.

On the morning of presentation to the ED, the patient had another large, watery stool and was unusually fussy. Her diaper was dry, with no urine output the night prior. The family could not accurately assess the number of wet diapers she had in the last 24 hours, given the difficulty distinguishing watery stool from urine. They also noted that her lips appeared dry and she had diminished tears.

### PMH

Lydia was born at 38 weeks via spontaneous vaginal delivery without complications. She required 1 day of phototherapy for hyperbilirubinemia. She was discharged from the nursery within 3 days of birth. She has experienced approximately six upper respiratory tract infections and two episodes of otitis media, all after introduction into daycare at 7 weeks of age. These illnesses have not resulted in hospitalization or ED visitation.

No sick contacts were noted until the day she presented to the ED, when the patient's mother developed abdominal discomfort and loose stools. In addition, multiple infants at the daycare Lydia attends were experiencing similar symptoms.

Immunizations are up-to-date. Development is normal. No medications have been given except for a daily multivitamin.

### All

NKDA

### FH

Lydia's mother and father are 29 years old and in good health. There are two older siblings ages 3 and 6, who have been well.

### SH

Lydia lives with her parents and siblings. There are two pet fish in the home but no reptile or other animal exposures. The patient attends daycare three times a week. The family uses city water and has not traveled out of state recently. Her diet consists of Enfamil Lipil and a myriad of solid foods. There has been no exposure to undercooked meats or fish.

### Physical Examination

*Gen*

Patient is ill-appearing but nontoxic. She is very fussy during the examination but consoled by her mother with some effort.

*VS*

T 38.4°C, P 145, RR 42, BP 92/50; Wt 8.2 kg (50–75%) (Wt 5 days earlier at well-child check 9.0 kg)

*Skin*

Pink, mild tenting noted, capillary refill 2–3 seconds

*HEENT*

Anterior fontanelle sunken, eyes moderately sunken, scant tears, nose with clear rhinorrhea, lips and tongue dry, TMs gray and translucent

*Neck/Lymph Nodes*

Normal

*Lungs/Thorax*

Tachypneic; no focal findings, including wheezes, rales, or rhonchi; no retractions or grunting

*Heart*

Tachycardic, 1/6 flow murmur, normal pulses

*Abd*

Distended, hyperactive bowel sounds; no focal tenderness, masses, or hepatosplenomegaly

*Genit/Rect*

Normal female genitalia, mild diaper dermatitis

*MS/Ext*

Normal

*Neuro*

Sleepy but arousable; very fussy when awake; no focal defects

### Labs

| | | |
|---|---|---|
| Na 137 mEq/L | Hgb 12.8 g/dL | WBC 14.0 × $10^3$/mm$^3$ |
| K 4.4 mEq/L | Hct 41% | 52% Polys |
| Cl 113 mEq/L | Plt 300 × $10^3$/mm$^3$ | Bands 5% |
| $CO_2$ 14 mEq/L | | Eos 0% |
| BUN 23 mg/dL | | Basos 3% |
| SCr 0.4 mg/dL | | Lymphs 24% |
| Glu 80 mg/dL | | Monos 16% |

### UA

Specific gravity 1.029; ketones 2+; otherwise negative

### Assessment

1. Typical viral gastroenteritis, likely rotavirus infection
2. Dehydration with metabolic acidosis

## QUESTIONS

### Problem Identification

1.a. Create a list of the patient's drug therapy problems.

1.b. What information (signs, symptoms, laboratory values) indicates the presence or severity of gastroenteritis?

### Desired Outcome

2. What are the goals of pharmacotherapy in this case?

### Therapeutic Alternatives

3.a. What nondrug therapies might be useful for this patient?

3.b. What feasible pharmacotherapeutic alternatives are available for treating this patient's diarrhea?

### Optimal Plan

4.a. What drug(s), dosage forms, schedule, and duration of therapy are best for this patient?

4.b. What is the efficacy and safety record of the available rotavirus vaccines, and what impact are they expected to have on preventing rotavirus-induced diarrhea?

### Outcome Evaluation

5. What clinical and laboratory parameters should be monitored to evaluate therapy for achievement of the desired therapeutic outcome?

### Patient Education

6. What information should be provided to the child's parents to enhance compliance, ensure successful therapy, and minimize adverse effects?

## SELF-STUDY ASSIGNMENTS

1. In what circumstances would antimicrobial therapy be considered for children with diarrhea and dehydration?
2. Explain the limitations of using probiotics for treating pediatric gastroenteritis including lack of FDA oversight, purity and standardization of products, lack of recognized treatment regimens, and safety concerns. Write a brief educational document explaining to parents why probiotics should not be used routinely.
3. What role does zinc supplementation have in the treatment of diarrhea in developing countries? Describe the rationale for its use and the most efficient way to administer it.
4. What is the efficacy of drug therapy in preventing diarrhea when traveling to foreign countries? What drugs are recommended, and what are the adult and pediatric doses?
5. What barriers exist to the widespread implementation of ORT, including parents and physicians? How can these barriers be overcome? (*Hint*: Explore the advantages of ORT vs. IV rehydration therapy, including ease of care at home vs. hospitalization, insurance issues, and physician reluctance.)
6. Write a two-page essay describing the role of the community-based practitioner in the care of patients with pediatric gastroenteritis and dehydration. Emphasize how you would monitor patient safety and outcome and what you would tell the parents to optimize treatment at home.

## CLINICAL PEARL

ORT is equivalent to IV therapy in rehydrating children with gastroenteritis and diarrhea with mild to moderate dehydration. It is the standard of care in the treatment of these patients and usually can be performed at home. Antidiarrheal, antiemetic, probiotic, and antimicrobial therapies are rarely necessary. IV rehydration is necessary only in patients with severe dehydration.

## REFERENCES


1. Elliot EJ. Acute gastroenteritis in children. BMJ 2007;334:35–40.
2. Kosek M, Bern C, Guerrant RL. The global burden of diarrhoeal disease, as estimated from studies published between 1992 and 2000. Bull World Health Organ 2003;81:197–204.

3. Mast TC, Walter EB, Bulotsky M, et al. Burden of childhood rotavirus disease on health systems in the United States. Pediatr Infect Dis J 2010;29:e19–e25.
4. Duggan C, Santosham M, Glass RI. The management of acute diarrhea in children: oral rehydration, maintenance, and nutritional therapy. MMWR Morb Mortal Wkly Rep 1992;41(RR-16):1–20.
5. Spandorfer PR, Alessandrini EA, Joffe MD, et al. Oral versus intravenous rehydration of moderately dehydrated children: a randomized, controlled trial. Pediatrics 2005;115:295–301.
6. Guarino A, Albano F, Ashkenazi S, et al. European Society for Paediatric Gastroenterology, Hepatology, and Nutrition/European Society for Paediatric Infectious Diseases evidence-based guidelines for the management of acute gastroenteritis in children in Europe. J Pediatr Gastroenterol Nutr 2008;46(Suppl 2):S81–S122.
7. Szajewska H, Dziechciarz P. Gastrointestinal infections in the pediatric population. Curr Opin Gastroenterol 2010;26:36–44.
8. DeCamp LR, Byerley JS, Doshi N, et al. Use of antiemetic agents in acute gastroenteritis: a systematic review and meta-analysis. Arch Pediatr Adolesc Med 2008;162:858–865.
9. Bhatnagar S, Bahl R, Sharma PK, et al. Zinc with oral rehydration therapy reduces stool output and duration of diarrhea in hospitalized children: a randomized controlled trial. J Pediatr Gastroenterol Nutr 2004;38:34–40.
10. Committee on Infectious Diseases, American Academy of Pediatrics. Prevention of rotavirus disease: updated guidelines for use of rotavirus vaccine. Pediatrics 2009;123:1412–1420.


# 43

# CONSTIPATION

All Bound Up . . . . . . . . . . . . . . . . . . . . . . . . . Level II


**Michelle Fravel, PharmD, BCPS**

**Beth Bryles Phillips, PharmD, FCCP, BCPS**


## LEARNING OBJECTIVES

After completing this case study, students should be able to:

- Identify medications that can exacerbate constipation.
- Describe the advantages and disadvantages of each class of laxatives and discuss the appropriate use of each class.
- Recommend an appropriate plan for the treatment of constipation, including lifestyle modifications and drug therapy.
- Educate patients regarding laxative therapy.

## PATIENT PRESENTATION

### Chief Complaint

"I feel just awful ever since starting these pain pills—I think I'd rather be in pain!"

### HPI

Kerry Reynolds is a 64-year-old woman who presents to the ED complaining of increasing abdominal cramping and nausea for several days and now vomiting for the past several hours. She says this all started when she began Percocet therapy 2 weeks ago for postprocedural pain in association with right TKA. Her last bowel movement was 6 days ago. She began "not feeling well" 4 days ago, with bloating, decreased appetite, decreased thirst, and fatigue. She reports that yesterday, when her cramping was at its worst, she even used a couple doses of Metamucil but it did not do a thing. She says she was almost to the point where she thought about trying some powerful laxatives, but she has heard about the addiction they can cause and the last thing she wants is to be addicted to a laxative. She has also tried to just quit taking the pain meds altogether, but she only makes it about halfway through the morning before the pain becomes unbearable. She reports that she has cut back on the pain pills and is only taking one pill four times a day now, compared to a week ago when she was taking two pills four times a day. On a scale of 1–10, with 1 being no pain and 10 being the worst pain ever experienced, she rates her pain at a 5 today. She does say the pain is improving every day. Her plan is to take one less pain pill every 3 days so that she can successfully taper the meds in about 2 weeks. She reports no fever, CP, or SOB. She states that she typically has daily bowel movements, with no straining, and spends less than 10 minutes, with little effort, having a bowel movement. Her last colonoscopy, performed 2 years ago, was unremarkable.

### PMH

Hypothyroidism
Diabetes mellitus, type 2—diet controlled
Hypertension
Dyslipidemia
Osteoarthritis

### FH

Her mother is in her 80s and is healthy. Her father died in his 60s from heart disease. She has three brothers and three sisters; one brother has type 2 diabetes. She has two sons who are healthy.

### SH

She is married and works as a social worker. She quit smoking >20 years ago. She does not drink alcohol and does not use illicit drugs.

### ROS

(+) For constipation, lower abdominal fullness, N/V, right knee pain, (–) for SOB, CP, or fever/chills

### Meds

Diltiazem CR 240 mg po daily
Chlorthalidone 25 mg po daily
Levothyroxine 50 mcg po daily
Simvastatin 20 mg po at bedtime
Multivitamin one tablet po daily
Warfarin 5 mg daily × 5 weeks for VTE prophylaxis as directed by Anticoagulation Clinic
Oxycodone/acetaminophen 5 mg/325 mg one to two tablets Q 4–6 h PRN

### All

NKDA

### Physical Examination

*Gen*

Pleasant woman in distress because of abdominal discomfort; is visibly uncomfortable and holding her stomach during the visit; appears tired

*VS*

BP 122/60, P 57, RR 16, T 36.2°C; Wt 112.4 kg, Ht 5′5″; waist circumference 37 in; pain rated 5 on scale of 1–10

*Skin*

Normal skin turgor and color

*HEENT*

PERRLA and EOM full without nystagmus; no scleral icterus; oral mucosa moist; no ulcerations noted

*Neck/Lymph Nodes*

Supple, no lymphadenopathy or JVD; no thyromegaly or bruits

*CV*

Regular, $S_1$ and $S_2$ without murmur

*Lungs*

Normal breath sounds; no crackles or wheezes

*Abd*

Soft, obese, tender; decreased bowel sounds; stool palpable on left side

*Rectal*

Stool present in rectal vault; no masses felt; tone fair; push strength fair; nontender

*MS/Ext*

S/P TKA right knee; surgical wound healing appropriately; no redness, swelling, exudation; range of motion within normal limits

*Neuro*

A & O × 3; CNs II–XII symmetric and intact; DTRs 2+

### Labs

| | | |
|---|---|---|
| Na 138 mEq/L | Glu 133 mg/dL (fasting) | RBC 6.05 × $10^6$/mm$^3$ |
| K 3.7 mEq/L | A1c 6.4% | Hgb 15.5 g/dL |
| Cl 101 mEq/L | Ca 9.3 mg/dL | Hct 48% |
| $CO_2$ 30 mEq/L | TSH 2.70 mIU/mL | MCV 79 μm$^3$ |
| BUN 14 mg/dL | INR 2.4 | MCH 26 pg |
| SCr 0.8 mg/dL | | MCHC 33% |
| | | RDW 15.4% |

### Assessment

Constipation with fecal impaction; secondary symptoms of abdominal discomfort, nausea, and vomiting; etiology likely drug-induced

### Plan

Obtain abdominal x-ray and CT scan to rule out other potential causes of constipation; perform disimpaction.

### Clinical Course

A plain x-ray of the abdomen showed gas-dilated loops in the colon. An abdominal CT scan was then performed and showed a large amount of stool in the colon and rectal vault. Disimpaction was successfully performed with no complications. A follow-up PEG-based bowel preparation was successful in clearing bowel and relieving the patient's abdominal pain. An appropriate medication regimen was recommended to maintain regular bowel function over the next 2 weeks while she continues her opioid therapy.

## QUESTIONS

### Identification

1.a. Develop a list of the potential therapy problems in this patient other than those related to her constipation.

1.b. What signs or symptoms are indicative of constipation in this patient?

1.c. What are some of the possible nonpharmacologic contributors to her constipation?

1.d. What are some of the possible pharmacologic contributors to constipation in this patient?

1.e. What information should be obtained from a patient who presents with a chief complaint of constipation?

### Desired Outcome

2. What are the goals of pharmacotherapy in treating constipation?

### Therapeutic Alternatives

3.a. What are some nonpharmacologic steps useful in treating constipation?

3.b. What are the pharmacologic options for the treatment of constipation?

3.c. Is this patient's current regimen for hypertension appropriate? If not, what recommendations can you make to optimize this regimen?

### Optimal Plan

4. After nonpharmacologic measures have been attempted, what would be the most appropriate choice of drug therapy for her, including dose and schedule? Provide the rationale for your answer.

### Outcome Evaluation

5.a. How would you monitor this patient to ensure that your pharmacotherapeutic goals have been achieved? How would you follow up with her to ensure resolution of the constipation?

## CLINICAL COURSE

The recommendations you made were implemented, and Ms Reynolds returns to your clinic 1 month later. She reports that the drug therapy you recommended resulted in regular bowel function throughout the last 2 weeks of her opioid therapy. She does report, however, that her orthopedic physicians have now recommended TKA on the opposite leg. She says that after the last episode with constipation, she just does not think she wants to go through with it.

5.b. You reassure the patient that this problem can be prevented with her next surgery and that you will discuss options with her physicians. What regimen would you recommend for preventing opioid-induced constipation in this patient if she chooses to go through with the second TKA procedure?

### Patient Education

6.a. What education would you provide to this patient who has concerns about recurrence of drug-induced constipation?

6.b. What education would you provide to this patient regarding her concerns about laxative addiction?

6.c. When instructing this patient on using a stimulant laxative, what information should you convey to ensure appropriate use of this product?

## SELF-STUDY ASSIGNMENTS

1. Suggest pharmacotherapeutic options for the treatment of opioid-induced constipation in a pediatric patient. How does this approach compare to that used in treatment of adults?
2. Perform a literature search to find medications under investigation for the treatment of constipation. What different types of constipation will these new entities be used to treat? What place in therapy will these medications have?

## CLINICAL PEARL

Although long-term or chronic use of stimulant laxatives is not recommended, stimulant use is appropriate for certain acute indications, such as opioid-induced constipation. The key to effective therapy is limited duration. Addiction or tolerance is not a concern with short-term use.

## REFERENCES


1. Lembo A, Camilleri M. Chronic constipation. N Engl J Med 2003;349:1360–1368.
2. Opioid Rx & Safety. Pain Treatment Topics Website. Available at: *http://pain-topics.org/opioid_rx/*. Accessed January 28, 2010.
3. Thorpe DM. Management of opioid-induced constipation. Curr Pain Headache Rep 2001;5:237–240.
4. Thomas J, Darver S, Cooney GA, et al. Methylnaltrexone for opioid-induced constipation in advanced illness. N Engl J Med 2008;358:2332–2343.


# 44

# ASCITES MANAGEMENT IN PORTAL HYPERTENSION AND CIRRHOSIS

Back to Drinking . . . . . . . . . . . . . . . . . . . . . . . . Level II


**Laurel Andrews, PharmD**

**Jeffery Evans, PharmD**


## LEARNING OBJECTIVES

After completing this case study, students should be able to:

- Identify signs and symptoms of cirrhosis and associated complications.
- Provide pharmacotherapeutic and lifestyle recommendations for managing ascites due to portal hypertension and cirrhosis.
- Develop a patient-specific regimen and monitoring parameters to meet the needs of a patient with ascites, esophageal varices, and hepatic encephalopathy.
- Interpret laboratory values associated with ascites.
- Provide appropriate patient education for the recommended pharmacologic and nonpharmacologic therapy to control complications of cirrhosis, as well as to prevent further complications.

## PATIENT PRESENTATION

### Chief Complaint

"I look like I'm pregnant and it is getting worse."

### HPI

Robert Smith is a 38-year-old man with a history of alcoholic cirrhosis who has been admitted to the hospital due to an unexplained 8-kg weight gain over the past 6 days, abdominal swelling and pain, shortness of breath, and mild confusion.

### PMH

Alcoholic cirrhosis diagnosed 2 years ago, Child–Pugh Grade A on diagnosis

EGD performed at time of cirrhosis diagnosis showed no esophageal varices

Allergic rhinitis

Hypertension

### FH

Father is alive and well at the age of 70 without significant disease. Mother died at age 47 due to complications of type 1 DM.

### SH

Recently separated from wife of 10 years and lives alone. Works as a plumber. History of extreme alcohol abuse but had quit drinking on cirrhosis diagnosis. Admits to heavy alcohol use over the last 2 months since separating from his wife and went on a drinking binge about 1 week ago.

### Meds

Fluticasone furoate two sprays per nostril once daily

Levocetirizine 5 mg once daily

Lisinopril 10 mg once daily

### All

NKDA

### ROS

Abdominal discomfort described as occurring throughout the abdomen, shortness of breath, and mild confusion. Patient denies chills or fevers.

### Physical Examination

*Gen*

Pleasant, chronically ill Caucasian man appearing to be in mild distress and fatigued

*VS*

BP 118/76, P 78, RR 27, T 37.2°C; Wt 94.2 kg, Ht 6′2″

*Skin*

(+) Palmar erythema, (+) spider angiomata, otherwise normal color

*HEENT*

PERRL, EOMI, clear sclerae, TMs normal, mucous membranes moist

*Neck/Lymph Nodes*

Supple, no thyroid nodules

*Lung/Thorax*

Mild bilateral crackles, decreased breath sounds in right lower lobe likely due to enlarged liver and ascites

*Breasts*

Nontender without masses

*CV*

RRR, $S_1$ and $S_2$ are normal, no MRG

*Abd*

Bulging, tender abdomen; hepatomegaly; (+) fluid wave; bowel sounds normal

*Genit/Rect*

Guaiac negative

*MS/Ext*

1+ pitting edema in both LE, palmar erythema; no clubbing or cyanosis

*Neuro*

Mildly confused, forgetful, A & O × 2 (oriented to person and time but does not know at which hospital he is)

### Labs

| | | | |
|---|---|---|---|
| Na 135 mEq/L | Hgb 16 g/dL | AST 88 IU/L | Ca 8.5 mg/dL |
| K 4.1 mEq/L | Hct 47% | ALT 116 IU/L | Mg 1.9 mEq/L |
| Cl 98 mEq/L | Plt 81 × $10^3$/mm$^3$ | LDH 167 IU/L | Phos 3.5 mg/dL |
| $CO_2$ 30 mEq/L | WBC 6.2 × $10^3$/mm$^3$ | T. bili 2.2 mg/dL | TSH 3.6 mIU/L |
| BUN 19 mg/dL | PT 14.3 sec | D. bili 0.7 mg/dL | $NH_3$ 94 mcg/dL |
| SCr 0.7 mg/dL | PTT 47 sec | T. prot 7.3 g/dL | HIV (–) |
| Glu 102 mg/dL | INR 1.33 | Alb 2.8 g/dL | |

### Assessment

Worsening cirrhosis; now presenting with ascites and acute encephalopathy
Perform diagnostic and therapeutic paracentesis
R/O spontaneous bacterial peritonitis (SBP)

### Clinical Course

After removal of 5 L of fluid by paracentesis, an analysis of the fluid was performed. The analysis reported a protein level of 1.4 g/dL, PMN 140 cells/mm$^3$, and SAAG 1.4 g/dL.
The culture results were negative after 3 days.
The patient's mental status began to improve after paracentesis and the administration of lactulose 30 mL po twice daily.

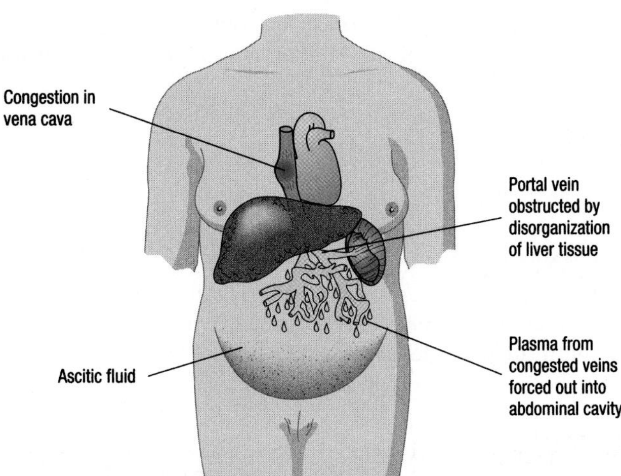


**FIGURE 44-1.** Development of ascites with portal hypertension due to cirrhosis. *(Reprinted with permission from Mulvihill ML. Human Diseases: A Systemic Approach, 4th ed. Norwalk, CT, Appleton & Lange, 1995:203.)*

Once stabilized, an EGD was performed, which showed small esophageal varices.

## QUESTIONS

### Problem Identification

1.a. Create a list of the patient's drug therapy problems.

1.b. What information (signs, symptoms, lab values) indicates the presence of ascites in this patient? (See Fig. 44-1.)

1.c. What information (signs, symptoms, lab values) indicates the presence or absence of hepatic encephalopathy and SBP in this patient?

1.d. What classification system is used to evaluate the prognosis of chronic liver disease? Use this system to calculate the score and grade for this patient.

### Desired Outcome

2. What are the goals of pharmacotherapy for managing ascites and related complications of cirrhosis?

### Therapeutic Alternatives

3.a. What nonpharmacologic therapies might be considered for this patient?

3.b. What pharmacologic therapies should be considered for this patient?

### Optimal Plan

4.a. Outline a suitable pharmaceutical care plan for the *acute* management of this patient. Include drug, dosage form, dose, dosing schedule, and duration of therapy.

4.b. Outline a suitable pharmacologic care plan for the *chronic* management of this patient. Include drug, dosage form, dose, dosing schedule, and duration of therapy.

4.c. If the initial therapy fails or is intolerable for the patient, what pharmacologic alternatives should be considered?

## Outcome Evaluation

5. How should the recommended therapy be monitored for efficacy and adverse effects?

## Patient Education

6. On discharge from the hospital, what information should be provided to the patient to enhance compliance, ensure successful treatment, and minimize or prevent adverse effects?

## ADDITIONAL CASE QUESTIONS

1. What other diseases should the patient be tested for that could impact his liver function?
2. What vaccinations should he receive on discharge, assuming that he has not had any vaccinations for over 20 years?

## SELF-STUDY ASSIGNMENTS

1. Identify which pain medications may be used safely in patients with cirrhosis and ascites.
2. Based on this patient's history, what 1-, 2-, and 5-year survival rates would be expected if the patient does not receive a liver transplant?

## CLINICAL PEARL

Angiotensin II increases portal pressure, and patients with cirrhosis often have elevated levels of angiotensin II. Losartan, an angiotensin II receptor blocker (ARB), has been studied in patients with portal hypertension and has shown some decrease in the hepatic venous pressure gradient (HVPG). However, due to inconsistent results from clinical trials, as well as the occurrence of hypotension and decreased glomerular filtration rate, the role of ARBs in patients with esophageal varices remains unclear.

## REFERENCES


1. Runyon BA, Practice Guidelines Committee, American Association for the Study of Liver Diseases (AASLD). Management of adult patients with ascites due to cirrhosis: an update. Hepatology 2009;49:2087–2107.
2. Dib N, Oberti F, Cales P. Current management of the complications of portal hypertension: variceal bleeding and ascites. CMAJ 2006;174:1433–1443.
3. Garcia-Tsao G. Current management of cirrhosis and portal hypertension: variceal hemorrhage, ascites, and spontaneous bacterial peritonitis. Gastroenterology 2001;120:726–748.
4. Garcia-Tsao G, Lim J, and Members of the Veterans Affairs Hepatitis C Resource Center Program. Management and treatment of patients with cirrhosis and portal hypertension: recommendations from the Department of Veterans Affairs Hepatitis C Resource Center Program and National Hepatitis C Program. Am J Gastroenterol 2009;104:1802–1829.
5. Gines P, Cardenas A, Arroyo V, et al. Management of cirrhosis and ascites. N Engl J Med 2004;350:1646–1654.
6. Han M, Hyzy R. Advances in critical care management of hepatic failure and insufficiency. Crit Care Med 2006;34(9 Suppl):S225–S231.
7. Moore KP, Aithal GP. Guidelines on the management of ascites in cirrhosis. Gut 2006;55(Suppl 6):vi1–vi12.


# 45

# ESOPHAGEAL VARICES

Where Low Class is Desired . . . . . . . . . . . . . . . Level I

**Cesar Alaniz, PharmD**

## LEARNING OBJECTIVES

After completing this case study, students should be able to:

- List nonpharmacologic options for managing patients with bleeding esophageal varices.
- Recommend appropriate pharmacologic therapy for controlling bleeding esophageal varices and adjunctive therapy in the setting of acute variceal bleeding.
- Provide appropriate education for patients receiving therapy for portal hypertension.

## PATIENT PRESENTATION

### Chief Complaint

"I've been throwing up blood, enough to fill my bathroom sink!"

### HPI

Ethyl Johnson is a 55-year-old woman who presents to the ED with complaint of vomiting blood and bright red blood per rectum. She was in her usual state of health, until shortly after taking a dose of lactulose when she began to feel sick and subsequently vomited a large amount of blood into the bathroom sink. She also reports a 2-day history of BRBPR.

### PMH

Cirrhosis secondary to hepatitis C (acquired from a blood transfusion in 1980s)
Hepatic encephalopathy
Peptic ulcer disease
Hypertension
Cellulitis (two admissions in past)

### FH

Father with CAD and CABG; no other history known

### SH

She lives alone and has been able to function independently. Quit smoking 10 years ago and does not drink alcohol. She works as an accountant.

### ROS

Negative except for complaints noted in HPI

### Meds

Sucralfate 1 g po BID
Omeprazole 20 mg po BID

Bumetanide 1 mg po BID
Spironolactone 50 mg po once daily
Propranolol 40 mg po BID (may not be taking)

## All

NKDA

## Physical Examination

*Gen*

Obese female looking older than stated age, looks somnolent but occasionally moves head

*VS*

BP 108/60, P 120, RR 14, T 37.8°C

*Skin*

Some spider angiomas on abdomen, thick skin, chronic venous stasis changes with lichenification

*HEENT*

PERRLA; icteric sclerae

*Neck/Lymph Nodes*

Neck supple; no masses

*Lungs/Thorax*

Clear to auscultation bilaterally

*Breasts*

No lumps or masses

*CV*

Tachycardia, RRR, no M/R/G

*Abd*

Obese, mildly distended, distant bowel sounds present, difficult to assess for hepatosplenomegaly

*Rect*

Frank blood

*Ext*

Bilateral 1+ pedal edema

*Neuro*

Sleepy, moves head occasionally; is arousable and oriented × 3; no asterixis

## Labs (on Admission)

| | | |
|---|---|---|
| Na 127 mEq/L | Hgb 7.8 g/dL | AST 104 IU/L |
| K 4.3 mEq/L | Hct 24.4% | ALT 49 IU/L |
| Cl 101 mEq/L | WBC 26.4 × $10^3$/mm$^3$ | Alk phos 114 IU/L |
| $CO_2$ 22 mEq/L | Neutros 59% | T. bili 4.3 mg/dL |
| BUN 57 mg/dL | Bands 17% | D. bili 3.3 mg/dL |
| SCr 1.9 mg/dL | Lymphs 23% | Protein 5.5 g/dL |
| Glu 155 mg/dL | Monos 1% | Alb 2.5 g/dL |
| | Plt 68 × $10^3$/mm$^3$ | Ca 8.4 mg/dL |
| | aPTT 42.1 sec | Phos 4.4 mg/dL |
| | PT 16.5 sec | |
| | INR 1.8 | |

## EGD

There is a large esophageal varix, with one large red spot and bulge that began spurting blood during the procedure. Two bands were applied to varices in that area but could not do more due to large amount of blood.

## Assessment

This is a 55-year-old woman with a history of alcohol abuse and chronic hepatitis C infection who presents to the ED acutely ill after hematemesis secondary to bleeding esophageal varices. Labs show severe anemia, leukocytosis with left shift, hyponatremia, renal dysfunction, hypoalbuminemia, increased serum aminotransferases, and coagulopathy. The patient presents with Child–Pugh class C severity of disease. Will admit to an intensive care unit for further management.

# QUESTIONS

## Problem Identification (Fig. 45-1)

1.a. Create a list of the patient's drug therapy problems.

1.b. What information supports the diagnosis of bleeding esophageal varices, and what indicates the relative severity of disease?

## Desired Outcome

2. What are the goals for managing this patient's clinical condition?

## Therapeutic Alternatives

3.a. What nonpharmacologic interventions should be considered for this patient?

3.b. What pharmacologic interventions should be considered for this patient?

## Optimal Plan

4. What pharmacotherapeutic plan should be implemented for managing the patient's current problems?

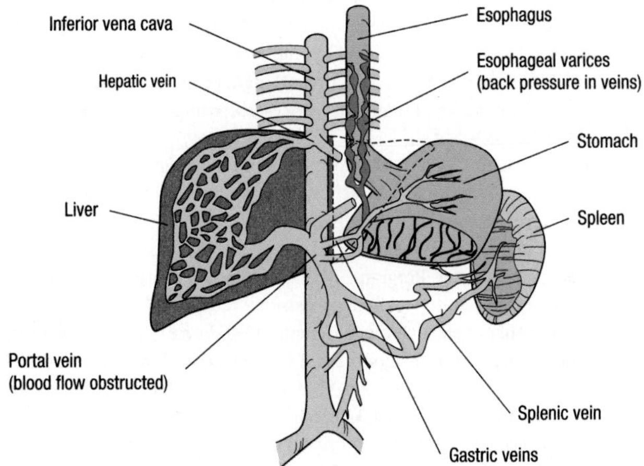


**FIGURE 45-1.** Anatomic relationships among intestinal veins affected by alcoholic cirrhosis. *(Reprinted with permission from Mulvihill ML. Human Diseases: A Systemic Approach, 4th ed. Norwalk, CT, Appleton & Lange, 1995:202.)*

## Outcome Evaluation

5. What clinical and laboratory parameters should be followed to evaluate the therapeutic interventions and to minimize the risk of adverse effects?

## Patient Education

6. What information should be provided to the patient about her medication therapy?

## CLINICAL PEARL

Although factor VII is often used in the setting of uncontrolled bleeding, it has not been shown to be of benefit in the management of variceal hemorrhage.

## SELF-STUDY ASSIGNMENTS

1. Examine the differences between octreotide and vapreotide for management of variceal hemorrhage.
2. Describe the effect of emerging fluoroquinolone resistance on use of antibiotics in patients presenting with variceal hemorrhage.
3. Describe the dose-related side effects in patients receiving combination β-blocker and isosorbide mononitrate therapy.

## REFERENCES


1. Garcia-Tsao G, Sanyal AJ, Grace ND, Carey W. Prevention and management of gastroesophageal varices and variceal hemorrhage in cirrhosis. Hepatology 2007;46:928–938.
2. Bosch J, Thabut D, Albillos A, et al. Recombinant factor VIIa for variceal bleeding in patients with advanced cirrhosis: a randomized, controlled trial. Hepatology 2008;47:1604–1614.
3. Tripathi D, Ferguson JW, Kochar N, et al. Randomized controlled trial of carvedilol versus variceal band ligation for the prevention of first variceal bleed. Hepatology 2009;50:825–833.
4. Alaniz C, Mohammad RA, Welage LS. Continuous infusion of pantoprazole with octreotide does not improve management of variceal hemorrhage. Pharmacotherapy 2009;29:248–254.
5. Ghassemi H, Garcia-Tsao G. Prevention and treatment of infections in patients with cirrhosis. Best Pract Res Clin Gastroenterol 2007;21:77–93.


# 46

# HEPATIC ENCEPHALOPATHY

State of Confusion . . . . . . . . . . . . . . . . . . . . . . . . Level I

**Carrie A. Sincak, PharmD, BCPS**

## LEARNING OBJECTIVES

After completing this case study, students should be able to:

- Identify and correct the precipitating factors associated with the development of hepatic encephalopathy in a cirrhotic patient.
- Recommend appropriate nonpharmacologic and pharmacologic intervention for a cirrhotic patient who develops hepatic encephalopathy.
- Design a plan for monitoring the efficacy and adverse effects of recommended treatments for hepatic encephalopathy.
- Provide patient education for those receiving treatment for hepatic encephalopathy.

## PATIENT PRESENTATION

### Chief Complaint (from Son)

"My mother says she is dizzy and has felt a little off over the last 2 days."

### HPI

Judy Sheddling is a 65-year-old woman who was brought to the ED by her son because of dizziness and confusion. Patient became increasingly confused over the last 2 days and on admission was alert to person only. The son states she is normally able to converse without difficulty but does require some assistance with ambulation. His mother had a scheduled endoscopy 2 days ago and did not take her lactulose the day prior to and the day of the test. She had also "retained a lot of water" and told her family that she was feeling bad. She began to decline further prior to admission with inability to answer questions properly.

### PMH

ESLD secondary to nonalcoholic steatohepatitis (NASH) cirrhosis diagnosed 5 years ago; complicated by ascites
Esophageal varices s/p band ligation (2 years ago)
TIPS procedure (1 year ago)
Hypothyroidism
Colon cancer s/p resection (15 years ago)

### FH

Not obtainable at this time

### SH

Retired; lives with her husband; they have one son and two daughters

### ROS

Constitutional: confused; weight gain
Eyes: no vision loss or pain
Ears, nose, mouth, throat: no hearing loss, nasal discharge, mouth or throat problems
Cardiovascular: no chest pains or palpitations
Respiratory: no shortness of breath, cough, or dyspnea on exertion
Gastrointestinal: (+) abdominal pain; no change in bowel habits, dysphagia, or odynophagia
Genitourinary: no dysuria or hematuria
Musculoskeletal: no joint pain or weakness
Neurologic: no weakness or headache
Psychiatric: no anxiety or depression
Endocrine: no diabetes; (+) thyroid disease
Hematologic: no enlarged lymph nodes

### Meds

Folic acid 1 mg po daily
Furosemide 40 mg po daily
Lactulose 10 g/15 mL, one tablespoonful po TID

Levothyroxine 100 mcg po daily
Multivitamin one tablet po daily
Pantoprazole 40 mg po daily
Tolvaptan 15 mg po daily
Thiamine 100 mg po daily

### All

No known allergies

### Physical Examination

*Gen*

Elderly woman in NAD who is disoriented to time and place

*VS*

BP 134/55, P 82, RR 20, T 36.7°C; Wt 79.4 kg, Ht 5′0″

*Skin*

Normal skin turgor

*HEENT*

PERRLA; dry mucous membranes; TMs intact; EOMI; fundi benign; anicteric sclerae; no sinus tenderness

*Lungs*

Chest symmetric; lungs CTA bilaterally; no wheezes or crackles

*CV*

$S_1$ and $S_2$ normal; RRR with no murmurs

*Abd*

Nontender; distended abdomen; no splenomegaly; liver edge not identifiable below the costal margin; hypoactive bowel sounds

*Rect*

Heme (–) stool; no masses

*Ext*

(+) LE edema; no clubbing or cyanosis

*Neuro*

Confused; oriented only to person; CNs II–XII intact; DTRs 2+; (+) asterixis

### Labs

| | | | |
|---|---|---|---|
| Na 135 mEq/L | Hgb 8.9 g/dL | WBC 5.2 × $10^3$/mm$^3$ | AST 63 IU/L |
| K 3.1 mEq/L | Hct 28% | 67% PMNs | ALT 23 IU/L |
| Cl 104 mEq/L | MCV 95 $\mu$m$^3$ | 3% Bands | Alk Phos 125 IU/L |
| $CO_2$ 25 mEq/L | MCHC 34 g/dL | 3% Eos | T. bili 1.2 mg/dL |
| BUN 10 mg/dL | Retic 1.1% | 25% Lymphs | D. bili 0.4 mg/dL |
| SCr 1.4 mg/dL | Plt 112 × $10^3$/mm$^3$ | 2% Monos | Alb 3.1 g/dL |
| Glu 123 mg/dL | | | $NH_3$ 70 mcg/dL |
| | | | Ca 9.4 mg/dL |
| | | | Mg 2.6 mg/dL |
| | | | Phos 3.5 mg/dL |
| | | | PT 15.2 sec |
| | | | aPTT 39.8 sec |
| | | | INR 1.5 |
| | | | TSH 10.38 $\mu$IU/mL |

### Assessment

Hepatic encephalopathy

## QUESTIONS

### Problem Identification

1.a. Create a list of the patient's drug therapy problems.

1.b. What information indicates the presence of hepatic encephalopathy in this patient?

1.c. What precipitating factors in this patient could potentially cause hepatic encephalopathy?

1.d. What additional information is needed to satisfactorily assess the hepatic encephalopathy of this patient?

### Desired Outcome

2. What are the general principles for the management of hepatic encephalopathy and desired therapeutic outcomes?

### Therapeutic Alternatives

3.a. What nondrug interventions are important before initiating pharmacotherapeutic agents for the treatment of hepatic encephalopathy?

3.b. What pharmacotherapeutic alternatives are available for the treatment of hepatic encephalopathy? Include the mechanism of action of each drug in your answer.

### Optimal Plan

4. Outline a pharmacotherapeutic plan for this patient's drug therapy problems. Include the drugs, dosage forms, doses, schedules, and duration of treatment for each problem.

### Outcome Evaluation

5. How would you monitor the efficacy and adverse effects of treatment that you recommended for this patient? (See Fig. 46-1.)

### Patient Education

6. What medication-related information should be provided to the patient about her therapy on discharge?

## CLINICAL COURSE

Two days after beginning treatment with the regimen you recommended, the patient is responding positively, and the dose has been titrated appropriately. She is oriented to time, place, and person, and no asterixis is detected. The plan is to discharge the patient home tomorrow.

## SELF-STUDY ASSIGNMENTS

1. Perform a literature search to assess the efficacy and the potential role of rifaximin in the treatment of hepatic encephalopathy.
2. List the potential advantages and disadvantages of using antibiotics for the treatment of hepatic encephalopathy.
3. Perform a literature search to determine if protein restriction is appropriate in patients with liver disease, particularly patients with cirrhosis.

Number Connection Test 1.

| Patient's Name | |
|---|---|
| Date | |
| Completion Time (seconds) | |
| Tester's Initials | |
| PT. Chart No. | |
| Patient's Signature | |

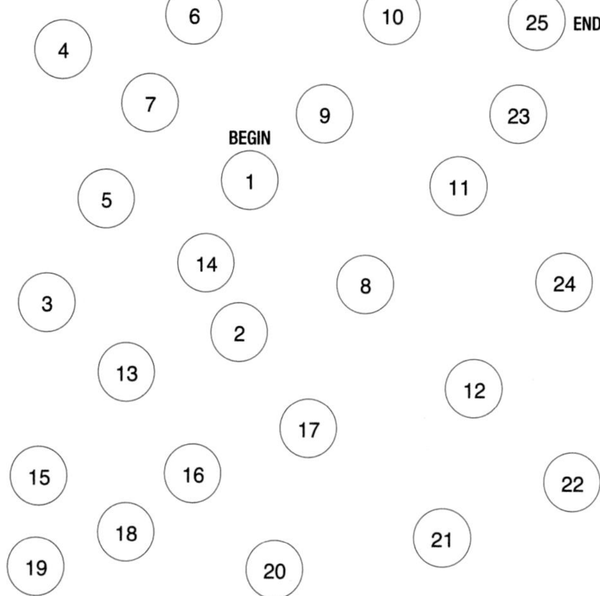


**FIGURE 46-1.** Number Connection Test Part A (NCT-A), which measures cognitive motor abilities. Subjects have to connect the numbers printed on paper consecutively from 1 to 25, as quickly as possible. Errors are not counted, but patients are instructed to return to the preceding correct number and then carry on. The test score is the time the patient needs to perform the test, including the time needed to correct all errors. A low score represents a good performance. *(Reprinted with permission from Quero JC, Schalm SW. Subclinical hepatic encephalopathy. Semin Liver Dis 1996;16:321–328.)*

## CLINICAL PEARL

Sedatives, tranquilizers, other CNS depressants, and medication noncompliance may precipitate episodic hepatic encephalopathy. A careful medication history is important in patients presenting with the disorder to identify and eliminate reversible causes.

## REFERENCES


1. Cordoba J, Minguez B. Hepatic encephalopathy. Semin Liver Dis 2008;28:70–80.
2. Sundaram V, Shaikh OS. Hepatic encephalopathy: pathophysiology and emerging therapies. Med Clin North Am 2009;93:819–836.
3. Riggio O, Ridola L. Emerging drugs for hepatic encephalopathy. Expert Opin Emerg Drugs 2009;14:537–549.
4. Blei AT, Cordoba J. Practice Parameters Committee of the American College of Gastroenterology. Hepatic encephalopathy. Am J Gastroenterol 2001;96:1968–1976.
5. Blei AT. Diagnosis and treatment of hepatic encephalopathy. Baillieres Best Pract Res Clin Gastroenterol 2000;14:959–974.
6. Mas A. Hepatic encephalopathy: from pathophysiology to treatment. Digestion 2006;73(Suppl 1):86–93.
7. Maclayton DO, Eaton-Maxwell A. Rifaximin for treatment of hepatic encephalopathy. Ann Pharmacother 2009;43:77–84.
8. Lawrence KR, Klee JA. Rifaximin for the treatment of hepatic encephalopathy. Pharmacotherapy 2008;28:1019–1032.
9. Bass NM, Mullen KD, Sanyal A, et al. Rifaximin treatment in hepatic encephalopathy. N Engl J Med 2010;362:1071–1081.


# 47

# ACUTE PANCREATITIS

A Sod Story. . . . . . . . . . . . . . . . . . . . . . . . . . . Level II


**Scott W. Mueller, PharmD, BCPS**

**Robert MacLaren, BSc, PharmD, FCCM, FCCP**


## LEARNING OBJECTIVES

After completing this case study, students should be able to:

- Evaluate precipitating factors associated with acute pancreatitis.
- Determine signs, symptoms, and laboratory abnormalities commonly associated with acute pancreatitis.
- Describe potential systemic complications associated with acute pancreatitis.
- Recommend appropriate pharmacologic and nonpharmacologic therapies for patients with acute pancreatitis.
- Develop monitoring parameters to assist in realizing desired therapeutic outcomes.

## PATIENT PRESENTATION

### Chief Complaint

"I've got a really bad pain in my stomach."

### HPI

Bill Jones is a 42-year-old man who presents to the ED shortly after midnight on a Friday night because of intense midepigastric pain radiating to his back. He states that the pain started shortly after dinner the night before but has progressively worsened. The pain is unrelated to physical activity, and he began vomiting around midnight tonight.

### PMH

Alcohol withdrawal seizures 5 months ago, which have not recurred. Hypertension, which is medically controlled.

### FH

Father died at age of 56 from an MVA; mother is 72 years old and has type 2 DM and "cholesterol issues," for which she is taking an unknown medication. One sister, also with "cholesterol issues," taking an unknown medication. The sister has a remote history of pancreatitis as well.

## SH

Divorced with three children. Employed as a groundskeeper at a golf course. Quit smoking 2 weeks ago, admits to a 40 pack-year history of smoking. He states that he used to consume 6–10 beers per day until 5 months ago when he had a withdrawal seizure but now drinks only on weekends a total of about 6 beers; he reports sharing a couple of pitchers with two friends last night with dinner. Drinks at least two cups of coffee each morning.

## Meds

Phenytoin 200 mg twice daily since his seizure
Hydrochlorothiazide 25 mg once daily for blood pressure
Doxycycline 100 mg twice daily for 10 days for "cellulitis" (now cleared as today is day 10)
Ibuprofen 200 mg OTC several doses per day PRN sore back muscles

## All

Amoxicillin/clavulanate makes his stomach upset.

## ROS

He states that he has been feeling well until last night. His back soreness from unloading pallets of heavy sod a week ago has resolved with occasional ibuprofen use. He just finished a course of antibiotics this morning for mild cellulitis that was limited to a 1 × 2-in area of the left lower tibia. He has vomited approximately six times since midnight tonight. No complaints of diarrhea or blood in the stool or vomitus. No knowledge of any prior history of uncontrolled blood sugars or cholesterol.

## Physical Examination

*Gen*

The patient is restless and in moderate distress but otherwise is a well-appearing, well-nourished male who looks his stated age.

*VS*

BP 99/56, P 124, RR 30, T 38.9°C; Wt 89 kg, Ht 5′10″

*HEENT*

PERRLA; EOMI; oropharynx pink and clear; oral mucosa dry

*Skin*

Dry with poor skin turgor; location of previous cellulitis appears healed; nontender, (–) erythema, swelling, or warmth

*Neck/Lymph Nodes*

Supple; no bruits, lymphadenopathy, or thyromegaly

*Cor*

Sinus tachycardia; no MRG

*Lungs/Thorax*

No external evidence of back injury; (–) spinal/CVA tenderness; normal range of motion; no abnormal breath sounds on auscultation

*Abd*

Moderately distended with active but diminished bowel sounds; (+) guarding; pain is elicited on light palpation of left upper and midepigastric region. No rebound tenderness, masses, or hepatosplenomegaly.

*Ext*

Extremities are warm and well perfused. Good pulses present in all extremities. No clubbing, palmar erythema, or spider angiomata.

*Rect*

Normal sphincter tone; no BRBPR or masses; stool is guaiac negative; prostate normal size.

*Neuro*

A & O × 3; neuro exam benign; CN II–XII intact; strength is equal bilaterally in all extremities. Normal tone and reflexes. No asterixis.

## Labs

| | | | |
|---|---|---|---|
| Na 128 mEq/L | Hgb 17 g/dL | AST 342 IU/L | Ca 7.2 mg/dL |
| K 3.4 mEq/L | Hct 50% | ALT 166 IU/L | Mg 1.7 mEq/L |
| Cl 105 mEq/L | WBC 15.2 × $10^3$/mm$^3$ | Alk phos 285 IU/L | Phos 2.2 mg/dL |
| $CO_2$ 18 mEq/L | Neutros 72% | LDH 255 IU/L | Trig 782 mg/dL |
| BUN 35 mg/dL | Bands 4% | T. bili 0.6 mg/dL | Repeat Trig 1,010 mg/dL |
| SCr 1.5 mg/dL | Eos 1% | Alb 3.2 g/dL | PT 12.8 s |
| Glu 375 mg/dL | Basos 1% | Prealb 25 mg/dL | INR 1.1 |
| | Lymphs 20% | Amylase 1,555 IU/L | aPTT 19.3 s |
| | Monos 2% | Lipase 2,220 IU/L | Phenytoin total 13 mg/L |
| | | | BAC 4 mg/dL |

## Other Tests

Negative for serum ketones, ASA, acetaminophen, all other alcohols, viral hepatitis titers, and HIV

## Arterial Blood Gases

pH 7.31, $PCO_2$ 38 mm Hg, $PO_2$ 88 mm Hg, $HCO_3^-$ 17 mEq/L, $O_2$ sat 98% in room air

## UA

Color yellow; turbidity clear; SG 1.010; pH 7.2; glucose >1,000 mg/dL; bilirubin (–); ketones (–); Hgb (–); protein (–); nitrite (–); crystals (–); casts (–); mucous (–); bacteria (–); urobilinogen: 0.25 EU/dL; WBC 0–5/hpf; RBC 0/hpf; epithelial cells: 0–10/hpf

## Chest X-Ray

AP view of chest shows the heart to be normal in size. The lungs are clear without any infiltrates, masses, effusions, or atelectasis. No notable abnormalities.

## Abdominal Ultrasound

Nonspecific gas pattern; no dilated bowel. Questionable opacity/abnormality of common bile duct. Cannot rule out gallstone/obstruction.

## ECG

Sinus tachycardia; rate 140 bpm. No changes from his last ECG (5 months ago), no evidence of myocardial ischemia.

## Assessment

Acute pancreatitis precipitating hyperglycemia, hypocalcemia, and nonanion gap metabolic acidosis

R/O choledocholithiasis

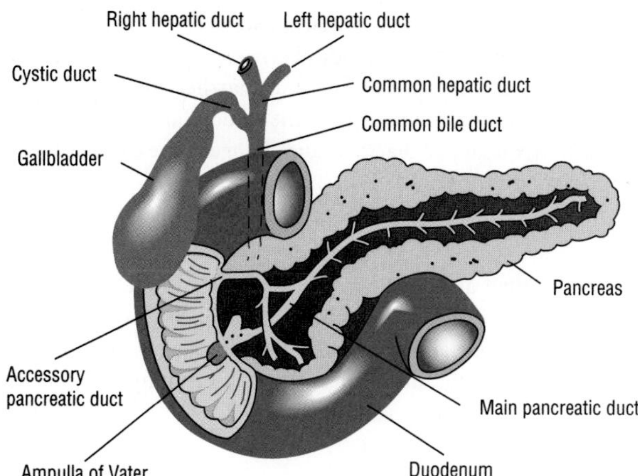


**FIGURE 47-1.** Anatomic structure of the pancreas and biliary tract. *(Reprinted with permission from DiPiro JT, Posey LM, Talbert RL, et al., eds. Pharmacotherapy: A Pathophysiologic Approach, 7th ed. New York, McGraw-Hill, 2008.)*

# QUESTIONS

## Problem Identification (Fig. 47–1)

1.a. What factors may have precipitated acute pancreatitis in this case?

1.b. What signs, symptoms, and laboratory tests are consistent with the diagnosis of acute pancreatitis?

1.c. Construct a drug therapy problem list for this patient.

## Desired Outcome

2. What are the goals of therapy for this patient?

## Therapeutic Alternatives

3. What therapies may be instituted to achieve the goals outlined above? Provide a rationale for each therapy.

## Optimal Plan

4. Develop a pharmacotherapeutic care plan for this patient, including duration of therapy.

## Outcome Evaluation

5. Outline the monitoring parameters for efficacy and adverse effects of therapy for pain management.

## Patient Education

6. When this patient is stable, what information should be provided to him to reduce the likelihood of recurrent pancreatitis?

# ■ CLINICAL COURSE

IV morphine is initiated for pain control. Partial parenteral nutrition (without lipids) is instituted after 24 hours and oral nutrition is started 24 hours later, at which time parenteral nutrition is discontinued. However, after several days of improvement in the hospital, the patient develops a WBC count of $23.4 \times 10^3/mm^3$ with neutrophils 77%, bands 15%, eosinophils 1%, basophils 0%, lymphocytes 3%, and monocytes 4%. He has a temperature of 39.8°C and is noted to be orthostatic (BP 128/76 sitting, 98/60 standing) with a glucose of 480 mg/dL. He has also experienced several episodes of diarrhea and steatorrhea.

Because of these setbacks in the patient's progress, a contrast-enhanced CT scan is obtained. The results demonstrate peripancreatic and retroperitoneal edema. The pancreas itself appears relatively normal with the exception of small nonenhancing areas around the neck of the pancreas, which are suggestive of necrosis.

## Follow-Up Questions

1.a. What potential etiologies might explain this patient's fever and relapsing acute pancreatitis?

1.b. What are the new treatment goals for this patient?

1.c. Given this new information, what therapeutic interventions should be considered for this patient?

1.d. How should these new therapies be monitored for efficacy and adverse effects?

# ■ SELF-STUDY ASSIGNMENTS

1. Describe the pathophysiology of autodigestion during acute pancreatitis.
2. Describe the controversies of early enteral nutrition, prophylactic antibiotics, and octreotide for management of acute pancreatitis.
3. Summarize published information regarding opioid effects on the sphincter of Oddi.
4. Review the Ranson scoring method for predicting the severity of acute pancreatitis, and outline its advantages and disadvantages when clinically applied.
5. Compose a list of drugs believed to aggravate or cause pancreatitis and assess the level of association for each agent.

# CLINICAL PEARL

More expensive microencapsulated pancreatic enzyme products have not consistently been shown to be superior to standard therapeutic doses of the less expensive, non–enteric-coated dosage forms.

# REFERENCES


1. Whitcomb DC. Acute pancreatitis. N Engl J Med 2006;354:2142–2150.
2. Kingsnorth A, O'Reilly D. Acute pancreatitis. BMJ 2006;332:1072–1076.
3. Frossard JL, Steer M, Pastor CM. Acute pancreatitis. Lancet 2008;371:143–152.
4. Skipworth JRA, Pereira SP. Acute pancreatitis. Curr Opin Crit Care 2008;14:172–178.
5. Talukdar R, Vege SS. Recent developments in acute pancreatitis. Clin Gastroenterol Hepatol 2009;7:S3–S9.
6. Balani AR, Grendall JH. Drug-induced pancreatitis: incidence, management, and prevention. Drug Saf 2008;31:823–837.
7. Al-Omran M, Albalawi ZH, Tashkandi MF, et al. Enteral versus parenteral nutrition for acute pancreatitis. Cochrane Database Syst Rev 2010;1:CD002837.
8. Petrov MS, Pylypchuk RD, Uchugina AF. A systematic review on the timing of artificial nutrition in acute pancreatitis. Br J Nutr 2009;101:787–793.

9. McClave SA, Martindale RG, Vanek VW, et al. Guidelines for the provision and assessment of nutrition support therapy in the adult critically ill patient: Society of Critical Care Medicine (SCCM) and American Society for Parenteral and Enteral Nutrition (A.S.P.E.N.). J Parenter Enteral Nutr 2009;33:277–316.
10. Forsmark CE, Baillie J. AGA Institute technical review on acute pancreatitis. Gastroenterology 2007;132:2022–2044.

# 48

# CHRONIC PANCREATITIS

Like a Shot to the Gut . . . . . . . . . . . . . . . . . . . Level II

**Joseph J. Kishel, PharmD, BCPS**

## LEARNING OBJECTIVES

After completing this case study, students should be able to:

- Identify subjective and objective findings consistent with chronic pancreatitis and acute exacerbations of chronic pancreatitis.
- Evaluate patient-specific data and develop a problem list for patients with acute exacerbations of chronic pancreatitis.
- Discuss therapeutic alternatives and outline a patient-specific plan for pain management during an acute exacerbation of chronic pancreatitis.
- Recommend appropriate pancreatic enzyme replacement therapy for management of steatorrhea in a patient with chronic pancreatitis.

## PATIENT PRESENTATION

### Chief Complaint

"I have had pain in my stomach for years, but now I just can't take it anymore. It feels like a shot to the gut."

### HPI

Madeline Jane is a 35-year-old woman who presents to the ED complaining of pain in her abdomen and with radiation to her back. She also has noticed an increase in loose, foul-smelling stools and has observed a fatty content and consistency to her stool. Ms Jane has experienced pain in her abdomen for several years; she has also experienced chronic diarrhea with newly increased frequency in the past week. Concurrent with the pain are nausea and vomiting, which have also increased in intensity and frequency in the past week. Ms Jane presents to the ED today because she finally found a job that provides health insurance. She did not seek medical attention previously due to the financial implications of being uninsured.

### PMH

There is no formal past medical history because the patient has not sought medical care since college due to being uninsured. Patient reports receiving the "usual" childhood vaccinations and medical care, but she has not seen a physician since college when she was dropped from her parent's medical coverage. Ms Jane states that she has had pain in her stomach and diarrhea for years but just dealt with it. Within the past week she noticed an increase in pain, increase in frequency of diarrhea, and change in the consistency and fatty content of her stool.

### SH

Parents are alive and healthy. She is an only child. Patient does not drink alcohol, smoke cigarettes, or use illicit drugs per patient report. She is single and not sexually active. Ms Jane just started a new job as a medical claims processor at St. Anthony's hospital; she has completed a college-level education.

### Meds

Multivitamin one tablet by mouth daily, has been taking for several years
Acetaminophen 500 mg by mouth Q 6 h PRN for abdominal pain; frequent daily use
Loperamide two tablets initially, and then one tablet by mouth PRN diarrhea; she usually takes two to four tablets per day
No prescription medications

### All

Amoxicillin → rash when she received it as a child for an ear infection, no use since

### ROS

Mild difficulty swallowing due to dry throat, (–) sore throat, or difficulty eating. No indigestion or bloating. Significant abdominal pain and diarrhea as described above. No constipation or fecal incontinence; normal flatus. No blood in the stool. No hemorrhoids. Urine is of normal color, volume, and odor.

### Physical Examination

*Gen*

Thin, ill-appearing Caucasian woman, appearing anxious

*VS*

BP 96/70, P 104, RR 18, T 37.8°C; Wt 55 kg, Ht 5′5″

*Skin*

Normal skin turgor

*HEENT*

PERRLA, EOMI, oropharynx clear, mucous membranes dry, eyes chronically dry

*Neck/Lymph Nodes*

Supple; (–) JVD, thyromegaly, lymphadenopathy, or bruits

*Lung/Thorax*

Audible breath sounds in all lung fields; trachea at midline; normal rate, rhythm, and effort of breathing; (–) vertebral tenderness or deformity

*CV*

Regular rate and rhythm without gallops or murmur

*Abd*

Sparse bowel sounds, (+) rebound and guarding

*Genit/Rect*

No masses, guaiac (–)

*MS/Ext*

Pulses intact bilaterally; good capillary refill; no cyanosis, clubbing, or edema

*Neuro*

A & O × 3, CN II–XII intact

### Labs

| | | | |
|---|---|---|---|
| Na 140 mEq/L | Hgb 12 g/dL | WBC 8.2 × $10^3$/mm$^3$ | T. bili 1.5 mg/dL |
| K 4.2 mEq/L | Hct 37% | Neutros 65% | Alk Phos 140 IU/L |
| Cl 95 mEq/L | RBC 4.0 × $10^6$/mm$^3$ | Bands 5% | Alb 4.4 g/dL |
| $CO_2$ 31 mEq/L | Plt 400 × $10^3$/mm$^3$ | Eos 0% | Prealb 20 mg/dL |
| BUN 8 mg/dL | MCV 85.1 μm$^3$ | Lymphs 28% | Lipase 100 IU/L |
| SCr 0.6 mg/dL | MCHC 35 g/dL | Monos 2% | Amylase 110 IU/L |
| | Glu 89 mg/dL | | |
| Antinuclear antibody pending | Antiplasminogen binding protein pending | Anti-SSA pending | IgG4 pending |

### ERCP

Changes consistent with chronic pancreatitis: inflammation of the common bile duct (Fig. 48-1)

### Assessment

1. Chronic pancreatitis, idiopathic etiology
2. Further workup planned

## QUESTIONS

### Problem Identification

1.a. Create a list of this patient's drug therapy problems.

1.b. What subjective and objective information is consistent with the diagnosis of chronic pancreatitis?

1.c. What signs, symptoms, and test results indicate that the patient is experiencing an acute exacerbation of chronic pancreatitis?

1.d. Which of the patient's problems are amenable to drug therapy?

1.e. What additional information is needed to satisfactorily assess the patient?

### Desired Outcome

2. What are the goals of pharmacotherapy in this case?

### Therapeutic Alternatives

3.a. What nondrug therapies could be useful in this patient?

3.b. What feasible pharmacotherapeutic alternatives are available for treating this acute exacerbation of chronic pancreatitis?

3.c. What additional care is required for a patient who has not seen a physician in about 15 years?

### Optimal Plan

4. What drug, dosage form, and duration of therapy are best for this patient?

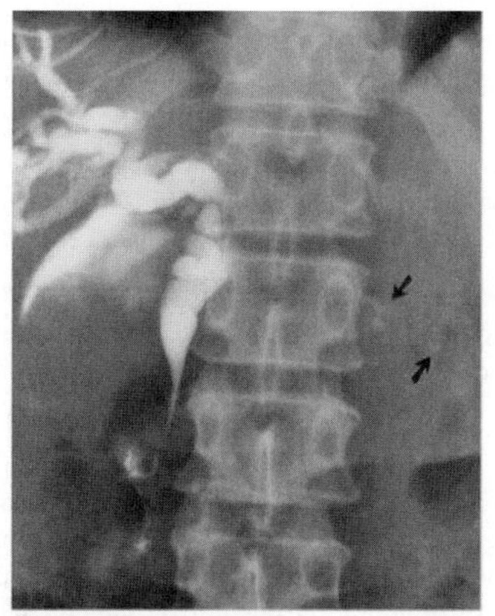


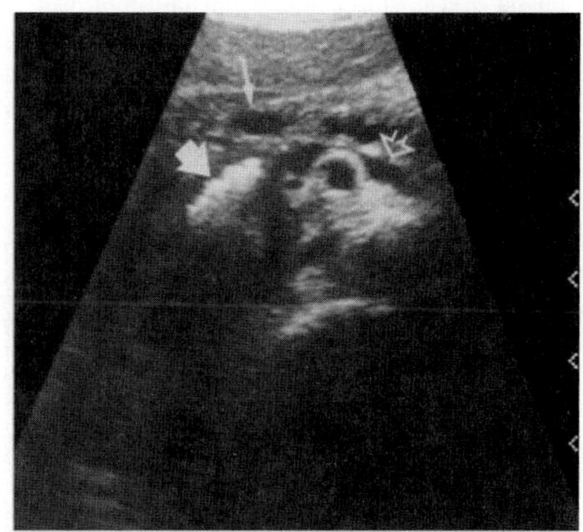


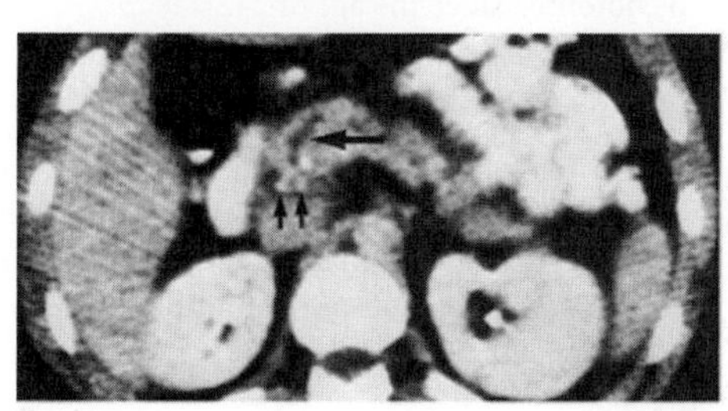


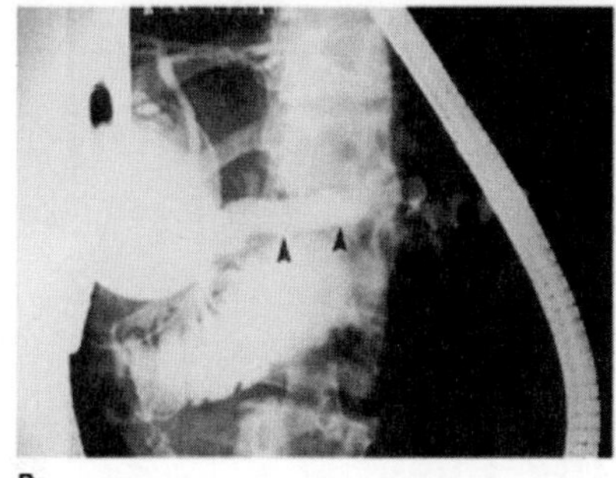


**FIGURE 48-1.** Example results of diagnosis testing. *A.* Percutaneous transhepatic cholangiography showing pancreatic calcification. *B.* Ultrasonography showing pancreatic calcification. *C.* CT scan with pancreatic calcification. *D.* Endoscopic retrograde cholangiogram showing dilation of pancreatic ducts. *(Reprinted with permission from Fauci AS, Braunwald E, Kasper DL, et al., eds. Harrison's Textbook of Internal Medicine, 17th ed. New York, McGraw-Hill: 2008.)*

## Outcome Evaluation

5. What clinical and laboratory parameters are necessary to evaluate the therapy for achievement of the desired therapeutic outcome and to detect or prevent adverse effects?

## Patient Education

6. Ms Jane wants information on her inpatient medication regimen and the nurse refers her to you, the floor-based pharmacist. What information will you provide to enhance her understanding of the medications, maximize compliance with the new medication regimen, enhance the chance of success, and minimize adverse effects?

## SELF-STUDY ASSIGNMENTS

1. Analyze the implication of an idiopathic diagnosis of disease. What other extrapancreatic diseases are associated with chronic pancreatitis?
2. What psychological factors will impact this patient's adherence to medical therapy or her willingness to seek further treatment given the patient's inattention to medical due diligence up to this point? How would this impact your ability to provide care for this patient?

## CLINICAL PEARL

Chronic pancreatitis is of idiopathic etiology in 30% of cases.

## REFERENCES

1. Pezzilli R. Etiology of chronic pancreatitis: has it changed in the last decade? World J Gastroenterol 2009;15(38):4737–4740.
2. Shafiq N, Rana S, Bhasin D, et al. Pancreatic enzymes for chronic pancreatitis. Cochrane Database Syst Rev 2009;(4):CD006302.
3. DiMagno MJ, DiMagno EP. Chronic pancreatitis. Curr Opin Gastroenterol 2009;25(5):454–459.
4. Winstead NS, Wilcox CM. Clinical trials of pancreatic enzyme replacement for painful chronic pancreatitis—a review. Pancreatology 2009;9(4):344–350 [Epub May 18, 2009].
5. Frulloni L, Lunardi C, Simone R, et al. Identification of a novel antibody associated with autoimmune pancreatitis. N Engl J Med 2009;361:2135–2142.
6. Kocher HM. Chronic pancreatitis. Am Fam Physician 2008;77(5):661–662.

# 49

# VIRAL HEPATITIS A VACCINATION

Forbid Dual Infections . . . . . . . . . . . . . . . . . . . Level II

**Juliana Chan, PharmD**

## LEARNING OBJECTIVES

After completing this case study, students should be able to:

- Determine which patient populations are at greatest risk for contracting hepatitis A.
- Recommend hepatitis A immunization for appropriate individuals based on current guidelines of the Centers for Disease Control and Prevention (CDC).
- Assess the efficacy and adverse effects of hepatitis A vaccines.
- Counsel eligible patients on the benefits of hepatitis A vaccination and the possible adverse effects associated with its use.

## PATIENT PRESENTATION

### Chief Complaint

"My doctor sent me to follow up on my liver disease."

### HPI

Hector is a 39-year-old Hispanic man, born and raised in Arizona, who will be visiting his family in Peru in the next 2 weeks. He will be seeing his grandmother for her 90th birthday with his wife and daughter. He was diagnosed with nonalcoholic fatty liver disease (NAFLD) at the age of 32. He also has hepatitis C secondary to several blood transfusions in 1991 after having multiple surgeries following a motorcycle accident. Hector's PCP referred him to see the hepatologist again before traveling for vaccinations and follow-up as he has not seen the specialist in the past 5 years.

### PMH

NAFLD diagnosed at age 32
Hepatitis C diagnosed in 1986
Hypercholesterolemia
HTN
Bipolar disorder

### Surgical History

Several surgeries after a motorcycle accident that required blood transfusions between 1991 and 1992

### FH

Mother died at 57 secondary to breast cancer and father is alive with liver disease; one brother with gout, HTN, and DM.

### SH

Married for 13 years and lives with wife and daughter. He smokes cigarettes one ppd and drinks two to three beers daily. He has several tattoos that were done professionally. There is no history of IV drug use, cocaine use, or body piercings. He has worked as a phlebotomist since the age of 24.

### ROS

Positive for fatigue, decrease in appetite. Denies any weight loss/gain, fevers, chills, headaches, shortness of breath, and coughing. He does have some abdominal pain intermittently, also constipation off and on. No black stools or obvious blood in stools.

### Meds

Multivitamin tablet po once daily
Simvastatin 40 mg po once daily
Lisinopril 40 mg po once daily
Lithium carbonate 300 mg po TID

## All

PCN

## Physical Examination

### Gen

The patient is a Hispanic-American man in no apparent distress.

### VS

BP 127/74, P 70, RR 22, T 36.9°C; Wt 143.8 kg, Ht 5′9″

### Skin

Warm and dry. Spider angiomas are not present.

### HEENT

PERRLA, EOMI; fundi normal; TMs clear. Head is normocephalic and atraumatic; sclerae anicteric.

### Neck/Lymph Nodes

Supple; no masses or JVD

### Chest

Clear without wheezes, rhonchi, or rales

### CV

RRR, $S_1$, $S_2$ normal

### Abd

(+) Bowel sounds, no masses, nontender, nondistended

### Genit/Rect

Rectal exam deferred

### MS/Ext

Normal range of motion throughout; no CCE

### Neuro

A & O × 3; CN II–XII intact; no focal deficits, negative for asterixis

## Labs (Nonfasting)

| | | | |
|---|---|---|---|
| Na 144 mEq/L | Hgb 15.6 g/dL | AST 31 IU/L | T. chol 245 mg/dL |
| K 5.0 mEq/L | Hct 45.0% | ALT 63 IU/L | Anti-HBs (+) |
| Cl 107 mEq/L | WBC 6.9 × $10^3$/mm$^3$ | Alk phos 67 IU/L | HBsAg (+) |
| $CO_2$ 30 mEq/L | Plt 305 × $10^3$/mm$^3$ | T. bili 1.0 mg/dL | Total anti-HAV (–) |
| BUN 16 mg/dL | | LDH 167 IU/L | |
| SCr 1.0 mg/dL | | PT 13.1 sec | |
| Glu 123 mg/dL | | Alb 4.5 g/dL | |
| HCV genotype 1a | | HCV RNA PCR 400,000 IU/mL | |

## Abdominal Ultrasound

### Findings

The liver has a course echotexture with smooth contour. No focal liver masses are seen. There is no intrahepatic biliary dilatation. The common bile duct measures 3 mm. Multiple shadowing stones are seen within the gallbladder. There is no gallbladder wall thickening or pericholecystic fluid. The head and body of the pancreas are grossly unremarkable; views of the tail are obscured by overlying bowel gas. A limited survey of the kidneys was performed. The right kidney measures 10.0 cm in length. The left kidney measures 11.6 cm. No hydronephrosis is seen in either kidney. The spleen is surgically absent. Visualized segments of the aorta and IVC are patent.

### Impression

1. Coarse heterogeneous appearance of the liver is consistent with patient's history of hepatitis. No evidence for focal liver mass.
2. Cholelithiasis without evidence for cholecystitis.

## Liver Biopsy

- Chronic hepatitis consistent with chronic hepatitis C virus (HCV) infection
- Minimal activity, grade 1 (0–4)
- No significant fibrosis, stage 0 (I–IV) by trichrome stain
- No significant steatosis
- Negative for dysplasia and negative for malignancy
- Hepatitis activity index:

  (Batts and Ludwig criteria; 0–4)

  Portal inflammation: 1

  Piecemeal necrosis: 1

  Lobular inflammation: 1

  Fibrosis: 0

## Assessment

This is a 39-year-old Hispanic male with a history of chronic hepatitis C who is immune to hepatitis B and NAFLD and is here to be evaluated for the hepatitis A vaccine prior to his Peru trip.

# QUESTIONS

## Problem Identification

1.a. Does this patient need to be vaccinated against hepatitis A? Please review the laboratory values to determine if the hepatitis A vaccine is needed.

1.b. What patient factors make this patient a candidate for the hepatitis A vaccination?

1.c. What other patient populations or environments present an increased risk for infection with hepatitis A?

## Desired Outcome

2. What are the goals of hepatitis A vaccination?

## Therapeutic Alternatives

3.a. What nonpharmacologic recommendations should be made to this patient and his family to minimize their risk of developing hepatitis A infection while in Peru?

3.b. What commercial products are available for vaccination against hepatitis A, and how effective are they in providing protective efficacy?

## Optimal Plan

4. Outline a vaccination regimen that includes dose, route of administration, and the number of doses required for the patient.

## Outcome Evaluation

5.a. How should the regimen you recommended be monitored for efficacy?

5.b. What adverse effects may be experienced with the regimen you recommended, and how may these events be treated?

## Patient Education

6. What information should be provided to the patient about the hepatitis A vaccine?

## ■ CLINICAL COURSE

Hector's wife and daughter (who is 6 months pregnant) returned to Arizona from Peru 8 days ago. His 41-year-old wife complains of nausea, weight loss, abdominal pain, and yellow eyes for 1 week. She was admitted to the hospital the following day for evaluation. His daughter is symptom free, but it was recommended that she follow up with her obstetrician as soon as possible. The following labs were obtained during the first day of hospitalization for Hector's wife:

| | | | |
|---|---|---|---|
| Na 137 mEq/L | Hgb 13.6 g/dL | AST 2,642 IU/L | Anti-HBs (+) |
| K 4.0 mEq/L | Hct 40.1% | ALT 2,166 IU/L | HBsAg (–) |
| Cl 100 mEq/L | WBC 7.7 × $10^3$/mm$^3$ | Alk phos 172 IU/L | Total anti-HAV (+) |
| $CO_2$ 26 mEq/L | Plt 422 × $10^3$/mm$^3$ | T. bili 20.5 mg/dL | Anti-HAV IgM (+) |
| BUN 6 mg/dL | | D. bili 12.9 mg/dL | Anti-HCV (–) |
| SCr 0.5 mg/dL | | PT 12.9 sec | Acetaminophen <10 mcg/mL |
| Glu (nonfasting) 143 mg/dL | | Alb 2.7 g/dL | |

## CT of the Abdomen With and Without IV Contrast

Clinical indication: 41 yo female with new hepatic failure

Impression:

1. Diffuse thickening of the transverse colon consistent with colitis, likely of infectious or inflammatory etiology
2. Diffuse low attenuation of the liver, perihepatic ascites, and edematous gallbladder wall consistent with underlying infectious/inflammatory process

## Follow-Up Questions

1. Based on the information provided, what medical condition does Hector's wife have?
2. What is your treatment recommendation for Hector's wife?
3. Hector's daughter is not experiencing any symptoms since returning from Peru. She visits her obstetrician the same day her mother was admitted to the hospital. She told her obstetrician that her mom is now hospitalized for acute hepatitis A. She will be 7 months pregnant in 1 week. What is your vaccination recommendation for Hector's daughter? When should the newborn be vaccinated?

## ■ SELF-STUDY ASSIGNMENTS

1. Compare and contrast the mechanism of action, immunogenicity rate, and adverse effects of the two commercially available hepatitis A vaccines.
2. Determine which vaccines can be given simultaneously with the hepatitis A vaccine.
3. Compare the cost of administering the Havrix and Engerix-B vaccines separately versus the combination product Twinrix for an adult.

## CLINICAL PEARL

The hepatitis A vaccine is highly effective in preventing hepatitis A infections when given immediately prior to departing to endemic areas.

According to the CDC, all children over 1 year of age should receive the hepatitis A vaccine in the United States.[1]

## REFERENCES


1. Update: prevention of hepatitis A after exposure to hepatitis A virus and in international travelers. Updated recommendations of the Advisory Committee on Immunization Practices (ACIP). MMWR Morb Mortal Wkly Rep 2007;56(RR41):1080–1084.
2. Prevention of hepatitis A through active or passive immunization. Recommendations of the Advisory Committee on Immunization Practices (ACIP). MMWR Morb Mortal Wkly Rep 2006;55(RR07):1–23.


# 50

# VIRAL HEPATITIS B

A Persistent Infection . . . . . . . . . . . . . . . . . . . . Level III

Juliana Chan, PharmD

## LEARNING OBJECTIVES

After completing this case study, students should be able to:

- Outline a pharmacologic and nonpharmacologic regimen for patients with chronic hepatitis B.
- Determine clinical and laboratory endpoints for treatment of chronic hepatitis B.
- Assess the efficacy and adverse effects of chronic hepatitis B treatment with interferon, pegylated interferon, lamivudine, adefovir dipivoxil, entecavir, telbivudine, and tenofovir.
- Recommend hepatitis B immunization for appropriate individuals based on current guidelines of the Centers for Disease Control and Prevention (CDC).
- Provide patient education on interferon, pegylated interferon, lamivudine, adefovir dipivoxil, entecavir, telbivudine, and tenofovir treatment.

## PATIENT PRESENTATION

### ■ Chief Complaint

"I'm here for my hepatitis B disease."

### ■ HPI

Trong Pan is a 21-year-old Chinese woman with no significant past medical history except for acquiring hepatitis B infection at birth from her mother. Over the summer, she was required to obtain a physical exam prior to entering her first year of nursing school. Laboratory test results indicated a positive HBsAg. She was referred to the liver clinic for further evaluation and possible treatment.

### ■ PMH

None

## Surgical History

None

## FH

Mother and father both positive for HBsAg. No siblings.

## SH

Single. She does not smoke or use IV drugs. She drinks socially on the weekends. She is in her first year of nursing school.

## Meds

Phenylephrine 10 mg po PRN for allergies
Calcium with vitamin D po daily

## All

None

## ROS

Denies any symptoms. Her weight is stable with no loss of appetite. No nausea, vomiting, diarrhea, abdominal pain, or constipation. No melena or hematochezia. No changes in urine or stool color and no history of icteric sclerae.

## Physical Examination

### *Gen*

The patient is not in acute distress.

### *VS*

BP 128/82, P 76, RR 20, T 37.6°C; Wt 52.1 kg, Ht 5′2″

### *Skin*

Warm and dry; no signs of jaundice. Good turgor.

### *HEENT*

Head is normocephalic, atraumatic. Sclerae are anicteric bilaterally. Neck is supple. No masses or palpable lymphadenopathy. PERRLA. Funduscopic exam normal.

### *Cor*

RRR, $S_1$, $S_2$ normal; no $S_3$ or $S_4$

### *Lungs*

Clear to P & A

### *Abd*

Good bowel sounds, soft, nontender; no evidence of ascites; no palpable hepatosplenomegaly

### *Rect*

Guaiac negative

### *Ext*

Normal range of motion throughout; no C/C/E, no gross lesions, ecchymosis, or peripheral edema

### *Neuro*

CN II–XII intact; DTRs 2+ throughout; negative Babinski

## Labs

| | | | |
|---|---|---|---|
| Na 139 mEq/L | Hgb 12.4 g/dL | AST 64 IU/L | HBsAg (+) |
| K 4.0 mEq/L | Hct 37.3% | ALT 111 IU/L | Anti-HBs (–) |
| Cl 104 mEq/L | Plt 272 × $10^3$/mm$^3$ | Alk phos 71 IU/L | HBeAg (+) |
| $CO_2$ 25 mEq/L | WBC 6.9 × $10^3$/mm$^3$ | T. bili 0.4 mg/dL | HBV DNA PCR Quant 6,368,844 IU/mL |
| BUN 12 mg/dL | TSH 1.96 μIU/mL | T. prot 7.2 g/dL | Anti-HBc IgM (–) |
| SCr 0.9 mg/dL | T. chol 132 mg/dL | Alb 4.2 g/dL | Anti-HBc (+) |
| Glu (nonfasting) 86 mg/dL | Trig 194 mg/dL | PT 10.8 s | HCV RNA quant <615 IU/mL |
| | | | Anti-HCV (–) |
| | | | Anti-HAV, total (+) |
| | | | Anti-HIV (–) |

## Other Tests

### *Complete Ultrasound of the Abdomen*

Findings: There is no ascites. The liver is normal in contour and echogenicity. There is no intrahepatic biliary dilatation; the common bile duct is not dilated and measures 0.5 cm. The gallbladder is unremarkable and without calculi, wall thickening, or pericholecystic fluid. The head and body of the pancreas are grossly unremarkable; views of the tail are obscured by overlying bowel gas.

A limited survey of the kidneys was performed. The kidneys are normal in size and echogenicity. The right kidney measures 9.5 cm in length. The left kidney measures 9.6 cm. No hydronephrosis is seen in either kidney. The spleen is normal in echotexture and size, measuring 9.4 cm. The visualized portions of the abdominal aorta and IVC are unremarkable.

Impression: Unremarkable ultrasound of the abdomen, including limited survey of both kidneys.

## Assessment

Ms Pan is a 21-year-old Chinese woman with elevated LFTs and chronic hepatitis B.

# QUESTIONS

## Problem Identification

1.a. Create a list of this patient's drug therapy problems.

1.b. Which clinical findings, laboratory values, and items in the medical history suggest the presence of chronic hepatitis B virus (HBV) infection?

## Desired Outcome

2. What are the goals of treatment for a chronic active HBV infection?

## Therapeutic Alternatives

3.a. What nonpharmacologic measures should be considered for this patient?

3.b. What pharmacotherapeutic alternatives are available for treatment of this patient?

## Optimal Plan

4. What drug, dose, dosage form, schedule, and duration of therapy should be recommended?

## Outcome Evaluation

5.a. How should the therapy you recommended be monitored for efficacy and adverse effects?

5.b. Which baseline parameters suggest that this patient may have a favorable or unfavorable response to treatment (i.e., sustained loss of HBeAg and HBV DNA)?

## Patient Education

6. What information should be provided to this patient regarding the treatment?

## ■ CLINICAL COURSE

The patient tolerated the initial therapy very well with minimal adverse effects. After 52 weeks of therapy, her physician stopped the medication. However, 3 months post-treatment, her serum HBV DNA was detectable. She also states that since finishing her hepatitis B therapy, she is in a relationship and sexually active. Her lab results for the last few months of treatment were as follows:

| Test | 12 Weeks After Therapy Started | 24 Weeks After Therapy Started | 52 Weeks After Therapy Started | 9 Months After Therapy Discontinued |
|---|---|---|---|---|
| AST (IU/L) | 54 | 39 | 21 | 55 |
| ALT (IU/L) | 78 | 30 | 25 | 84 |
| Alk phos (IU/L) | 76 | 80 | 83 | 73 |
| T. bili (mg/dL) | 0.5 | 0.9 | 0.9 | 0.8 |
| PT (sec) | 11.2 | 11.2 | 10.7 | 10.1 |
| Alb (g/dL) | 3.9 | 4.8 | 4.8 | 4.2 |
| HBsAg | (+) | (+) | (+) | (+) |
| Anti-HBs | (-) | (-) | (-) | (-) |
| HBeAg | (+) | (+) | Nonreactive | (+) |
| HBeAb | (-) | (+) | (+) | (-) |
| HBV DNA (IU/mL) | 904 | <29[a] | <29[a] | 1,122,971 |

[a]<29 IU/mL indicates undetectable HBV DNA level.

## Follow-Up Questions

1. Based on these results, what therapy would you recommend, if any? Include the drug name, dose, dosage form, schedule, and duration of therapy.
2. What adverse effects may occur with this new therapy, and how would you monitor for them?
3. What information should be provided to this patient about the new treatment?
4. What information or therapeutic intervention do you need to provide to the patient and for her new boyfriend?

## ■ CLINICAL COURSE

Eighteen months after the completion of her initial course of therapy, Mrs Pan is now married and is 23 years old. She is 6 months pregnant and is due to give birth at 36 weeks. The patient continues to be on hepatitis B therapy, and her HBsAg status is positive.

## Follow-Up Questions (continued)

5. Would you recommend hepatitis B vaccination to Mrs Pan's newborn? If yes, include the doses and dosage schedule.

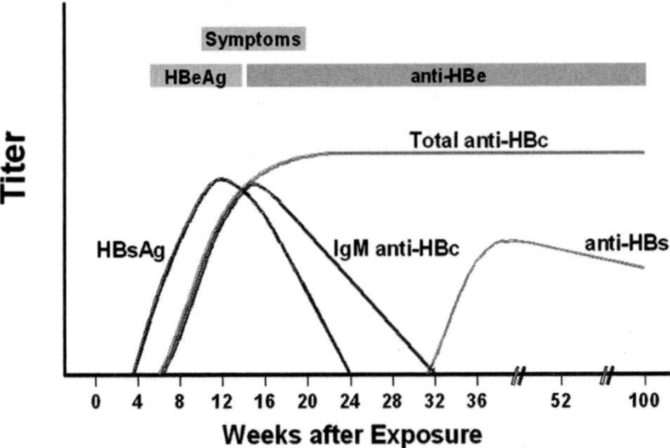


**FIGURE 50-1.** Typical serologic course of acute hepatitis B virus infection with recovery. *Note:* Serologic markers of infection vary depending on whether the infection is acute or chronic. *(Source: Centers for Disease Control and Prevention. Viral Hepatitis Resource Center. http://www.cdc.gov/HEPATITIS/Resources/Professionals/Training/Serology/gr_hbv_acute.htm.)*

## ■ SELF-STUDY ASSIGNMENTS

1. Describe the ideal hepatitis B candidate to respond to antiretroviral HBV therapy and what you would monitor for therapeutic efficacy and adverse effects.
2. Compare and contrast the mechanism of action, immunogenicity rate, and adverse effects of the two available hepatitis B vaccines.
3. Survey several pharmacies to estimate the approximate retail cost of the antiretroviral HBV agents and pegylated interferon therapy for the treatment of hepatitis B.
4. Review the time course of serologic markers after an acute HBV infection and explain their significance to one of your peers (Fig. 50-1).

## CLINICAL PEARL

To eliminate HBV transmission that occurs during infancy and childhood, the Immunization Practices Advisory Committee of the Centers of Disease Control and Prevention recommends that all newborn infants be vaccinated regardless of the hepatitis B status of the mothers.[6,7]

## REFERENCES

1. Lok AS, McMahon BJ. Chronic hepatitis B: update 2009. Hepatology 2009;50:1–6.
2. Keeffe EB, Dieterich DT, Han SH, et al. A treatment algorithm for the management of chronic hepatitis B virus infection in the United States: 2008 update. Clin Gastroenterol Hepatol 2008;6:1315–1341.
3. Keeffe EB, Dieterich DT, Pawlotsky J, et al. Chronic hepatitis B: preventing, detecting, and managing viral resistance. Clin Gastroenterol Hepatol 2008;6:268–274.
4. Marcellin P, Heathcote EJ, Buti M, et al. Tenofovir disoproxil fumarate versus adefovir dipivoxil for chronic hepatitis B. N Engl J Med 2008;359:2442–2455.
5. ter Borg MJ, van Zonneveld M, Zeuzem S, et al. Patterns of viral decline during PEG-interferon alpha-2b therapy in HBeAg-positive chronic hepatitis B: relation to treatment response. Hepatology 2006;44:721–727.

6. Centers for Disease Control and Prevention. Hepatitis virus B: a comprehensive immunization strategy to eliminate transmission of hepatitis B virus infection in the United States: recommendations of the Advisory Committee on Immunization Practices (ACIP) part 1: immunization of infants, children, and adolescents. MMWR Morb Mortal Wkly Rep 2005;54(RR16):1–31.
7. Centers for Disease Control and Prevention. Hepatitis virus B: a comprehensive immunization strategy to eliminate transmission of hepatitis B virus infection in the United States: recommendations of the Advisory Committee on Immunization Practices (ACIP) part II: immunization of adults. MMWR Morb Mortal Wkly Rep 2006;55(RR16):1–33.

# 51

# VIRAL HEPATITIS C

## Guidelines for Optimal Care De-LIVER-y . . . . Level II

**Randolph E. Regal, BS, PharmD**

## LEARNING OBJECTIVES

After completing this case study, students should be able to:

- Know and evaluate the clinical manifestations and laboratory parameters relevant to the assessment and treatment of chronic hepatitis C.
- Design a patient-specific pharmaceutical care plan for a patient with chronic hepatitis C, including drugs, doses, and duration of therapy.
- Develop a plan for monitoring efficacy and adverse effects of the pharmacologic agents used in the management of chronic hepatitis C.
- Provide patient education for patients with chronic hepatitis C regarding their medications, nonpharmacologic interventions/behaviors, and vaccinations.

## PATIENT PRESENTATION

### Chief Complaint

"About a month ago, my family doctor told me that my liver tests were abnormal. He sent me to your specialty GI clinic for assessment and follow-up. I was worried because I just have not been feeling very well for the last several months. I had my first liver clinic visit last week, and I'm here today to talk about treatment options."

### HPI

Timothy Riggs is a 45-year-old man who has been referred by his family physician to the GI/liver clinic for assessment of his abnormal liver enzymes. After a conversation between the family physician and the one of the clinic specialists, Mr Riggs had a battery of labs drawn and a liver biopsy done last week, and he returns to the clinic today for a complete physical and further workup.

About 5 weeks ago, he went to his family physician because of a rash that slowly developed on both his lower extremities and to talk about a prescription for Viagra because of a recent decline in sexual function. Since he was about 25 year old, he has worked out with weights about 3–4 days a week and runs two to three times a week. Although he continues to maintain his regimen despite working long hours, he has noticed a progressive decline in his stamina over the last year, and he more frequently experiences dizziness on exertion. He says he is slowly losing "bulk" and has lost about 10 lb in the last 6 months. He also reports an increased incidence of headaches, mild RUQ abdominal pain (especially toward the end of running sessions), and muscle and joint pain that persists between weight and running sessions.

He reports frequent use of recreational drugs in high school and up to about his mid-20s, including marijuana, alcohol, and intranasal cocaine. He denies using IV drugs at any point in his life. He has had three female sexual partners in the past 25 years, all fairly long-term relationships. In the last 10 years, after going about 10 years without a drink, his consumption of alcohol had gone from just an occasional social drink to drinking one to two drinks about four to five nights a week. At least once a week, he reported that he actually drinks until he was "drunk," usually on Saturday night "because he does not work on Sundays." However, since he found out his liver enzymes were elevated, he has cut down alcohol consumption to "almost nothing."

He does not recall ever having a blood transfusion.

### PMH

Depression: States treated with Prozac and later Wellbutrin for about 1 year at age 25, no reported depression since
Hypothyroidism: Under treatment and well controlled on Synthroid with minor dose adjustments for the past 20 years
GERD: Began several years ago, is often exacerbated by exercise and alcohol
Gastritis: Complaints of intermittent epigastric pain, increased in last 10 years (PUD never confirmed by EGD)
Early osteoarthritis treated with PRN Darvocet and acetaminophen

### FH

No known family history of liver disease. Both parents are alive, still living independently, and doing reasonably well considering they are in their early 80s. Has one brother and one sister, both older in their early 50s. The brother suffers from chronic alcoholism, HTN, and survived an MI last year. The sister has been treated for hypothyroidism for the last 25 years.

### SH

Patient earned bachelor's degree in business administration after high school. After being laid off as a customer service representative/mechanic at a local car dealer where he had worked since his college graduation, he eventually found a job as a car sales manager where he has been employed for the last 10 years. He was divorced after 4 years of marriage at age 25 with no children. He has since had two long-term relationships but never remarried, currently living with his girlfriend of the last 5 years.

This is a nonsmoker who drank and used recreational drugs, including cocaine, up until about age 25, when he began counseling for his substance abuse, depression, and his impending divorce. He was clean for about 10 years until he was laid off from his first job and has gradually increased his alcohol consumption over the last 10 years.

## Meds

MVI one tablet po daily × 1 year

Cimetidine 400 mg po BID × 10 years

Levothyroxine 100 mcg po once daily × 20 years

Ripped Ma Huang Herbal Remedy capsules twice daily for last 2 years

Darvocet-N 100 one to two tablets up to three times daily PRN for bone and joint aches (averages three to four tablets per day) for last year

## Allergies and Intolerances

Fluoxetine: Reduced libido

## ROS

Ten of 14 systems reviewed; all negative except for the following: (+) increased headaches and fatigue, weight loss, loss of libido, and dizziness; (+) joint discomfort but no apparent effect on ROM

## Physical Examination

### Gen

Tired-appearing but well nourished, fairly muscular and well-built Caucasian man in NAD

### VS

BP 120/68, P 65, RR 18, T 37.0°C; Wt 95 kg, Ht 5′9″

### Skin

No jaundice or palmar erythema. Slight vascular spider angiomata on posterior LE. A few palpable purpuric lesions on bilateral anterior aspects of shins.

### HEENT

PERRLA; EOMI; sclerae anicteric; funduscopic exam normal; TMs intact

### Neck/Lymph Nodes

Neck supple; no lymphadenopathy or thyromegaly; no carotid bruits

### Lungs/Thorax

Normal breath sounds; mild gynecomastia

### CV

RRR, $S_1$, $S_2$ normal; no $S_3$ or $S_4$

### Abd

Liver slightly enlarged (span 13 cm); mild splenomegaly; no evidence of ascites; RUQ tender to palpation

### MS/Ext

No edema in LE bilaterally; peripheral pulses 2+ throughout; normal ROM. Some discomfort with movement in knees, elbows, and hands. Mild tenderness, pain elicited by local pressure to knees and elbows.

### Neuro

A & O × 3; CN II–XII intact; DTRs 2+

## Labs Obtained 5 Weeks Ago from Patient's PCP

| | | |
|---|---|---|
| Na 140 mEq/L | Hgb 14.2 g/dL | AST 49 IU/L |
| K 4.2 mEq/L | Hct 42.6% | ALT 42 IU/L |
| Cl 98mEq/L | Plt 170 × $10^3$/mm$^3$ | Alk phos 116 IU/L |
| $CO_2$ 28 mEq/L | WBC 7.7 × $10^3$/mm$^3$ | T. bili 0.9 mg/dL |
| BUN 11 mg/dL | 67% PMNS | Alb 3.8 g/dL |
| SCr 1.1 mg/dL | Bands 1% | PT 12.0 sec |
| Glu 111 mg/dL | Lymphs 22% | HBsAg (–) |
| TSH 7.32 μIU/mL | Monos 10% | Anti-HAV (–) |
| | | Anti-HCV (+) |

## Labs Obtained at Preclinic Lab Drawn About 1 Week Ago

| | | | |
|---|---|---|---|
| Na 142 mEq/L | Hgb 14.0 g/dL | AST 58 IU/L | HBsAg (–) |
| K 4.4 mEq/L | Hct 42.0% | ALT 48 IU/L | Anti-HAV (–) |
| Cl 96 mEq/L | Plt 151 × $10^3$/mm$^3$ | Alk phos 98 IU/L | Anti-HCV (+) |
| $CO_2$ 28 mEq/L | WBC 9.7 × $10^3$/mm$^3$ | T. bili 1.1 mg/dL | HCV RNA (bDNA assay) 2 × $10^6$ copies/mL; 1 × $10^6$ IU/mL |
| BUN 15 mg/dL | 70% PMNS | Alb 3.6g/dL | HCV genotype 1 |
| SCr 1.2 mg/dL | Bands 1% | PT 12.0 s | HIV (–) |
| Glu 100 mg/dL | Lymphs 22% | ANA (+) | |
| TSH 8.04 μIU/mL | Monos 7% | Serum iron: 50 mcg/dL | |
| | | Ferritin: 283 ng/mL | |
| | | TIBC: 251 mcg/dL | |
| | | T. sat. 20% | |

## Liver Biopsy (Performed After Liver Clinic Visit 1 Week Ago)

Moderate fibrosis and inflammation consistent with chronic hepatitis

## Assessment/Diagnosis

Newly diagnosed hepatitis C, likely chronic

R/O cryoglobulinemia secondary to hepatitis C virus (HCV) (recently converted to positive ANA)

# QUESTIONS

## Problem Identification

1.a. Create a list of the patient's drug therapy problems. Prioritize the problems from most urgent to least urgent for addressing at this initial presentation. Other than the need for treating hepatitis C, are any adjustments needed in his current medication regimen?

1.b. What physical findings and laboratory values indicate the presence of chronic HCV infection?

1.c. What risk factor(s) for HCV infection does the patient have?

1.d. What are the compelling reasons to treat this patient for chronic HCV?

## Desired Outcome

2. What are the goals of treatment for chronic HCV infection?

## Therapeutic Alternatives

3.a. What nonpharmacologic treatment measures should be implemented for this patient?

3.b. What pharmacotherapeutic alternatives are available for treatment of HCV infection in this patient?

3.c. Does this patient have any medical conditions that are considered at least relative contraindications to receiving the treatments discussed in the previous question?

## Optimal Plan

4. Design a pharmacotherapeutic plan for this patient. Include the drug, dose, schedule, and duration of therapy.

## Outcome Evaluation

5.a. How should the therapy you recommended for HCV infection be monitored for efficacy and adverse effects?

5.b. Which baseline patient parameters may be predictors of poor response to the treatment you recommended?

5.c. What actions can be taken if the patient develops intolerable adverse effects to the treatment you recommended?

## Patient Education

6. What information should be provided to this patient regarding his treatment?

## ■ CLINICAL COURSE: 4-WEEK VISIT

At his 4-week visit, Mr Riggs reports feeling just a bit more fatigue than at baseline; his AST and ALT are mildly increased to 74 and 90 IU/L, but his HCV RNA value is now at 20,000 copies/mL (10,000 IU/mL). The chills, extreme fatigue, and diffuse muscle aches that plagued him around the time of his 2-week visit just abated this week. He reports no SOB, DOE, or orthostatic symptoms. Other labs are similar to the initial presentation except for hemoglobin 11.6 g/dL, WBC 4.8 × $10^3/mm^3$, platelets 130 × $10^3/mm^3$, and TSH 4.14 μIU/mL.

## Follow-Up Questions

1. Based on this information, should the therapy continue as planned? Why or why not?
2. What likely caused his chills and muscle aches early in therapy?
3. What is the likely cause of his anemia?
4. What other laboratory tests would help you to monitor his drug therapy tolerance?

## ■ CLINICAL COURSE: 12-WEEK VISIT

At his 12-week visit, Mr Riggs reports feeling better; lab values include AST 50 IU/L, ALT 65 IU/L, and HCV RNA 1,000 copies/mL (500 IU/mL). Other labs are similar to the previous visit with the exception of hemoglobin 11.0 g/dL, WBC 4.5 × $10^3/mm^3$, platelets 180 × $10^3/mm^3$, and TSH 1.01 μIU/mL. He is beginning to exercise a bit more and has put on about 5 lb in the last month or so.

## Follow-Up Question

5. Based on this information, should the therapy continue as planned? Why or why not?

## ■ CLINICAL COURSE: 24-WEEK VISIT

At his 24-week visit, he is feeling much better, although he has noticed a bit more fatigue on exertion when using his treadmill, even compared to last month.

Laboratory tests include: AST 21 IU/L, ALT 30 IU/L, qualitative HCV RNA test (–), hemoglobin 10.2 g/dL, WBC 4.2 × $10^3/mm^3$ (ANC ~3.0 × $10^3/mm^3$), and platelets 120 × $10^3/mm^3$.

## Follow-Up Questions

6. Based on this new information, what changes would you recommend for the treatment of chronic hepatitis C for this patient, and for how long?
7. Outline a plan for vaccinating this patient against other forms of viral hepatitis.

## ■ SELF-STUDY ASSIGNMENTS

1. Telaprevir is a promising investigational drug for treatment of chronic HCV, especially for genotype 1 disease, when used in combination with peginterferon and ribavirin. Review the PROVE 1 and PROVE 2 trials and summarize the advantages and disadvantages of adding this third drug to the two established agents.
2. Perform a literature search to compare the differences in pharmacokinetic properties and tolerance between interferon and each of the two peginterferon products
3. The guidelines in this chapter address the current standards for treating *chronic* hepatitis C. Perform a literature search on the latest recommendations for treatment of *acute* hepatitis C.

## CLINICAL PEARL

The course of chronic hepatitis C infection and treatment response can be adversely affected by alcohol consumption. Patients should be advised to stop all alcohol ingestion.

## REFERENCES


1. Ghany MG, Strader DB, Thomas DL, Seef LB, American Association for the Study of Liver Diseases. Diagnosis, management, and treatment of hepatitis C: an update. Hepatology 2009;49:1335–1374.
2. Chronic Hepatitis C: Current Disease Management. National Digestive Diseases Information Clearinghouse. NIH Publication No. 07-4230. November 2006. Available at: *http://www.digestive.niddk.nih.gov/ddiseases/pubs/chronichepc/*. Accessed April 5, 2010.
3. Smith JP. Treatment options for patients with hepatitis C: role of pharmacists in optimizing treatment response and managing adverse events. Pharmacotherapy 2008;28(9):1151–1161.
4. Benson GD, Koff RS, Tolman KG. Therapeutic use of acetaminophen in patients with liver disease. Am J Ther 2005;12:133–141.
5. Long RG. Endocrine aspects of liver disease. Br Med J 1980;280: 225–228.
6. Dara L, Hewett J, Lim JK. Hydroxycut hepatotoxicity: a case series and review of liver toxicity from herbal weight loss supplements. World J Gastroenterol 2008;14:6999–7004.
7. Manns MP, McHutchinson JG, Gordon SC, et al. Peginterferon alfa-2b plus ribavirin compared with interferon alfa-2b plus ribavirin for initial treatment of chronic hepatitis C: a randomised trial. Lancet 2001;358:958–965.
8. Fried MW, Shiffman ML, Reddy KR, et al. Peginterferon alfa-2a plus ribavirin for chronic hepatitis C virus infection. N Engl J Med 2002;347:975–982.
9. Jacobson IM, Brown RS Jr, Freilich B, et al. Peginterferon alfa-2a and weight based or flat-dose ribavirin in chronic hepatitis C patients: a randomized trial. Hepatology 2007;46:971–981.
10. Kramer ES, Hofmann C, Smith PG, Shiffman ML, Sterling RK. Response to hepatitis A and B in patients with chronic hepatitis C virus and advanced fibrosis. Dig Dis Sci 2009;54;2016–2025.

# SECTION 5
# RENAL DISORDERS

## 52

## DRUG-INDUCED ACUTE KIDNEY INJURY

Not a Cute Consequence . . . . . . . . . . . . . . . . Level II

Mary K. Stamatakis, PharmD

### LEARNING OBJECTIVES

After completing this case study, students should be able to:

- Evaluate clinical and laboratory findings in a patient with AKI.
- Select pharmacotherapy for treatment of complications associated with AKI.
- Assess appropriateness of aminoglycoside serum concentrations in relation to efficacy and toxicity.
- Develop strategies to prevent drug-induced AKI, including the selection of pharmacologic alternatives that do not adversely affect kidney function.
- Adjust drug dosages based on a patient's estimated kidney function to maximize efficacy and minimize adverse events.

### PATIENT PRESENTATION

#### Chief Complaint

Not available.

#### HPI

Wilbur Elliott is a 79-year-old man who originally presented to the hospital 1 month ago with symptoms of heart failure that culminated in mitral valve replacement surgery. His surgery was complicated by a 1-hour hypotensive episode, with BP of 70/50 mm Hg during surgery. Three days postoperation, purulent drainage was noted from the surgical site, and he was subsequently diagnosed with mediastinitis. At that time, he was also found to have *Serratia* bacteremia (blood cultures × 4 positive for *Serratia marcescens*, sensitive to gentamicin, piperacillin, ceftazidime, ceftriaxone, and ciprofloxacin; resistance was noted to ampicillin). Therapy was initiated with gentamicin and ceftazidime. Thus far, he has completed day 21 of a 6-week course of antibiotics. A gradual increase in his BUN and serum creatinine concentrations from baseline and signs of volume overload have been noted since admission (see Table 52-1).

#### PMH

Type 2 DM
CKD
Dyslipidemia
Osteoarthritis
HTN
Heart failure
Depression

#### PSH

Mechanical mitral valve replacement surgery 28 days ago

#### FH

Father had type 2 DM.

#### SH

Denies smoking or alcohol; retired coal miner (11 years ago)

#### Current Meds

Gentamicin (see Table 52-1 for dosages and serum drug concentrations; currently on hold)
Ceftazidime 1 g IVPB Q 12 h
Warfarin 5 mg po once daily
Enalapril 5 mg po once daily
Colace 100 mg po twice daily
Furosemide 80 mg po Q 12 h × 2 days
Atorvastatin 20 mg po daily
Escitalopram 10 mg po daily
Glipizide 10 mg po daily
Ibuprofen 400 mg po Q 4–6 h PRN pain (started today for joint pain)

#### All

NKDA

#### ROS

Currently complains of trouble breathing, weakness, general malaise, and pain in right hand. No fever or chills.

#### Physical Examination

*Gen*

Confused-appearing man in mild distress

*VS*

BP 152/90, P 80, RR 26, T 37.7°C; current Wt 80 kg (admission Wt 75 kg), Ht 5′9″

*Skin*

Normal skin turgor, surgical incision site healing with no drainage

*HEENT*

PERRLA, EOMI, poor dentition

*Neck/Lymph Nodes*

(+) JVD

**TABLE 52-1 Serum Creatinine, BUN, and Serum Gentamicin Concentrations During Hospitalization**

| Postoperative Day | SCr (mg/dL) | BUN (mg/dL) | Gentamicin (mcg/mL) | | Gentamicin Dosages |
|---|---|---|---|---|---|
| | | | Peak[a] | Trough[b] | |
| 3 | 1.5 | 15 | | | 140 mg × 1, and then 120 mg Q 12 h |
| 5 | 1.5 | 22 | 6.3 | 1.1 | Continue current regimen |
| 7 | 1.7 | 21 | | | |
| 10 | 2.1 | 22 | 6.9 | 1.8 | Continue current regimen |
| 14 | 2.7 | 21 | 8.3 | 2.5 | Decrease to 120 mg Q 24 h |
| 17 | 3.0 | 26 | | | |
| 21 | 3.2 | 27 | 9.4 | 2.7 | Gentamicin on hold |

BUN, blood urea nitrogen; SCr, serum creatinine.
[a]Serum drug concentrations drawn 30 minutes after a 30-minute infusion.
[b]Serum drug concentrations drawn immediately before a dose.

*Chest*

Basilar crackles, inspiratory wheezes

*CV*

$S_1$, $S_2$ normal, no $S_3$, irregular rhythm

*Abd*

Soft, nontender, (+) BS, (−) HSM

*Genit/Rect*

(−) Masses

*MS/Ext*

2+ ankle/sacral edema; some tenderness and limited motion in right hand

*Neuro*

A & O to person and place, but not to time

### Labs (Current)

| | | |
|---|---|---|
| Na 139 mEq/L | Hgb 9.7 g/dL | Ca 8.6 mg/dL |
| K 3.7 mEq/L | Hct 29.5% | Mg 2.1 mg/dL |
| Cl 103 mEq/L | Plt 303 × 10³/mm³ | Phos 4.4 mg/dL |
| $CO_2$ 24 mEq/L | WBC 8.6 × 10³/mm³ | INR 2.7 |
| BUN 50 mg/dL | (BUN 19 mg/dL on admission) | |
| SCr 3.2 mg/dL | (SCr 1.5 mg/dL on admission) | |
| Glu 119 mg/dL | | |

### UA

Color, yellow; character, hazy; glucose (−); ketones (−); SG 1.010; pH 5.0; protein 30 mg/dL; coarse granular casts 5–10/lpf; WBC 0–3/hpf; RBC 0–2/hpf; no bacteria; nitrite (−); osmolality 325 mOsm; urinary sodium 45 mEq/L; creatinine 33 mg/dL, $FE_{NA}$ = 3.1%.

### Repeat Blood Cultures Today

Negative

### Fluid Intake/Output and Daily Weights

| Day | I/O | Weight (kg) |
|---|---|---|
| 3 days ago | 3,200 mL/900 mL | N/A |
| 2 days ago | 2,600 mL/1,000 mL | 76 |
| Yesterday | 2,800 mL/1,300 mL | N/A |
| Today | N/A | 80 |

### Assessment

AKI with extracellular fluid expansion

# QUESTIONS

## Problem Identification

1.a. Create a list of the patient's drug therapy problems.

1.b. What information (signs, symptoms, laboratory values) indicates the presence or severity of the patient's problem(s)?

1.c. Based on the patient's estimated creatinine clearance and clinical presentation, do any of his medications require dosage adjustment? If so, what adjustment would you recommend?

1.d. What additional laboratory information would assist in the assessment of this patient?

1.e. Could any of the patient's problems have been caused by drug therapy?

1.f. What risk factors did the patient have for gentamicin-induced AKI?

1.g. What therapeutic interventions could have been initiated to decrease the likelihood of developing drug-induced AKI?

1.h. Could extended-interval gentamicin dosing have minimized the likelihood of nephrotoxicity?

## Desired Outcome

2. What are the goals of pharmacotherapy in this case?

## Therapeutic Alternatives

3.a. What nondrug therapies might be useful for this patient?

3.b. What feasible pharmacotherapeutic alternatives are available for treating AKI in this patient?

## Optimal Plan

4. What drugs, dosage forms, doses, schedules, and duration of therapy are best for this patient?

## Outcome Evaluation

5. What clinical and laboratory parameters are necessary to evaluate therapy for achievement of the desired therapeutic outcomes and to detect or prevent adverse effects?

## Patient Education

6. What information should be provided to the patient to enhance compliance, ensure successful therapy, and minimize adverse effects?

## ■ CLINICAL PEARL

Furosemide administration enhances sodium excretion, which results in an elevated $FE_{NA}$, and limits the utility of the $FE_{NA}$ calculation to assess AKI. To avoid misinterpretation of the $FE_{NA}$ results, the clinician should delay obtaining an $FE_{NA}$ until the effect of the furosemide dose is complete (up to 10 hours in patients with kidney disease).

## ■ SELF-STUDY ASSIGNMENTS

1. Based on the patient's change in serum creatinine or urine output, classify the patient's AKI based on the RIFLE criteria.
2. Identify other drugs that may potentiate the patient's AKI and should be avoided in this patient.
3. Assume that Mr Elliott's serum creatinine is 1.4 mg/dL at 1 month after discharge. At what point would you consider restarting the ACE inhibitor? Justify the use of ACE inhibitors in patients with chronic kidney disease.
4. What is the target INR in this patient, and do any of his medications interact with warfarin?

## REFERENCES


1. Bellomo R, Ronco C, Kellum JA, Mehta RL, Palevsky P, ADQI Workgroup. Acute renal failure—definition, outcome measures, animal models, and information technology needs: the Second International Consensus Conference of the Acute Dialysis Quality Initiative (ADQI) Group. Crit Care 2004;8:R204–R212.
2. Bellomo R, Kellum JA, Ronco C. Defining and classifying acute renal failure: from advocacy to consensus and validation of the RIFLE criteria. Intensive Care Med 2007;33:409–413.
3. Jelliffe R. Estimation of creatinine clearance in patients with unstable renal function, without a urine specimen. Am J Nephrol 2002;22:320–324.
4. Oliveira JF, Silva CA, Barbieri CD, Oliveira GM, Zanetta DMT, Burdmann EA. Prevalence and risk factors for aminoglycoside nephrotoxicity in intensive care units. Antimicrob Agents Chemother 2009:53:2887–2891.
5. Bentley ML, Corwin HL, Dasta J. Drug-induced acute kidney injury in the critically ill adult: recognition and prevention strategies. Crit Care Med 2010:38(6 Suppl):S169–S174.
6. Shankar SS, Brater DC. Loop diuretics: from the Na–K–2Cl transporter to clinical use. Am J Physiol Renal Physiol 2003;284:F11–F21.
7. Bellomo R, Chapman M, Finfer S, Hickling K, Myburgh J. Low-dose dopamine in patients with early renal dysfunction: a placebo-controlled randomized trial. Australian and New Zealand Intensive Care Society (ANZICS) Clinical Trials Group. Lancet 2000;356:2139–2143.


# 53

# ACUTE KIDNEY INJURY

## What We Used to Call Acute Renal Failure. . . Level II

**Scott Bolesta, PharmD, BCPS**

## LEARNING OBJECTIVES

After completing this case study, the reader should be able to:

- Assess a patient with AKI using clinical and laboratory data.
- Classify AKI in a patient.
- Distinguish between AKI resulting from prerenal and that from intrinsic injury.
- Recommend changes to the pharmacotherapeutic regimen of a patient with AKI.
- Justify appropriate therapeutic interventions for a patient with AKI.

## PATIENT PRESENTATION

### ■ Chief Complaint

"I feel really weak."

### ■ HPI

Everit Mitchell is a 72-year-old man who presents to the ED with complaints of severe weakness that started this morning and recent stomach pain for the past week. He was feeling normal until he developed stomach pain 1 week ago that worsened with meals. The pain subsided 2 days ago, but last evening he felt more tired than usual and went to bed early. Since waking this morning, he has been too weak to perform his normal ADLs. His wife brought him to the ED because his physician is away on vacation.

### ■ PMH

HTN × 30 years
CAD × 20 years
MI × 2 with most recent 2 months ago s/p PCI with drug-eluting stent placement
s/p CABG 20 years ago
CHF × 4 years
RA × 1 year

### ■ FH

Father died of an acute MI at age 52; mother had diabetes mellitus and died of a stroke at the age of 65.

### ■ SH

Retired and living at home with his wife. Before retirement, the patient was employed as an accountant. No alcohol, no tobacco use.

### ■ Meds

Aspirin 81 mg po daily
Amlodipine 10 mg po once daily
Furosemide 40 mg po once daily
Metoprolol succinate 50 mg po once daily
Enalapril 20 mg po once daily
Clopidogrel 75 mg po daily
Naproxen 500 mg po BID

### ■ All

NKA

### ■ ROS

In addition to weakness and stomach pain, the patient complains of feeling cold but denies chills or fever. No changes in vision. Denies SOB, CP, and cough. Complains of feeling lightheaded. Has been having frequent black diarrhea over the last 3 days but denies current abdominal pain. Has noted a decrease in the frequency of his urination over the last 24 hours. Denies musculoskeletal pain or cramping.

## Physical Examination

*Gen*

Pale, elderly Caucasian man who appears generally weak and lethargic

*VS*

BP 89/43 (77/32 on standing), P 123, RR 25, T 36.1°C; Wt 78 kg, Ht 5′9″

*Skin*

Pale and cool with poor turgor

*HEENT*

PERRLA; EOMI; fundi normal; conjunctivae pale and dry; TMs intact; tongue and mouth dry

*Neck/Lymph Nodes*

No JVD or HJR; no lymphadenopathy or thyromegaly

*Lungs*

No crackles or rhonchi

*CV*

Tachycardic with regular rhythm; normal $S_1$, $S_2$; no $S_3$; faint $S_4$; no MRG

*Abd*

Soft, NT/ND; no HSM; hyperactive BS

*Genit/Rect*

Stool heme (+); slightly enlarged prostate

*MS/Ext*

Weak pulses; no peripheral edema; mild swelling of MCP joints of both hands

*Neuro*

A & O × 3; CNs intact; DTRs 2+; Babinski (–)

## Labs

| | |
|---|---|
| Na 139 mEq/L | Ca 8.6 mg/dL |
| K 5.6 mEq/L | Mg 2.1 mg/dL |
| Cl 103 mEq/L | Phos 4.3 mg/dL |
| $CO_2$ 22 mEq/L | WBC 8.6 × $10^3$/mm$^3$ |
| BUN 53 mg/dL | Hgb 7.6 g/dL |
| SCr 1.8 mg/dL | Hct 22.5% |
| Glu 123 mg/dL | Plt 96 × $10^3$/mm$^3$ |

## Assessment

A 72-year-old man with a suspected acute UGI bleed secondary to combined antiplatelet and NSAIDs use that has resulted in anemia and AKI from hypovolemia

# QUESTIONS

## Problem Identification

1.a. Create a list of the patient's drug therapy problems as they relate to his AKI.

1.b. What information (signs, symptoms, laboratory values) indicates the presence or severity of hypovolemia and AKI in this patient?

## Desired Outcome

2. What are the goals of pharmacotherapy in this case?

# CLINICAL COURSE

On admission, the patient was resuscitated aggressively with IV normal saline and multiple transfusions (4 units of PRBCs). His home medications were held, and he underwent an emergent EGD. During endoscopy, a large ulcer in the gastric antrum was found with an exposed spurting artery. Endoscopic therapy was unsuccessful, and the patient was taken to the OR for surgical intervention. He was hypotensive in the OR (BP 70 mm Hg systolic on average) and was ved on a norepinephrine infusion to maintain a stable BP. Postoperatively he remained on mechanical ventilation, and his urine output was <100 mL total over the first 12 postoperative hours despite continued aggressive IV hydration and repeated transfusions in the OR. He also remained on norepinephrine for a continued low BP. On the morning of postoperative day 1, his labs were as follows:

| | |
|---|---|
| Na 132 mEq/L | Ca 8.2 mg/dL |
| K 5.4 mEq/L | Mg 2.2 mg/dL |
| Cl 111 mEq/L | Phos 4.7 mg/dL |
| $CO_2$ 19 mEq/L | WBC 14.6 × $10^3$/mm$^3$ |
| BUN 49 mg/dL | Hgb 10.3 g/dL |
| SCr 2.5 mg/dL | Hct 29.8% |
| Glu 145 mg/dL | Plt 112 × $10^3$/mm$^3$ |

Urinalysis also showed muddy brown casts, urine sodium of 72 mEq/L, and specific gravity of 1.004. A diagnosis of ATN was made, and the patient was started on furosemide 80 mg IV Q 8 h. On postoperative day 2, the patient remained on mechanical ventilation and norepinephrine, his urine output had not improved, and his chest radiograph showed diffuse bilateral pulmonary edema with a decrease in $O_2$ saturation to 86%. An echocardiogram revealed hypokinesis of the anterior portion of the left ventricle and an EF of 25%. The patient was started on dobutamine, and a femoral vein catheter was inserted and CVVH-DF was begun. On postoperative day 5, his heart failure had resolved, norepinephrine and dobutamine had been weaned off, and the catheter was removed. His subsequent hospital course was uneventful, and his kidney function gradually improved.

## Therapeutic Alternatives

3.a. What nondrug therapies were used to manage this patient's AKI? Discuss the evidence that supports their use.

3.b. What pharmacotherapeutic alternatives have been studied for the treatment of AKI?

## Optimal Plan

4. Design an optimal therapeutic plan for managing this patient's AKI postoperatively.

## Outcome Evaluation

5. What clinical and laboratory parameters are necessary to evaluate the therapy for achievement of the desired therapeutic outcome and to detect or prevent adverse effects?

## Patient Education

6. What information should be provided to the patient to help avoid future episodes of AKI?

## CLINICAL PEARL

Patients in the recovery (or "diuretic") phase of ATN produce large amounts of dilute urine due to resolution of tubular obstruction from sloughed tubular epithelial cells and inability of the recovering tubular cells to reabsorb sodium. This return of urine output does not signal complete recovery of kidney function, and medications eliminated to a large extent by active tubular secretion may still accumulate and require dosage adjustment.

## SELF-STUDY ASSIGNMENTS

1. Compare and contrast the RIFLE criteria for defining and classifying AKI to that published by the Acute Kidney Injury Network.
2. Write a brief paper that discusses the pharmacotherapeutic interventions that have been studied for the prevention of AKI from causes other than IV contrast agents.

## REFERENCES


1. Lameire N, Van Biesen W, Vanholder R. Acute renal failure. Lancet 2005;365:417–430.
2. Gill N, Nally JV Jr, Fatica RA. Renal failure secondary to acute tubular necrosis: epidemiology, diagnosis, and management. Chest 2005;128:2847–2863.
3. Uchino S, Doig GS, Bellomo R, et al. Diuretics and mortality in acute renal failure. Crit Care Med 2004;32:1669–1677.
4. Ho KM, Sheridan DJ. Meta-analysis of furosemide to prevent or treat acute renal failure. BMJ 2006;333:420–425.
5. Sampath S, Moran JL, Graham PL, et al. The efficacy of loop diuretics in acute renal failure: assessment using Bayesian evidence synthesis techniques. Crit Care Med 2007;35:2516–2524.
6. Friedrich JO, Adhikari N, Herridge MS, et al. Meta-analysis: low-dose dopamine increases urine output but does not prevent renal dysfunction or death. Ann Intern Med 2005;142:510–524.
7. Bellomo R, Wan L, May C. Vasoactive drugs and acute kidney injury. Crit Care Med 2008;36(Suppl):S179–S186.


# 54

# PROGRESSIVE RENAL DISEASE

It Was Only a Matter of Time . . . . . . . . . . . . . Level III

**Michelle D. Furler, BSc Pharm, PhD**

## LEARNING OBJECTIVES

After completing this case study, students should be able to:

- Understand various methods for estimating creatinine clearance and glomerular filtration rate.
- Differentiate AKI from CKD.
- Identify risk factors for progression of renal disease.
- Recommend nonpharmacologic and pharmacologic interventions to alter the rate of progression of renal disease.
- Recognize and treat potential comorbid or pathologic conditions that are frequently associated with chronic renal insufficiency.
- Educate patients about the common medications prescribed for chronic renal insufficiency.
- Provide recommendations for renal disease therapy during pregnancy.

## PATIENT PRESENTATION

### Chief Complaint

"I'm here to check the results of my labs."

### HPI

Christine Karter-Davis is a 35-year-old woman with type 2 diabetes mellitus who returns to her PCP for a follow-up visit. Her last visit was 3 months ago for a routine physical examination and her annual kidney screening (last year's screening revealed SCr elevation of 1.2 mg/dL and microalbuminuria). A spot urine conducted at that time revealed 3+ protein and ACR was 659 mg/g. A follow-up appointment was scheduled 6 weeks ago, and a second spot urine test showed persistent elevation of ACR 615 mg/g. Complete laboratory workup was scheduled at that time along with a 24-hour urine collection. She has returned to the office today to review the results of this testing.

A pleasant woman with no current medical complaints, Ms Karter-Davis arrives in the office today with a printout of her home blood glucose monitor readings. Review of the report shows only six tests in the last month, all between 6:00 and 7:00 AM. From her past pregnancy she is known to have an aversion to needles, and on questioning reveals that she hates the lancing device, and the finger pricks really hurt so she does not test very often. She has started a new regimen of daily vitamin D and aspirin because she heard that it was good for her (a friend saw it on TV). She also shows you her new pill organizer (dosette pack) that she picked up at the pharmacy on the way to the office. She says that with the new vitamins she has been forgetting to take some of her medications but feels that the pill organizer will help her remember.

### PMH

Type 2 DM × 8 years (history of gestational diabetes with use of insulin required)
HTN × 6 years
Dyslipidemia × 5 years
Gastric ulcer treated several years ago with *H. pylori* regimen (antibiotics and PPI)
Appendectomy at age 16

### FH

Father had DM and CHD and died at age 50 secondary to MI; mother (age 62) has HTN and dyslipidemia. Brother (age 31) has DM, and two sisters (age 27 and 29) have no known medical problems other than obesity.

### SH

The patient is an administrative assistant, married for 6 months with one child (age 10) from a past relationship. Her job provides medical coverage and prescription drug benefits. She reports occasional alcohol consumption on weekends or when out with friends (one to two alcoholic beverages per month). She is a one-ppd smoker; this is a decrease from her reported use of two ppd last year. No history of illicit drug use.

The patient admits to a somewhat sedentary lifestyle but says her husband and son have been trying to interest her in family outings with their new puppy. She drinks three to four cups of coffee per day. She tends to have fast food on her lunch hour but has begun making her lunches in an effort to save money for her belated honeymoon. Her husband is a weekend basketball player, and they have recently set up a home gym with a weight set that she has "played around with" but has not used in any serious way. She mentions that her husband enjoys protein shakes and bars that she has started taking occasionally in her lunches. She enjoys fried foods but indicates that her husband is now doing most of the cooking, barbequing several times per week. She has lost 4 kg since last year.

## All

NKDA, seasonal allergies to grass and pollen

## Meds

Metformin 500 mg po TID × 2 years; prescription reads 1,000 mg AM, 500 mg lunch, and 1,000 mg supper
Hydrochlorothiazide 50 mg po daily × 1 year, increased last year from 25 mg daily
Atorvastatin 10 mg po at bedtime × 1 year
Nasonex two sprays in each nostril BID (seasonal—not using currently)
Cetirizine 10 mg po daily PRN allergies
Aleve po PRN headaches
Omeprazole OTC 20 mg po PRN "indigestion"
Multivitamin po daily
Vitamin $D_3$ 1,000 IU po daily × 2 weeks
ASA 325 mg po daily × 2 weeks

## ROS

Occasional headaches, generally associated with menstruation; no c/o polyuria, polydipsia, polyphagia, sensory loss, or visual changes
No dysuria, flank pain, hematuria, pedal edema, chest pain, or SOB

## Physical Examination

### Gen

The patient is a moderately obese African-American woman in NAD.

### VS

BP 162/94 sitting and standing in both arms, HR 82, RR 18, T 37.5°C; Wt 93 kg, Ht 5′6″

### Skin

Warm, dry, no rashes

### HEENT

PERRLA, EOMI, fundi have microaneurysms consistent with diabetic retinopathy; no retinal edema or vitreous hemorrhage. TMs intact. Oral mucosa moist with no lesions.

### Neck/Lymph Nodes

Supple without adenopathy or thyromegaly

### Lungs/Thorax

Clear, breath sounds normal

### CV

Heart sounds normal, no murmurs, no bruits

### Abd

Soft NT/ND

### Genit/Rect

Rectal exam deferred; recent Pap smear negative

### MS/Ext

No CCE, normal ROM

### Neuro

A & O × 3; CNs intact; normal DTRs

## Labs (1 Week Ago, Fasting)

| | | |
|---|---|---|
| Na 140 mEq/L | Hgb 12.2 g/dL | *Fasting lipid profile:* |
| K 3.1 mEq/L | Hct 36.1% | T. chol 213 mg/dL |
| Cl 107 mEq/L | WBC 9.5 × $10^3$/mm$^3$ | Trig 149 mg/dL |
| $CO_2$ 26 mEq/L | Plt 148 × $10^3$/mm$^3$ | LDL 141 mg/dL |
| BUN 29 mg/dL | Ca 9.4 mg/dL | HDL 42 mg/dL |
| SCr 1.4 mg/dL | Phos 2.7 mg/dL | Alb 3.4 g/dL |
| Glu 196 mg/dL | Uric acid 6.2 mg/dL | |
| A1C 10.4% | $eGFR_{MDRD}$ 41.2 mL/min/1.73 m$^2$ | |

## UA (1 Week Ago)

pH 5.2, 1+ glucose, (–) ketones, 3+ protein, (–) leukocyte esterase and nitrite; (–) RBC; 3–4 WBC/hpf, ACR 673 mg/g

## 24-Hour Urine Collection

Total urine volume 2.2 L, urine creatinine 66 mg/dL, urine albumin 873 mg/24 hours

## Assessment

A 35-year-old woman recently diagnosed with diabetic nephropathy and overt albuminuria complicated by inadequately controlled comorbid conditions

# QUESTIONS

## Problem Identification

1.a Create a list of the patient's drug therapy problems and include the evidence to support your assessment.

1.b. What signs, symptoms, or laboratory values indicate the presence, severity, and nature of renal disease in this patient?

1.c. What other risk factors for renal disease are present in this patient?

1.d. Are there alterative explanations for kidney disease in diabetic patients, and are additional laboratory evaluations indicated?

1.e. Discuss the value of the urine ACR. Calculate the ACR from the reported 24-hour urine and compare it to the spot urine results. Was collection of a 24-hour urine necessary in this patient?

1.f. What is the GFR in this patient both last year and last week, estimated using the 24-hour urine collection and the Cockcroft–Gault, MDRD, and CKD-EPI equations? Which of these estimates provides the best information for adjustment of drug dosing?

1.g. What degree of renal failure does this patient have?

1.h. Compare the definition, classification, and prognosis of CKD to AKI.

## Desired Outcome

2. What are the goals of pharmacotherapy for the patient's medical conditions? Focus on renal insufficiency, diabetes, hypertension, and dyslipidemia.

## Therapeutic Alternatives

3.a. What nonpharmacologic therapies might be useful to control this patient's medical conditions?

3.b. What are the pharmacotherapeutic alternatives for preventing renal disease progression and managing this patient's diabetes mellitus, hypertension, and dyslipidemia?

## Optimal Plan

4. What drug regimens would provide optimal therapy for this patient's medical problems?

## Outcome Evaluation

5. Outline the clinical and laboratory parameters necessary to evaluate the efficacy and safety of the recommended regimens for the patient's nephropathy, diabetes mellitus, hypertension, and dyslipidemia.

## Patient Education

6. Based on the regimen you recommended, what information should be provided to the patient to ensure successful therapy and minimize adverse effects?

# ■ CLINICAL COURSE

The patient is started on the medications you recommended for renal protection, diabetes, hypertension, dyslipidemia, and cardiovascular protection. The patient returns to clinic 4 weeks later. She has a bit of a cough but reports tolerating her new medications well. She states that she is watching her diet and has been enjoying more outings with her family, exercising before work three times per week in the family weight room, and walking the dog for 20–30 minutes each evening after work with her husband and son. On evaluation, the following results are obtained: BP sitting and standing 150/87, HR 80, and ACR 420 mg/g. Fasting labs: BUN 29 mg/dL, SCr 1.6 mg/dL, Glu 146 mg/dL, A1C 10.2%, K 4.3 mEq/L, Na 140 mEq/L, Alb 3.2 g/dL, Hct 36.1%, eGFR 42.2 mL/min/1.73 m$^2$, T. chol 203 mg/dL, TG 147 mg/dL, LDL 132 mg/dL, and HDL 42 mg/dL.

## Follow-Up Questions

1. Is the patient experiencing any adverse effects from her new medication regimen?
2. What additional information would be beneficial to you in evaluating her response to therapy?
3. For each of the major medical problems, describe any adjustments in pharmacotherapy that are required and outline a follow-up plan.

# ■ CLINICAL COURSE

After several months, the patient presents to the pharmacy for a refill of her medications. While speaking with the pharmacist, she asks for a recommendation regarding prenatal vitamins, indicating that she and her husband have recently discovered that she is pregnant.

## Follow-Up Questions

4. What impact, if any, will pregnancy have on the management and progression of nephropathy in this patient?
5. Are any changes required in her drug therapy at this time? If so, which ones and why?

# ■ SELF-STUDY ASSIGNMENTS

1. Discuss the role of diuretic therapy in patients with normal renal function compared to those with creatinine clearance values <20 mL/min.
2. Review and compare the effects of antihypertensive agents on renal blood flow and glomerular filtration rate in patients with hypertension and diabetic nephropathy.

# CLINICAL PEARL

Both normotensive and hypertensive patients with type 2 diabetes and persistent albuminuria should be treated with either an ACE inhibitor or ARB to slow the progression of diabetic nephropathy and other microvascular and macrovascular diseases. A comprehensive treatment plan must include comorbid illnesses, with a particular focus on glycemic control and cardiovascular disease. Effective disease management must be tailored to patient needs and modified according to patient preferences and lifestyle.

# REFERENCES


1. American Diabetes Association. Standards of medical care in diabetes—2010. Diabetes Care 2010;33(Suppl 1):S11–S61.
2. National Kidney Foundation. K/DOQI clinical practice guidelines and clinical practice recommendations for diabetes and chronic kidney disease. Am J Kidney Dis 2007;49(Suppl 2):S1–S180.
3. Canadian Diabetes Association Clinical Practice Guidelines Expert Committee. Canadian Diabetes Association 2008 clinical practice guidelines for the prevention and management of diabetes in Canada. Can J Diabetes 2008;32(Suppl 1):S1–S201.
4. National Kidney Foundation. KDOQI clinical practice guidelines for chronic kidney disease: evaluation, classification, and stratification. Am J Kidney Dis 2002;39(2 Suppl 1):S1–S266.
5. International Diabetes Federation. Self-monitoring of blood glucose in non-insulin-treated type 2 diabetes recommendations based on a workshop of the International Diabetes Federation Clinical Guidelines Taskforce in collaboration with the SMBG International Working Group. International Diabetes Federation, 2009. Available at: *http://www.idf.org/webdata/docs/SMBG_EN2.pdf*. Accessed March 1, 2010.
6. National Kidney Foundation. K/DOQI clinical practice guidelines for nutrition in chronic renal failure. Am J Kidney Dis 2000;35 (6 Suppl 2):S1–140.
7. Stevens LA, Levey AS. Frequently asked questions about GFR estimates. National Kidney Foundation, 2007. Available at: *http://www.kidney.org/professionals/kls/pdf/faq_gfr.pdf*. Accessed March 1, 2010.
8. Levey AS, Stevens LA, Schmid CH, et al. A new equation to estimate glomerular filtration rate. Ann Intern Med 2009;150:604–612.
9. The ADVANCE Collaborative Group. Intensive blood glucose control and vascular outcomes in patients with type 2 diabetes. N Engl J Med 2008;358:2560–2572.
10. Ramin SM, Vidaeff AC, Yeomans ER, et al. Chronic renal disease in pregnancy. Obstet Gynecol 2006;108:1531–1539 [erratum in: Obstet Gynecol 2007;109:788].

*Note*: All NKF K/DOQI clinical practice guidelines are available online at *www.kidney.org/professionals/kdoqi/guidelines.cfm*.

# 55

# END-STAGE KIDNEY DISEASE

Urine Trouble . . . . . . . . . . . . . . . . . . . . . . . . . . Level II

Katie E. Cardone, PharmD

## LEARNING OBJECTIVES

On completing this case study, students should be able to:

- Identify medication-related problems in a patient with end-stage kidney disease maintained on chronic hemodialysis.
- State the desired therapeutic outcomes of each problem.
- List therapeutic alternatives for managing each problem.
- Develop a plan for managing each problem that includes plans for monitoring patient response to interventions.
- Outline a plan for helping the patient understand and effectively implement medication-related interventions.

## PATIENT PRESENTATION

### Chief Complaint

"I feel tired, nauseated, and constipated."

### HPI

Jane Lopez is a 42-year-old woman who presents to the outpatient dialysis center for her routine hemodialysis treatment. She has ESKD secondary to hypertension and has been on hemodialysis for 4 years. She has a failed AV fistula and graft and is currently dialyzed via central venous catheter. She has an upcoming appointment with the vascular surgeon to reevaluate her HD access. She also frequently leaves HD 30–60 minutes early against medical advice.

### PMH

ESRD secondary to HTN
HTN
Anemia
Secondary hyperparathyroidism
H/O gestational diabetes 12 years ago
GERD

### PSH

Cesarean section 12 years ago
Tubal ligation 10 years ago
AV fistula creation 5 years ago (failed)
AV graft creation 3 years ago (failed)

### FH

Father died of MI at age 60. Mother deceased due to breast cancer. No siblings. Has a 12 yo son in good health.

### SH

Married, lives with husband and 12 yo son. Occasional social alcohol use. Smokes 1/2 pack per day (decreased from one ppd × 10 years). Denies caffeine consumption.

### ROS

Complains of feeling tired and weak over the past several weeks. Report some swelling in feet and lower legs. Also reports constipation, nausea, and heartburn.

### Meds

Furosemide 80 mg po daily
Metoprolol tartrate 50 mg po BID
Lisinopril 20 mg po daily
Calcium acetate 667 mg three caps po TID with meals
Cinacalcet 60 mg po daily (increased from 30 mg 2 weeks ago)
Nephro-Vite po daily
Omeprazole 20 mg po daily
Zolpidem 10 mg po at bedtime PRN
Ferrous sulfate 325 mg po TID
Docusate 100 mg po daily PRN
Calcium carbonate po PRN heartburn
Epoetin alfa 10,000 units IV three times weekly with dialysis (dose stable for 3 months)
Iron sucrose 50 mg IV once weekly

### All

NKDA

### Physical Examination

*Gen*

The patient is a WDWN Hispanic woman in NAD who appears her stated age.

*VS*

BP 175/88 (predialysis); 149/89 (postdialysis)
Wt 88.6 kg (predialysis); 84.0 kg (postdialysis)
P 91, RR 16, T 36.5°C, Ht 5′4″

*Skin*

Dry, scaly arms and legs

*Ext*

Mild bilateral lower extremity edema.
Remainder of the PE was WNL.

### Labs

| | | | |
|---|---|---|---|
| Na 143 mEq/L | Hgb 9.8 g/dL | AST 21 IU/L | *Fasting lipid profile:* |
| K 4.3 mEq/L | Hct 27.5% | ALT 4 IU/L | T. chol 123 mg/dL |
| Cl 95 mEq/L | RBC 2.84 × $10^6$/$mm^3$ | LDH 139 IU/L | HDL 37 mg/dL |
| $CO_2$ 26 mEq/L | MCV 81.8 $m^3$ | Alk phos 175 IU/L | Trig 113 mg/dL |
| BUN 59 mg/dL | MCHC 32.4 g/dL | T. bili 0.3 mg/dL | iPTH 655 pg/mL |
| SCr 12.9 mg/dL | | Alb 3.0 g/dL | T. sat 12% |
| Glu 88 mg/dL | WBC 5.7 × $10^3$/$mm^3$ | Ca 9.0 mg/dL | Ferritin 185 ng/mL |
| | | Phos 6.7 mg/dL | |

Mrs Lopez's nephrologist provided the following dialysis prescription:
Dialyze 3.5 hours per session, three times per week (T, Th, Sat, morning shift)
Dry weight: 83.5 kg
Dialyzer: F180 (high flux)
Blood flow rate: 400 mL/min
Dialysate flow rate: 800 mL/min
Dialysate: Bicarbonate
Na 145 mEq/L, K 2.0 mEq/L, Ca 2.5 mEq/L, $HCO_3$ 35 mEq/L
Heparin: 5,000 unit IV bolus, and then 1,000 units/h until 1 hour before termination

## QUESTIONS

### Problem Identification

1.a. Create a list of the patient's drug therapy problems.

1.b. Could any of these problems have been caused or exacerbated by medications?

### Desired Outcome

2. State the goal of pharmacotherapy for each problem identified.

### Therapeutic Alternatives

3. What therapeutic options are available for each of this patient's drug therapy problems? Indicate the advantages and disadvantages of each option.

### Optimal Plan

4. Which of the available therapeutic options identified in question 3 would you recommend for this patient? Provide a rationale for each recommendation. Include the name, dosage form, dose, schedule, and duration of therapy for any drugs recommended.

### Outcome Evaluation

5. What clinical and laboratory parameters would you recommend to evaluate the desired and undesired consequences of each of your recommended interventions?

### Patient Education

6. What information should be provided to the patient to enhance compliance, ensure successful therapy, and minimize adverse effects?

## ■ SELF-STUDY ASSIGNMENTS

1. Mrs Lopez develops a sinus infection for which she goes to an urgent care clinic. She is prescribed levofloxacin 500 mg po daily ×14 days. Evaluate the appropriateness of this prescription for Mrs Lopez. What changes, if any, would you suggest regarding this prescription?
2. Mrs Lopez would like a kidney transplant but must first quit smoking to become eligible for transplant. Create a smoking cessation plan for her.

## CLINICAL PEARL

The dose of ESAs should always be minimized. In the face of iron deficiency and low hemoglobin, iron should be replenished before increasing the ESA dose.

## REFERENCES


1. Alborzi P, Patel N, Agarwal R. Home blood pressures are of greater prognostic value than hemodialysis unit recordings. Clin J Am Soc Nephrol 2007;2:1228–1234.
2. National Kidney Foundation. K/DOQI clinical practice guidelines for cardiovascular disease in dialysis patients. Am J Kidney Dis 2005;45:S1–S153.
3. National Kidney Foundation. KDOQI clinical practice guideline and clinical practice recommendations for anemia in chronic kidney disease: 2007 update of hemoglobin target. Am J Kidney Dis 2007;50:471–530.
4. Pfeffer MA, Burdmann EA, Chen C-Y, et al. A trial of darbepoetin alfa in type 2 diabetes and chronic kidney disease. N Engl J Med 2009;361:2019–2032.
5. Epogen (Epoetin Alfa) Package Insert. Amgen Inc, 2010.
6. National Kidney Foundation. K/DOQI clinical practice guidelines and clinical practice recommendations for anemia in chronic kidney disease. Am J Kidney Dis 2006;47:S11–S145.
7. Kidney Disease: Improving Global Outcomes (KDIGO) CKD-MBD Work Group. KDIGO clinical practice guideline for the diagnosis, evaluation, prevention, and treatment of chronic kidney disease-mineral and bone disorder (CKD-MBD). Kidney Int Suppl 2009;113:S1–S130.
8. National Kidney Foundation. K/DOQI clinical practice guidelines for bone metabolism and disease in chronic kidney disease. Am J Kidney Dis 2003;42:S1–S201.
9. Feraheme (Ferumoxytol) Package Insert. AMAG Pharmaceuticals Inc, 2009.


# 56

# SYNDROME OF INAPPROPRIATE ANTIDIURETIC HORMONE RELEASE

Lodging a Complaint . . . . . . . . . . . . . . . . . . . . Level I

**Jane Gervasio, PharmD, FCCP, BCNSP**

**Sarah A. Nisly, PharmD, BCPS**

## LEARNING OBJECTIVES

After completing this case study, readers should be able to:

- Identify the etiologies of hyponatremia and specifically the syndrome of inappropriate antidiuretic hormone (SIADH) release.
- Assess risk factors for developing hyponatremia and SIADH.
- Evaluate osmotic and fluid status in patients with hyponatremia.
- Recommend and monitor appropriate therapy and alternative treatments for SIADH.
- Discuss treatment options for SIADH, proper administration of selected treatments, and potential side effects.

## PATIENT PRESENTATION

### ■ Chief Complaint

"There's nothing wrong with me, I don't know why she made me come here!"

### ■ HPI

Gerald O'Flannery is a 73-year-old man who presents to the ED after several episodes of "weird" behavior, according to his family and friends. He is accompanied by his wife who stated that Gerald had been the unrestrained driver in a car accident 3 days earlier.

Gerald was driving himself home from the Caribou Lodge when he swerved off the road and hit a tree. His wife indicates that he hit his head on the steering wheel and lost consciousness for approximately 2 minutes but appeared otherwise unharmed except for a cut on his forehead. The paramedics cleaned and bandaged the patient's lesion and noted that he was combative and disoriented but refused to go to the hospital. The wife states that Gerald has not been "acting like himself" since the accident and she had observed him displaying worsening confused and disoriented behavior in the last 24 hours.

■ PMH

Exercise-induced asthma since childhood
Depression for 7 years

■ SH

Lives at home with wife; has two children, both living out of state. Employed part time as a cab driver. Social alcohol use, mostly at the lodge. Denies smoking and use of illicit substances.

■ Meds

Albuterol inhaler PRN
Fluoxetine 20 mg po daily for 6 years

■ All

Penicillin (reaction unknown)

■ ROS

Difficult to obtain because of decreased mental status. Wife states that he has no medical problems except asthma and depression.

■ Physical Examination

*Gen*

A & O × 3 but disoriented about recent events. Patient is agitated and confused.

*VS*

BP 142/94, P 110, RR 24, T 35.9°C; Wt 95kg, Ht 5′9″

*Skin*

Diaphoretic centrally and very warm; small lesion above left eye

*HEENT*

NC/AT; EOMI; PERRL; TMs WNL bilaterally

*Neck/Lymph Nodes*

Supple without lymphadenopathy, masses, goiter, or bruits

*Lung/Thorax*

Clear to A & P bilaterally

*CV*

RRR; no MRG

*Abd*

Soft, NT/ND w/o masses or organomegaly; decreased bowel sounds in all four quadrants

*Genit/Rect*

Deferred

*MS/Ext*

Normal ROM; muscle strength 5/5 and equal bilaterally; pulses 2+ throughout; no CCE; capillary refill <2 seconds

*Neuro*

CN II–XII intact; DTRs 2/4 and equal bilaterally; sensory intact; (–) Babinski

■ Labs

| | | |
|---|---|---|
| Na 112 mEq/L | Ca 9.2 mg/dL | T. chol 177 mg/dL |
| K 3.2 mEq/L | Phos 2.9 mg/dL | TSH 5.12 μIU/mL |
| Cl 90 mEq/L | Uric acid 3.2 mg/dL | Serum osm 238 mOsm/kg |
| $CO_2$ 27 mEq/L | AST 87 IU/L | |
| BUN 16 mg/dL | ALT 59 IU/L | |
| SCr 0.9 mg/dL | T. bili 0.7 mg/dL | |
| Glu 115 mg/dL | LDH 256 IU/L | |

■ UA

SG 1.008, pH 6.8, leukocyte esterase (–), nitrite (–), protein (–), ketones (–), urobilinogen nl, bilirubin (–), blood (–), glucose 80 mg/dL, spot urine sodium 125 mEq/L, osmolality 420 mOsm/kg

■ CT Head

Closed head injury (head trauma)

■ Assessment

1. Closed head injury
2. SIADH
3. Electrolyte disturbances

## QUESTIONS

### Problem Identification

1.a. Create a list of the patient's drug therapy problems.

1.b. What information (signs, symptoms, laboratory values) indicates the presence or severity of SIADH as the cause of his hyponatremia?

1.c. Could any of the patient's problems have been caused by drug therapy?

### Desired Outcome

2. What are the goals of pharmacotherapy in this case?

### Therapeutic Alternatives

3.a. What nondrug therapies might be useful for this patient?

3.b. What pharmacotherapeutic alternatives are available for the treatment of hyponatremia?

### Optimal Plan

4. What drug, dosage form, dose, schedule, and duration of therapy are most appropriate for initial treatment of this patient?

### Outcome Evaluation

5. What clinical and laboratory parameters are necessary to evaluate the therapy for achievement of the desired therapeutic outcome and to detect or prevent adverse effects?

## Patient Education

6. What information should be provided to the patient to enhance compliance, ensure successful therapy, and minimize adverse effects?

## CLINICAL COURSE

After Mr O'Flannery's serum sodium returned to baseline, the team began to discuss his discharge regimen. What should his discharge medication list include?

## Follow-Up Question

1. Is discontinuation of the patient's SSRI warranted?

## SELF-STUDY ASSIGNMENTS

1. Calculate this patient's serum osmolality.
2. What are the risk factors for selective serotonin reuptake inhibitors (SSRIs) to cause hyponatremia?
3. Perform a literature search to determine which SSRIs are most commonly associated with SIADH. Identify the general progression of SSRI-induced SIADH.

## CLINICAL PEARL

Cerebral salt wasting (CSW) is another potential cause of hyponatremia, especially if the patient has had a head injury such as subarachnoid hemorrhage or stroke. It is often difficult to differentiate CSW from SIADH due to the overlap in their clinical features. Both CSW and SIADH present with inappropriately high urine osmolality and high urine sodium (usually >40 mEq/L). One difference is that CSW is associated with extracellular fluid depletion, whereas SIADH is associated with normal or slightly increased extracellular fluid volume. CSW can only be diagnosed in patients with clear evidence of volume depletion (hypotension, decreased skin turgor, elevated hematocrit). SIADH is usually corrected through fluid restriction; however, establishing euvolemia through volume repletion with normal saline usually corrects CSW.

## REFERENCES


1. Sterns RH. Severe symptomatic hyponatremia: treatment and outcome. A study of 64 cases. Ann Intern Med 1987;107:656–664.
2. Adrogue HJ, Madias NE. Hyponatremia. N Engl J Med 2000;342:1581–1589.
3. Fried LF, Palevsky PM. Hyponatremia and hypernatremia. Med Clin North Am 1997;81:585–609.
4. Siragy HM. Hyponatremia, fluid–electrolyte disorders, and the syndrome of inappropriate antidiuretic hormone secretion: diagnosis and treatment options. Endocr Pract 2006;12:446–457.
5. Finfgeld DL. SSRI-related hyponatremia among aging adults. J Psychosoc Nurs Ment Health Serv 2003;41:12–16.
6. Liu BA, Mittmann N, Knowles SR, et al. Hyponatremia and the syndrome of inappropriate secretion of antidiuretic hormone associated with the use of selective serotonin reuptake inhibitors: a review of spontaneous reports. CMAJ 1996;55:519–527.
7. Munger MA. New agents for managing hyponatremia in hospitalized patients. Am J Health Syst Pharm 2007;64:253–265.
8. Thompson CA. FDA approves oral vasopressin antagonist. Am J Health Syst Pharm 2009;66:1154.
9. Jacob S, Spinler SA. Hyponatremia associated with selective serotonin-reuptake inhibitors in older adults. Ann Pharmacother 2006;40:1618–1622.


# 57

# ELECTROLYTE ABNORMALITIES IN CHRONIC KIDNEY DISEASE

Turn Down the 'Lytes. . . . . . . . . . . . . . . . . . . . Level II


**Lena M. Maynor, PharmD, BCPS**

**Mary K. Stamatakis, PharmD**


## LEARNING OBJECTIVES

After completing this case study, students should be able to:

- Interpret clinical and biochemical findings in patients with CKD.
- Recommend a patient-specific therapeutic plan for treating electrolyte abnormalities and secondary hyperparathyroidism in CKD.
- Monitor the effectiveness of the pharmacotherapeutic plan for treating electrolyte abnormalities in CKD.
- Educate patients with CKD on nonprescription medications that can worsen electrolyte abnormalities in CKD.

## PATIENT PRESENTATION

### Chief Complaint

"I'm not quite feeling like myself."

### HPI

Robert Wolfe is a 67-year-old man with type 2 DM, HTN, and stage 5 CKD. He receives hemodialysis three times a week with a high-flux hemodialysis membrane. His wife brought him into the ED this morning after she noticed increased confusion and lethargy, worsening over the last 2–3 days. According to his wife, the patient missed his HD session 2 days ago. She reports no other new symptoms except for increased pain from his neuropathy for which his PCP increased his gabapentin dose last week.

### PMH

Type 2 DM × 20 years
HTN × 30 years
Stage 5 CKD; he has been receiving HD for the past 5 years with a high-flux cellulose triacetate membrane; he has no residual renal function
Diabetic neuropathy
Anemia of CKD
Dyslipidemia
Secondary hyperparathyroidism

### FH

Father with CAD; mother with DM and HTN

### SH

Retired from a glass factory; on disability; past history of smoking, quit 3 years ago; (–) ETOH for the past 7 years

## Meds

Calcium acetate 667 mg, 2 po TID
Gabapentin 300 mg po BID (increased last week from 300 mg po at bedtime)
Nephrocaps 1 po daily
Sodium ferric gluconate 62.5 mg IV once weekly with HD
Metoprolol 25 mg po BID
Procardia XL 60 mg po daily
Lipitor 10 mg po daily
Pioglitazone 30 mg po daily
Sitagliptin 25 mg po daily
Epogen 6,000 IU IV three times a week with HD
Calcijex 2 mcg IV three times a week with HD
Ensure nutritional supplement, one bottle (240 mL) po TID

## All

NKDA

## ROS

Increase fatigue and confusion; reduced sensation in lower extremities

## Physical Examination

*Gen*

Patient somnolent; does not appear to be in distress

*VS*

BP 168/82, P 82, RR 14, T 36.8°C; dry body Wt 68 kg, Ht 5′11″

*Skin*

Normal; intact, warm and dry

*HEENT*

NC/AT, PERRLA, EOMI, funduscopy WNL, oropharyngeal mucosa clear

*Neck/Lymph Nodes*

Positive JVD; no lymphadenopathy, normal thyroid

*Lungs*

Crackles in bases bilaterally

*CV*

Normal $S_1$ and $S_2$; no $S_3$ or $S_4$

*Abd*

Soft, NT/ND, no HSM

*Genit/Rect*

Normal prostate, guaiac-negative stool

*MS/Ext*

1+ bilateral pedal edema, no clubbing or cyanosis

*Neuro*

A & O to person only, CN II–XII intact, normal DTRs bilaterally

## Labs

| | | | | |
|---|---|---|---|---|
| Na 140 mEq/L | Hgb 11.2 g/dL | Ca 9.8 mg/dL | BUN 82 mg/dL | ALT 8 IU/L |
| K 6.1 mEq/L | Hct 34.5% | Mg 2.4 mg/dL | SCr 8.2 mg/dL | T. bili 0.9 mg/dL |
| Cl 99 mEq/L | Plt 182 × $10^3$/mm$^3$ | Phos 7.6 mg/dL | Glu 118 mg/dL | Alk phos 34 IU/L |
| $CO_2$ 18 mEq/L | WBC 7.8 × $10^3$/mm$^3$ | AST 12 IU/L | | Alb 2.2 g/dL |
| | | | | Intact PTH 140 pg/mL (last month 172 pg/mL) |

## ABG

pH 7.35, $pO_2$ 94, $pCO_2$ 38, $HCO_3$ 20 on room air

## Chest X-Ray

No infiltrates or effusions

## ECG

Sinus rhythm

## Assessment

67-year-old man with type 2 DM, CKD on HD with altered mental status, hyperkalemia, hyperphosphatemia, and H/O secondary hyperparathyroidism

## Plan

Patient missed HD session yesterday. Will dialyze now to correct some of the electrolyte abnormalities.
Patient with altered mental status following missed HD session; likely worsened by increased dose of gabapentin. Will dialyze and change gabapentin dose to 300 mg po at bedtime.

# QUESTIONS

## Problem Identification

1.a. Create a list of the patient's drug therapy problems.

## Problem 1—Hyperkalemia

1.b. What information (signs, symptoms, laboratory values) indicates the presence or severity of hyperkalemia?

1.c. Could any medications the patient is receiving be contributing to his hyperkalemia?

1.d. What is the pathophysiology of the patient's hyperkalemia?

1.e. What are the clinical consequences of hyperkalemia?

### Desired Outcome

2. What are the goals for treating this patient's hyperkalemia?

### Therapeutic Alternatives

3.a. What nondrug therapies are available for treating hyperkalemia?

3.b. What feasible pharmacotherapeutic alternatives are available for treating hyperkalemia?

### Optimal Plan

4. What drug, dosage form, dose, schedule, and duration of therapy are best for treating hyperkalemia in this patient?

### Outcome Evaluation

5. What clinical and laboratory parameters are necessary to evaluate the therapy for achievement of the desired therapeutic outcomes and to detect or prevent adverse effects?

### Patient Education

6. What information should be provided to the patient regarding over-the-counter medications that may increase the risk of hyperkalemia?

## Problem 2—Hyperphosphatemia, Hypercalcemia, and Secondary Hyperparathyroidism

1.b. What information (signs, symptoms, laboratory values) indicates the presence or severity of hyperphosphatemia and hypercalcemia?

1.c. Could any of the patient's medications be contributing to his hyperphosphatemia and hypercalcemia?

1.d. What is the pathophysiology of the patient's hyperphosphatemia and hypercalcemia?

1.e. What are the clinical consequences of hyperphosphatemia and hypercalcemia?

### *Desired Outcome*

2. What are the goals of pharmacotherapy for treating this patient's hyperphosphatemia and hypercalcemia?

### *Therapeutic Alternatives*

3.a. What nondrug therapies might be useful for treating this patient's hyperphosphatemia and hypercalcemia?

3.b. What pharmacotherapeutic alternatives are available for treating hyperphosphatemia?

3.c. What pharmacotherapeutic options are available for treating hypercalcemia?

### *Optimal Plan*

4. What drugs, dosage forms, schedules, and duration of therapy are best for treating this patient's hyperphosphatemia and hypercalcemia?

### *Outcome Evaluation*

5. What clinical and laboratory parameters are necessary to evaluate the therapy for achievement of the desired therapeutic outcome and to detect or prevent adverse effects?

### *Patient Education*

6. What information should be provided to the patient regarding the administration of his phosphate binder to ensure an optimal outcome?

## ■ ADDITIONAL CASE QUESTIONS

1. What alternative regimens could be considered for this patient's painful diabetic neuropathy (include drug[s], dose, route of administration, and frequency)?
2. One month later, the following laboratory values and erythropoietin dosages were available from the outpatient hemodialysis unit. Formulate a treatment plan for the patient's anemia of CKD.

| Time | Hgb (g/dL) | Ferritin (ng/mL) | Transferrin Saturation (%) | Erythropoietin Dosage |
|---|---|---|---|---|
| 1 month ago | 11.2 | - | - | 6,000 IU IV 3 × per week |
| Current | 9.2 | 210 | 25 | 6,000 IU IV 3 × per week |

## CLINICAL PEARL

Sodium polystyrene sulfonate (SPS) is an ion-exchange resin commonly prescribed to patients with hyperkalemia to bind potassium in the colon. Commonly used preparations are available as premixed suspensions in sorbitol. In 2009, the US Food and Drug Administration issued a warning regarding the use of SPS in combination with sorbitol following multiple case reports of colonic necrosis. The concomitant use of SPS and sorbitol is not recommended.

## ■ SELF-STUDY ASSIGNMENT

Compare the cost of a 1-month supply of calcium carbonate, calcium acetate, sevelamer carbonate, and lanthanum carbonate using usual doses for treatment of hyperphosphatemia.

## REFERENCES


1. Putcha N, Allon M. Management of hyperkalemia in dialysis patients. Semin Dial 2007;20:431–439.
2. Sterns RH, Rojas M, Bernstein P, Chennupati S. Ion-exchange resins for the treatment of hyperkalemia: are they safe and effective? J Am Soc Nephrol 2010;21:733–735.
3. Noordzij M, Korevaar J, Boeschoten E, et al. Netherlands Cooperative Study (NECOSAD) Study Group. The Kidney Disease Outcomes Initiative (K/DOQI) guideline for bone metabolism and disease in CKD: association with mortality in dialysis patients. Am J Kidney Dis 2005:46:925–932.
4. National Kidney Foundation. K/DOQI clinical practice guidelines for bone metabolism and disease in chronic kidney disease. Am J Kidney Dis 2003;42(4 Suppl 3):S1–S201.
5. Tonelli M, Pannu N, Manns B. Oral phosphate binders in patients with kidney failure. N Engl J Med 2010;362:1312–1324.
6. Sprague SM, Llach F, Amdahl M, et al. Paricalcitol versus calcitriol in the treatment of secondary hyperparathyroidism. Kidney Int 2003;63:1483–1490.
7. Pop-Busui R, Roberts L, Pennathur S, et al. The management of diabetic neuropathy in CKD. Am J Kidney Dis 2010;55:365–385.
8. Phrommintikul A, Haas SJ, Elsik M, et al. Mortality and target haemoglobin concentrations in anaemia patients with chronic kidey disease treated with erythropoietin: a meta-analysis. Lancet 2007;369:381–388.


# 58

# HYPERCALCEMIA OF MALIGNANCY

Up, Up, and Away . . . . . . . . . . . . . . . . . . . . . . . Level I


**Laura L. Jung, PharmD**

**Lisa M. Holle, PharmD, BCOP**


## LEARNING OBJECTIVES

After completing this case study, students should be able to:

- Recognize the signs and symptoms of hypercalcemia.
- Evaluate laboratory data and clinical symptoms for assessment and monitoring of hypercalcemia, hypercalcemia treatment, and complications of hypercalcemia.
- Recommend a pharmacotherapeutic plan for the initial treatment of cancer-related hypercalcemia.
- Recognize and develop management strategies for toxicities associated with treatment options for hypercalcemia.

## PATIENT PRESENTATION

### Chief Complaint

"I can't stop throwing up."

### HPI

Mary Krupp is a 62 yo woman who presented to her family practitioner today with a 2-day history of nausea and vomiting. She states that her stomach has not felt normal for the past 3–4 days and is painful. Her daughter states that for the past several days she has complained of constipation, nausea, and extreme thirst, but because she has been vomiting, it has been hard to keep her mother drinking enough liquids. She also reports that her mother stopped taking the sustained-release morphine that was started last week because she thought these were side effects of the morphine. The daughter states that her mom's last bowel movement was 3 days ago despite administration of a stool softener daily. Daughter also reports her mother has gone "downhill" over the last month and spends 80% of her day in bed and the remainder in the recliner.

### PMH

Stage IV non-small cell lung cancer diagnosed 1.5 years ago. At time of diagnosis, a CT scan revealed a 3-cm mass in the hilum of the right lung, extensive mediastinal lymphadenopathy, and a moderate right pleural effusion with pleural studding. A transbronchial biopsy identified the mass as adenocarcinoma. Cytology of the pleural effusion also revealed adenocarcinoma. She was treated with the following regimens: (1) carboplatin/paclitaxel × 4 cycles; (2) pemetrexed monotherapy × 6 cycles; and (3) erlotinib monotherapy. Erlotinib was discontinued 1 week ago because of grade 4 skin rash. The last CT scan performed 1 month ago revealed a new tumor 3.5 × 4.2 mm in the left lower lobe and liver metastases.

COPD × 4 years

Dyslipidemia

### FH

Mother died of NSCLC at age 80 years; father died of MI at 64 years; one sister died of breast cancer at 69 years; one sister and three brothers alive.

### SH

Tobacco: 2 ppd × 30 years; chronic alcohol use × 30 years EtOH (three to four drinks per day). Worked as an office assistant × 25 years. Lives at home with boyfriend of 16 years; has four grown daughters, ages 47, 44, 39, and 34 years. Had her first child at age 15.

### ROS

No fever or chills. Daughter has noted that the patient is more tired than usual and is extremely thirsty, which she believes has affected her appetite over the past week. She denies polyuria, chest pain, unusual shortness of breath, dyspnea, or cough. Ms Krupp states her pain is 8/10 throughout the day.

### Medications

Morphine sulfate sustained-release 30 mg po Q 12 h (started 1 week ago)

Morphine sulfate oral solution 5 mg po Q 2 h PRN pain (estimated use two times in the 24 hours before she stopped taking sustained-released)

Docusate sodium 200 mg po at bedtime PRN

Simvastatin 20 mg po daily

### All

Cephalosporins, penicillin

### Physical Examination

*Gen*

Thin Caucasian woman in obvious discomfort

*VS*

BP 95/70, P 105, RR 16, T 38°C; Wt 50 kg; Ht 5 1

*Skin*

Slightly warm to touch, fair skin turgor (mild tenting noted)

*HEENT*

PERRLA, EOMI, fundi benign; nonerythematous TMs; oropharynx clear; mucous membranes dry

*Neck/LN*

Neck supple, slight axillary lymphadenopathy

*Heart*

RRR, $S_1$, $S_2$ normal; without MRG

*Lungs*

Decreased breath sounds; bilateral wheezes

*Abd*

Firm, distended, tender; decreased bowel sounds; stool palpable on left side

*Genit/Rect*

Normal female genitalia; stool heme (–)

*Neuro*

A & O × 3; sensory and motor intact; strength 5/5 upper, 4/5 lower; CN II–XII intact; Babinksi (–)

### Labs

| | | | |
|---|---|---|---|
| Na 142 mEq/L | Glu 100 mg/dL | AST 63 IU/L | Ca 13.0 mg/dL |
| K 3.5 mEq/L | Hgb 12.7 g/dL | ALT 35 IU/L | Mg 1.5 mEq/L |
| Cl 109 mEq/L | Hct 40% | Alk phos 200 IU/L | Phos 3.5 mEq/L |
| $CO_2$ 22 mEq/L | Plt 174 × $10^3$/mm$^3$ | LDH 160 IU/L | T. prot 5.1 g/dL |
| BUN 40 mg/dL | WBC 6.8 × $10^3$/mm$^3$ | T. bili 1.6 mg/dL | Alb 2.2 g/dL |
| SCr 0.9 mg/dL | | D. bili 0.7 mg/dL | |

### Chest X-Ray

Osteolytic lesions on the right and left clavicles, masses in right and left lower lobes consistent with NSCLC

### Assessment/Plan

62 yo woman with metastatic NSCLC s/p three different treatment regimens. Poor performance status. Presenting with first episode of possible tumor-induced hypercalcemia and associated complications and uncontrolled pain.

Admit to inpatient oncology service for further management of hypercalcemia, related complications, and pain control.

## QUESTIONS

### Problem Identification

1.a. Create a list of the patient's drug therapy problems.

1.b. What information (signs, symptoms, laboratory values) indicates the presence or severity of hypercalcemia?

1.c. What is the patient's corrected serum calcium level based on her serum albumin level?

1.d. Could any of the patient's problems have been exacerbated by her current drug therapy?

1.e. What are the possible etiologies of hypercalcemia in this patient?

1.f. What additional information is needed to satisfactorily assess this patient?

## Desired Outcome

2. What are the goals of pharmacotherapy for this patient?

## Therapeutic Alternatives

3.a. What nondrug therapies might be useful for this patient?

3.b. What feasible pharmacotherapeutic alternatives are available for treatment of hypercalcemia in this patient?

## Optimal Plan

4.a. What drug, dosage form, dose, schedule, and duration of therapy are best for treating hypercalcemia in this patient?

4.b. What alternatives would be appropriate if the initial therapy fails or cannot be used?

## Outcome Evaluation

5. What clinical and laboratory parameters are necessary to evaluate the therapy for achievement of the desired outcome and to detect or prevent adverse effects?

## Patient Education

6. What information should be provided to the patient and her family to enhance compliance, ensure successful therapy, and minimize adverse effects?

## CLINICAL COURSE

An initial decrease in the serum calcium level occurred with initial treatment you recommended. However, the normalization of her calcium level slowed and reversed within 3 days. The calcium level today is 18 mg/dL. She is very somnolent and lethargic.

## Follow-Up Questions

1. What pharmacologic and nonpharmacologic options might be considered at this time and why?
2. How would you monitor the therapy you recommended for efficacy and adverse effects?

## SELF-STUDY ASSIGNMENTS

1. What are the roles of oral bisphosphonates and intranasal calcitonin in the treatment of hypercalcemia?
2. What nonmalignant disease states can induce hypercalcemia?
3. What treatment(s) can decrease the risk of developing hypercalcemia in patients receiving calcitriol for anticancer therapy?

## CLINICAL PEARL

When evaluating a patient for hypercalcemia, a corrected calcium must be used to account for the patient's albumin level.

## REFERENCES


1. National Cancer Institute. Hypercalcemia (PDQ®) supportive care—health professionals. Available at: *www.cancer.gov/cancertopics/pdq/supportivecare/hypercalcemia/healthprofessional.* Accessed February 9, 2010.
2. Leyland-Jones B. Treating cancer-related hypercalcemia with gallium nitrate. J Support Oncol 2004;2:509–516.
3. Leyland-Jones B. Treatment of cancer-related hypercalcemia: the role of gallium nitrate. Semin Oncol 2003;30(2 Suppl 5):13–19.
4. Stewart AF. Hypercalcemia associated with cancer. N Engl J Med 2005;352:373–379.
5. Fojo AT. Metabolic emergencies. In: DeVita VT Jr, Lawrence S, Rosenberg SA, eds. DeVita, Hellman and Rosenberg's Cancer Principles & Practice of Oncology, 8th ed. Philadelphia, PA, Lippincott Williams & Wilkins, 2008.
6. Saunders Y, Ross JR, Broadley KE, et al. Systematic review of bisphosphonates for hypercalcemia of malignancy. Palliat Med 2004;18:418–431.
7. McMahan J, Linneman T. A case of resistant hypercalcemia of malignancy with a proposed treatment algorithm. Ann Pharmacother 2009;43:1532–1538.
8. Davidson TG. Conventional treatment of hypercalcemia of malignancy. Am J Health Syst Pharm 2001;58(Suppl 3):S8–S15.
9. Tanvetyanon T, Stiff PJ. Management of the adverse effects associated with intravenous bisphosphonates. Ann Oncol 2006;17:897–907.
10. Ruggiero S, Gralow J, Marx RE, et al. Practical guidelines for the prevention, diagnosis, and treatment of osteonecrosis of the jaw in patients with cancer. J Oncol Pract 2006;2:7–14.
11. Zojer N, Keck AV, Pecherstorfer M. Comparative tolerability of drug therapies for hypercalcaemia of malignancy. Drug Saf 1999;21:389–406.
12. Major P, Lortholary A, Hon J, et al. Zoledronic acid is superior to pamidronate in the treatment of hypercalcemia of malignancy: a pooled analysis of two randomized, controlled clinical trials. J Clin Oncol 2001;19:558–567.
13. Zometa [package insert]. East Hanover, NJ, Novartis Pharmaceuticals Corporation, 2009.
14. Cancer Statistics. Surveillance Epidemiology and Results. National Cancer Institute. Available at: *http://seer.cancer.gov/statfacts/html/lungb.html.* Accessed February 16, 2010.
15. Non–Small Cell Lung Cancer NCCN Clinical Practice Guidelines in Oncology. V.2.2009. 2009 National Comprehensive Cancer Network Inc. Available at: *NCCN.org.* Accessed February 16, 2010.


# 59

# HYPOKALEMIA AND HYPOMAGNESEMIA

A Super Bowl Party. . . . . . . . . . . . . . . . . . . . . . Level III

**Denise R. Sokos, PharmD, BCPS**

**W. Greg Leader, PharmD**

## LEARNING OBJECTIVES

After completing this case study, the reader should be able to:

- Analyze a patient case history and identify potential causes of electrolyte disorders.
- Select the appropriate route of administration and dose of electrolyte replacement therapy specific for a patient.
- Develop a monitoring plan for efficacy and toxicity in patients receiving electrolyte replacement therapy.

## PATIENT PRESENTATION

### Chief Complaint

"I'm short of breath."

### HPI

Dorothy Snow is a 45-year-old woman with a history of dilated cardiomyopathy who presents to the ED with a 3-day history of shortness of breath with mild to moderate exertion. She reports two- to three-pillow orthopnea × 2 days and cough during sleep. Denies chest pain; positive occasional palpitations. Reports a 10-lb weight gain in the last week and an increase in her lower extremity edema.

### PMH (Per Patient Report and Medical Records)

Dilated cardiomyopathy—echo LVEF 25% (11 months ago)
ICD placement—primary prevention (3 weeks ago)
Pulmonary hypertension—secondary left heart disease
Hypertriglyceridemia
HTN
Asthma
Sleep apnea
Type 2 DM with peripheral neuropathy
Obesity
Chronic sinusitis
Anxiety disorder
Hypothyroidism

### FH

Both parents are deceased.

### SH

Lives with husband. No alcohol use. Former smoker—quit 8 years ago. No illicit drugs.

### Meds

Valsartan 160 mg po BID
Omeprazole 20 mg po daily
Carvedilol 25 mg po BID
Digoxin 0.25 mg po daily
Spironolactone 25 mg po daily
Furosemide 80 mg po daily
Citalopram 20 mg po daily
Simvastatin 80 mg po daily
Insulin glargine 30 units SC Q 12 h
Insulin aspart 20 units SC TID with meals
Pregabalin 50 mg po BID
Metolazone 5 mg po daily
Loratadine 10 mg po daily
Tiotropium one puff daily
Fluticasone/salmeterol 500/50 one puff BID
Mometasone one spray each nostril daily
Meclizine 12.5 mg po BID
Magnesium oxide 400 mg po TID
Potassium chloride 80 mEq po BID
Levothyroxine 75 mcg po daily
ASA 81 mg po daily
Lorazepam 0.5 mg po TID
Fenofibrate 48 mg po daily
Folic acid 1 mg po daily

### ALL

NKDA

### ROS

Patient reports becoming short of breath for the last 3 days while walking up one flight of stairs or if she walks too quickly on a flat surface. Previously she could walk two flights of stairs before becoming short of breath. She uses several pillows at night to sleep but does not report PND symptoms. She reports increased swelling in her lower extremities. States that she has not changed her diet, but did attend an all-day Super Bowl party the previous weekend and ate foods that were not part of her normal diet (e.g., chili, buffalo wings, veggies and dip, pizza). Denies ever having an ICD discharge.

### Physical Examination

*Gen*

Appears older than her stated age; obese; mild dyspnea at rest

*VS*

P 112, RR 22, BP 110/60, T 35.8°C, weight 192 lb (baseline weight 184 lb), height 5′5″, $O_2$ sat 88% room air

*Skin*

Skin warm, dry

*HEENT*

PERRLA; conjunctivae clear; moist mucous membranes; tongue midline

*Neck/Lymph Nodes*

Supple; JVP estimated at 13 cm; no carotid bruit; no lymphadenopathy; (+) thyroid nodules

*Lungs*

Bibasilar rales R > L; occasional wheezes

*CV*

Tachycardic; normal $S_1$, $S_2$; $+S_3$; $-S_4$; 2/6 holosystolic murmur best heard at second left intercostal space

*Abd*

Obese; good bowel sounds; no bruits; no hepatosplenomegaly, (+) hepatojugular reflux; no evidence of ascites

*Genit/Rect*

Deferred

*Ext*

No cyanosis; 3+ pitting edema to knees bilaterally; 2+ pulses bilaterally in upper and lower extremities

*Back*

No CVA tenderness

*Neuro*

Alert & oriented × 3; no focal deficits; mild sensory deficit in feet bilaterally; CN II–XII grossly intact

### Labs

| | | | |
|---|---|---|---|
| Na 133 mEq/L | Hgb 10.4 g/dL | Ca 8.3 mg/dL | Alb 3.0 g/dL |
| K 2.8 mEq/L | Hct 29.3% | Mg 1.3 mEq/L | PT 14 s |
| Cl 93 mEq/L | WBC 4.5 × $10^3$/mm$^3$ | Phos 3.1 mEq/L | INR 1.2 |
| $CO_2$ 30 mEq/L | Plt 165× $10^3$/mm$^3$ | AST 100 IU/L | aPTT 21 s |
| BUN 17 mg/dL | BNP 1,027 pg/mL | ALT 110 IU/L | T. chol 144 mg/dL |
| SCr 0.8 mg/dL | | Troponin I < 0.01 ng/mL | |
| Glu 143 mg/dL | | CK 30 IU/L | |

■ Chest X-Ray

Bilateral pulmonary edema; moderate R pleural effusion; small L pleural effusion; (+) cardiomegaly

■ 12-Lead ECG

Sinus tachycardia; LBBB; no evidence of acute ischemia

■ Assessment

Admit to inpatient monitored bed.

1. Acute on chronic systolic heart failure
2. NYHA class III symptoms, ACC stage C
3. Volume overload
4. Electrolyte abnormalities
5. Hyperglycemia

## QUESTIONS

### Problem Identification

1.a. Create a list of the patient's drug therapy problems.

1.b. What information (signs, symptoms, laboratory values) indicates the presence and severity of the electrolyte abnormalities?

1.c. What are the potential causes of the electrolyte disorders in this patient?

1.d. What additional information is needed to satisfactorily assess this patient's electrolyte disorders?

### Desired Outcome

2. What are the goals of pharmacotherapy in this patient?

### Therapeutic Alternatives

3. What feasible pharmacotherapeutic alternatives are available for treatment of hypervolemia, hypokalemia, and hypomagnesemia in this patient?

### Optimal Plan

4. Given the therapeutic alternatives outlined above, what is the most appropriate therapy?

### Outcome Evaluation

5. What clinical and laboratory parameters are necessary to evaluate the therapy for the desired therapeutic outcome and prevention of adverse effects?

### Patient Education

6. What information should be provided to the patient to enhance adherence, ensure successful therapy, and minimize adverse effects?

## ■ CLINCIAL COURSE

Five months ago, Mrs Snow was hospitalized briefly with atypical chest pain and had persistent hypokalemia for which the metolazone was discontinued. She subsequently developed significant fluid retention and her PCP restarted metolazone 5 mg po daily. She had a recent ED visit where it was found that her potassium was 7.2 mEq/L. A repeat serum potassium level was 5.5 mEq/L. During that visit, her potassium supplement was reduced from 80 mEq po QID to 80 mEq po BID.

### Follow-Up Questions

1. Develop a plan to monitor this patient's electrolytes in the long term.
2. What changes should be made to the patient's medication regimen to prevent future electrolyte imbalances?
3. What changes should be made in the therapy for the patient's other medical conditions?
4. What vaccinations should this patient receive?

## CLINICAL PEARL

Hypokalemia and hypomagnesemia often coexist. In patients refractory to potassium replacement, magnesium concentrations should be evaluated, and any magnesium deficit must be corrected before potassium can be appropriately replaced.

## ■ SELF-STUDY ASSIGNMENTS

1. Outline a therapeutic plan for the treatment of pulmonary hypertension in this patient.
2. Describe how a patient's acid–base status can affect serum electrolyte concentrations.

## REFERENCES


1. Weiner ID, Wingo CS. Hypokalemia—consequences, causes and correction. J Am Soc Nephrol 1997;8(7):1179–1188.
2. Gennari FJ. Hypokalemia. N Engl J Med 1998;339(7):451–458.
3. Agus ZS. Hypomagnesemia. J Am Soc Nephrol 1999;10(7):1616–1622.
4. Jessup M, Abraham WT, Casey DE, et al. 2009 focused update: ACCF/AHA guidelines for the diagnosis and management of heart failure in adults: a report of the American College of Cardiology Foundation/American Heart Association Task Force on Practice Guidelines: developed in collaboration with the International Society for Heart and Lung Transplantation. Circulation 2009;119:1977–2016.
5. Kruse JA, Carlson RW. Rapid correction of hypokalemia using concentrated intravenous potassium chloride infusions. Arch Intern Med 1990;150(3):613–617.
6. Hamill RJ, Robinson LM, Wexler HR, et al. Efficacy and safety of potassium infusion therapy in hypokalemic critically ill patients. Crit Care Med 1991;19(5):694–699.


# 60

# METABOLIC ACIDOSIS

Oh, My Aching Acidosis . . . . . . . . . . . . . . . . . . Level II

**Brian M. Hodges, PharmD, BCPS, BCNSP**

## LEARNING OBJECTIVES

After completing this case study, students should be able to:

- Recognize the clinical and laboratory manifestations of metabolic acidosis.
- Differentiate among different causes of metabolic acidosis.

- Develop a patient-specific pharmacotherapeutic plan for treating chronic metabolic acidosis.
- Provide medication education for patients with chronic metabolic acidosis.

## PATIENT PRESENTATION

### Chief Complaint

"I just feel so weak all the time."

### HPI

Sue Rider is a 67-year-old woman with progressively declining renal function, due to hypertension, who is being seen in the nephrology clinic for management of fatigue, dyspnea, somnolence, and lethargy. She further reports that over the last few months she has experienced a decrease in appetite and occasionally feels nauseated without vomiting. She reports frequent nonadherence to her antihypertensive regimen "when I feel good." She also reports no history of diarrhea.

### PMH

HTN
Declining renal function due to HTN
Seasonal allergic rhinitis

### SH

She is a retired schoolteacher who lives with her husband of 38 years and has three grown children. She denies alcohol use. There is no history of tobacco habituation or recreational drug use.

### FH

History of CAD in her mother's family

### ROS

As per HPI

### Meds

Amlodipine 5 mg po daily
Metoprolol succinate 25 mg po daily
Metolazone 2.5 mg po daily, taken intermittently for lower extremity edema (reports that she has not taken any for the last few months)

### ALL

NKDA

### Physical Examination

*Gen*

Pleasant African-American woman in NAD

*VS*

BP 145/85, P 78, RR 22, T 37.2°C; Wt 75 kg, Ht 5′4″

*HEENT*

No hemorrhages or exudates on funduscopic examination

*Neck/Lymph Nodes*

JVP was 5 cm; carotid pulses were 2+ bilaterally; no thyromegaly or lymphadenopathy

*Lungs*

CTA and P

*CV*

Unable to palpate PMI; regular rate and rhythm; normal $S_1$ and $S_2$; no murmurs

*Abd*

Obese, soft, nontender; normoactive bowel sounds; no organomegaly

*MS/Ext*

Minimal sternal and quadriceps tenderness

*Neuro*

No focal cranial nerve deficits; strength 5/5 in all extremities. DTRs are 1+ brachioradialis, 2+ biceps, 2+ quadriceps, 1+ ankle jerks, toes downgoing bilaterally.

### Labs

| | | |
|---|---|---|
| Na 132 mEq/L | Hgb 12.2 g/dL | AST 13 IU/L |
| K 4.4 mEq/L | Hct 37% | ALT 7 IU/L |
| Cl 98 mEq/L | Plt 225 × $10^3$/mm$^3$ | Alk phos 113 IU/L |
| $CO_2$ 16 mEq/L | WBC 7.6 × $10^3$/mm$^3$ | GGT 14 IU/L |
| BUN 37 mg/dL | Ca 7.4 mg/dL | T. bili 0.4 mg/dL |
| SCr 2.9 mg/dL | Mg 2.2 mg/dL | Alb 3.6 g/dL |
| Glu 89 mg/dL | Phos 4.3 mg/dL | |

### ABG on RA

pH 7.28; $pCO_2$ 34 mm Hg; $pO_2$ 106 mm Hg; bicarbonate 15.5 mEq/L

### UA

SG 1.025; pH 5.0

### KUB

No nephrocalcinosis

### Assessment

1. Acidosis
2. CKD
3. Hypertension
4. Hyponatremia
5. Hypocalcemia

## QUESTIONS

### Problem Identification

1.a. Identify the type of acidosis (metabolic vs. respiratory) this patient exhibits, calculate the anion gap, and identify the potential causes.

1.b. What medical conditions present in this patient are either untreated or inadequately treated?

1.c. Which information obtained from the patient's symptoms, physical examination, and laboratory analysis indicates the presence of a chronic metabolic acidosis due to CKD?

1.d. What are the proposed mechanisms of metabolic acidosis in patients with CKD?

1.e. What are the complications associated with prolonged acidosis in patients with CKD?

## Desired Outcome

2. What are the pharmacotherapeutic goals for this patient?

## Therapeutic Alternatives

3. What treatment alternatives are available to achieve the desired therapeutic outcomes?

## Optimal Plan

4. Design a pharmacotherapeutic plan for the management of metabolic acidosis and its complications in this patient.

## Outcome Evaluation

5. Outline a clinical and laboratory monitoring plan to assess the patient's response to the pharmacotherapeutic regimen you recommended.

## Patient Education

6. How should the patient be counseled about the drug therapy to treat chronic metabolic acidosis?

## ■ CLINICAL COURSE

At the patient's 3-month clinic visit, 2+ pedal edema is noted. During the patient interview, she states that her adherence to her medications has improved. Labs are as follows:

| | |
|---|---|
| Na 135 mEq/L | Ca 8.6 mg/dL |
| K 3.9 mEq/L | Mg 1.9 mg/dL |
| Cl 101 mEq/L | Phos 5.0 mg/dL |
| $CO_2$ 22 mEq/L | Alb 3.0 g/dL |
| BUN 36 mg/dL | |
| SCr 3.0 mg/dL | |
| Glu 99 mg/dL | |

## Follow-Up Case Questions

1. How might the patient's buffer therapy requirement change if she is started on sevelamer to prevent dietary phosphorus absorption?
2. What clinical and laboratory parameters should be monitored to assess the adequacy of the patient's ACE inhibitor dosing to slow the progression of her CKD?

## ■ SELF-STUDY ASSIGNMENTS

1. Differentiate between the bone disease of metabolic acidosis and that associated with chronic renal failure and osteoporosis.
2. Discuss the types of metabolic acidosis that may be present in patients with CKD and how they may be differentiated.

## CLINICAL PEARL

While the chronic metabolic acidosis associated with CKD is usually not progressive, there is increasing evidence that correction of the acidosis is related to decreased progression of CKD. Appropriate sodium bicarbonate therapy may result in improved nutritional status, renal function, and quality of life for patients with CKD.

## REFERENCES


1. Uribarri J. Acidosis in chronic renal insufficiency. Semin Dial 2000;13:232–234.
2. Kraut JA, Kurtz I. Metabolic acidosis of CKD: diagnosis, clinical characteristics, and treatment. Am J Kidney Dis 2005;45:978–993.
3. Mandayam S, Mitch WE. Dietary protein restriction benefits patients with chronic kidney disease. Nephrology (Carlton) 2006;11:53–57.
4. National Kidney Foundation. K/DOQI clinical practice guidelines on hypertension and antihypertensive agents in chronic kidney disease. Am J Kidney Dis 2004;43(Suppl 1):S1–S290.
5. Mathur RP, Dash SC, Gupta N, et al. Effects of correction of metabolic acidosis on blood urea and bone metabolism in patients with mild to moderate chronic kidney disease: a prospective randomized single blind controlled trial. Ren Fail 2006;28:1–5.
6. National Kidney Foundation. K/DOQI clinical practice guidelines for bone metabolism and disease in chronic kidney disease. Am J Kidney Dis 2003;42(Suppl 3):S1–S201.

*Note:* All NKF K/DOQI clinical practice guidelines are available online at *www.kidney.org/professionals/kdoqi/guidelines.cfm*.


# 61

# METABOLIC ALKALOSIS

Keep Me in the Loop. . . . . . . . . . . . . . . . . . . . Level I

**Jennifer Confer, PharmD, BCPS**

## LEARNING OBJECTIVES

After completing this case study, students should be able to:

- Recognize the signs and symptoms of metabolic alkalosis.
- Describe patient-specific factors that contribute to the development of metabolic disorders.
- Recommend appropriate first-line treatment regimens and alternatives for metabolic alkalosis.
- Formulate a patient-specific pharmacotherapeutic plan for the treatment and monitoring of metabolic alkalosis.

## PATIENT PRESENTATION

### ■ Chief Complaint

"I feel very weak and tired."

### ■ HPI

Lois Strickland is a 60-year-old woman who presents to the ED with complaints of generalized weakness, fatigue, myalgias, and polyuria over the past 2 days. She states that recently she has felt bloated and has been taking an extra dose of her "water pill" every day for the past week and a half. She also mentioned that she may have eaten something bad because she has thrown up three times since dinner last night.

### ■ PMH

Hypertension × 15 years
CHF diagnosed 2 years ago

Diabetes, type 2—diet controlled
Dyslipidemia

## FH

Mother is alive with a history of HTN and dyslipidemia. Father is alive with HTN. Younger sister is alive with dyslipidemia.

## SH

Patient reports she does not consume alcohol except a glass of wine "at special occasions." She denies tobacco or illicit drug use. Lives at home with her husband of 35 years and their two dogs.

## Meds

Lisinopril 10 mg po once daily
Carvedilol 3.125 mg po BID
Furosemide 40 mg po once daily
Simvastatin 10 mg po at bedtime
Last dose of all meds was this morning 3 hours before arriving at the ED (except simvastatin, which was taken yesterday evening)

## All

Codeine—patient reports "I get short of breath"

## ROS

Denies unusual weight gain or loss. She denies fever, chills, or night sweats, but reports dizziness that has occurred off and on over the past week in addition to the generalized fatigue and weakness. No reported chest pain, palpitations, shortness of breath, or cough. She denies diarrhea, constipation, or change in bowel habits. She reports a recent increase in thirst and urination, but no change in urine color. She reports myalgias and perioral numbness that began recently with the fatigue and weakness.

## Physical Examination

*Gen*

The patient is ill-appearing and feels warm to the touch.

*VS*

BP 93/62, HR 101, RR 20, T 37.9°C; Wt 80 kg, Ht 5′7″; $O_2$ sat 96% on RA

*Skin*

Soft, intact, warm, dry

*HEENT*

EOMI; PERRLA; no sinus tenderness; dry mucous membranes; no oral lesions; no nasal congestion present

*Neck/Lymph Nodes*

No JVD or bruits; no lymphadenopathy or thyromegaly

*Chest*

CTA bilaterally

*Breasts*

Deferred

*CV*

RRR; normal $S_1$, $S_2$; no $S_3$ or $S_4$; no murmurs, rubs, gallops

*Abd*

Soft, NTND; (+) bowel sounds

*GU/Rect*

WNL

*Ext*

No CCE; feet are dry and wrinkled

*Neuro*

A & O × 3. CN II–XII intact.

## Labs

| | | |
|---|---|---|
| Na 132 mEq/L | Hgb 12.4 g/dL | Alb 3.8 g/dL |
| K 2.9 mEq/L | Hct 36.7% | AST 19 IU/L |
| Cl 85 mEq/L | Plt 324 × $10^3/mm^3$ | ALT 16 IU/L |
| $CO_2$ 39 mEq/L | WBC 12.1 × $10^3/mm^3$ | Alk phos 62 IU/L |
| BUN 24 mg/dL | Mg 1.7 mEq/L | T. bili 0.4 mg/dL |
| SCr 1.1 mg/dL | Phos 3.6 mg/dL | PT 11.3 s |
| Glu 118 mg/dL | Ca 7.6 mg/dL | INR 0.96 |

## ABG

pH 7.54, $pCO_2$ 46 mm Hg, $pO_2$ 86 mm Hg, $HCO_3$ 38.3 mEq/L on RA

## UA

Urine sodium 18 mEq/L; potassium 33 mEq/L; chloride 13 mEq/L, urine pH 6.6

## Chest X-Ray

Mild pulmonary congestion, otherwise unremarkable

## ECG

Sinus tachycardia, rate 101, no acute ST-segment or T-wave changes

## Assessment

Admit patient for hypotension, flulike symptoms, electrolyte abnormalities, and metabolic alkalosis.

# QUESTIONS

## Problem Identification

1.a. Identify the type of acid–base disturbance present in this patient. Explain the patient's arterial blood gas results and identify potential causes to support your response.

1.b. Create a list of this patient's drug therapy problems.

1.c. Describe the physical exam and laboratory findings that are consistent with metabolic alkalosis and those that are inconsistent with this acid–base disorder.

1.d. What is the pathophysiology underlying this patient's metabolic alkalosis?

1.e. What medications, dietary supplements, and medical procedures could contribute to metabolic alkalosis? Include those that may not apply to this patient.

## Desired Outcome

2. What are the desired therapeutic outcomes for this patient?

## Therapeutic Alternatives

3. What pharmacologic and nonpharmacologic alternatives should be considered for the treatment of metabolic alkalosis in this patient?

## Optimal Plan

4.a. What drug, dosage form, dose, schedule, and duration of therapy are best for this patient?

4.b. What other modifications in the patient's current drug regimen are warranted? Include your rationale.

## Outcome Evaluation

5.a. What clinical and laboratory parameters are necessary to evaluate the therapy for achievement of the desired outcome and to detect or prevent adverse effects?

# CLINICAL COURSE

The patient was started on IV fluids, and 24 hours later the patient is observed to have 1+ pitting edema in her lower extremities. Laboratory values are as follows:

| | | |
|---|---|---|
| Na 140 mEq/L | BUN 14 mg/dL | ABG |
| K 3.8 mEq/L | SCr 0.9 mg/dL | pH 7.46 |
| Cl 103 mEq/L | Mg 2.1 mEq/L | $pCO_2$ 42 mm Hg |
| $CO_2$ 30 mEq/L | | $pO_2$ 92 mm Hg |
| | | $HCO_3$ 31 mEq/L |

5.b. What is your assessment of the patient's response to the IV fluids? What modifications in therapy are warranted, if any?

## Patient Education

6. What information should be provided to the patient to help enhance adherence, ensure successful outcomes, and prevent future complications?

# SELF-STUDY ASSIGNMENTS

1. Prepare a paper on the three phases (initiation, maintenance, and compensation) of the pathogenesis of metabolic alkalosis. Describe the mechanisms behind each phase and the treatments, if appropriate.
2. Describe how assessment of urine electrolytes is useful in the diagnosis and treatment of metabolic alkalosis.

## CLINICAL PEARL

Although most cases of metabolic alkalosis are asymptomatic, the disorder can lead to serious complications from electrolyte abnormalities (e.g., tetany, arrhythmias, mental status changes). In addition to assessing arterial blood gas and laboratory tests, it is important to obtain a thorough patient history to identify underlying cause of metabolic alkalosis and treat it appropriately.

## REFERENCES


1. Galla JH. Metabolic alkalosis. J Am Soc Nephrol 2000;11:369–375.
2. Gennari FJ, Weise WJ. Acid–base disturbances in gastrointestinal disease. Clin J Am Soc Nephrol 2008;3:1861–1868.
3. Richardson RMA, Forbath N, Karanicolas S. Hypokalemic metabolic alkalosis caused by surreptitious vomiting: report of four cases. CMAJ 1983;129:142–146.
4. Adrogue HJ, Madias NE. Management of life-threatening acid–base disorders: second of two parts. NEJM 1998;338(1):107–111.
5. Dellinger RP, Levy MM, Carlet JM, et al. Surviving Sepsis Campaign: international guidelines for management of severe sepsis and septic shock. Crit Care Med 2008;36:296–327.
6. Moviat M, Pickkers P, van der Hoeven PHJ, et al. Acetazolamide-mediated decrease in strong ion difference accounts for the correction of metabolic alkalosis in critically ill patients. Crit Care 2006;10(1):R14.

SECTION 6
# NEUROLOGIC DISORDERS

## 62

## ALZHEIMER'S DISEASE

Not Going Gentle Into That Good Night. . . . . . . . . . . . . . . . . . . . . . . Level II

**Carol A. Ott, PharmD, BCPP**

**Leticia K. Jones, PharmD, BCPP**

### LEARNING OBJECTIVES

After completing this case study, the reader should be able to:

- Recognize cognitive deficits and noncognitive/behavioral symptoms of AD.`
- Evaluate the drug therapy regimens for medications that could interfere with the AD process, as well as future drug therapy recommendations.
- Recommend pharmacotherapy to manage the cognitive and behavioral symptoms of AD.
- Provide education and counseling to patients and caregivers about AD, the possible benefits and adverse effects of pharmacotherapy for the disorder, and the importance of adherence to therapy.
- List at least three theories of AD etiologies and agents under investigation based on those theories.

### PATIENT PRESENTATION

#### Chief Complaint

"Mom has become apathetic and tearful in the past month. She complains that someone is stealing from her and she is not always cooperative. She lives on her own, but I am considering moving her to a nursing home."

#### HPI

Norma Dale is a 74-year-old woman who presents to the geriatric care clinic for a routine visit accompanied by her daughter Ann. Norma was diagnosed with AD 6 years ago. Her initial symptoms included forgetting times and dates easily, misplacing and losing items, repeating questions and current events, inability to answer questions, and increasing difficulty with managing finances. She was initially treated with rivastigmine, which was eventually discontinued due to intolerable side effects, although it worked well to slow her decline. Treatment with Aricept 10 mg at bedtime has been well tolerated for the past 4 years, and Norma has been participating more actively in family and social functions. Behavioral problems have been infrequent since diagnosis and have not been treated in the past. Since her last clinic visit, Norma began using Depend undergarments as extra protection for urinary incontinence.

Norma lives on her own; her daughter and son share the duties of visiting her twice a day. They have been able to maintain a regular routine with her mother's daily activities, nutrition, and financial responsibilities, using lists and notes to help Norma orient herself. Ann sets up a medication box weekly for Norma. Ann is moving in 1 month to live closer to her own daughter to help with grandchildren and has asked her youngest unmarried brother, Sam, to help take care of their mother. Sam has agreed to be his mother's caregiver. He lives and works across town and is not sure if he wants to move his mother into his home. There has been discussion about placing Norma in a long-term care facility. Norma displays lack of interest, apathy, and tearfulness lately, especially when Ann and Sam are talking about her care. Ann asks about Norma's current Alzheimer's medication and her recent lack of cooperation and mood.

#### PMH

Osteoarthritis in hands and hip × 6 years
Hypertension × 15 years
Dyslipidemia × 6 years
AD diagnosed 6 years ago
Urinary incontinence × 6 months

#### FH

Noncontributory, both parents deceased. Five children, four who live nearby.

#### SH

Lives at home; has been widowed for 10 years (husband died of cancer)

#### Meds

Aricept 10 mg po at bedtime
Vitamin E 400 IU po once daily
Lisinopril 10 mg po once daily
Simvastatin 20 mg po every evening
Aspirin 81 mg po once daily
Oxybutynin 5 mg po twice daily (×2 months)
Ensure drinks PRN
Acetaminophen PRN

#### All

NKDA

#### ROS

Reports occasional bladder incontinence and knee pain; no c/o heartburn, chest pain, or shortness of breath

## Physical Examination

*Gen*

WD woman who appears her stated age

*VS*

BP 144/82, P 76, RR 18, T 37°C; Wt 165 lb, Ht 5′6″

*Skin*

Normal texture and color

*HEENT*

WNL, TMs intact

*Neck/Lymph Nodes*

Neck supple without thyromegaly or lymphadenopathy

*Lungs/Thorax*

Clear, normal breath sounds

*Breasts*

No masses or tenderness

*CV*

RRR, no murmurs or bruits

*Abd*

Soft, NTND

*Genit/Rect*

Normal external female genitalia

*MS/Ext*

No CCE, Heberden's nodes on both hands, decreased ROM (L) hip

*Neuro*

Motor, sensory, CNs, cerebellar, and gait normal. Folstein MMSE score 16/30, compared to a score of 19/30 and 24/30, last year and at the initial diagnosis, respectively. Disoriented to season, month, date, and day of week. Disoriented to country. Good registration but impaired attention and very poor short-term memory. Unable to remember any of three items after 3 minutes. Able to follow commands. Displayed apathy, tearfulness, and frustration during MMSE.

## Labs (Fasting)

| | | | |
|---|---|---|---|
| Na 139 mEq/L | Hgb 13.5 g/dL | T. bili 0.9 mg/dL | *Fasting lipid panel* |
| K 3.7 mEq/L | Hct 39.0% | D. bili 0.3 mg/dL | T. chol 212 mg/dL |
| Cl 108 mEq/L | AST 25 IU/L | T. prot 7.5 g/dL | LDL 130 mg/dL |
| $CO_2$ 25.5 mEq/L | ALT 24 IU/L | Alb 4.5 g/dL | HDL 45 mg/dL |
| BUN 16 mg/dL | Alk phos 81 IU/L | Ca 9.7 mg/dL | TG 180 mg/dL |
| SCr 1.4 mg/dL | GGT 22 IU/L | Phos 4.5 mg/dL | |
| Glu 102 mg/dL | LDH 85 IU/L | Vit $B_{12}$ 430 pg/mL | Free T4 0.9 ng/dL |
| | | TSH 2.5 mIU/L | UA 6.8 mg/dL |

## Urinalysis

| | |
|---|---|
| Specific gravity | 1.010 |
| Color | Dark yellow |
| Appearance | Clear |
| Glucose | Pos |
| Bilirubin | Neg |
| Ketones | Neg |
| pH | 7.4 |
| Protein | Neg |
| Blood | Neg |
| Nitrite | Pos |
| WBC/HPF | 25–50 |
| RBC/HPF | 0 |
| Leukocyte esterase | 2+ |
| Bacteria | 1+ |

## CT Scan (Head, 4 Years Ago)

Mild to moderate generalized cerebral atrophy

## Assessment

1. AD, stage 5 on the Global Deterioration Scale (moderate AD—early dementia)
2. Behavioral problems reported by caregiver as lack of interest, apathy, uncooperative behavior, and tearfulness
3. Occasional urinary incontinence
4. Occasional hip and hand pain secondary to osteoarthritis; generally well controlled with acetaminophen PRN
5. Dyslipidemia not optimally controlled with current drug therapy
6. Possible urinary tract infection

# QUESTIONS

## Problem Identification

1.a. Create a list of the patient's drug therapy problems.

1.b. What information (signs, symptoms, laboratory values) indicates the presence or severity of the cognitive and noncognitive problems of this patient with AD?

1.c. Rank the drug therapy problems according to the urgency of need to address.

## Desired Outcome

2.a. What are the goals of pharmacotherapy in this case?

2.b. What drugs or disease states may interfere with achieving these goals?

## Therapeutic Alternatives

3.a. What nondrug therapies might be useful for this patient?

3.b. What feasible pharmacotherapeutic alternatives are available for the treatment of the cognitive deficits of AD?

3.c. What pharmacologic treatments may be useful to treat the noncognitive symptoms and behaviors of this patient?

3.d. What economic and psychosocial considerations are applicable to this patient?

## Optimal Plan

4.a. What drug, dosage form, dose, schedule, and duration of therapy are best for the cognitive and noncognitive symptoms of this patient?

4.b. What alternatives would be appropriate if the initial therapy fails or cannot be used?

## Outcome Evaluation

5. What clinical and laboratory parameters are necessary to evaluate the therapy for achievement of the desired therapeutic outcome and to detect or prevent adverse effects?

## Patient Education

6. What information should be provided to the patient to enhance compliance, ensure successful therapy, and minimize adverse effects?

## ■ CLINICAL COURSE

Norma's uncooperative behavior and apathy improve with your recommended drug therapy changes. She remains tearful at times and is now not sleeping well at night. She continues to be fearful of someone coming into her house and insists that some of her things are missing.

## Follow-Up Questions

1. What further evaluation should be done to address the patient's continued tearfulness and sleep problems?
2. Discuss the use of antipsychotic medications for the treatment of psychiatric and behavioral problems in AD. Include a discussion of the pros and cons of treatment.
3. What is the impact of vitamin $B_{12}$ and thyroid function on the presentation and progression of dementia symptoms?
4. What options are available for the treatment of urinary incontinence in this patient after discontinuation of oxybutynin?
5. Discuss the treatment of medical conditions, including hypertension and dyslipidemia, in the patient with progressing dementia. What are the pros and cons of treatment relative to the patient's quality of life; cost, side effects, and complexity of the drug regimen; and ethical treatment?

## ■ CLINICAL COURSE: ALTERNATIVE THERAPY

Mrs Dale's son, Sam, is concerned about his increasing role in his mother's care, and he has been reading everything he can find about potential treatments for AD. He has read that *Ginkgo* has improved some symptoms, including apathy and depression, and asks if adding it to her medicines might help her current issues. See Section 19 in this casebook for questions about the use of *Ginkgo biloba* for treatment of AD.

## ■ SELF-STUDY ASSIGNMENTS

1. Describe neurofibrillary tangles and neuritic plaques and their roles in AD development.
2. List at least three theories of the etiology of AD. What therapies are under investigation to support these theories?
3. Characterize the stages of cognitive decline as described by the global deterioration scale and define the stage where AD may be identified.
4. Differentiate cognitive deficits from noncognitive/psychiatric symptoms and behaviors of AD.
5. Evaluate potential therapies under investigation for Alzheimer's dementia.

## CLINICAL PEARL

The elderly, especially those with dementia, can develop delirium very easily, and it may appear acutely as a behavioral problem. Causes may include medications (e.g., anticholinergic agents) and medical conditions (e.g., a UTI); therefore, a thorough assessment should be performed.

## REFERENCES


1. Rabins PV, Blacker D, Rovner BW, et al. American Psychiatric Association practice guideline for the treatment of patients with Alzheimer's disease and other dementias. 2nd edition. Am J Psychiatry 2007;164(Suppl 12):5–56.
2. Birks J. Cholinesterase inhibitors for Alzheimer's disease. Cochrane Database Syst Rev 2006;1:CD005593.
3. vanMarnum RJ. Update on the use of memantine in Alzheimer's disease. Neuropsychiatr Dis Treat 2009;5:237–247.
4. Vogel T, Dali-Youcef N, Kaltenbach G, Andrés E. Homocysteine, vitamin $B_{12}$, folate and cognitive functions: a systematic and critical review of the literature. Int J Clin Pract 2009;63(7);1061–1067.
5. ADAPT Research Writing Committee. Naproxen and celecoxib do not prevent AD in early results from a randomized controlled trial. Neurology 2007;68:1800–1818.
6. Shah K, Qureshi SU, Johnson M, et al. Does use of antihypertensive drugs affect the incidence or progression of dementia? A systematic review. Am J Geriatr Pharmacother 2009;7:250–261.
7. Beier MT. Pharmacotherapy for behavioral and psychological symptoms of dementia in the elderly. Am J Health Syst Pharm 2007;64(Suppl 1):S9–S17.
8. Jeste DV, Blazer D, Casey D, et al. ACNP white paper: update on use of antipsychotic drugs in elderly persons with dementia. Neuropsychopharmacology 2008;33:957–970.
9. Caraci F, Copani A, Nicoletti F, Drago F. Depression and Alzheimer's disease: neurobiological links and common pharmacological targets. Eur J Pharmacol 2010;626(1):64–71.
10. Cancelli I, Valentis L, Merlino G, et al. Drugs with anticholinergic properties as a risk factor for psychosis in patients affected by Alzheimer's disease. Clin Pharmacol Ther 2008;84(1):63–68.


# 63

# MULTIPLE SCLEROSIS

White Dots and Black Holes . . . . . . . . . . . . . . . Level I

**Jacquelyn L. Bainbridge, BS Pharm, PharmD, FCCP**

**John R. Corboy, MD**

**Michael D. Egeberg, PharmD**

## LEARNING OBJECTIVES

After completing this case study, students should be able to:

- Describe the signs and symptoms of MS that often mimic those of other neurologic diseases.
- Design a pharmacotherapeutic regimen for treating an acute exacerbation of MS.
- Identify patients for whom disease-modifying therapy would be appropriate and recommend the most appropriate alternative for an individual patient.
- Implement a pharmacotherapeutic plan for a patient with worsening MS.
- Educate a patient on the proper dosing, self-administration, adverse effects, and storage of interferon β-1a (Avonex, Rebif), interferon β-1b (Betaseron), glatiramer acetate (Copaxone), mitoxantrone, and natalizumab.

## PATIENT PRESENTATION

### Chief Complaint

"My legs are numb and weak, and I'm having trouble walking and urinating."

### HPI

Loretta Mansfield is a 24-year-old woman who was in excellent health until 4 days ago, when she developed numbness and tingling in her left foot. Over the course of the next 4 days, the numbness extended higher up her leg to her lower abdomen, stopping at the umbilicus, and then going down the right leg. She also developed weakness in both legs, trouble walking, and urinary urgency.

### PMH

Frequent migraine headaches since adolescence that have been difficult to control despite therapy with acetaminophen, aspirin, and caffeine (Excedrin) and sumatriptan
Mild recurrent bouts of depression that have not been treated pharmacologically
Obesity most of her life

### FH

The patient is of English descent. She was born in Arizona and moved at the age of 12 to Ohio. She has no siblings, and both parents are alive and well. There is no family history of neurologic disease.

### SH

The patient is married and is employed as an accountant. She has smoked one pack per day for 8 years. Her use of alcohol is limited to an occasional glass of wine or beer on weekends.

### Meds

Acetaminophen, aspirin, and caffeine (Excedrin) two tablets po PRN headache
Sumatriptan 50 mg po PRN migraine

### Allergies

NKDA

### ROS

Unremarkable except that she reports feeling run down and tired. No previous history of visual disturbance (e.g., pain, blurred or double vision), sensory, motor, bowel, bladder, or gait disturbance.

### Physical Examination

*Gen*

The patient is a Caucasian woman who appears to be slightly anxious but is otherwise in NAD.

*VS*

BP 120/72, P 88 and regular, RR 20, T 36.6°C; Wt 86.4 kg, Ht 5′2″, BMI 34.7

*Skin*

Normal turgor; no obvious lesions, tumors, or moles

*HEENT*

NC/AT, TMs clear

*Neck/Lymph Nodes*

Supple, without lymphadenopathy or thyromegaly

*CV*

RRR; $S_1$, $S_2$ normal; no MRG

*Lungs*

Clear to A & P

*Abd*

NTND

*Genit/Rect*

Deferred

*MS/Ext*

Normal ROM; pulses 2+ throughout

*Neuro*

The patient is alert, oriented, and cooperative. No Lhermitte's sign is noted.

CNs II–XII are intact with the exception of abnormal saccadic movements on horizontal gaze; no signs of optic neuropathy.

Motor: Tone, bulk, and strength are 5/5 in both arms, with good fine motor movements. In the legs, she has 4/5 strength in an upper motor neuron pattern, with normal tone and bulk.

Sensory: Moderately diminished light touch, pain, and temperature in both legs with a cord level at the umbilicus, and decreased vibratory sensation in both great toes. (+) Romberg sign.

Coordination: Finger-to-nose and alternating movements with the hands are normal, as is heel to shin bilaterally.

Gait: Mildly unsteady on tandem walking. Timed 25-foot walk was 5.2 seconds.

Reflexes: 2/2 in UE, 3/3 in LE; (+) Babinski bilaterally.

### Labs

| | |
|---|---|
| Na 145 mEq/L | AST 12 IU/L |
| K 4.1 mEq/L | ALT 40 IU/L |
| Cl 99 mEq/L | GGT 33 IU/L |
| $CO_2$ 23 mEq/L | Wintrobe ESR 20 mm/h |
| BUN 11 mg/dL | TSH 1.0 μIU/mL |
| SCr 0.9 mg/dL | ANA negative |
| Glu 109 mg/dL | CRP 1.0 mg/dL |
| 25(OH) vitamin D 17 ng/mL | Lyme serology negative |

### Lumbar Puncture

CSF analysis shows opening pressure 140 mm $H_2O$, 10 WBC/μL, 97% lymphocytes; protein 30 mg/dL, glucose 65 mg/dL; IgG index 1.7; 12 oligoclonal bands unique to CSF.

### MRI Scan

Thoracic spine MRI with and without injection of contrast material reveals a one-segment long enhancing lesion in the posterior thoracic spine at level T10.

Brain MRI shows multiple areas of T2 and FLAIR hyperintense lesions; four were periventricular, one was in the left cerebellum, two were juxtacortical; none of the areas enhance after injection of contrast material. A total of 12 T2 and FLAIR lesions were seen in the brain; see Figure 63-1.

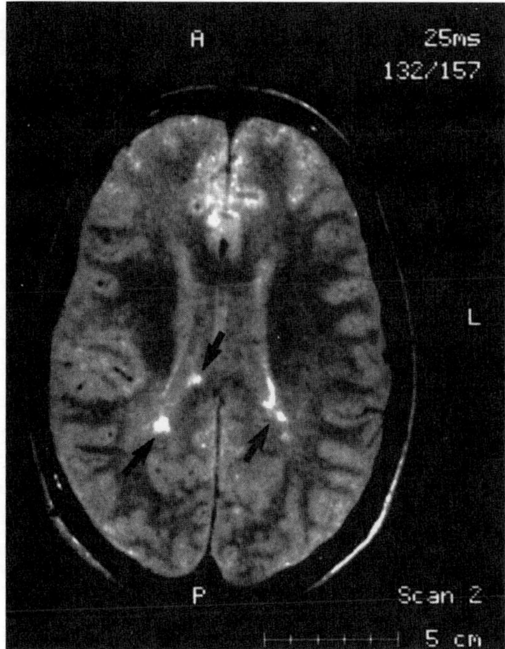


**FIGURE 63-1.** Brain MRI scan. Arrows highlight typical periventricular white matter lesions seen in multiple sclerosis.

### Assessment/Plan

Medical history, physical exam findings, and other diagnostic tests are consistent with MS. Because this is her first episode of MS-like symptoms, diagnosis is CIS. Diagnostic tests suggest high risk of recurrent disease activity over 5–20 years.

Plan to initiate therapy to treat acute signs/symptoms. Will consider long-term therapy with a disease-modifying agent and symptomatic therapies.

Will provide patient counseling on lifestyle and dietary modifications that may help improve quality of life and slow or prevent disease progression.

# QUESTIONS

## Problem Identification

1.a. What clinical information (patient demographics, signs, symptoms, lab values) suggests the diagnosis of clinically isolated syndrome (CIS) in this patient?

1.b. What additional information (laboratory tests, diagnostic procedures) may be useful in assessing this patient?

## Desired Outcome

2. What are the goals of therapy for this patient?

## Therapeutic Alternatives

3.a. What pharmacotherapeutic options are available to treat this patient's acute neurologic signs and symptoms?

3.b. What pharmacotherapeutic options are available to reduce the risk of recurrent disease activity in this patient?

3.c. What symptomatic treatments may be indicated for this patient?

3.d. What behavioral or dietary changes may be beneficial?

## Optimal Plan

4. Design a comprehensive pharmacotherapeutic plan for this patient on her initial presentation.

## Outcome Evaluation

5. What clinical and laboratory parameters are necessary for assessment of both efficacy and toxicity?

## Patient Education

6. What information would you provide to this patient about her initial therapy?

# CLINICAL COURSE

The patient was treated with the regimen you recommended, with gradual resolution of her symptoms. Six months after the initial presentation, she returns to clinic with complaints of painful loss of vision in her left eye, which evolved over 3 days. On exam, she has visual acuity of 20/200 in the left eye and 20/20 in the right eye. Visual fields are normal, but she has loss of color sensitivity in the left eye. There is a left relative afferent pupillary defect (Marcus Gunn pupil). There is no disc swelling or atrophy in either eye on funduscopic examination. The remainder of the physical exam is notable only for a mild Romberg sign and increased reflexes in the lower extremities. Her affect is sad, and she is tearful during the examination. She is concerned that she has now progressed to a diagnosis of clinically definite MS.

## Follow-Up Question

1. Would you consider the new information gathered at the follow-up visit to be evidence of significant disease progression that would prompt you to change your treatment strategy? If so, what therapies would be appropriate for the patient?

# SELF-STUDY ASSIGNMENTS

1. Obtain relevant information and formulate an opinion on the role of plasmapheresis in the treatment of MS.
2. Review the clinical studies evaluating comparative trials of disease-modifying therapies for MS. How does glatiramer acetate compare to interferon β-1b and interferon β-1a in terms of both efficacy and toxicity?
3. Outline a plan for providing patient education on the dosing, administration, monitoring, and storage of interferon β-1b, interferon β-1a, and glatiramer acetate.
4. Identify recent clinical trials assessing the efficacy and toxicity of natalizumab, rituximab, alemtuzumab, fingolimod, and cladribine for MS. Considering the data available, define the potential role(s) of these agents for patients with MS.

## CLINICAL PEARL

Many patients do not feel better with interferon therapy and may experience unpleasant adverse effects. It is important to reinforce that the ABC-R (Avonex, Betaseron, Copaxone, Rebif) medications do not reduce disease symptoms but will reduce attacks and progression of disability over time. Adequate counseling about the potential benefits and expected side effects is essential to ensuring adherence to the therapy.

## REFERENCES


1. Healy BC, Ali EN, Guttmann CR, et al. Smoking and disease progression in multiple sclerosis. Arch Neurol 2009;66:858–864.
2. Goodin DS, Frohman EM, Garmany GP, et al. Disease modifying therapies in multiple sclerosis. Report of the Therapeutics and Technology Assessment Subcommittee of the American Academy of Neurology and the MS Council for Clinical Practice Guidelines. Neurology 2002;58:169–178.
3. Kaufman DI, Trobe JD, Eggenberger ER, Whitaker JN. Practice parameter: the role of corticosteroids in the management of acute monosymptomatic optic neuritis. Report of the Quality Standards Subcommittee of the American Academy of Neurology. Neurology 2000;54:2039–2044.
4. Martinelli V, Rocca MA, Annovazzi P, et al. A short-term randomized MRI study of high-dose oral vs intravenous methylprednisolone in MS. Neurology 2009;73(22):1842–1848.
5. Comi G, Martinelli V, Rodegher M, et al. Effect of glatiramer acetate on conversion to clinically definite multiple sclerosis in patients with clinically isolated syndrome (PreCISe study): a randomised, double-blind, placebo-controlled trial. Lancet 2009;374:1503–1511.
6. Schapiro RT. Managing symptoms of multiple sclerosis. Neurol Clin 2005;23(1):177–187, vii.
7. Mikol DD, Barkhof F, Chang P, et al. Comparison of subcutaneous interferon beta-1a with glatiramer acetate in patients with relapsing multiple sclerosis (the REbif vs Glatiramer Acetate in Relapsing MS Disease [REGARD] study): a multicentre, randomised, parallel, open-label trial. Lancet Neurol 2008;7:903–914.
8. Polman CH, O'Connor PW, Havrdova E, et al. A randomized, placebo-controlled trial of natalizumab for relapsing multiple sclerosis. N Engl J Med 2006;354:899–910.
9. Corboy JR, Goodin DS, Frohman EM. Disease-modifying therapies for multiple sclerosis. Curr Treat Options Neurol 2003;5:35–54.
10. Hauser SL, Waubant E, Arnold DL, et al. B-cell depletion with rituximab in relapsing-remitting multiple sclerosis. N Engl J Med 2008;358:676–688.


# 64

# COMPLEX PARTIAL SEIZURES

An Overdue Visit to a Neurology Clinic . . . . . . Level I

**James W. McAuley, RPh, PhD, FAPhA**

## LEARNING OBJECTIVES

After completing this case study, students should be able to:

- Identify necessary data to collect for patients with complex partial seizures.
- Define potential drug-related problems for established and new antiepileptic drugs.
- List desired therapeutic outcomes for patients with complex partial seizures.
- Based on patient characteristics, choose appropriate pharmacotherapy for treatment of partial seizures and develop a suitable care plan.
- Identify key issues for a woman of childbearing potential taking antiepileptic drugs.

## PATIENT PRESENTATION

### Chief Complaint

"My family doctor told me I should see a neurologist about my seizures."

### HPI

Peggy Livingston is a 36-year-old woman referred to the neurology clinic by her PCP for evaluation of her seizures and anticonvulsant therapy. She is enduring quite a heavy seizure burden. Her last seizure was 10 days ago, which resulted in her falling down her basement stairs. Her seizures started at a very early age, and she said no one has been able to identify why she started having seizures. She remembers having them in grade school and being confused a lot throughout her schooling. She was briefly tried on phenobarbital initially but has been on phenytoin most of her life. She has poor seizure control with no extended seizure-free periods. She has not seen a neurologist for years, if ever. She has not had any neuroimaging studies and provides no previous EEG results.

On speaking with the patient and her husband of 2.5 years, most of her events involve "blackouts" and losing track of time. Occasionally, she has "grand mal" seizures. She is more likely to have a seizure if she gets overly tired or stressed. She has no history of severe head injury with loss of consciousness, or other significant risk factors for seizures. She states that at some time in her past, she "felt really bad, almost drunk" on higher doses of phenytoin. She states that she is very adherent, although she has run out of medication more than once. Because she is having seizures, she does not drive and therefore must rely on others for transportation. This lack of independence is a major concern for Peggy.

Data gathered from reviewing her seizure calendar over the last 2 months (Fig. 64-1) suggest that she is experiencing approximately eight "small" seizures per month (complex partial seizures with no secondary generalization) and one "big" seizure per month (a secondarily generalized tonic–clonic seizure). Her interview details and her overall score on her responses to the QOLIE-31 questions show a significant impact of the seizures on her quality of life. Her scores on the energy/fatigue, seizure worry, and social function domains are especially low in comparison with a cohort of other patients with epilepsy. The score on her NDDI-E was 11, indicating that she had some mood issues, but she was not depressed. On asking if there is anything else the patient would like to discuss, Mrs Livingston and her husband state they desire to start a family in the near future.

### PMH

Noncontributory, except as described previously

### FH

Both parents deceased; one younger brother in good health; no seizure disorder, cancer, or CV disease

### SH

Married; works in a local restaurant; denies tobacco and alcohol use; finished high school with a "C" average; no children

### ROS

Tired a lot, but no problems with balance or double vision

### Meds

Phenytoin (Dilantin) 300 mg po at bedtime

### All

NKDA

**Patient Instructions:** Please record the number and type of seizures you have each day.

**S = Small, B = Big, ? = Possible seizure** **Patient: P. Livingston**

March

| Sunday | Monday | Tuesday | Wednesday | Thursday | Friday | Saturday |
|---|---|---|---|---|---|---|
| | | 1 | 2 | 3 | 4 | 5<br>S |
| 6 | 7 | 8 | 9 | 10 | 11<br>S | 12<br>S |
| 13 | 14<br>S ➤ B | 15 | 16 | 17 | 18 | 19 |
| 20 | 21 | 22<br>S, S | 23<br>S | 24 | 25 | 26 |
| 27 | 28 | 29 | 30<br>S | 31 | | |

April

| Sunday | Monday | Tuesday | Wednesday | Thursday | Friday | Saturday |
|---|---|---|---|---|---|---|
| | | | | | 1 | 2 |
| 3 | 4<br>S | 5 | 6<br>S | 7<br>S | 8 | 9 |
| 10 | 11 | 12 | 13 | 14 | 15<br>S | 16<br>S, S ➤ B |
| 17 | 18 | 19<br>S | 20 | 21 | 22 | 23 |
| 24 | 25<br>? S | 26 | 27 | 28 | 29<br>S | 30 |

**FIGURE 64-1.** Seizure calendar (S, small; B, big; ?, possible seizure).

## Physical Examination

*Gen*

Pleasant woman showing some anxiety during this initial visit

*VS*

BP 132/87, P 72, RR 18, T 36.2°C; Wt 66.8 kg, Ht 5′1″

*Skin*

Normal color, hydration, and temperature

*HEENT*

Mild hirsutism; (+) gingival hyperplasia

*Neck/Lymph Nodes*

(–) JVD; (–) lymphadenopathy

*Lungs/Thorax*

CTA

*Breasts*

Deferred

*CV*

Normal $S_1$ and $S_2$, RRR, NSR, normal peripheral pulses

*Abd*

NTND, (+) BS, no HSM

*Genit/Rect*

Deferred

*MS/Ext*

Significant burn on palm of right hand. This happened within the last week or so, when she had a seizure while frying eggs on the stovetop. Her husband stated that she put her hand directly in the frying pan.

*Neuro*

CNs II–XII intact; slight lateral gaze nystagmus noted. Motor: 4/5 muscle strength on left side, 5/5 on right side. DTRs: 2+ RUE, 1+ LUE, 0 RLE, 0 LLE. Sensory: normal light touch and pinprick. Station: normal.

## Labs

| | | |
|---|---|---|
| Na 137 mEq/L | Hgb 14.5 g/dL | AST 31 IU/L |
| K 4.1 mEq/L | Hct 41.7% | ALT 22 IU/L |
| Cl 100 mEq/L | RBC 4.71 × $10^6$/mm$^3$ | Alk phos 187 IU/L |
| $CO_2$ 29 mEq/L | MCV 88.6 μm$^3$ | GGT 45 IU/L |
| BUN 9 mg/dL | MCHC 34.7 g/dL | Ca 7.3 mg/dL |
| SCr 0.6 mg/dL | Plt 212 × $10^3$/mm$^3$ | Alb 3.9 g/dL |
| Glu 107 mg/dL | WBC 5.4 × $10^3$/mm$^3$ | |

## EEG

Abnormal for bitemporal slowing, which is more significant in the left temporal region, as characterized by polymorphic and epileptiform discharges consistent with a history of seizure disorder

## Assessment

Uncontrolled complex partial seizures, with occasional secondary generalization

# QUESTIONS

## Problem Identification

1.a. Create a list of the patient's drug therapy problems.

1.b. Which information (signs, symptoms, laboratory values) indicates the presence or severity of complex partial seizures?

## Desired Outcome

2. What are the goals of pharmacotherapy in this case?

## Therapeutic Alternatives

3.a. What nonpharmacologic therapies might be useful for this patient?

3.b. What feasible pharmacotherapeutic alternatives are available for treatment of complex partial seizures in this patient?

3.c. What economic and psychosocial considerations are applicable to this patient?

## Optimal Plan

4. What drug, dosage form, dose, schedule, and duration of therapy are best for this patient?

## Outcome Evaluation

5. Which clinical and laboratory parameters are necessary to evaluate the therapy for achievement of the desired therapeutic outcome and to detect or prevent adverse effects?

## Patient Education

6. What information should be provided to the patient to enhance adherence, ensure successful therapy, and minimize adverse effects?

# CLINICAL COURSE

A collective decision was made among the health care practitioners, the patient, and her husband to add one of the newer antiepileptic drugs to her current drug regimen and to see her back in 6 weeks. She was given written and verbal information on this new drug and instructed to call with any questions, problems, or concerns. She and her husband verbalized an understanding. At her next visit, the patient reported that there had been an initial response to the addition of the new antiepileptic drug (i.e., fewer seizures), but she still has some "small" seizures and one "big" seizure per month. There are no recent laboratory data. Her neurologic examination is unchanged. She and her husband would like to discuss further their desire to start a family.

## Follow-Up Question

1. What is known about long-term effects on cognition and behavior in children exposed to antiepileptic drugs in utero?

# CLINICAL PEARL

Although epilepsy affects men and women equally, there are many women's health issues, including menstrual cycle influences on seizure activity, contraceptive–antiepileptic drug interactions, teratogenicity of antiepileptic drugs, and influence of hormone replacement therapy in postmenopausal women with epilepsy.

## SELF-STUDY ASSIGNMENTS

1. Outline a plan for assessing this patient's compliance with her medication regimen.
2. What risk factors does this patient have for osteoporosis? What interventions should be made?
3. Would switching this patient from brand Dilantin to generic phenytoin be an appropriate alternative? What are the ramifications of making this change?
4. What role can community pharmacists play in the care of patients with epilepsy?

## REFERENCES


1. Jacoby A, Snape D, Baker GA. Determinants of quality of life in people with epilepsy. Neurol Clin 2009;27:843–863.
2. Gilliam FG, Barry JJ, Hermann BP, Meador KJ, Vahle V, Kanner AM. Rapid detection of major depression in epilepsy: a multicentre study. Lancet Neurol 2006;5:399–405.
3. Mohanraj R, Brodie MJ. Measuring the efficacy of antiepileptic drugs. Seizure 2003;12:413–443.
4. Pennell PB. Hormonal aspects of epilepsy. Neurol Clin 2009;27: 941–965.
5. Holmes LB, Baldwin EJ, Smith CR, et al. Increased frequency of isolated cleft palate in infants exposed to lamotrigine during pregnancy. Neurology 2008;70:2152–2158.
6. Labiner DM, Ettinger AB, Fakhoury TA, et al. Effects of lamotrigine compared with levetiracetam on anger, hostility, and total mood in patients with partial epilepsy. Epilepsia 2009;50:434–442.
7. Meador KJ, Baker GA, Browning N, et al. Cognitive function at 3 years of age after fetal exposure to antiepileptic drugs. N Engl J Med 2009;360:1597–1605.
8. McAuley JW, Chen AY, Elliott JO, Shneker BF. An assessment of patient and pharmacist knowledge of and attitudes toward reporting adverse drug events due to formulation switching in patients with epilepsy. Epilepsy Behav 2009;14:113–117.
9. Hermann B, Jacoby A. The psychosocial impact of epilepsy in adults. Epilepsy Behav 2009;15(Suppl 1):S11–S16.
10. Hesdorffer DC, Kanner AM. The FDA alert on suicidality and antiepileptic drugs: fire or false alarm? Epilepsia 2009;50:978–986.


# 65

# GENERALIZED TONIC–CLONIC SEIZURES

Senior Seizures. . . . . . . . . . . . . . . . . . . . . . . . . Level II

**Sharon M. Tramonte, PharmD**

## LEARNING OBJECTIVES

After completing this case study, students should be able to:

- Define epilepsy.
- Differentiate seizure types based on clinical presentation and description.
- Recommend drugs of choice and alternative therapies for different types of seizures.
- Identify appropriate dosing, the most common adverse effects, and monitoring parameters for anticonvulsants.
- Develop an appropriate pharmaceutical care plan for a patient with epilepsy.

## PATIENT PRESENTATION

### Chief Complaint

"I had a seizure a few weeks ago and banged up my head."

### HPI

Carter McNeely is a 68-year-old man whose seizures are well controlled with carbamazepine monotherapy. The seizure 2.5 weeks ago was the first seizure in 20 months. During the seizure, he fell to the floor and sustained a laceration to his occipital region that required staples for closure. The description of his seizures is vague because there have been only six seizures documented since he developed epilepsy 3 years ago. Because Mr McNeely lives alone in an assisted living facility, only half of the documented seizures have been witnessed by another individual who could provide a description. Two seizures were witnessed by other residents who described him as "falling to the ground and starting to shake." One seizure occurred in the day room when a facility nurse was in the room, and he documented that Mr McNeely fell to the ground, developed rhythmic extensions to both his legs, became incontinent of urine, and was sleepy and disoriented for 2 hours after the episode.

He has only been treated with carbamazepine. This was started by his family practice physician after his second seizure. An EEG was obtained at that time and was unremarkable. Because the seizures are so infrequent, the dose of carbamazepine has never been adjusted.

### PMH

Tonic–clonic seizures diagnosed 3 years ago
HTN adequately controlled with lisinopril monotherapy
Dyslipidemia controlled with atorvastatin and low-cholesterol diet
BPH, currently symptom-free on dutasteride

### FH

Mother died at age 74 of "natural causes"; had HTN for many years. Father died at age 70 of "natural causes"; did not have any known medical illnesses. All of his children and grandchildren are alive and well. One son and one daughter have HTN.

### SH

Retired factory worker; resides in an assisted living facility. He is widowed and has six children and nine grandchildren, whom he sees frequently. He denies past or present tobacco and illicit drug use. He reports a history of regular alcohol use but now only drinks one beer that his grandson brings to him every Saturday evening.

### Meds

Aspirin 81 mg orally once daily
Atorvastatin 40 mg orally once daily
Carbamazepine XR 200 mg orally twice daily
Dutasteride 0.5 mg orally once daily
Lisinopril 20 mg orally once daily
Multivitamin with minerals one tablet orally once daily

### All

NKDA
Adverse drug effect history—none

### Physical Examination

*Gen*

Exam reveals an elderly Caucasian man who appears his stated age in NAD.

*VS*

BP 126/78, HR 72, RR 16, temperature not measured; Ht 5′10″, Wt 72.5 kg

*HEENT*

Normocephalic; scalp: healing 3-cm lesion in the occipital region with corresponding mild tenderness and bruising; PERRL

*Neck/LN*

No thyromegaly, lymphadenopathy, or carotid bruits

*Chest/Lungs*

Lungs CTA

*CV*

RRR, no m/r/g

*Abd*

Soft, nontender; no HSM; (+) BS

*MS/Ext*

Normal tone; 5/5 strength in all extremities

*Neuro*

Awake; A & O × 3; CN II–XII intact, reflexes 2+ and symmetric throughout

### Labs

| | | |
|---|---|---|
| Na 127 mEq/L | Hgb 13.5 g/dL | Cholesterol 155 mg/dL |
| K 4.7 mEq/L | Hct 41% | Triglyceride 123 mg/dL |
| Cl 90 mEq/L | RBC 3.9 × $10^6$/mm$^3$ | HDL cholesterol 39 mg/dL |
| $CO_2$ 25 mEq/L | WBC 5.1 × $10^3$/mm$^3$ | LDL cholesterol 91 mg/dL |
| BUN 10 mg/dL | Diff WNL | |
| SCr 0.6 mg/dL | MCV 97 μm$^3$ | |
| Glu 100 mg/dL | Carbamazepine 6 mcg/mL | |

### EEG

Sleep-deprived EEG unremarkable. Photic stimulation failed to produce any other changes.

### Assessment

68 yo man with fairly well-controlled seizures on carbamazepine monotherapy

## QUESTIONS

### Problem Identification

1.a. What are this patient's drug therapy problems?

1.b. What additional information is needed to fully assess the patient's problems related to epilepsy or his drug therapy?

1.c. What are the age-specific management issues for this patient?

### Desired Outcome

2. What are the goals of pharmacotherapy in this case?

### Therapeutic Alternatives

3.a. What nonpharmacologic interventions may be helpful for this patient?

3.b. What pharmacotherapeutic options are available to treat his epilepsy?

### Optimal Plan

4. What is the best pharmacotherapeutic plan for this patient?

### Outcome Evaluation

5. Which clinical and laboratory parameters are needed to evaluate the therapy to ensure the best possible outcome?

### Patient Education

6. What information should the patient receive to ensure successful therapy and to minimize adverse effects?

## SELF-STUDY ASSIGNMENTS

1. Smoking can affect serum concentrations of drugs. Perform a literature search to determine why this occurs and what effect it might have on anticonvulsants.
2. Perform a literature search to identify articles that have concluded that seizure medications can be withdrawn after a certain seizure-free interval.
3. Write a concise paper outlining the current recommendations for assisting a person who is having a seizure.
4. Assume that a patient taking valproic acid has poorly controlled seizures and a decision is made to add lamotrigine. What precautions, if any, should be taken? How should you initiate lamotrigine therapy?

## CLINICAL PEARL

Many important historical figures had epileptic seizures, including Buddha, Socrates, Alexander the Great, Julius Caesar, St. Paul the Apostle, Mohammed, Peter the Great, Handel, Napoleon, Paganini, Kierkegaard, Alfred Nobel, and Dostoyevsky. It may be useful to share some of these names with patients to break the stigma of mental illness associated with epilepsy.

## REFERENCES

1. Commission on Classification and Terminology of the International League Against Epilepsy. Proposal for revised classification of epilepsies and epileptic syndromes. Epilepsia 1989;30:389–399.
2. Garnett WR. Antiepileptic drug treatment: outcomes and adherence. Pharmacotherapy 2000;20(8 Pt 2):191S–199S.
3. Forcadas MI, Mayor PP, Puig JS. Special situations in epilepsy: women and the elderly. Neurologist 2007;13(6S):S52–S61.
4. Baker GA, Jacoby A, Buck D, et al. The quality of life of older people with epilepsy: findings from a UK community study. Seizure 2001;10:92–99.
5. Waterhouse E, Towne A. Seizures in the elderly: nuances in presentation and treatment. Cleve Clin J Med 2005;72(Suppl 3):S26–S37.
6. Hope OA, Zeber JE, Kressin NR, et al. New-onset geriatric epilepsy care: race, setting of diagnosis, and choice of antiepileptic drug. Epilepsia 2009;50:1085–1093.

# 66

# STATUS EPILEPTICUS

Tempest in a Tom Collins . . . . . . . . . . . . . . . . . Level I

**Sharon M. Tramonte, PharmD**

## LEARNING OBJECTIVES

After completing this case study, students should be able to:

- Define status epilepticus and its precipitating causes.
- Identify measures that should be taken in the ED for a patient in status epilepticus.
- Recommend appropriate drug treatment for status epilepticus.
- Recommend an appropriate pharmaceutical care plan for a patient with status epilepticus.

## PATIENT PRESENTATION

### Chief Complaint

As given by a friend of the patient: "I walked back into the room after getting breakfast and Josh was having a seizure. He kept shaking for a couple of minutes so I went to get the RA and he said we needed to get him to the ED."

### HPI

Joshua Banch is a 20 yo man brought to the university ED by his college roommate and dormitory RA. The roommate reported that he and Joshua went out partying the night before because all the fraternities were throwing rush parties. The roommate left Joshua partying at the Delta Tau Chi fraternity house at about 2 AM. He heard Joshua return to the room at approximately 4:30 AM and he was clearly intoxicated.

### PMH

Medical records revealed that the patient developed generalized tonic–clonic seizures in childhood. Phenobarbital was initiated and controlled the seizures for many years. Withdrawal of phenobarbital was attempted 10 years ago after several years of being seizure-free. The drug was restarted when seizures occurred during the attempted taper. Phenobarbital was replaced with carbamazepine because of sedation and lethargy. Phenytoin was added 8 years ago because of frequent and prolonged breakthrough seizures. He has had occasional breakthrough seizures since his admission to the university 2 years ago. Breakthrough seizures are typically associated with Joshua's noncompliance with medications or sleep deprivation due to prolonged study sessions. He is routinely followed in the university neurology clinic.

### FH

Negative for epilepsy; the patient has two siblings, all alive and well. No other information on family history was obtained.

### SH

Single with no children; no tobacco use; reports drinking up to six beers per week

### Meds

Carbamazepine 500 mg po TID

Phenytoin 100 mg po BID

### All

NKDA

### ROS

Unobtainable

### Physical Examination

*Gen*

WDWN Caucasian man who is unarousable; clothes are wet from urinary incontinence.

*VS*

BP 150/90, P 150, RR 25, T 37.5°C; Ht 5′7″, Wt 68.3 kg

*Skin*

Warm, dry, and pale; nail beds are pale

*HEENT*

Mucous membranes are dry

*Neck/Lymph Nodes*

Supple; no thyromegaly or lymphadenopathy

*Lungs/Chest*

Symmetric, lungs CTA

*CV*

RRR, no m/r/g

*Abd*

Soft, no HSM, BS normal in all four quadrants

*MS/Ext*

Muscle mass normal, full ROM

*Neuro*

Unarousable; reflexes 3+ bilaterally

### Labs

| | | |
|---|---|---|
| Na 136 mEq/L | Hgb 12.8 g/dL | Drug screen: pending |
| K 4.5 mEq/L | Hct 41% | Carbamazepine: pending |
| Cl 97 mEq/L | Plt 320 × $10^3$/mm$^3$ | Phenytoin: pending |
| $CO_2$ 28 mEq/L | WBC 9.0 × $10^3$/mm$^3$ | |
| BUN 16 mg/dL | Diff WNL | |
| SCr 1.0 mg/dL | | |
| Glu 60 mg/dL | | |

### EEG

Baseline from medical record: Diffuse background slowing; no focal changes or epileptiform activity present; photic stimulation failed to produce other changes.

### Assessment

20 yo man with a history of tonic–clonic seizures now in status epilepticus

## QUESTIONS

### Problem Identification

1.a. What are this patient's drug therapy problems?

1.b. What steps should be taken when the patient is first seen in the ED?

### Desired Outcome

2. What are the goals of pharmacotherapy in this case?

### Therapeutic Alternatives

3. What pharmacotherapeutic options are available to treat status epilepticus?

### Optimal Plan

4. What is the best pharmacotherapeutic plan for this patient?

### Outcome Evaluation

5. What clinical and laboratory parameters are needed to evaluate the therapy to ensure the best possible outcome?

### Patient Education

6. What information should the patient receive to ensure successful therapy and to minimize adverse effects?

### SELF-STUDY ASSIGNMENTS

1. There are several drug interactions with phenytoin and carbamazepine. Describe the effects that these drugs have on each other. What, if anything, should be done to compensate for these drug interactions?
2. There are several sports that patients with epilepsy should not participate in. What are some of these sports, and why should these individuals not participate in them?
3. Finger-stick assays are available for phenytoin, carbamazepine, and phenobarbital. What role might they play in the emergent therapy of status epilepticus? Characterize the accuracy of these tests.
4. Prepare a two-page paper summarizing the hematologic adverse effects of all of the anticonvulsants.

## CLINICAL PEARL

EEG studies have demonstrated that benign self-limited tonic/clonic seizures in adults last about 1 minute on average and rarely last more than 2 minutes.

## REFERENCES


1. Bone RC, ed. Treatment of convulsive status epilepticus. Recommendations of the Epilepsy Foundation of America's Working Group on Status Epilepticus. JAMA 1993;270:854–859.
2. Meierkord H, Boon P, Engelsen B, et al. EFNS guideline on the management of status epilepticus. Eur J Neurol 2006;13:445–450.
3. Kinirons P, Doherty CP. Status epilepticus: a modern approach to management. Eur J Emerg Med 2008;15:187–195.
4. Appleton R, Macleod S, Marland T. Drug management for acute tonic–clonic convulsions including convulsive status epilepticus in children. Cochrane Database Syst Rev 2008;(3). Art. no.: CD001905. DOI: 10.1002/14651858.CD001905.pub2.
5. Trinka E. What is the relative value of the standard anticonvulsants: phenytoin and fosphenytoin, phenobarbital, valproate, and levetiracetam? Epilepsia 2009;50(Suppl 12):40–43.


# 67

# ACUTE MANAGEMENT OF THE BRAIN INJURY PATIENT

The Agony of Defeat . . . . . . . . . . . . . . . . . . . . Level III

Denise H. Rhoney, PharmD, FCCP, FCCM

Dennis Parker, Jr., PharmD

## LEARNING OBJECTIVES

After completing this case study, students should be able to:

- Discuss the goals of cerebral resuscitation.
- Interpret parameters beneficial in assessing the severity of the brain injury.
- Describe the impact of prior antithrombotic therapy on traumatic brain injury and devise an appropriate treatment plan for patients with traumatic brain injury while on antithrombotic therapy.
- Discuss the therapeutic management of traumatic brain injury and increased intracranial pressure associated with acute brain injury.
- Recommend appropriate therapy to prevent medical complications after brain injury.

## PATIENT PRESENTATION

### Chief Complaint

Not available—the patient was brought to the ED by EMS as a trauma code.

### HPI

Oliver Johnson is a 55-year-old man who was brought to the ED after suffering a ski accident while on vacation with his wife. His wife reports that he was unarousable at the scene of the accident.

### PMH (As Per Patient's Wife)

Dyslipidemia
NSTEMI (1 year ago)

### FH

Unknown

### SH

Unknown

## CHAPTER 67

### ROS

Unobtainable

### Meds

Aspirin 325 mg po daily
Clopidogrel 75 mg po daily
Simvastatin 40 mg po daily

### All

No known drug allergies

### Physical Examination

*Gen*

WDWN man who does not speak, open his eyes, or move on verbal stimuli. On painful stimuli, he does not speak or open his eyes but does exhibit flexor posturing.

*VS*

BP 87/60, P 126, RR 30, T 38.3°C; Wt 85 kg, Ht 6′0″

*Skin*

Multiple bruises on the face and extremities bilaterally

*HEENT*

The patient has multiple soft tissue injuries to the face. The left pupil is 5 mm and nonreactive to direct light, and the right pupil is 2 mm and slowly reactive to light. EOMs are not reactive and not moving. External inspection of ears and nose reveals no acute abnormalities. There is some dried blood in the mouth. The head has a large open scalp laceration on the forehead with surrounding ecchymoses. Neck is in a cervical collar; therefore, movement was not attempted. There are no gross masses in the neck.

*Lungs*

Rhonchi and crackles present bilaterally with thick secretions

*Heart*

Sinus tachycardia with $S_1$ and $S_2$ present

*Abd*

Soft with no masses or tenderness but decreased bowel sounds. There is no gross hepatosplenomegaly.

*Ext*

No nontraumatic edema is noted.

*Neuro*

There is no response other than flexor posturing to pain. The Glasgow Coma Scale score is 5.

### Labs

| | | | |
|---|---|---|---|
| Na 140 mEq/L | Hgb 13.8 g/dL | Ca 8.4 mg/dL | ABG |
| K 3.7 mEq/L | Hct 40.9% | Mg 1.8 mg/dL | pH 7.49 |
| Cl 106 mEq/L | Plt 166 × $10^3$/mm$^3$ | Phos 2.4 mEq/L | $HCO_3$ 22 mEq/L |
| $CO_2$ 20 mEq/L | WBC 26.0 × $10^3$/mm$^3$ | Alb 3.4 g/dL | $pCO_2$ 33 mm Hg |
| BUN 15 mg/dL | Diff N/A | | $pO_2$ 66 mm Hg |
| SCr 1.1 mg/dL | | | $O_2$ sat 86% on RA |
| Glu 285 mg/dL | | | Urine drug screen (–) |
| | | | Blood alcohol (<20 mg/dL) |

### Portable Chest X-Ray

Right upper lobe atelectasis. No rib fractures. The ET tube is above the carina.

### Head CT

There is a left parietal open depressed skull fracture. There is an area of hemorrhagic contusion in the left frontal region. There are multiple left temporal and parietal epidural hematomas with midline shift.

### Assessment

1. S/P head trauma secondary to ski accident
2. Skull fracture and temporal and parietal epidural hematomas with midline shift
3. Coma
4. Respiratory distress
5. Hyperglycemia

### Clinical Course

On arrival in the ED, IV access was initiated, and the patient was intubated orally using a rapid sequence intubation technique (fentanyl 200 mcg IV followed by lidocaine 100 mg IV, midazolam 2 mg IV, and rocuronium 5 mg IV). The patient was started on 3% sodium/acetate solution at 75 mL/h and midazolam infusion at 12 mg/h. Other medications include levetiracetam 2 g IV load followed by 1g IV Q 12 h, fentanyl 25 mcg IV Q 1 h PRN, and insulin aspart correction dose protocol as needed hourly. A ventriculostomy was placed for monitoring of ICP with an initial ICP reading of 18 mm Hg. The patient was then transferred to the neurointensive care unit for monitoring.

Over the next 48 hours, pertinent laboratory measurements included serum sodium 158 mEq/L, serum osmolality 290 mOsm/L, urine osmolality 250 mOsm/L, and urine specific gravity 1.010 g/cm$^3$. See ICU Flowsheet at the end of the chapter for other important parameters for the first 24 hours (Fig. 67-1) and second 24 hours (Fig. 67-2) in the ICU.

## QUESTIONS

### Problem Identification

1.a. Could any of the patient's prehospital medications have contributed to the extent of the brain injury?

1.b. What information (signs, symptoms, laboratory values) indicates the severity of this patient's brain injury?

1.c. What patient factors may complicate assessment of the neurologic examination?

1.d. What poor prognostic indicators does this patient exhibit?

### Desired Outcome

2.a. What are the immediate goals of therapy for this patient?

2.b. What are the goals of fluid resuscitation and hemodynamic monitoring for this patient?

2.c. What are the goals of therapy for patients with traumatic brain injury and prehospital use of antiplatelet medications?

### Therapeutic Alternatives

3.a. What therapeutic alternatives are available for reversal of the antiplatelet effects of clopidogrel and aspirin?

3.b. What therapeutic alternatives are available for fluid resuscitation, and which would be the most appropriate for this patient?

| Time | Temp (°C) | HR (bpm) | BP (mm Hg) | ICP (mm Hg) | CPP (mm Hg) | BG (mg/ dL) | Fluid A (mL) | Fluid B (mL) | Fluid C (mL) | Nutrition | UOP (mL) | Meds given |
|---|---|---|---|---|---|---|---|---|---|---|---|---|
| 0600 | 37.6 | 85 | 120/86 | 18 | 79 | 306 | 80 | | 12 | NPO | 60 | Insulin aspart 8 units |
| 0700 | | 88 | 128/88 | 22 | 77 | | 80 | | 12 | | 105 | |
| 0800 | | 89 | 119/67 | 15 | 69 | | 80 | | 12 | NPO | 100 | |
| 0900 | | 85 | 125/89 | 16 | 70 | | 80 | 100 | 12 | | 60 | Levetiracetam 1000mg IV |
| 1000 | 38.2 | 86 | 110/65 | 20 | 60 | 288 | 80 | | 12 | NPO | 55 | Insulin aspart 6 units<br>APAP 325 mg |
| 1100 | | 92 | 115/79 | 22 | 71 | | 80 | | 12 | | 60 | Fentanyl 25 mcg × 2 |
| 1200 | | 94 | 129/55 | 18 | 62 | | 80 | | 12 | NPO | 67 | |
| 1300 | | 100 | 100/68 | 19 | 60 | | 80 | | 12 | | 100 | |
| 1400 | 38.1 | 92 | 113/70 | 17 | 67 | 270 | 80 | | 12 | NPO | 55 | Insulin aspart 6 units<br>APAP 325 mg |
| 1500 | | 98 | 130/85 | 21 | 79 | | 80 | | 12 | | 70 | |
| 1600 | | 89 | 129/75 | 18 | 75 | | 80 | | 12 | NPO | 60 | |
| 1700 | | 94 | 119/88 | 20 | 76 | | 80 | | 12 | | 60 | |
| 1800 | 37.5 | 85 | 115/66 | 22 | 75 | 240 | 80 | | 12 | NPO | 60 | Aspart 2 units |
| 1900 | | 86 | 124/50 | 22 | 53 | | 80 | | 12 | | 80 | |
| 2000 | | 83 | 144/54 | 16 | 68 | | 80 | | 12 | NPO | 60 | |
| 2100 | | 89 | 140/87 | 24 | 81 | | 80 | 100 | 12 | | 70 | Levetiracetam 1000mg IV |
| 2200 | 38.6 | 86 | 139/84 | 24 | 78 | 220 | 80 | | 12 | NPO | 75 | Aspart 2 units<br>APAP 325 mg |
| 2300 | | 90 | 120/86 | 20 | 77 | | 80 | | 12 | | 60 | |
| 2400 | | 70 | 132/75 | 12 | 82 | | 80 | | 12 | NPO | 50 | |
| 0100 | | 78 | 140/70 | 20 | 73 | | 80 | | 12 | | 110 | |
| 0200 | 37.5 | 72 | 135/68 | 20 | 70 | 190 | 80 | | 12 | NPO | 120 | |
| 0300 | | 79 | 149/75 | 19 | 81 | | 80 | | 12 | | 80 | |
| 0400 | | 75 | 137/68 | 28 | 63 | | 80 | | 12 | NPO | 110 | |
| 0500 | | 77 | 130/68 | 27 | 62 | | 80 | | 12 | | 60 | |

Fluid A = 3% sodium chloride/acetate; Fluid B = levetiracetam IVPB; Fluid C = midazolam infusion (concentration = 1 mg/mL).
*HR= heart rate; BP= blood pressure; ICP = intracranial pressure; CPP = cerebral perfusion pressure; BG = blood glucose; UOP = urine output; IVPB = intravenous piggy bag.*

**FIGURE 67-1.** Neurointensive care unit flowsheet. Day 1 (0–24 hours postadmission).

3.c. What nondrug therapies may be useful for preventing or treating increased ICP?

3.d. What pharmacotherapeutic alternatives are available for treating increased ICP?

## Optimal Plan

4.a. Develop an optimal pharmacotherapeutic plan to treat the patient's increased ICP.

4.b. Outline a pharmacotherapeutic plan for prevention of medical complications that may occur in this patient.

## Outcome Evaluation

5. What monitoring parameters should be instituted to ensure efficacy and prevent toxicity for the therapy recommended for increased ICP and other medical issues?

## Patient Education

6. What medication education should this patient receive if he is discharged on clopidogrel and aspirin?

## SELF-STUDY ASSIGNMENTS

1. Review the different types of neurologic monitoring devices that are available and how drug therapy might influence these monitoring parameters.
2. Review paroxysmal autonomic instability or "sympathetic storming" and its treatment options and monitoring parameters.
3. Evaluate the role of serum biomarkers in predicting outcome after traumatic brain injury.
4. Review the guidelines for managing the neurobehavioral sequelae of traumatic brain injury.

## CLINICAL PEARL

There are only three standards of care for severe brain injury patients: (1) use of corticosteroids is not recommended for improving outcome or reducing ICP; (2) in the absence of increased ICP, chronic prolonged hyperventilation (pa$CO_2$ <25 mm Hg) should be avoided; and (3) prophylactic use of antiepileptic drugs is not recommended for preventing late post-traumatic seizures (>7 days).

| Time | Temp (°C) | HR (bpm) | BP (mm Hg) | ICP (mm Hg) | CPP (mm Hg) | BG (mg/ dL) | Fluid A (mL) | Fluid B (mL) | Fluid C (mL) | Nutrition | UOP (mL) | Meds given |
|---|---|---|---|---|---|---|---|---|---|---|---|---|
| 0600 | 37.4 | 85 | 121/76 | 19 | 72 | 226 | 80 | | 12 | NPO | 70 | Insulin aspart 4 units IV |
| 0700 | | 78 | 125/80 | 20 | 75 | | 80 | | 12 | | 150 | |
| 0800 | | 80 | 129/66 | 25 | 62 | | 80 | | 12 | NPO | 100 | |
| 0900 | | 82 | 135/87 | 26 | 77 | | 80 | 100 | 12 | | 200 | Levetiracetam 1000 mg IV |
| 1000 | 38.2 | 86 | 120/60 | 20 | 60 | 188 | 80 | | 12 | NPO | 350 | Insulin aspart 2 units IV APAP 325 mg |
| 1100 | | 95 | 110/70 | 28 | 55 | | 125 | | 12 | | 300 | Fentanyl 25 mcg × 2 |
| 1200 | | 98 | 119/65 | 28 | 55 | | 125 | | 12 | NPO | 150 | |
| 1300 | | 97 | 110/78 | 29 | 60 | | 125 | | 12 | | 350 | |
| 1400 | 38.3 | 90 | 118/77 | 35 | 55 | 286 | 125 | | 12 | NPO | 300 | Insulin aspart 8 units IV APAP 325 mg |
| 1500 | | 88 | 135/80 | 31 | 67 | | 125 | | 12 | | 500 | |
| 1600 | | 89 | 129/85 | 28 | 72 | | 125 | | 12 | NPO | 350 | |
| 1700 | | 77 | 120/87 | 20 | 78 | | 125 | | 12 | | 200 | |
| 1800 | 38.1 | 80 | 135/68 | 23 | 67 | 240 | 125 | | 12 | NPO | 250 | Aspart 2 units IV APAP 325 mg |
| 1900 | | 76 | 128/60 | 24 | 59 | | 125 | | 12 | | 200 | |
| 2000 | | 80 | 141/70 | 26 | 68 | | 125 | | 12 | NPO | 150 | |
| 2100 | | 78 | 140/86 | 14 | 90 | | 125 | 100 | 12 | | 250 | Levetiracetam 1000 mg IV |
| 2200 | 37.8 | 80 | 129/89 | 24 | 78 | 220 | 125 | | 12 | NPO | 300 | Aspart 4 units IV |
| 2300 | | 80 | 130/76 | 18 | 84 | | 125 | | 12 | | 300 | |
| 2400 | | 76 | 137/70 | 25 | 80 | | 125 | | 12 | NPO | 250 | |
| 0100 | | 78 | 140/80 | 17 | 83 | | 125 | | 12 | | 250 | |
| 0200 | 37.9 | 78 | 145/78 | 22 | 78 | 190 | 125 | | 12 | NPO | 100 | Aspart 2 units IV |
| 0300 | | 88 | 145/70 | 28 | 77 | | 125 | | 12 | | 250 | |
| 0400 | | 80 | 127/78 | 25 | 76 | | 125 | | 12 | NPO | 300 | |
| 0500 | | 75 | 138/69 | 27 | 75 | | 125 | | 12 | | 250 | |

Fluid A = 3% sodium chloride/acetate; Fluid B = levetiracetam IVPB; Fluid C = midazolam infusion (concentration = 1 mg/mL).
*HR = heart rate; BP = blood pressure; ICP = intracranial pressure; CPP = cerebral perfusion pressure; BG = blood glucose; UOP = urine output; IVPB = intravenous piggy bag.*

**FIGURE 67-2.** Neurointensive care unit flowsheet. Day 2 (24–48 hours postadmission).

## REFERENCES


1. McMillian WD, Rogers FB. Management of prehospital antiplatelet and anticoagulant therapy in traumatic head injury: a review. J Trauma 2009;66:942–950.
2. Wong DK, Lurie F, Wong LL. The effects of clopidogrel on elderly traumatic brain injured patients. J Trauma 2008;65:1303–1308.
3. Clifton GL, Miller ER, Choi SC, Levin HS. Fluid thresholds and outcome from severe brain injury. Crit Care Med 2002;30:739–745.
4. Forsyth LL, Liu-DeRyke X, Parker D Jr, Rhoney DH. Role of hypertonic saline for the management of intracranial hypertension after stroke and traumatic brain injury. Pharmacotherapy 2008;28:469–484.
5. Guidelines for the management of severe traumatic brain injury. J Neurotrauma 2007;24(Suppl 1):S1–S106.
6. Polderman KH. Mechanisms of action, physiological effects, and complications of hypothermia. Crit Care Med 2009;37:S186–S202.
7. Corbett SM, Montoya ID, Moore FA. Propofol-related infusion syndrome in intensive care patients. Pharmacotherapy 2008;28:250–258.
8. Pandharipande PP, Pun BT, Herr DL, et al. Effect of sedation with dexmedetomidine vs lorazepam on acute brain dysfunction in mechanically ventilated patients: the MENDS randomized controlled trial. JAMA 2007;298:2644–2653.
9. Riker RR, Shehabi Y, Bokesch PM, et al. Dexmedetomidine vs midazolam for sedation of critically ill patients: a randomized trial. JAMA 2009;301:489–499.
10. Martindale RG, McClave SA, Vanek VW, et al. Guidelines for the provision and assessment of nutrition support therapy in the adult critically ill patient: Society of Critical Care Medicine and American Society for Parenteral and Enteral Nutrition: executive summary. Crit Care Med 2009;37:1757–1761.
11. Rhoney DH, Parker D Jr. Considerations in fluids and electrolytes after traumatic brain injury. Nutr Clin Pract 2006;21:462–478.

# 68

# PARKINSON'S DISEASE

Slow and Shaky . . . . . . . . . . . . . . . . . . . . . . . Level III

Mary Louise Wagner, PharmD, MS

Margery H. Mark, MD

## LEARNING OBJECTIVES

After completing this case study, students should be able to:

- Recognize motor and nonmotor symptoms of PD.
- Develop an optimal pharmacotherapeutic plan for a patient with PD as he or she progresses through different stages of the disease.
- Recommend alterations in therapy for a patient experiencing adverse drug effects, drug–drug interactions, and drug–food interactions.
- Educate patients with PD about the disease, its drug therapy, and nonpharmacologic treatments.

## PATIENT PRESENTATION

### Chief Complaint

"My work performance has declined because my tremor makes it difficult to type on the computer, and I am slower with most tasks."

### HPI

Lisa Farmer is a 53-year-old, right-handed woman who presents to the neurology clinic because of a mild tremor in her right hand that has worsened over the last 6 months. It takes her longer to do things because it takes more effort to get movement started, and her muscles feel stiff. For the last few months, she feels that she has not been thinking as quickly and that it takes her longer to remember things. The stiffness, slowness, tremor, and sleep problems have affected her job performance as a graphic designer, resulting in her contemplating early retirement. She also complains of constipation, loss of sense of smell for about 2 years, decreased libido for 6–8 months, night sweats that cause nighttime awakenings, and very irregular menstrual periods for the last year.

### PMH

HTN × 1 year

Broken left wrist after fall 2 years ago

### FH

Mother died at age 89 of complications associated with a hip fracture, osteoporosis, and Alzheimer's disease; father died from an ischemic stroke; two daughters are in good health.

### SH

(–) Alcohol, (–) tobacco, married for 23 years

### ROS

No complaints other than those noted in the HPI. She denies any other symptoms of autonomic dysfunction such as problems with swallowing, urination, drooling, or dizziness. She also denies any psychological problems such as depression, panic attacks, vivid dreams, acting out dreams, hallucinations, or paranoia.

### Meds

Verapamil SR 180 mg every morning for 1 year

Calcium carbonate 600 mg every morning and night

### All

None

### Physical Examination

*Gen*

The patient is a Caucasian woman who appears to be her stated age but with minimal hypomimia.

*VS*

BP 118/74 sitting, 116/70 standing; P 70; RR 13; T 36.8°C; Wt 53 kg, Ht 5′2″

*Skin*

Small amount of dry yellow scales in her eyebrows

*HEENT*

Decreased facial expression, decreased eye blinking; PERRLA; EOMI

*Neck/Lymph Nodes*

Supple, no masses, normal thyroid, no bruits

*Lungs/Thorax*

Clear, normal breath sounds, CTA

*CV*

RRR, no murmurs, no bruits

*Abd*

Soft, nontender, no palpable masses

*Genit/Rect*

No nodules palpated; no rectal polyps

*MS/Ext*

Normal peripheral pulses and postural stability. No CCE.

*Neuro*

General neurologic exam intact, Folstein MMSE 30/30, Hamilton Depression Scale 3/66 (sleep and libido problems)

UPDRS: Total 19

*Part 1:* Mentation, behavior, and mood score 0/16.

*Part 2:* ADL score 5/52 (mild trouble with handwriting, cutting food, tremor, and dressing [putting on nylon stockings and buttoning small buttons]). She has no problems with gait, but her right arm is flexed at elbow and does not swing when she walks. She has no problems with speech, salivation, swallowing, hygiene, turning in bed, falling, freezing, walking, or sensory effects.

*Part 3:* Motor exam 14/108 (mild problems with facial expression and overall bradykinesia). She has right-sided rigidity and rest tremor, appearing like classic pill-rolling tremor. She has problems with fine motor coordination on her right side noted by the rapid alternating movements, finger taps, hand movements, and foot tap tests. She has no problems arising from a chair or problems with posture or postural stability.

Handwriting sample: Somewhat slow and progressively smaller in size indicating signs of micrographia

### Labs

| | | |
|---|---|---|
| Na 136 mEq/L | Hgb 13.5 g/dL | AST 20 IU/L |
| K 4.3 mEq/L | Hct 40.5% | ALT 24 IU/L |
| Cl 101 mEq/L | RBC 4.42 × $10^6$ | Alk phos 80 IU/L |
| $CO_2$ 23 mEq/L | WBC 5.0 × $10^3$/mm$^3$ | GGT 18 IU/L |
| BUN 12 mg/dL | Plt 395 × $10^3$/mm$^3$ | Ferritin 100 ng/mL |
| SCr 0.73 mg/dL | Homocysteine 6 μmol/L | TSH 2.0 mIU/L |
| Glu 83 mg/dL | Vitamin D, 25-hydroxy 25 ng/mL | T4 total 7.5 mcg/dL |

### Assessment

Based on the HPI and UPDRS, the patient's symptoms are consistent with early, mild PD.

## CLINICAL COURSE

The patient is told that she has PD, and the various treatment options are presented to her. She asks about treatment options that may delay disease progression.

## QUESTIONS

### Problem Identification

1.a. List and assess each one of the patient's complaints. Determine if there are multiple potential etiologies that could account for the symptoms.

1.b. Assess the abnormalities in the physical examination and laboratory findings.

1.c. List the cardinal motor and nonmotor symptoms of PD, and describe which signs and symptoms of PD are present in this patient.

1.d. According to the Hoehn–Yahr Scale, what stage is the patient's disease?

### Desired Outcome

2. What are the goals of therapy for patients with PD?

### Therapeutic Alternatives

3.a. What nonpharmacologic alternatives may be beneficial for the treatment of PD in this patient both now and in the future?

3.b. Based on the patient's signs and symptoms, what pharmacotherapeutic alternatives are viable options for her at this time?

### Optimal Plan

4. What drug, dosage form, dose, schedule, and duration of therapy are best for this patient's current problems?

### Outcome Evaluation

5. Which monitoring parameters should be used to evaluate the patient's response to medications and to detect adverse effects?

### Patient Education

6. What information should be provided to the patient to ensure successful therapy, enhance compliance, and minimize adverse effects?

## CLINICAL COURSE—6 MONTHS LATER

Six months later, Ms Farmer returns to the clinic. After taking rasagiline for 3 months, her PD symptoms did not improve as much as she wanted them to, so she started pramipexole, which was gradually increased to 1 mg three times a day. Her slowness, stiffness, tremor, and thinking have improved since then. She is better able to perform her job, enjoys the work, and is no longer planning her retirement. Her constipation has improved only marginally with the increased fluids and addition of the Metamucil that she takes one tablespoonful twice daily. Her libido and night sweats improved after starting conjugated equine estrogens 0.45 mg per day and medroxyprogesterone acetate 1.5 mg per day. She now complains of itchy eyebrows and scalp. She continues to take verapamil SR, multivitamin, calcium carbonate 600 mg, and vitamin D and rasagiline 1 mg daily. The patient reports no side effects from the medicine. However, her husband complains that her personality has changed because she shops excessively, often buying duplicates of things, which is straining their budget.

*Vitals:* BP 116/70 sitting; P 70

*UPDRS* (patient states she is "on"): Mental 0, ADLS = 3 and motor = 6, total 9

*Medications:*

Verapamil SR 180 mg every morning
Multivitamin one daily
Calcium carbonate 600 mg every morning and night
Vitamin D 1,000 IU daily
Conjugated equine estrogens 0.45 mg daily
Medroxyprogesterone acetate 1.5 mg daily
Metamucil one tablespoonful twice daily
Pramipexole 1 mg three times daily
Rasagiline 1 mg daily

### Follow-Up Questions

1. What is your assessment of the effectiveness of the PD therapy the patient is now receiving?
2. What potential side effects from therapy is the patient now experiencing?
3. What adjustments in drug therapy do you recommend for each of the patient's problems?
4. What information should the patient receive about her medical problems and therapy at this visit?
5. What additional tests could be ordered to assess comorbid conditions?

## CLINICAL COURSE—7 YEARS LATER

Ms Farmer returns to the neurology clinic for a routine follow-up visit. She is now 60 years old and still working with reduced hours. She no longer has trouble with compulsive behaviors. Her constipation initially improved with a bowel regimen but now has worsened since starting supplements that she purchased over the Internet. Her symptoms are now bilateral and include tremor, rigidity, stiffness, and gait problems. She also reports that she is slower and clumsier in almost all activities but especially when driving, handling utensils, dressing, turning in bed, and getting out of a chair. She still has good postural stability without falls. There are no difficulties with mood, autonomic symptoms, or hallucinations. She started an exercise program, converted to organic food, reads extensively about her symptoms on the Internet, and purchases various treatments that she hears about from her friends in the local PD support group. About a month prior to the visit, she purchased coenzyme Q10 and cowage (a herbal supplement that contains natural levodopa) thinking they would be a natural way to help her PD. She read about RLS and, thinking that her nighttime restlessness, trouble falling asleep, and daytime fatigue were related to RLS, she started iron supplements and kava several months ago and was planning to tell her doctor about her findings at the next visit.

She claims that the restlessness occurs only at night after dinner when she is sitting. She notes that she has a bubbling feeling in her veins that leads to restlessness, which is relieved by walking or movement. Her husband says that she kicks him at night and the bed covers are quite tousled in the morning.

BP 120/74 and weight 50 kg.

She has a positive glabellar reflex (Myerson's sign).

Hamilton Psychiatric Rating Scale for Depression 3/66.

Folstein MMSE 29/30.

UPDRS scores while "on" are: mood 3, ADL 12, and motor 43.

Laboratory values are normal and similar to previous labs. Ferritin 150 ng/mL.

DXA scan (6 years ago) T-score spine –1.0 and left hip –1.4

Patient diary (day prior to visit):

## Follow-Up Questions

1. List the patient's problems at this visit.
2. List and explain any drugs or foods that could be causing any drug–drug or drug–food interactions.
3. For each of the problems identified, what adjustments in drug therapy do you recommend?
4. What information should be provided to the patient to ensure successful therapy, enhance compliance, and minimize adverse effects with medications that have been added since the last visit?

## ■ CLINICAL COURSE: ALTERNATIVE THERAPY

Ms Farmer has been taking coenzyme Q10 for about a month before coming in for reevaluation. Unlike the kava and cowage, which could be actively worsening her symptoms or posing other safety problems, coenzyme Q10 might actually have some benefit for PD. The question is whether Ms Farmer should continue taking the supplement. See Section 19 in this casebook for questions about the use of coenzyme Q10 for treatment of PD.

## ■ SELF-STUDY ASSIGNMENTS

1. Review the pharmacology and efficacy reports of investigational drugs for PD.
2. Investigate the treatment of other nonmotor symptoms of PD such as autonomic dysfunction, depression, anxiety, and psychosis.
3. Investigate the use of deep brain stimulation for the treatment of advanced PD.

| Time | Meds | Symptoms | Comments |
|---|---|---|---|
| 7 AM | Carbidopa/levodopa 25/100 | Mild stiffness and slowness | Med onset 30 min |
| 8 AM | Verapamil SR 180<br>Cowage (*Mucuna pruriens*) 30 g<br>Calcium 600 mg<br>Benefiber one tablespoon<br>Rasagiline 1 mg<br>Coenzyme Q10 100 mg | Good control of symptoms | Breakfast |
| 8:30–10 AM | | Dancelike movements in extremities (chorea) | Noted this since I started supplements |
| 11:30 AM | Carbidopa/levodopa 25/100<br>Ferrous sulfate 300 mg<br>Benefiber one tablespoon<br>MVI<br>Colace 100 mg | "On" without chorea | Onset 30 min but does not take full effect. It feels like half a dose since supplements started |
| Noon | | | Lunch |
| 4:30 pm | | "Off" with tremor, stiffness, and slowness | 11:30 dose wearing off earlier since supplements started |
| 5:30 pm | Carbidopa/levodopa 25/100<br>Coenzyme Q10 100 mg | "Off" with tremor, stiffness, and slowness | Dinner<br>Delayed onset 60 min |
| 10 pm | Carbidopa/levodopa 25/100 calcium 600 mg<br>Vitamin D 1,000 IU<br>Kava 100 mg<br>Coenzyme Q10 100 mg | "On" without chorea | I fall asleep between 10:30 and 11:30 PM depending on restlessness and funny sensations in my legs |
| 10 pm–7 AM | | | My husband says that I have restless sleep and kick him during the night. I wake up between 1 and 2 AM to go to the bathroom and have a hard time going back to sleep because of feeling stiff all over and restlessness in my legs |

## CLINICAL PEARL

As PD progresses, the timing of medication needs to coincide with symptoms. Evaluate the onset and duration of each dose and make modifications accordingly. Symptoms may worsen when patients are forced to receive medications at predetermined dosing times such as those used in hospitals and nursing homes. Thus, let the patient's symptoms guide the dosing times.

## REFERENCES


1. Lees AJ, Hardy J, Revesz T. Parkinson's disease. Lancet 2009;373: 2055–2066.
2. Nutt JG, Wooten GF. Diagnosis and initial management of Parkinson's disease. N Engl J Med 2005;353:1021–1027.
3. Olanow CW, Stern MB, Sethi K. The scientific and clinical basis for the treatment of Parkinson's disease (2009). Neurology 2009;72(21 Suppl 4):S1–S136.
4. Zesiewicz TA, Sullivan KL, Arnulf I, et al. Practice parameter: treatment of nonmotor symptoms of Parkinson disease: report of the Quality Standards Subcommittee of the American Academy of Neurology. Neurology 2010;74:924–931.
5. Aarsland D, Marsh L, Schrag A. Neuropsychiatric symptoms in Parkinson's disease. Mov Disord 2009;24:15:2175–2186.
6. Natural Standard: The Authority on Integrative Medicine. Available at: *www.naturalstandard.com*. Accessed on April 22, 2010.
7. Anonymous. Drugs for Parkinson's disease. Treat Guidel Med Let 2007;5(62):89–94.
8. Olanow CW, Rascol O, Hauser R, et al. A double-blind, delayed-start trial of rasagiline in Parkinson's disease. N Engl J Med 2009;361: 1268–1278.
9. Katzenschlager R, Evans A, Manson A, et al. *Mucuna pruriens* in Parkinson's disease: a double blind clinical and pharmacological study. J Neurol Neurosurg Psychiatry 2004;75:1672–1677.


# 69

# CHRONIC PAIN MANAGEMENT

A Different Kind of Pain . . . . . . . . . . . . . . . . . . . Level I

**Christine K. O'Neil, PharmD, BCPS, FCCP, CGP**

## LEARNING OBJECTIVES

After completing this case study, students should be able to:

- Define the goals for pain management in a patient with chronic nonmalignant pain.
- Define a pharmacotherapeutic pain management plan.
- Understand the use of NSAIDs, other nonopioids, and opioid analgesics in the treatment of chronic nonmalignant pain.
- Establish monitoring parameters for safety and efficacy when managing analgesic therapy.

## PATIENT PRESENTATION

### Chief Complaint

"The pain in my hips was bad, but this pain in my feet is really different. The medication does not seem to make a difference."

### HPI

Olivia Adams is 65-year-old woman who has had a 10-year history of osteoarthritis, primarily affecting her hips and knees. She has frequent complaints of joint pain after walking or other activities and experiences stiffness in the morning when she awakes or after sitting during bridge games. Recently, she has had difficulty walking and has had several near falls. She states that her feet feel very heavy, numb, and tingly. She describes the feeling as like pins and needles.

### PMH

Type 2 diabetes mellitus × 10 years
HTN × 15 years
Osteoarthritis × 10 years

### SH

Ms Adams is a retired university professor. She lives at a retirement community that has multiple levels of care, from independent living to skilled nursing care. She lives alone in an apartment. She is independent but has assistance with housekeeping and laundry. She enjoys cooking for herself but frequently participates in social events and dining at the community's social center. She has two sisters and one brother and numerous nieces and nephews. She volunteers at the local library as a storyteller.

### FH

Noncontributory

### Meds

Aspirin 325 mg po once daily
Lisinopril 20 mg po once daily
Metformin 500 mg po BID × 2 years
Acetaminophen 500 mg two tablets po BID

### All

Meperidine → bronchospasm, hives
PCN → allergy as a child
Flurbiprofen → GI intolerance

### ROS

Positive for mild to moderate hip pain. Tingling and numbness in feet—reports 8 out of 10 level of discomfort. No other complaints.

### Physical Examination

*Gen*

Patient is a 65-year-old woman in no obvious distress.

*VS*

BP 104/72, P 72, RR 15, T 37.4°C; Wt 68 kg, Ht 5′0″

*HEENT*

PERRLA, EOMI, TMs intact

*Neck*

Supple, no JVD, no bruits

*Resp*

CTA and P; no crackles or wheezes

*CV*

NSR without MRG

*Breasts*

Negative

*Abd*

Soft, NT, liver and spleen not palpable, (+) BS

*Genit/Rect*

Heme (–) stool, pelvic exam deferred

*MS/Ext*

Both hips tender to palpation; right hip pain with flexion >90° and with internal and external rotation >45°; diminished hair growth on toes, and reduced peripheral pulses in lower extremities

*Neuro*

CN II–XII intact, A & O × 3; diminished ankle and knee jerks, decreased sensation to monofilament testing and decreased vibratory sensation

### Labs

Na 144 mEq/L
K 3.9 mEq/L
Cl 103 mEq/L
$CO_2$ 31 mEq/L
BUN 16 mg/dL
SCr 1.0 mg/dL
Glu 95 mg/dL (fasting)

CBC and diff: WNL
A1C 8.0%
Ca 9.8 mg/dL
T. bili 0.2 mg/dL
T. prot 8.1 g/dL
Alb 3.8 g/dL

AST 30 IU/L
ALT 15 IU/L
Alk phos 182 IU/L

### MRI of Spine

Slight degenerative disc disease; no evidence of spinal stenosis or herniated disc

### DEXA Scan

Lumbar spine T score: –0.8
Left hip T score: –0.5

### Assessment

Diabetic peripheral neuropathy
Chronic mild–moderate hip pain due to osteoarthritis
Type 2 diabetes mellitus
HTN—controlled

# QUESTIONS

## Problem Identification

1.a. Create a list of the patient's drug therapy problems.

1.b. What information indicates the presence or severity of chronic nonmalignant pain?

1.c. Could any of the patient's problems have been caused by drug therapy?

1.d. What additional information is needed to satisfactorily assess this patient's pain?

## Desired Outcome

2. What are the goals of pharmacotherapy in this case?

## Therapeutic Alternatives

3.a. What nondrug therapies might be useful for this patient?

3.b. Compare the pharmacotherapeutic alternatives available for treatment of this patient's pain.

## Optimal Plan

4.a. What drug, dosage, form, schedule, and duration of therapy are best for treating this patient's pain?

4.b. What alternatives would be appropriate if the initial therapy fails or cannot be used?

## Outcome Evaluation

5. What clinical and laboratory parameters are necessary to evaluate the therapy for achievement of the desired therapeutic outcome and to detect or prevent adverse effects?

## Patient Education

6. What information should be provided to the patient to enhance compliance, ensure successful therapy, and minimize adverse effects?

# CLINICAL COURSE

The physician elected to use gabapentin at the recommended initial dosing of 300 mg po TID. At her 2-week follow-up appointment, the patient reported minimal pain relief. She describes the pain in her feet as 7 on a scale of 1–10. Her hip pain is bearable and does not affect her activities.

## Follow-Up Questions

1. Based on this new information, how would you alter your treatment plan?
2. If this patient were to require an alternative therapy for osteoarthritis, what would you recommend?
3. What changes or additions to her diabetes regimen would you suggest?

# CLINICAL COURSE: ALTERNATIVE THERAPY

At Ms Adams' next follow-up appointment, she is not completely satisfied with her response to the prescription therapy for her neuropathic pain, although she states that her pain has decreased somewhat. She reports that she read an article on α-lipoic acid in a health magazine last week and wonders if it might be a good product to try. All other disease states are stable on current therapies. See Section 19 in this casebook for questions about the use of α-lipoic acid for treatment of diabetic neuropathy.

# SELF-STUDY ASSIGNMENTS

1. Prepare a list of opioids and their corresponding equianalgesic dosing.
2. Prepare a set of guidelines for managing chronic malignant cancer pain.

## CLINICAL PEARL

Antidepressants, particularly tricyclic antidepressants, are effective first-line therapy for neuropathic pain.

## REFERENCES


1. American Geriatrics Society Panel on Persistent Pain in Older Persons. Pharmacological management of persistent pain in older persons. J Am Geriatr Soc 2009;57:1331–1346.
2. American College of Rheumatology Subcommittee on Osteoarthritis. Recommendations for the medical management of osteoarthritis of the hip and knee. Arthritis Rheum 2000;43:1905–1915.
3. Zhang W, Moskowitz RW, Nuki G, et al. OARSI recommendations for the management of hip and knee osteoarthritis, part II: OARSI evidence-based, expert consensus guidelines. Osteoarthritis Cartilage 2008;16:137–162.
4. American Pain Society. Principles of Analgesic Use in the Treatment of Acute Pain and Cancer Pain, 5th ed. Glenview, IL, American Pain Society, 2003:13–41.
5. Ballantyne JC, Mao J. Medical progress: opioid therapy for chronic pain. N Engl J Med 2003;349:1943–1953.
6. Rowbotham MC, Twilling L, Davies PS, et al. Oral opioid therapy for chronic peripheral and central neuropathic pain. N Engl J Med 2003;348;1223–1232.
7. Maizels M, McCarberg B. Antidepressants and antiepileptic drugs for chronic non-cancer pain. Am Fam Physician 2005;71:483–490.
8. Zin CS, Nissen LM, Smith MT, et al. An update on the pharmacological management of post-herpetic neuralgia and painful diabetic neuropathy. CNS Drugs 2008;22:417–442.
9. Gilron I, Watson CP, Cahill CM, Moulin DE. Neuropathic pain: a practical guide for the clinician. CMAJ 2006;175:265–275.
10. Dworkin RH, O'Connor AB, Audette J, et al. Recommendations for the pharmacological management of neuropathic pain: an overview and literature update. Mayo Clin Proc 2010;85(3 Suppl): S3–S14.


# 70

# ACUTE PAIN MANAGEMENT

## No Pain, Much Gain. . . . . . . . . . . . . . . . . . . . . . Level I

**Gina M. Carbonara Baugh, PharmD**

**Charles D. Ponte, BS, PharmD, BC-ADM, BCPS, CDE, CPE, FAPhA, FASHP, FCCP**

## LEARNING OBJECTIVES

After completing this case study, students should be able to:

- Differentiate acute pain from chronic pain.
- Describe the typical clinical findings associated with acute pain.
- Describe the subjective and objective assessment of pain.
- Identify appropriate nonopioid and opioid analgesics for selected patients with acute pain.
- Choose suitable drug and nondrug therapy for the management of common opioid analgesic side effects.
- Develop an appropriate therapeutic plan (including monitoring parameters) for a patient with acute pain.

## PATIENT PRESENTATION

### Chief Complaint

"My belly hurts, and I can't stand the sight of food."

### HPI

Charles Porter is a 58-year-old man who presents to the Family Practice Center with a 2-day history of nausea, vomiting, and epigastric and RUQ abdominal pain. The patient states that the pain began several hours after eating a large platter of cheese ravioli with sausage and meatballs at a local restaurant. The pain intensified and was associated with escalating nausea followed by several episodes of vomiting. The vomiting finally ceased but the abdominal pain has persisted and is made worse after meals. The pain is now dull, constant, and "bores" to his back. Lying up in bed or sitting in a chair seems to relieve some of the pain. Since the initial episode, his appetite has decreased and he has been avoiding fried or fatty foods. He denies any change in stool color or consistency.

### PMH

HTN × 18 years; poorly controlled
Type 2 DM × 23 years; under fair control
History of gout; last attack 15 years ago
Dyslipidemia × 23 years
Alcoholic hepatitis without cirrhosis × 5 years

### FH

Father deceased (esophageal varices), age 76; mother deceased (MI), age 83; brother alive and well, age 65; sister with breast cancer and gallbladder disease, age 48

### SH

Is a retired bar owner. He lives with his wife (married for 25 years) on a 10-acre farm a few miles from town. He has two dogs and a cat. He has a 50 pack-year history of smoking and a history of chronic alcohol abuse.

### ROS

As per HPI; otherwise negative

### Meds

Atorvastatin 20 mg po once daily
Hydrochlorothiazide 25 mg po once daily
Losartan 100 mg po once daily
Glipizide 10 mg po BID
Metformin 500 mg po BID
Aspirin 81 mg po once daily
Insulin glargine 10 units subQ at bedtime
Pepcid AC 20 mg po PRN heartburn
MVI one po once daily

### All

Erythromycin—abdominal pain
Morphine—hives and mild wheezing

### Physical Examination

*Gen*

A pleasant, middle-aged white man in mild to moderate acute distress; appears his stated age

*VS*

BP 160/95 (sitting), P 84, RR 20, T 37.8°C; pain6/10; Wt 90 kg, Ht 5′10″

*HEENT*

PERRLA, fundi with mild AV nicking; TMs intact; mucous membranes moist

*Chest*

Clear to A & P

*Heart*

Normal $S_1$ and $S_2$; without murmur, rub, or gallop

*Abd*

Normal bowel sounds, without organomegaly, moderate diffuse epigastric pain with deep palpation with mild guarding

*Genit/Rect*

Slightly enlarged prostate; guaiac (−) stool

*Ext*

Good strength throughout, reflexes intact, mild decreased pinprick sensation to both lower extremities; no CCE

### Labs

| | | |
|---|---|---|
| Na 138 mEq/L | Hgb 12.6 g/dL | AST 98 units/L |
| K 3.3 mEq/L | Hct 36% | ALT 77 units/L |
| Cl 97 mEq/L | Platelets 340 × $10^3$/mm$^3$ | Alk phos 200 units/L |
| $CO_2$ 23 mEq/L | WBC 14.0 × $10^3$/mm$^3$ | T. bili 3.4 mg/dL |
| BUN 15 mg/dL | Neutros 76% | D. bili 2.6 mg/dL |
| SCr 1.3 mg/dL | Bands 4% | Amylase 435 units/L |
| Glu 210 mg/dL | Eos 2% | Lipase 367 units/L |
| | Lymphs 18% | *Fasting lipid profile* |
| | | T. chol 210 mg/dL |
| | | HDL 30 mg/dL |
| | | LDL 120 mg/dL |
| | | Trig 300 mg/dL |

### Assessment

Acute epigastric abdominal pain; R/O cholelithiasis, acute cholecystitis, ascending cholangitis, acute pancreatitis, hepatitis

# QUESTIONS

## Problem Identification

1.a. Create a list of the patient's drug therapy problems.

1.b. What clinical information indicates the presence of an acute pain syndrome?

1.c. What is the pathophysiologic basis for the development of acute pain?

1.d. Could the patient's problem have been caused by drug therapy?

## Desired Outcome

2. What are the goals of pharmacotherapy in this case?

## Therapeutic Alternatives

3.a. What feasible pharmacotherapeutic alternatives are available for the treatment of acute pain?

3.b. What economic, psychosocial, and ethical considerations are applicable to this patient?

## Optimal Plan

4.a. What drug, dosage form, dose, schedule, and duration of therapy are best for this patient?

4.b. What alternatives would be appropriate if the initial therapy fails or cannot be used?

## Outcome Evaluation

5. What clinical and laboratory parameters are necessary to evaluate the therapy for achievement of the desired therapeutic outcome and to detect or prevent adverse effects?

## Patient Education

6. What information should be provided to the patient to enhance adherence, ensure successful therapy, and minimize adverse effects?

## CLINICAL COURSE

The patient was admitted to the inpatient service for presumed cholecystitis/acute pancreatitis/hepatitis and pain control. An abdominal ultrasound and abdominal CT were ordered. Blood cultures were obtained. Gastroenterology and general surgery services were consulted. The patient was made NPO except for his home medications. A sliding scale insulin regimen was also ordered.

The drug therapy regimen that you recommended for the patient was initiated. At the end of the first hospital day, the patient states that the medication "eases the pain some" but the pain is inadequately controlled. The pain is rated as an 8/10 using a single-dimensional visual analog pain scale. The patient also complains of some nausea and urinary hesitancy.

## Follow-Up Questions

1. What is the most likely cause of this patient's inadequate pain control?
2. What are the revised management goals for this patient?
3. What therapeutic alternatives would be appropriate for this patient?
4. What clinical and laboratory parameters are necessary to evaluate the therapy for achievement of the desired therapeutic outcome and to detect or prevent adverse effects?
5. What is the role of the pharmacist in the management of patients with acute pain?

## SELF-STUDY ASSIGNMENTS

1. Describe the role of NMDA antagonists in the management of pain.
2. Describe the pathophysiology and management of opioid-induced respiratory depression.
3. What types of pain do *not* typically respond to opioid analgesics?
4. Explain the pathophysiology behind the development of opioid tolerance.
5. Explain the concepts of equianalgesic doses and relative analgesic potency.

6. Explain the WHO analgesic ladder and list representative analgesic classes (or individual agents) associated with each step of the ladder.
7. Describe the advantages and disadvantages of single- and multidimensional pain assessment instruments.

## CLINICAL PEARL

Analgesic tolerance can be overcome by switching from one opioid to another. Because cross-tolerance is not complete among opioids, use only 50–75% of the equianalgesic dose of an opioid when changing from one drug to another and titrate accordingly.

## REFERENCES


1. American Medical Association. Pain management: pathophysiology of pain and pain assessment. Module 1. Chicago, IL: American Medical Association, 2003. Available at: *http://www.ama-cmeonline.com/pain_mgmt/module01/03patho/index.htm*. Accessed February 25, 2010.
2. Institute for Clinical Systems Improvement (ICSI) Healthcare Guideline. Assessment and management of acute pain. Bloomington, MN, Institute for Clinical Systems Improvement (ICSI), March 2008:59 pp. Available at: *http://www.icsi.org/pain_acute/pain_acute_assessment_and_management_of_3.html*. Accessed February 25, 2010.
3. National Institutes of Health. Pathophysiology of alcohol and drug-induced pancreatitis. Available at: *http://www.grants.nih.gov/grants/guide/rfa-files/RFA-DK-94-022.html*. Accessed February 25, 2010.
4. American Diabetes Association. Standards of medical care in diabetes—2010. Diabetes Care 2010:33(S1):S11–S61. Available at: *http://care.diabetesjournals.org/content/33/Supplement_1/S11.full*. Accessed February 24, 2010.
5. American Pain Society. Principles of Analgesic Use in the Treatment of Acute Pain and Cancer Pain, 6th ed. Glenview, IL, American Pain Society, 2008.
6. American Medical Association. Pain management: pathophysiology of pain and pain assessment. Module 2. American Medical Association, 2003. Available at: *http://www.ama-cmeonline.com/pain_mgmt/module02/index.htm*. Accessed April 12, 2010.
7. Thompson DR. Narcotic analgesic effects on the sphincter of Oddi: a review of the data and therapeutic implications in treating pancreatitis. Am J Gastroenterol 2001;96:1266–1272.
8. Spiegel B. Meperidine or morphine in acute pancreatitis? Am Fam Physician 2001;64:219–220.


# 71

# MIGRAINE HEADACHE

Oh, My Aching Head! . . . . . . . . . . . . . . . . . . . . Level II

**Susan R. Winkler, PharmD, BCPS**

## LEARNING OBJECTIVES

After completing this case study, students should be able to:

- Develop pharmacotherapeutic goals for treating and preventing migraine headaches.
- Make recommendations regarding pharmacotherapeutic regimens for an individual patient based on information concerning the patient's headache type and severity, medical history, previous drug therapy, concomitant problems, and pertinent laboratory data.
- Provide information to patients on the use of abortive and prophylactic agents for migraine headaches and menstrual migraines.
- Describe the appropriate use of a headache diary and how it may be used to refine headache treatment.

## PATIENT PRESENTATION

### Chief Complaint

"This new medication is not working for my migraines. My headaches are worse around my period and I have gained 10 pounds!"

### HPI

Sarah Miller is a 34-year-old woman who presents to the Neurology Clinic for follow-up of migraine headaches. She states that she used to get about two migraines every month; however, she recently went back to work full-time and has two young children, ages 3 and 5, to care for. Since then, the frequency of her migraines has increased to about four to five per month. She states her migraines usually occur in the morning and are more frequent around her menses. Her typical headache evolves quickly (within 1 hour) and involves severe throbbing pain, which is unilateral and temporal in distribution. Her headaches are preceded by an aura, which consists of nausea and pastel lights flashing throughout her visual field. Photophobia occurs frequently, and vomiting may occur with an extreme headache. She reports experiencing severe migraine attacks that cause her to miss 1 day of work each month. She is unable to complete household chores and has a difficult time caring for her children on the days she has severe migraine attacks. She also complains of having mild migraine attacks lasting 3 days per month during which her productivity at work and at home is reduced by half. She typically has to retreat to a dark room and avoid any noise, or the severity of the migraine increases. She rates her migraines as 7–8 on a headache scale of 1–10, with 10 being the worst. At her previous visit to the Neurology Clinic 3 months ago, she was prescribed naratriptan 2.5 mg orally to be taken at the onset of headache. However, naratriptan has not been effective for half of the migraines she has had in the last 3 months. During two of the attacks, she experienced partial pain relief, with the pain returning later in the day. She mentions that she was prescribed naratriptan when the Cafergot she was taking stopped working. She states she has taken her medications exactly as advised. She prefers to use medications that can be taken orally. She was started on valproic acid at her last clinic visit for headache prophylaxis and has noticed a 10-lb weight gain. She inquires about switching from valproic acid to another medication.

### PMH

Migraine with aura since age 29; previous medical workup, including an EEG and a head MRI, demonstrated no PVD, CVA, brain tumor, infection, cerebral aneurysm, or epileptic component. Drug therapies have included the following:

- Abortive therapies:
  1. Simple analgesics, NSAIDs, and Cafergot (good efficacy until 3 months ago)

2. Narcotics (good efficacy, but puts her "out of commission for days")
3. Midrin (no efficacy)
4. Naratriptan (minimal efficacy)

- Prophylactic therapies:
  1. Valproic acid 500 mg daily (weight gain)
  2. Propranolol 20 mg BID (increased episodes of dizziness and lightheadedness; patient self-discontinued medication)
- Mild depression for 8 months, treated with:
  1. Phenelzine 15 mg po TID (minimal efficacy, discontinued 2 months ago)
  2. Sertraline 50 mg po at bedtime (recently started 1 month ago)

## FH

Positive for migraines (both parents); hypertension and type 2 diabetes (mother)

## SH

Secretary; recently changed jobs to a full-time position. Mother of two boys, ages 5 and 3. Denies alcohol use; started smoking cigarettes again 3 months ago due to stress, one ppd. Occasional caffeine intake.

## ROS

Complains of increased frequency of migraine headaches starting about 6 months ago; increased frequency around menses. Limited efficacy with naratriptan; no nausea, vomiting, diarrhea, or flashing lights at present.

## Meds

Naratriptan 2.5-mg tablets, one tablet po at onset of migraine, repeat dose of 2.5 mg po in 4 hours if partial response or if headache returns. Maximum dose 5 mg per 24 hours.
Metoclopramide 10 mg po at onset of migraine.
Valproic acid 500 mg po at bedtime.
Sertraline 50 mg po at bedtime.

## All

NKDA

## Physical Examination

*Gen*

WDWN woman in mild distress

*VS*

BP 142/86, HR 76, RR 18, T 37.2°C; Wt 75 kg, Ht 5′3″

*Skin*

Normal skin turgor; no diaphoresis

*HEENT*

PERRLA; EOMI; no funduscopic exam performed

*Neck*

Supple; no masses, thyroid enlargement, adenopathy, bruits, or JVD

*Chest*

Good breath sounds bilaterally; clear to A & P

*CV*

RRR; $S_1$, $S_2$ normal; no murmurs, rubs, or gallops

*Abd*

Soft, NT/ND, no hepatosplenomegaly; (+) BS

*Genit/Rect*

Deferred

*MS/Ext*

UE/LE strength 5/5 with normal tone; radial and femoral pulses 3+ bilaterally; no edema; no evidence of thrombophlebitis; full ROM

*Neuro*

A & O × 3; no dysarthria or aphasia; memory intact; no nystagmus; no fasciculations, tremor, or ataxia; (–) Romberg; CN II–XII intact; sensory intact; DTRs: 2+ throughout; Babinski (–) bilaterally

## Labs

| | | |
|---|---|---|
| Na 142 mEq/L | Hgb 13 g/dL | AST 23 IU/L |
| K 4.2 mEq/L | Hct 40% | ALT 25 IU/L |
| Cl 101 mEq/L | Plt 302 × $10^3$/mm$^3$ | Alk phos 35 IU/L |
| $CO_2$ 23 mEq/L | WBC 8 × $10^3$/mm$^3$ | Urine pregnancy test (–) |
| BUN 12 mg/dL | Differential WNL | |
| SCr 0.8 mg/dL | | |
| Glu 95 mg/dL | | |

## Assessment

1. Increase in frequency of migraines related to menses and increased stress.
2. Minimal efficacy of naratriptan 2.5 mg po as an abortive treatment.
3. Previous prophylactic treatments have been unsuccessful and cause unwanted adverse effects.

# QUESTIONS

## Problem Identification

1.a. Create a list of the patient's drug therapy problems at this clinic visit.

1.b. Calculate the patient's MIDAS score and describe the severity of her migraine headaches. (See Figure 71-1 for MIDAS questionnaire.)

1.c. What clinical information is consistent with a diagnosis of migraines in this patient?

1.d. Could any of the patient's problems have been caused or exacerbated by her drug therapy?

## Desired Outcomes

2. What are the goals of therapy for this patient?

## Therapeutic Alternatives

3.a. What pharmacotherapeutic alternatives are available for treatment of the patient's nausea, and how will they impact potential abortive therapies?

3.b. What pharmacotherapeutic alternatives are available for the abortive treatment of this patient's migraine attacks?

**INSTRUCTIONS:** Please answer the following questions about ALL the headaches you have had over the last 3 months. Write your answer in the box next to each question. Write zero if you did not do the activity in the last 3 months.

**Days**

1. How many days in the last 3 months did you miss work or school because of your headaches? ☐

2. How many days in the last 3 months was your productivity at work or school reduced by half or more because of headaches? *(Do not include days you counted in question 1 where you missed work or school.)* ☐

3. How many days in the last 3 months did you NOT do household work because of your headaches? ☐

4. How many days in the last 3 months was your productivity in household work reduced by half or more because of your headaches? *(Do not include days you counted in question 3 where you did not do household work.)* ☐

5. On how many days in the last 3 months did you miss family, social, or leisure activities because of your headaches? ☐

**MIDAS Score**: Add the total number of days from questions 1–5. **Total** ☐

**NOTE:** Scores from A and B below are not included in the MIDAS score, but are used to assess frequency and intensity of pain.

A. How many days in the last 3 months did you have a headache? *(If a headache lasted more than 1 day, count each day.)* ☐

B. On a scale of 0–10, on average how painful were these headaches? *(0 = no pain, and 10 = pain as bad as it can be.)* ☐

**Interpretation**

The MIDAS questionnaire is scored in units of lost days. Depending on the MIDAS score, patients are assigned to 1 of 4 grades:

| MIDAS Grade | Definition | Score |
|---|---|---|
| I | Minimal or infrequent disability | 0–5 |
| II | Mild or infrequent disability | 6–10 |
| III | Moderate disability | 11–20 |
| IV | Severe disability | ≥ 21 |

**FIGURE 71-1.** MIDAS questionnaire. *(Reprinted with permission from Bigal ME, Lipton RB, Krymchantowski AV. The medical management of migraine. Am J Ther 2004;11:130–140. Lippincott Williams & Wilkins, www.lww.com.)*

3.c. What pharmacotherapeutic alternatives are available for prophylaxis of this patient's migraine attacks?

## Optimal Plan

4.a. Considering this patient's past successes and failures in treating her migraine attacks, design an optimal pharmacotherapeutic plan for aborting her migraine headaches.

4.b. Design an optimal pharmacotherapeutic plan for prophylaxis of her migraine headaches.

## Outcome Evaluation

5. What clinical and/or laboratory parameters should be assessed regularly to evaluate the therapy for achievement of the desired therapeutic outcome and to detect or prevent adverse effects?

**Name:** ______________________ **Month:** ________ **Year:** ________

| Date of Headache | | | | | | | | | | | | | | |
|---|---|---|---|---|---|---|---|---|---|---|---|---|---|---|
| **Headache Intensity** | | | | | | | | | | | | | | |
| Excruciating pain | 10 | 10 | 10 | 10 | 10 | 10 | 10 | 10 | 10 | 10 | 10 | 10 | 10 | 10 |
| | 9 | 9 | 9 | 9 | 9 | 9 | 9 | 9 | 9 | 9 | 9 | 9 | 9 | 9 |
| Severe pain | 8 | 8 | 8 | 8 | 8 | 8 | 8 | 8 | 8 | 8 | 8 | 8 | 8 | 8 |
| | 7 | 7 | 7 | 7 | 7 | 7 | 7 | 7 | 7 | 7 | 7 | 7 | 7 | 7 |
| Severe pain | 6 | 6 | 6 | 6 | 6 | 6 | 6 | 6 | 6 | 6 | 6 | 6 | 6 | 6 |
| | 5 | 5 | 5 | 5 | 5 | 5 | 5 | 5 | 5 | 5 | 5 | 5 | 5 | 5 |
| Moderate pain | 4 | 4 | 4 | 4 | 4 | 4 | 4 | 4 | 4 | 4 | 4 | 4 | 4 | 4 |
| | 3 | 3 | 3 | 3 | 3 | 3 | 3 | 3 | 3 | 3 | 3 | 3 | 3 | 3 |
| Mild pain | 2 | 2 | 2 | 2 | 2 | 2 | 2 | 2 | 2 | 2 | 2 | 2 | 2 | 2 |
| Aura only | 1 | 1 | 1 | 1 | 1 | 1 | 1 | 1 | 1 | 1 | 1 | 1 | 1 | 1 |
| **Headache Duration (hours)** | | | | | | | | | | | | | | |
| **Level of Disability** | | | | | | | | | | | | | | |
| Hospitalized | | | | | | | | | | | | | | |
| Treatment by health care professional | | | | | | | | | | | | | | |
| Bedrest required | | | | | | | | | | | | | | |
| Decrease in activity by 50% | | | | | | | | | | | | | | |
| Decrease in activity by 25% | | | | | | | | | | | | | | |
| Normal activity | | | | | | | | | | | | | | |
| Other (comment below) | | | | | | | | | | | | | | |
| **Associated Symptoms** | | | | | | | | | | | | | | |
| Nausea | | | | | | | | | | | | | | |
| Vomiting | | | | | | | | | | | | | | |
| Visual disturbances | | | | | | | | | | | | | | |
| Menstrual period | | | | | | | | | | | | | | |
| Neurological | | | | | | | | | | | | | | |
| Other (comment below) | | | | | | | | | | | | | | |
| **Medications Taken** | | | | | | | | | | | | | | |
| 1. | | | | | | | | | | | | | | |
| 2. | | | | | | | | | | | | | | |
| 3. | | | | | | | | | | | | | | |
| 4. | | | | | | | | | | | | | | |
| 5. | | | | | | | | | | | | | | |
| **Treatment Results** | | | | | | | | | | | | | | |
| Complete relief | | | | | | | | | | | | | | |
| 75% relief | | | | | | | | | | | | | | |
| 50% relief | | | | | | | | | | | | | | |
| 25% relief | | | | | | | | | | | | | | |
| No relief | | | | | | | | | | | | | | |
| Other (comment below) | | | | | | | | | | | | | | |
| **General Comments** | | | | | | | | | | | | | | |

Note: A normal diary includes space to record a full month of headache activity. This form has been truncated for space purposes.

**FIGURE 71-2.** A headache diary.

## Patient Education

6.a. What information should be provided to the patient regarding migraine triggers?

6.b. What information should be provided to the patient regarding her new abortive and prophylactic therapies?

## ■ CLINICAL COURSE: ALTERNATIVE THERAPY

While discussing possible changes from her valproic acid therapy, Ms Miller says that a friend who also has migraines had read about some herbal remedies used for migraine prevention. She asks whether any products like that could be used instead of or along with her prescription medications. Ms Miller is very interested in a more "natural" therapy, but only if it could really reduce the number of her migraines. For questions related to the use of Butterbur and feverfew for the prevention of migraine headaches, please see Section 19 of this casebook.

## Follow-Up Question

1. Describe how a headache diary could help the treatment of this patient's migraine headaches. (See Figure 71-2 for headache diary.)

## ■ SELF-STUDY ASSIGNMENTS

1. Review the literature regarding IV agents (e.g., dihydroergotamine, valproate sodium) that are used for aborting migraines.

2. Prepare a report highlighting the antiepileptic drugs that are used for the prophylaxis of migraines.
3. Review the literature on the efficacy of the calcitonin gene–related peptide receptor antagonists, telcagepant and olcegepant, for acute treatment of migraines.

## CLINICAL PEARL

Migraines are three times more prevalent in women and are associated with estrogen levels. Sixty percent of women migraineurs report menstrually associated migraines, and 7–14% have migraines exclusively with menses.

## REFERENCES


1. Bigal ME, Lipton RB, Krymchantowski AV. The medical management of migraine. Am J Ther 2004;11:130–140.
2. Smith TR, Stoneman J. Medication overuse headache from antimigraine therapy. Drugs 2004;64:2503–2514.
3. FDA Public Health Advisory. Combined use of 5-hydroxytryptamine receptor agonists (triptans), selective serotonin reuptake inhibitors (SSRIs) or selective serotonin/norepinephrine reuptake inhibitors (SNRIs) may result in life-threatening serotonin syndrome. Available at: *http://www.fda.gov/Drugs/DrugSafety/PublicHealthAdvisories/ucm124349.htm*. Accessed February 26, 2010.
4. Shapiro RE, Tepper SJ. The serotonin syndrome, triptans, and the potential for drug–drug interactions. Headache 2007:47:266–269.
5. Silberstein SD. Preventive migraine treatment. Neurol Clin 2009: 27:429–443.
6. Schrader H, Stovner LJ, Helde G, et al. Prophylactic treatment of migraine with angiotensin converting enzyme inhibitor (lisinopril): randomised, placebo controlled, crossover study. BMJ 2001;322: 19–22.
7. Tronvik, E, Stovner LJ, Helde G, et al. Prophylactic treatment of migraine with an angiotensin II receptor blocker: a randomized controlled trial. JAMA 2003;289:65–69.
8. Rothrock JF. Menstrual migraine. Headache 2009;49:1399–1400.
9. Mathew NT, Loder EW. Evaluating the triptans. Am J Med 2005;118:28S–35S.
10. Silberstein SD. Practice parameter: evidence-based guidelines for migraine headache (an evidence-based review): report of the Quality Standards Subcommittee of the American Academy of Neurology. Neurology 2000;55:754–762.

SECTION 7
# PSYCHIATRIC DISORDERS

# 72

## ATTENTION-DEFICIT HYPERACTIVITY DISORDER

He Is So Energized, He Keeps Going and Going and .................... Level I

**Darin C. Ramsey, PharmD, BCPS**

**Laura F. Ruekert, PharmD, BCPP**

## LEARNING OBJECTIVES

After completing this case study, the reader should be able to:

- Recognize and describe the signs and symptoms of ADHD as defined by DSM-IV-TR.
- Apply the diagnostic criteria for ADHD and differentiate between symptoms of inattention and hyperactivity/impulsivity.
- Differentiate treatment options for ADHD with regard to effectiveness, tolerability, safety, monitoring parameters, and potential for drug interactions.
- Compare the advantages and disadvantages of once-daily stimulant preparations to immediate-release stimulants.
- Develop useful dosing schedule strategies that may be employed in the management of patients with ADHD to enhance medication adherence.
- Perform patient assessment to determine efficacy with selected therapy and appropriate monitoring for any adverse effects.

## PATIENT PRESENTATION

### Chief Complaint

"My son has trouble focusing and sitting still while completing his afternoon homework."

### HPI

David Handlon is a 10-year-old boy who returns for a routine visit to his psychiatrist with his mother. He was diagnosed 2 years ago with ADHD and is currently being treated with Adderall XR 20 mg every morning. His mother states that during the last parent–teacher meeting, his teacher indicated that David's behavior is well controlled during the day. Despite David's good behavior during the day, his mother reports difficulty getting David to complete any afternoon tasks or assignments after school. David's rules include no playtime activities until he has completed his afternoon homework assignments. Instead of focusing on homework, David insists on playing Guitar Hero® in his room, and he sometimes carelessly throws his guitar. David has also exhibited impulsive and reckless behavior when interacting with his younger 8-year-old brother. Initially David's mother thought the medication was working. However, within the past year, David's afternoon antics have progressively gotten worse. Mrs Handlon is afraid that uncontrolled afternoon antics will have serious repercussions on David's daytime behavior and grades. She questions, "What are my options?"

### PMH

Asthma × 3 years  
ADHD × 2 years  
Tonsillectomy (1 year ago)  
Broken wrist at age 8 (fell from tree)  
Vaccinations are up to date

### FH

Both father and uncle have a history of hyperactivity and are currently receiving treatment as adults.

### SH

Lives with both parents and younger brother in the suburbs

### Meds

Adderall XR 20 mg daily (given every morning at 7 AM)  
Albuterol inhaler two puffs Q 4–6 h PRN shortness of breath  
Singulair 5 mg po daily

### All

NKDA

### ROS

Physical assessment was difficult to assess in David as he could not sit still for more than 30 seconds and was jumping off of the exam table. Asthma symptoms appear controlled with PRN inhaler use at bedtime only and daily Singulair.

### Physical Examination

*Gen*

Well-nourished, healthy-appearing male child, normal physical development

*VS*

BP 110/72, P 82, RR 25, T 37.5°C; Wt 50 kg, Ht 5′2″

*Skin*

No signs of rash, skin irritation, or bruising noted. Scar noticed on left wrist from where he fell from tree. Minor cuts on knees from frequent falls on school playground.

*HEENT*

Unable to assess

*Neck/Lymph Nodes*

Unable to assess

*Lungs/Thorax*

No rales, rhonchi, or wheezing

*CV*

RRR

*Abd*

Deferred

*Genit/Rect*

Deferred

*MS/Ext*

Unable to assess

*Neuro*

A & O × 3; no underlying tics noted

### Labs

| | | | |
|---|---|---|---|
| Na 138 mEq/L | Hgb 14 g/dL | WBC 9 × $10^3$/mm$^3$ | Mag 1.8 mg/dL |
| K 3.8 mEq/L | Hct 44.5% | Neutros 66% | Serum iron 95 mcg/dL |
| Cl 106 mEq/L | RBC 4.6 × $10^6$/mm$^3$ | Bands 2% | TSH 3.6 mIU/L |
| $CO_2$ 23 mEq/L | Plt 278 × $10^3$/mm$^3$ | Eos 3% | |
| BUN 18 mg/dL | MCV 85 μm$^3$ | Lymphs 24% | |
| SCr 0.8 mg/dL | MCHC 33 g/dL | Monos 5% | |
| Glu 110 mg/dL | | | |

### Other

**ECG:** NSR; changes not clinically significant

### Assessment

1. ADHD
2. Mild-persistent asthma, well controlled with PRN albuterol and daily Singulair

## QUESTIONS

### Problem Identification

1.a. Create a list of the patient's drug therapy problems.

1.b. What information (signs, symptoms, laboratory values) indicates the presence or severity of ADHD?

### Desired Outcome

2. What are the goals of treatment (pharmacotherapy and nonpharmacotherapy) for a patient diagnosed with ADHD?

### Therapeutic Alternatives

3.a. What nondrug therapies might be beneficial for patients diagnosed with ADHD?

3.b. What pharmacotherapeutic stimulant and nonstimulant dosage formulations are available for the treatment of ADHD?

### Optimal Plan

4.a. What drug, dosage form, dose, schedule, and duration of therapy are best for this patient?

4.b. What therapeutic alternatives would be appropriate if the patient fails to respond to stimulant therapy?

### Outcome Evaluation

5. What clinical and laboratory parameters are necessary to evaluate the therapy for achievement of the desired therapeutic outcome and to detect or prevent adverse effects?

### Patient Education

6. What information, specific to this case, should be provided to the patient and his family to enhance adherence, ensure successful therapy, and minimize adverse effects?

## SELF-STUDY ASSIGNMENTS

1. Many parents are apprehensive about starting stimulants in children with the fear of the potential for stimulant abuse when they become older. After performing a literature search, prepare an educational brochure addressing the question, "Does stimulant treatment of ADHD increase the risk for drug abuse?"
2. Provide a summary that addresses the long-term effect stimulants have on growth and appetite.
3. Review the "black box" warning that the Drug Safety and Risk Management Advisory Committee of the FDA recommended to be added to the product labeling of stimulants used to treat ADHD. What patient population does this "black box" warning affect, and what events prompted this recommendation by the FDA?
4. Develop an appropriate recommendation for product conversion in a patient who is switching from oral methylphenidate (Concerta®) 36 mg po daily to methylphenidate (Daytrana®) transdermal patch. Also, be able to convert doses of mixed amphetamine salts (Adderall IR/Adderall XR®) to lisdexamfetamine (Vyvanse®).
5. Perform a literature search and defend or refute the role of modafinil, selective serotonin reuptake inhibitors, tricyclic antidepressants, and atypical antipsychotics in the treatment of ADHD.

## CLINICAL PEARL

Stimulant medications are considered first-line therapy in children with ADHD. The American Academy of Pediatrics reports at least an 80% response rate when these agents are used appropriately in the management of ADHD. If a patient does not respond adequately to initial stimulant therapy, a second or even third stimulant should be tried before initiating a nonstimulant medication. Most patients will be successfully treated by an alternative stimulant.

## REFERENCES

1. Pliszka S, Bernet W, Bukstein O, et al, for the American Academy of Child and Adolescent Psychiatry Work Group on Quality Issues. Practice parameter for the assessment and treatment of children and adolescents with attention-deficit-hyperactivity disorder. J Am Acad Child Adolesc Psychiatry 2007;46:894–921.
2. Dopheide JA, Pliszka SR. Attention-deficit-hyperactivity disorder: an update. Pharmacotherapy 2009;29(6):656–679.

## CHAPTER 73

3. American Academy of Pediatrics, Subcommittee on Attention-Deficit/Hyperactivity Disorder, Committee on Quality Improvement. Clinical practice guideline: treatment of the school-aged child with attention-deficit/hyperactivity disorder. Pediatrics 2001;108:1033–1044.
4. Institute for Clinical Systems Improvement. Health Care Guideline: Diagnosis and Management of Attention Deficit Hyperactivity Disorder in Primary Care for School-Age Children and Adolescents, 8th ed. March 2010. Available at: *http://www.icsi.org/adhd/adhd_2300.html*. Accessed May 14, 2010.
5. Rappley MD. Attention deficit-hyperactivity disorder. N Engl J Med 2005;352:165–173.
6. Abramowicz M, Zuccotti G, Pflomm JM, et al. Drugs for treatment of ADHD. Treat Guidel Med Lett 2006;4:77–82.
7. Culpepper L. Primary care treatment of attention-deficit/hyperactivity disorder. J Clin Psychiatry 2006;67:51–58.
8. Allen AJ, Kurlan RM, Gilbert DL, et al. Atomoxetine treatment in children and adolescents with ADHD and comorbid tic disorders. Neurology 2005;65:1941–1949.


# 73

# EATING DISORDERS: BULIMIA NERVOSA

Self-Conscious Socialite . . . . . . . . . . . . . . . . . . . Level I


**Laura F. Ruekert, PharmD, BCPP**

**Cheen Lum, PharmD, BCPP**


## LEARNING OBJECTIVES

After completing this case study, the reader should be able to:

- Define Bulimia Nervosa (BN) according to DSM-IV criteria, and classify the disorder as either purging or nonpurging.
- Recognize and assess signs and symptoms commonly associated with the presentation of longstanding BN.
- Name effective pharmacologic and nonpharmacologic treatment options for the management of BN.
- Recommend a therapeutic treatment plan for comprehensive inpatient management and outpatient interdisciplinary follow-up of BN.
- Specify monitoring parameters and counseling points for a patient with BN.

## PATIENT PRESENTATION

### Chief Complaint

"I am worried about my daughter."

### HPI

Sara Witter is a 17-year-old female presenting to her PCP with her mother, who has noticed abnormal behavior by her daughter. The physician provides a definitive diagnosis of bulimia (the purging type) after documenting Sara's reports of self-induced vomiting several times a week following binges on large quantities of food. She also admits to using laxatives approximately three times a week. Her mother states she has overheard Sara's purging behaviors for approximately 3 months now. Sara reports extreme guilt after eating, which is why she purges. She claims it is extremely important to her to keep her figure and not gain any weight. Sara has had a history of depression that she feels has not gotten any better. She takes her medication every morning but only on the days after she eats a large breakfast.

### PMH

Depression × 2 years
Seasonal allergies

### FH

Parents divorced 2 years ago. Father is an alcoholic and lives out of state. He does not currently receive treatment or counseling. Sara lives alone with her mother.

### SH

Denies tobacco use
Drinks three to four mixed drinks 3 days a week (prefers rum and diet cola)

### Meds

Fluoxetine 20 mg daily (admits she is only adherent to her medication regimen when she eats)
Singulair 10 mg daily

### All

NKDA

### ROS

Sara expresses feelings of hopelessness and frustration with her life in general. She seems to be craving attention from anyone who will listen. She reports baseline fatigue and low energy. She denies being sexually active.

### Physical Examination

*Gen*

Pale, normal weight, depressed Caucasian female

*VS*

BP 98/72, P 52, RR 20, T 36.4°C; Wt 55 kg, Ht 5′4″

*HEENT*

Normocephalic; brittle/coarse hair; PERRLA, EOMI; mild parotid gland enlargement

*Neck/Lymph Nodes*

No JVD

*Lungs/Thorax*

Lungs CTA; no rales, rhonchi, wheezes

*CV*

Hypotensive; bradycardic

*Abd*

Slightly distended, (–) BS

*Genit/Rect*

Unremarkable

*MS/Ext*

No cyanosis, clubbing, edema; abrasions on palmar surface of hands (Russell's sign)

*Neuro*

A & O × 3

## Labs

| | | | |
|---|---|---|---|
| Na 137 mEq/L | Hgb 14 g/dL | WBC 7.3 × $10^3$/mm$^3$ | AST 20 IU/L |
| K 3.8 mEq/L | Hct 39% | | ALT 15 IU/L |
| Cl 100 mEq/L | RBC 5 × $10^6$/mm$^3$ | Neutros 60% | Ca 8.9 mg/dL |
| $HCO_3$ 22 mEq/L | Plt 247 × $10^3$/mm$^3$ | Bands 3% | Mg 1.8 mg/dL |
| BUN 17 mg/dL | MCV 83 fL | Eos 2% | Serum iron 96 mcg/dL |
| SCr 1.0 mg/dL | MCHC 34 g/dL | Lymphs 31% | Folic acid 9.3 ng/mL |
| Glu 74 mg/dL | Albumin 4.1 g/dL | Monos 4% | Ferritin 110 ng/mL |

## Assessment

1. BN, purging type
2. Depression
3. Alcohol abuse

# QUESTIONS

## Problem Identification

1.a. Create a list of the patient's drug therapy problems.

1.b. What signs, symptoms, and laboratory values indicate the severity of the BN, secondary complications, and depression?

## Desired Outcome

2. What are the goals of therapy for this patient?

## Therapeutic Alternatives

3.a. What nonpharmacologic treatment strategies would be beneficial for this patient?

3.b. What pharmacologic treatment strategies are available for the treatment of eating disorders?

## Optimal Plan

4.a. What drug, dosage form, route, schedule, and duration of therapy are best for comprehensive management of this patient?

4.b. What pharmacologic alternatives would be appropriate if initial treatment interventions fail or are insufficient to achieve desired outcomes?

## Outcome Evaluation

5. What clinical and laboratory parameters are necessary to evaluate the therapy for achievement of the desired therapeutic outcome and to detect or prevent adverse effects?

## Patient Education

6. What information should be provided to the patient to enhance adherence, ensure successful therapy, and minimize adverse effects?

# SELF-STUDY ASSIGNMENTS

1. Compare and contrast the differences in the etiologies and presentations of the various eating disorders.
2. Prepare a one-page patient information handout to aid in counseling the patient on various pharmacologic treatment options if he or she were diagnosed with an eating disorder.
3. Prepare a table highlighting the different laboratory parameters seen in a patient presenting with acidosis secondary to laxative abuse versus a patient presenting with alkalosis secondary to excessive purging.
4. Review the literature and prepare a one-page paper describing the complications of eating disorders and the overall implications of eating disorders on long-term health.

# CLINICAL PEARL

Comprehensive management of both longstanding anorexia nervosa and BN involves intensive pharmacologic and nonpharmacologic treatment of complications such as metabolic alkalosis with respiratory compensation, electrolyte imbalances with EKG changes, low bone mineral density, acute renal insufficiency, anemia, thrombocytopenia, amenorrhea, substance abuse issues, and psychiatric disorders.

# REFERENCES

1. American Psychiatric Association (APA). Practice Guidelines for the Treatment of Patients with Eating Disorders, 3rd ed. Washington, DC, American Psychiatric Association (APA), June 2006.
2. Becker AE, Eddy KT, Perloe A. Clarifying criteria for cognitive signs and symptoms for eating disorders in DSM-V. Int J Eat Disord 2009;42:611–619.
3. Finzi-Dottan R, Zubery E. The role of depression and anxiety in impulsive and obsessive–compulsive behaviors among anorexic and bulimic patients. Eat Disord 2009;17:162–182.
4. Whitaker JS, Sware RD, Hards L. Anorexia nervosa. In: Merritt R, DeLegge MH, Holcombe BH, et al, eds. A.S.P.E.N. Nutrition Support Manual, 2nd ed. Silver Spring, MD, A.S.P.E.N., 2005:349–354.
5. Drug treatment for eating disorders. Pharm Lett Prescriber's Lett 2006;22:220811.
6. Fluoxetine Bulimia Nervosa Collaborative Study Group. Fluoxetine in the treatment of bulimia nervosa: a multicenter, placebo-conrolled, double-blind trial. Arch Gen Psychiatry 1992;49:139–147.

# 74

# ALCOHOL WITHDRAWAL

## Economic Hardship Can Result in Unexpected Problems . . . . . . . . Level I

**Kevin M. Tuohy, PharmD, BCPS**

# LEARNING OBJECTIVES

After completing this case study, the reader should be able to:

- Recognize the signs and symptoms of acute alcohol withdrawal syndrome.

- Recognize the common laboratory abnormalities seen in alcohol-dependent patients.
- Develop a treatment plan for acute alcohol withdrawal and alcohol-related seizures.
- Recommend an appropriate regimen for electrolyte replacement in an alcohol-dependent patient.

## PATIENT PRESENTATION

### Chief Complaint

"My husband has been acting strange, sweating, and shaking all day. I think he had a seizure an hour ago."

### HPI

Brian Johnson is a 54-year-old man who is brought to the ED by his wife. She states that her husband has abused alcohol since she met him while in college. She states that his typical daily consumption for the past 25 years has averaged about 14–18 alcoholic beverages. She reports that he has not been able to afford to drink recently due to a recent layoff from his job. He has not had any alcohol to drink in the previous 48 hours.

### PMH

Alcohol abuse and dependence
Alcohol withdrawal with seizure 4 years prior
Hypertension × 10 years
GERD × 4 years

### SH

The patient is an unemployed construction worker. He has not worked for the past 6 months. He has been married for 22 years. He has been a heavy drinker for past 25 years. Drinks an average of 16 drinks (usually beer- or vodka-containing drinks) per day. (+) Tobacco history—quit 5 years ago. Denies any illicit drug use.

### Meds

Hydrochlorothiazide 25 mg po daily
Amlodipine 5 mg po daily
OTC omeprazole 20 mg po as needed for heartburn symptoms

### All

NKDA

### ROS

The patient exhibits overall confusion and is not responsive to questions. Wife states his mental status was normal until this afternoon when his confusion, sweating, and shakiness started.

### Physical Examination

*Gen*

Thin, undernourished-appearing male, in mild distress who is acutely confused and tremulous

*VS*

BP 162/85, P 107, RR 20, T 38.3°C; Wt 62 kg, Ht 5′10″

*Skin*

Moist, diaphoretic

*HEENT*

Head—atraumatic, icteric sclera, PERRLA, EOMI, mild AV nicking seen on funduscopic exam

*Neck/Lymph Nodes*

Supple, no thyromegaly or lymphadenopathy

*Lungs/Thorax*

Symmetric, lungs CTA

*CV*

RRR, no MRG

*Abd*

Soft, nontender; (+) bowel sounds; (+) hepatomegaly

*Genit/Rect*

(–) Occult blood in stool

*MS/Ext*

Confused, tremor in both hands

*Neuro*

A & O only to person, DTRs exaggerated

### Labs

| | | |
|---|---|---|
| Na 139 mEq/L | Phos 2.8 mg/dL | PT 14.5 sec |
| K 3.2 mEq/L | Ca 9.5 mg/dL | INR 1.30 |
| Cl 88 mEq/L | GGT 310 IU/L | ETOH (–) |
| $CO_2$ 26 mEq/L | AST 250 IU/L | |
| BUN 14 mg/dL | ALT 120 IU/L | |
| SCr 1.1 mg/dL | T. bili 1.7 mg/dL | |
| Glu 99 mg/dL | D. bili 1.1 mg/dL | |
| Mg 1.6 mg/dL | Alb 2.4 g/dL | |

### Assessment

Alcohol withdrawal with possible seizure

## QUESTIONS

### Problem Identification

1.a. Create a list of patient's drug therapy problems.

1.b. What information (signs, symptoms, laboratory values) indicates that this patient is experiencing alcohol withdrawal?

1.c. What signs, symptoms, and history are consistent with alcohol dependence in this patient?

1.d. What laboratory abnormalities may be expected in a patient with a history of alcohol abuse?

### Desired Outcome

2. What are the goals of pharmacotherapy in this case?

### Therapeutic Alternatives

3.a. What pharmacotherapeutic alternatives are available for the treatment of alcohol withdrawal?

3.b. How should alcohol withdrawal seizures be managed pharmacologically?

3.c. What electrolyte imbalances need to be corrected in this patient, and what vitamin deficiencies should be corrected?

3.d. What pharmacotherapeutic agent can be recommended to treat this patient's acutely elevated blood pressure and heart rate?

## Optimal Plan

4. Design an appropriate pharmacotherapy regimen for the treatment of alcohol withdrawal in this patient. Include recommendations for electrolyte replacement and correction of vitamin deficiencies, as well as for the management of the patient's other medical problems.

## Outcome Evaluation

5. What clinical and laboratory parameters are necessary to evaluate your therapy for the achievement of desired therapeutic outcome and to detect or prevent adverse effects?

## Patient Education

6. What information should be provided to the patient to enhance adherence, ensure successful therapy, and minimize adverse effects?

## SELF-STUDY ASSIGNMENTS

1. Research alcohol-related treatment Web sites that can be recommended to patients with alcohol dependence.
2. Discuss the pharmacologic options that are currently marketed in the United States (FDA-approved drugs) for the treatment of alcohol dependence.

## CLINICAL PEARL

All benzodiazepines appear similarly efficacious in reducing signs and symptoms of alcohol withdrawal. The choice of the agent should be determined based on patient-specific factors and the pharmacokinetic profile of the drug.

## REFERENCES


1. Mayo-Smith MF. Pharmacological management of alcohol withdrawal: a meta-analysis and evidence-based practice guideline. American Society of Addiction Medicine Working Group on Pharmacological Management of Alcohol Withdrawal. JAMA 1997;278:144–151.
2. Holbrook AM, Crowther R, Lotter A, Cheng C, King D. Meta-analysis of benzodiazepine use in treatment of acute alcohol withdrawal. CMAJ 1999;160:649–655.
3. Saitz R, O'Malley SS. Pharmacotherapies for alcohol abuse. Withdrawal and treatment. Med Clin North Am 1997;81:881–907.
4. Martinotti G, diNicola M, Frustaci A, et al. Pregabalin, tiapride, and lorazepam in alcohol withdrawal syndrome: a multi-centre, randomized, single-blind comparison trial. Addiction 2010:105:288–299.
5. Mayo-Smith MF, Beecher LH, Fischer TL, et al. Management of alcohol withdrawal delirium: an evidence-based practice guideline. Arch Intern Med 2004;164:1405–1412.
6. Rathlev NK, Ulrich AS, Delanty N, D'Onofrio G. Alcohol-related seizures. J Emerg Med 2006;31:157–163.
7. Hillbom M, Pieninkeroinen I, Leone M. Seizures in alcohol-dependent patients. Epidemiology, pathophysiology and management. CNS Drugs 2003;17:1013–1030.
8. Sullivan JT, Sykora K, Schniederman J, Naranjo CA, Sellers EM. Assessment of alcohol withdrawal: the revised Clinical Institute Withdrawal Assessment for Alcohol scale (CIWA-Ar). Br J Addict 1989;84:1353–1357.


# 75

# NICOTINE DEPENDENCE

What's That Smell? . . . . . . . . . . . . . . . . . . . . . . Level II

Julie C. Kissack, PharmD, BCPP

## LEARNING OBJECTIVES

After completing this case study, the reader should be able to:

- Explain the adverse effects to people exposed to secondhand smoke.
- Interpret the stage of change exhibited by a specific patient, and prepare an action plan to promote smoking cessation and nicotine abstinence based on the 5A plan.
- Design patient-specific recommendations for initiating lifestyle modifications and pharmacologic treatment to encourage reduction or elimination of cigarette smoke exposure.
- Recommend alternative treatments for nicotine dependence if an initial plan fails.
- Develop patient counseling on the use of pharmacotherapeutic agents used to treat nicotine dependence for a specific patient.

## PATIENT PRESENTATION

### Chief Complaint

"I don't know why I'm feeling so bad, but giving up these coffin sticks might be a good thing to do."

### HPI

PHIL Morris is a 32-year-old man who presents to the charitable care clinic complaining of extreme thirst, excessive urination, and generally feeling unwell for the past 2 weeks. "I have missed 2–3 days of work each week in the past month so there is less money to stretch for our expenses. My wife and 3 kids are hungry and I can only afford to buy one cigarette at a time. And one more thing, it is so hard to remember to take that medication that was prescribed to control my sugar the last time I came to this clinic. Can you help me get right so I can get back to work?"

### PMH

Diabetes mellitus (diagnosed at age 29)

### FH

Mother (age 52) has history of type 2 diabetes and ovarian cancer. Father (age 57) has history of hypertension, myocardial infarction, and obesity. Patient is the oldest child of six siblings. All siblings have smoked cigarettes, but in the past 5 years, two of the siblings have quit smoking. Wife is a nonsmoker and son has asthma; one daughter has ADHD, and one daughter has no identified health problems.

■ SH

Works at a local convenience store. Smokes a pack of cigarettes daily, when he can afford to buy them, and has smoked for the past 18 years. Drinks 10 cans of Mountain Dew a day when he is working. States that he only drinks a six pack of beer on Friday nights after he gets paid. Lives with his wife of 14 years and their three children who are 12, 9, and 3 years old. Wife is a stay-at-home mother. Children have insurance coverage through a state program; however, neither parent has insurance coverage.

■ Meds

Metformin 500 mg po BID with meals

■ All

NKDA

■ ROS

General feeling of being unwell. Denies history of goiter; has no intolerance to heat or cold. Has had polyuria for the past week.

■ Physical Examination

*Gen*

Heavy-set African-American man who has dark circles under his eyes, looks sad, and appears his stated age. Strong odor of cigarette smoke. Yellowed skin on fingers. Yellow teeth.

*VS*

BP 128/85, P 89 obtained by pharmacist reviewing his medication history at the clinic; Wt 125 kg, Ht 5′8″

■ Labs

FBG 150 mg/dL; A1C 7.5% (documented in clinic chart 1 month prior to this visit)

■ Assessment

Nicotine dependence—patient may be ready to quit smoking
Type 2 diabetes—not adequately controlled
Prehypertension
Obesity
Poor adherence to medication regimen—lack of insurance coverage may adversely impact ability to comply with pharmacotherapy
Compromised quality of life secondary to work absences

**A Cigarette and Select Smoke Components**

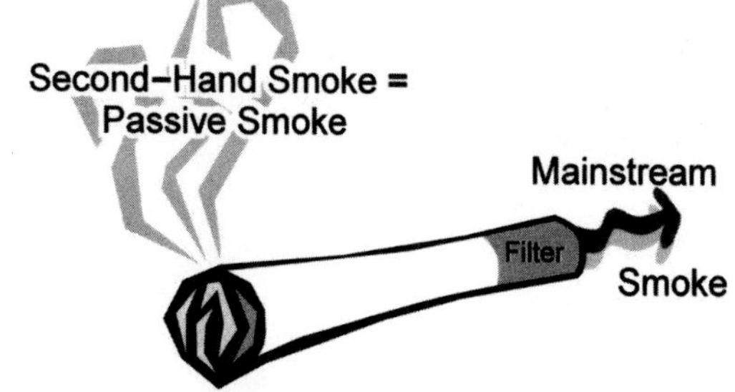


**Cigarette Smoke**

| *Gaseous Component* | *Particulate Component* |
|---|---|
| Carbon monoxide | Nicotine |
| Hydrogen cyanide | Tobacco alkaloids |
| Toluene | Tar |
| Methanol | Polynuclear Aromatic |
| Acetone | Hydrocarbons (PAH) |

**FIGURE 75-1.** A cigarette and select smoke components.

# QUESTIONS

## Problem Identification

1.a. Create a list of this patient's drug therapy problems.

1.b. What information in the patient's history can be identified as disease or symptoms directly related to the patient's smoking history (Fig. 75-1)?

1.c. Identify the stage of change that the patient is currently in at this time of his life, and describe your intervention plan using one of the A's from the 5A intervention plan for smokers (Table 75-1). State monitoring parameters that indicate uncontrolled disease states in addition to the nicotine dependence.

1.d. Describe aspects of the case that reveal the severity of nicotine dependence.

## Desired Outcome

2. What are the goals of smoking cessation pharmacotherapy and disease state management for this patient?

## Therapeutic Alternatives

3.a. Describe nondrug therapies that may help this patient reach treatment goals and improve work attendance.

**TABLE 75-1** Stages of Change and Smoking Cessation Counseling

| Stage of Change | Patient's Mindset | Response |
|---|---|---|
| Precontemplation | Not interested in quitting, fails to recognize smoking as a problem | Provide concise and relevant statement about why the smoker should think about quitting smoking |
| Contemplation | Smoking is a problem and might consider quitting | State that there is good evidence that cigarette smoke and secondhand smoke are dangerous. Encourage smoker to quit |
| Preparation | Cigarette smoking is problematic and now ready to think about quitting | Discuss options for treatment–both pharmacotherapeutic and nonpharmacotherapeutic |
| Action | Motivated to quit, instituting a plan with an identified quit date and developing a plan to cope with stressors | Encourage quit attempt, offer to be a resource during the quit attempt, and praise former smokers' abstinent status |
| Maintenance | Former smokers who have not smoked for a period of time | Great job staying quit. Continued cessation is a positive move in becoming healthier |

3.b. What pharmacotherapeutic alternatives are available for the treatment of the nicotine dependence and other disease states, and which would be an acceptable recommendation to make to this patient?

3.c. What economic, psychosocial, racial, and ethical issues need to be considered in this patient's treatment?

## Optimal Plan

4. What drug, dosage form, dose, schedule, and duration of therapy to control all disease states are best for this patient?

## Outcome Evaluation

5. What clinical and laboratory parameters are necessary to evaluate the therapy for achievement of the desired therapeutic outcome and to detect or prevent adverse effects?

## Patient Education

6. What information should be provided to the patient about the medications you recommended to enhance adherence, ensure successful outcome, and minimize adverse effects?

## SELF-STUDY ASSIGNMENTS

1. Evaluate current literature concerning the use of quitlines to enhance quit-smoking attempts. What is the status of quitlines in your state? In a one-page paper, explain how you could educate your community about quitlines.
2. Visit the *smokefree.gov* Web site and select three studies that are currently enrolling smokers to help them quit smoking. Compare and contrast the three studies. Create a flyer that could be used to recruit patients to one of the three studies.
3. Review the Surgeon General's report about secondhand smoke found at *http://www.surgeongeneral.gov/library/secondhandsmoke.* Develop a 10-item list stating how secondhand smoke acts as a toxin to cause disease. Write a two-page paper delineating how you could use this information to encourage parents and other caregivers to quit smoking.
4. Could smoking intervention be successful in a barbershop? Explore current medical literature to answer this question. Write a one-page paper identifying three intervention settings where a health care professional could creatively partner with others to help people think about a quit-smoking attempt.

## CLINICAL PEARL

No secondhand smoke exposure is safe. An intervention with a smoker must be personalized and relevant to the smoker's current stage of change status (see Table 75-1). Smoking cessation is achieved through a dynamic process involving pharmacotherapy and nonpharmacotherapy treatments. Health care professionals need to consider creative options for outreach to nicotine-dependent patients to help them in their quit attempts.

## REFERENCES


1. Fiore MC, Jaén CR, Baker TB, et al. Treating Tobacco Use and Dependence: 2008 Update. Clinical Practice Guideline. Rockville, MD, U.S. Department of Health and Human Services. Public Health Service, 2008. Available at: *http://surgeongeneral.gov/tobacco/.* Accessed April 15, 2010.
2. U.S. Department of Health and Human Services. The Health Consequences of Involuntary Exposure to Tobacco Smoke: A Report of the Surgeon General—Executive Summary. U.S. Department of Health and Human Services, Centers for Disease Control and Prevention, Coordinating Center for Health Promotion, National Center for Chronic Disease Prevention and Health Promotion, Office on Smoking and Health, 2006. Available at: *http://www.surgeongeneral.gov/library/secondhandsmoke.* Accessed April 15, 2010.
3. Chandler MA, Rennard SI. Smoking cessation. Chest 2010;137:428–435.
4. Smith SS, McCarthy DE, Japuntich S, et al. Comparative effectiveness of 5 smoking cessation pharmacotherapies in primary care clinics. Arch Intern Med 2009:169:2148–2155.
5. Chemla D, Antony I, Plamann K, Abastado P, Nitenberg A. Hypertension, prehypertension and blood pressure related diseases. Immunol Endocr Metabol Agents Med Chem 2006;6:319–330.
6. Willi C, Bodenmann P, Ghali WA, Faris PD, Cornuz J. Active smoking and the risk of type 2 diabetes: a systematic review and meta-analysis. JAMA 2007;298(22):2654–2664.
7. Mills AM, Rhodes KV, Follansbee CW, Shofer FS, Prusakowski M, Bernstein ST. Effect of household children on adult ED smokers' motivation to quit. Am J Emerg Med 2008;26:757–762.
8. Hartz SM, Bierut LJ. Genetics of addictions. Psychiatr Clin North Am 2010;33:107–124.
9. Benowitz NL. Nicotine addiction. N Engl J Med 2010;362:2295–2303.
10. Centers for Disease Control and Prevention. Cigarette smoking among adults and trends in smoking cessation—United States, 2008. MMWR 2009;58(44):1227–1232.


# 76

# SCHIZOPHRENIA

A Thousand Worms Inside My Body. . . . . . . . . Level I

**Lawrence J. Cohen, PharmD, BCPP, FASHP, FCCP**

## LEARNING OBJECTIVES

After completing this case study, the reader should be able to:

- Identify the target symptoms of schizophrenia.
- Manage an acutely psychotic patient with appropriate pharmacotherapy.
- Manage adverse effects of the antipsychotics.
- Discuss the role of atypical antipsychotics in the treatment of schizophrenia.

## PATIENT PRESENTATION

### Chief Complaint

"I want to see my lawyer."

### HPI

This is the first admission for Anita Gonzalez, a 32-year-old woman who was brought to the state hospital by the police. Earlier today she was brought to the Crisis Center by a friend in her apartment building after the landlord threatened to call the police since Anita was creating a disturbance. At the Crisis Center Anita became increasingly agitated and suspicious; the police were called; however, she left before being seen by staff. The patient apparently has been delusional and believes people sneak into her room at night when she is asleep and place a thousand worms inside her body. She also believes that she is being raped by passing men on the street. She is quite preoccupied about having massive wealth. She claims to have bought some gold and left it at the grocery store. She believes that her ideas have been given to a Cuban communist who has had plastic surgery to look like her and is using her ID to take possession of all of her property. She states that she is having difficulty getting her property back.

Apparently, the precipitating event today that eventually resulted in her hospitalization was that she created a disturbance at a local fast food restaurant, claiming that she owned it. Because of the disturbance, police were called, and she subsequently was sent here on an order of protective custody. According to the patient, she bought a hamburger and sat down to eat it, and for some reason somebody called the police and charged her with illegal trespassing. She claims that 6 years ago she was raped by a relative of a sister and broke her hip in the process. She states that her feet were cut off because she would not do what her impostors wanted her to do, and her feet were subsequently sent back to her from Central America and were reattached.

Her speech is quite rambling. She speaks of having been part of an experiment in Monterey, Mexico, in which 38 eggs were taken from her body, and children were produced from them and then killed by the government. She claims that she has worms in her that are the type that kill dogs and horses and says that they have been put there by the government. She also claims that at one time she had transmitters in her backbone and that it took 3 years to have them taken out by the government. She claims to have had surgery in the past, and the surgeon did not know what he was doing and took out her gallbladder and put it in the intestines, where it exploded. The patient also states that on one occasion a physician was removing the snakes from her abdominal cavity, and the snakes killed the doctor and a nurse. She also claims that she worked as a surgeon herself before 1963.

## Past Psychiatric History

The patient denies any prior hospitalization for mental problems and denies any street drugs or significant substance use. There is some history of her having frequent visits to the local hospital. She denies any drug or alcohol use. She smokes two packs of cigarettes per day.

## PMH

The patient's past records indicate that she did have gallbladder surgery (cholecystectomy) 2 months ago.

There is no record of her ever being raped or having a broken hip. No further medical history is known.

## Family Psychiatric History

The patient claims that her alleged family is not really her family and that she is not sure who is her family.

## Meds

None noted

## All

Penicillin → rash

## Legal/Social Status

Divorced; heterosexual; lives in an apartment alone; employment history unknown

## Mental Status Examination

The patient is a white female of Hispanic ethnicity, modestly dressed, with some disarray. She is morbidly obese. Her hair is black and unwashed. She is alert, is oriented, and in no acute distress. Her speech is clear, constant, and pressured, with many grandiose delusions and illogical thoughts. She is quite rambling, going from one subject to the other without interruption. Her affect is mood-congruent, her mood is euphoric, and there is a marked degree of grandiosity. Her thought processes are quite illogical, with marked delusional thinking. There is no current evidence of auditory hallucinations, and she denies visual hallucinations. She denies any suicidal or homicidal ideation, but she is quite verbal and pressured in her thought content, verbalizing a great deal about the things that have been taken away from her illegally by people impersonating her. She has marked delusional symptoms, with paranoid ideation prominent. Her memory (immediate, recent, and remote) is fair. Her cognition and concentration are adequate. Her intellectual functioning is within the average range. Insight and judgment are markedly impaired.

## ROS

Reports occasional GI upset; complains that worms are inside her stomach; otherwise negative

## Physical Examination

### *VS*

BP 140/85, P 80, RR 17, T 37.1°C; Wt 97 kg; Ht 5′3″

### *HEENT*

PERRLA; EOMI; fundi benign; throat and ears clear; TMs intact

### *Skin*

Scratches on both hands

### *Neck*

Supple, no nodes; normal thyroid

### *Lungs*

CTA & P

### *CV*

RRR, normal $S_1$ and $S_2$

### *Abd*

(+) BS, nontender

### *Ext*

Full ROM, pulses 2+ bilaterally

### *Neuro*

A & O × 3; reflexes symmetric; toes downgoing; normal gait; normal strength; sensation intact; CNs II–XII intact

## Labs

See Table 76-1.

## UA

Color yellow; appearance slightly cloudy; glucose (–); bili (–); ketones, trace; SG 1.025; blood (–); pH 6.0; protein (–); nitrites (–); leukocyte esterase (–)

**TABLE 76-1 Lab Values**

| | | | | |
|---|---|---|---|---|
| Na 140 mEq/L | Hgb 14.6 g/dL | WBC 11.0 × $10^3$/mm$^3$ | AST 34 IU/L | Ca 9.6 mg/dL |
| K 3.9 mEq/L | Hct 45.7% | Neutros 66% | ALT 22 IU/L | Phos 5.1 mg/dL |
| Cl 104 mEq/L | RBC 4.7 × $10^6$/mm$^3$ | Lymphs 24% | Alk phos 89 IU/L | TSH 4.5 μIU/mL |
| $CO_2$ 22 mEq/L | MCV 90.2 μm$^3$ | Monos 8% | GGT 38 IU/L | RPR negative |
| BUN 19 mg/dL | MCH 31 pg | Eos 1% | T. bili 0.9 mg/dL | Urine pregnancy (−) |
| SCr 1.1 mg/dL | MCHC 34.5 g/dL | Basos 1% | Alb 3.6 g/dL | |
| Glu 100 mg/dL | | Plt 232 × $10^3$/mm$^3$ | T. chol 208 mg/dL | |

## ASSESSMENT

Axis I: schizophrenia, paranoid type, acute exacerbation

Axis II: none

Axis III: patient allergic to penicillin by history; S/P gallbladder surgery 2 months ago; obesity

Axis IV: unemployment

Axis V: GAF Scale = 32

## QUESTIONS

### Problem Identification

1.a. Create a list of the patient's drug therapy problems.

1.b. Which information (signs, symptoms, laboratory values) indicates the presence or severity of an acute exacerbation of schizophrenia, paranoid type?

### Desired Outcome

2. What are the goals of pharmacotherapy in this case?

### Therapeutic Alternatives

3.a. What nondrug therapies might be useful for this patient?

3.b. What pharmacotherapeutic options are available for the treatment of this patient?

### Optimal Plan

4.a. What drug, dosage form, dose, schedule, and duration of therapy are best for this patient?

4.b. What alternatives would be appropriate if the initial therapy fails or cannot be used?

### Outcome Evaluation

5. What clinical and laboratory parameters are necessary to evaluate the therapy for achievement of the desired therapeutic outcome and to detect or prevent adverse effects?

### Patient Counseling

6. What information should be provided to the patient to enhance adherence, ensure successful therapy, and minimize adverse effects?

## SELF-STUDY ASSIGNMENTS

1. Perform a literature search regarding weight gain with each of the atypical antipsychotics currently marketed. Which ones are more likely to cause weight gain? Which ones are less likely to cause weight gain?
2. Perform a literature search regarding QTc changes with both typical and atypical antipsychotics. Which antipsychotics are more likely to alter the QT interval?
3. Review the pharmacoeconomic literature for the atypical antipsychotics. For your geographic area, compare costs for the average daily doses of haloperidol, aripiprazole, clozapine, olanzapine (oral, rapid-dissolving formulation, and injectable formulation), risperidone (oral, rapid-dissolving formulation, and injectable formulation), quetiapine, ziprasidone (oral and injectable formulation), paliperidone (oral and injectable formulation), asenapine, and iloperidone.

## CLINICAL PEARL

A benzodiazepine (e.g., lorazepam) may be used during the initiation of an antipsychotic to minimize agitation or aggression and allow time for the antipsychotic to take effect. The addition of lorazepam may also allow lower dosages to be used initially and during the maintenance phase of treatment.

## REFERENCES

1. Marder SR. Facilitating compliance with antipsychotic medication. J Clin Psychiatry 1998;59(Suppl 3):21–25.
2. Freedman R. Schizophrenia. N Engl J Med 2003;349:1738–1749.
3. Expert Consensus Panel for Optimizing Pharmacologic Treatment of Psychotic Disorders. Expert consensus guideline series. Optimizing pharmacologic treatment of psychotic disorders. J Clin Psychiatry 2003;64(Suppl 12):2–97.
4. Revicki DA. Methods of pharmacoeconomic evaluation of psychopharmacologic therapies for patients with schizophrenia. J Psychiatry Neurosci 1997;22:256–266.
5. Conley RR, Kelly DL, Richardson CM, Tamminga CA, Carpenter WT Jr. The efficacy of high-dose olanzapine versus clozapine in treatment-resistant schizophrenia: a double-blind crossover study. J Clin Psychopharmacol 2003;23:668–671.
6. Citrome L. Paliperidone palmitate—review of the efficacy, safety and cost of a new second-generation depot antipsychotic medication. Int J Clin Pract 2010;64(2):216–239.
7. Nelson MW, Reynolds R, Kelly DL, et al. Safety and tolerability of high dose quetiapine in treatment refractory schizophrenia: preliminary results from an open-label trial. Schizophr Res 2003;60(Suppl):363 [abstract].
8. Sharma T, Mockler D. The cognitive efficacy of atypical antipsychotics in schizophrenia. J Clin Psychopharmacol 1998;18(Suppl 1):12S–19S.
9. Citrome L. Asenapine for schizophrenia and bipolar disorder: a review of the efficacy and safety profile for the newly approved sublingually absorbed second-generation antipsychotic. Int J Clin Pract 2009;63(12):1762–1784.
10. Citrome L. Iloperidone for schizophrenia: a review of the efficacy and safety profile for this newly commercialized second-generation antipsychotic. Int J Clin Pract 2009;63(8):1237–1248.

## ADDITIONAL RESOURCES

1. Texas Medication Algorithm Project (TMAP). Available at: *http://www.dshs.state.tx.us/mhprograms/disclaimer.shtm*. Accessed February 4, 2011.
2. Lieberman JA, Stroup TS, McEvoy JP, et al., for the Clinical Antipsychotic Trials of Intervention Effectiveness (CATIE) Investigators. Effectiveness of antipsychotic drugs in patients with chronic schizophrenia. N Engl J Med 2005;353:1209–1223.
3. Lehman AF, Kreyenbuhl J, Buchanan RW, et al. The Schizophrenia Patient Outcomes Research Team (PORT): updated treatment recommendations 2003. Schizophr Bull 2004;30(2):193–217.
4. Dixon LB, Dickerson F, Bellack AS, et al. The 2009 Schizophrenia PORT psychosocial treatment recommendations and summary statements. Schizophr Bull 2010;36(1):48–70.

# 77

# MAJOR DEPRESSION

A Life Worth Living . . . . . . . . . . . . . . . . . . . . . . . Level I

**Brian L. Crabtree, PharmD, BCPP**

**Victor G. Dostrow, MD**

## LEARNING OBJECTIVES

After completing this case study, the reader should be able to:

- Identify the signs and symptoms of depression.
- Develop a pharmacotherapy plan for a patient with depression.
- Compare side-effect profiles of various antidepressant drugs.
- Discuss pharmacoeconomic considerations that must be taken into account when selecting antidepressant therapy.

## PATIENT PRESENTATION

### Chief Complaint

"I don't know if I can handle this anymore."

### HPI

Geneva Flowers is a 41-year-old woman who is referred by her family physician to an outpatient mental health clinic. She c/o feeling down and sad, with crying spells, trouble sleeping, increased eating, depression, impaired concentration, and fatigue. She has not worked in over 2 months and has used up her vacation and sick leave.

She went through treatment for alcoholism over a year ago. Things were going fairly well for her after her treatment and she remarried approximately 8 months ago. Arguments with her teenage sons about family issues and past incidents have made her increasingly depressed over the last few months. Her older son, 17, moved out to live with his father. Her younger son, 12, moved to live with his paternal grandparents.

She divorced the boys' father after approximately 10 years of marriage when she discovered he was having an affair with another woman. She left her second husband after approximately 2 years because of problems involving his children that caused increasing conflict with her then-husband. Without a second income in the household, she accumulated large credit card debts. She began drinking and soon developed a pattern of using alcohol to relieve stress. Just before entering alcoholism treatment, there was a sexual fondling incident involving one of her son's friends while the friend was visiting her son at her house, but she was amnestic for the incident the next day. Her present husband, her third, has been supportive of her, but she feels guilty about her failed previous marriages and her sons, worries about her debt, and has become more despondent. She has taken a leave of absence from her job as an administrative assistant at an elementary school.

The patient sought treatment for depression 3 months ago from her family physician, who prescribed mirtazapine. Her spirits have not improved, and she says the medication made her gain weight. Because of vague references the physician believed could possibly indicate suicidal ideas, she has been referred for psychiatric evaluation.

### PMH

Childhood illnesses—she has had all of the usual childhood illnesses. She was hospitalized at age 3 for bacterial meningitis but knows of no residual effects.

Adult illnesses—no current nonpsychiatric adult illnesses; no previous psychiatric treatment.

Trauma—fractured arm due to bicycle accident at age 9, otherwise unremarkable.

Surgeries—Hx childbirth by C-section; tonsillectomy at age 6.

Travel—no significant travel history.

Diet—no dietary restrictions. Despite not having much of an appetite, reports eating more since taking mirtazapine.

Exercise—no regular exercise program.

Immunizations—no personal records of childhood vaccinations; had tetanus booster 9 years ago.

### FH

Father is deceased, had coronary artery disease, but ultimately died of colon cancer. Mother has well-controlled HTN. A sister has depression and anxiety, takes antidepressant medication (G.F. does not know its name). A second sister committed suicide.

### SH

High school graduate; works as an administrative assistant but on leave for approximately 2 months. Married approximately 8 months, two previous divorces. Lived with husband and sons until sons moved out in the last few weeks. Health insurance is through the school district where she is employed; includes adjusted copay on prescriptions. Reports heavy credit card debt. Attended church regularly in the past (Protestant), but not recently. Attends AA weekly.

Denies drinking alcohol since chemical dependence treatment. Denies smoking. Drinks three to four cups of caffeinated coffee per day; usually drinks iced tea with evening meal; drinks colas as leisure beverage. Used marijuana a few times after high school, denies use in more than 10 years; denies present or past use of other illicit substances.

### Meds

Mirtazapine 30 mg po QHS (started on mirtazapine 15 mg po QHS approximately 3 months ago)

Ortho-Novum 1/35-28, one po daily; has not taken for 2 months

St. John's wort 300 mg po TID for the last 2 weeks at suggestion of husband (purchased at health food store)

APAP 1,000–1,500 mg po PRN headaches, two or three times a week
Uses OTC antihistamines and decongestants for colds or allergies; none in recent months

## All

NKDA

## ROS

General appearance—pt c/o feeling tired much of the time
HEENT—wears contact lenses; no tinnitus, ear pain, or discharge; no c/o nasal congestion; Hx of dental repair for caries
Chest—no Hx of asthma or other lung disease
CV—reports occasional feelings of "pounding heart"; no Hx of heart disease
GI—reports infrequent constipation; takes MOM PRN; has gained 9 lb in last 2 months
GU—has regular menses; LMP ended a week ago
Neuromuscular—occasional headaches, worse over the past few months; no syncope, vertigo, weakness or paralysis, numbness or tingling
Skin—no complaints

## Physical Examination

Performed by nurse practitioner

### *Gen*

Overweight WF, slightly unkempt

### *VS*

BP 132/78, P 88, RR 22, T 36.9°C; Wt 187 lb, Ht 5′8″

### *Skin*

Normal skin, hair, and nails

### *HEENT*

PERRLA; EOM intact, no nystagmus. Fundus—disks sharp, no retinopathy; no nasal discharge or nasal polyps; TMs gray and shiny bilaterally; minor accumulation of cerumen

### *Neck/Lymph Nodes*

Supple without thyromegaly or lymphadenopathy

### *Chest/Lungs*

Frequent sighing during examination, but no tachypnea or SOB; chest CTA

### *Breasts*

No masses, tenderness, or discharge

### *Heart*

RRR without murmur

### *Abd*

Soft, nontender; (+) BS; no organomegaly

### *Genit/Rect*

Deferred

### *Ext*

Unremarkable

### *Neuro*

CN—EOM intact, no nystagmus, no weakness of facial or tongue muscles. Casual gait normal. Finger-to-nose normal. Motor—normal symmetric grip strength. DTRs 2+ and equal. Sensory—intact bilaterally.

### *Mental Status*

When seen in the clinic, the patient is pale and appears moderately overweight, dressed in casual slacks and sweater. Grooming is fair and without makeup. She speaks slowly, often not responding to questions for approximately 30 seconds before beginning answers. She describes depressed mood and lack of energy and says she feels no pleasure in life. Her husband is good to her, but she feels everyone else she loves has left her. She has no social contacts other than occasional visits by her parents. She spends most of her time in bed. She feels worthless and blames herself for her problems. She feels particularly anguished about the incident with her son's friend even though she does not remember it. She is often anxious and worries about the future. She wonders if her sons love her and if they will ever return. She worries how she will repay her financial debts. Her speech is logical, coherent, and goal-oriented. She denies suicidal intent but says the future seems dim to her, and she wonders sometimes if life is worth living. She admits she sometimes wishes she could just go to sleep and not wake up. She denies hallucinations. Paranoid delusions, FOI, IOR, and LOA are absent. There is no dysarthria or anomia.

## Labs (Collected 11:45 am)

| | | |
|---|---|---|
| Na 139 mEq/L | Hgb 14.0 g/dL | AST 34 IU/L |
| K 4.2 mEq/L | Hct 46.2% | ALT 42 IU/L |
| Cl 102 mEq/L | MCV 92 μm$^3$ | GGT 38 IU/L |
| $CO_2$ 24 mEq/L | MCH 29 pg | T. bili 0.8 mg/dL |
| BUN 12 mg/dL | Plt 234 × 10$^3$/mm$^3$ | T. prot 7.0 g/dL |
| SCr 0.9 mg/dL | WBC 7.3 × 10$^3$/mm$^3$ | Alb 4.4 g/dL |
| Glu 98 mg/dL | Segs 49% | CK 57 IU/L |
| Ca 9.5 mg/dL | Bands 1% | $T_4$ 8.6 mcg/dL |
| Mg 1.7 mEq/L | Lymphs 42% | $T_3$ uptake 29% |
| Uric acid 4.0 mg/dL | Monos 2% | TSH 2.8 mIU/L |
| | Eos 6% | |

## UA

Glucose (–); ketones (–); pH 5.8; SG 1.016; bilirubin (–); WBC 1/hpf, protein (–), amorphous—rare, epithelial cells 1/hpf; color yellow; blood (–), RBC 0/hpf; mucus—rare; bacteria—rare; casts 0/lpf; appearance clear

## Assessment

Major depressive disorder, single episode, with melancholic features

## Plan

Refer for support group, psychotherapy; begin antidepressant medication

# QUESTIONS

## Problem Identification

1.a. Create a list of this patient's drug therapy problems.

1.b. What signs, symptoms, and laboratory values indicate the presence and severity of depression in this patient?

1.c. What factors in the family history support a diagnosis of depression?

1.d. Is there anything in the patient's medication history that could cause or worsen depression?

## Desired Outcome

2. What are the goals of pharmacotherapy in this case?

## Therapeutic Alternatives

3.a. What nonpharmacologic treatments are important in this case? Should nonpharmacologic treatments be tried before beginning medication?

3.b. What pharmacotherapeutic options are available for the treatment of depression?

## Optimal Plan

4.a. What drug regimen (drug, dosage, schedule, and duration) is best for this patient?

4.b. How should the patient be advised about the herbal therapy, St. John's wort?

4.c. What alternatives would be appropriate if the patient fails to respond to initial therapy?

## Outcome Evaluation

5. What clinical and laboratory parameters are necessary to evaluate the therapy for efficacy and adverse effects?

## Patient Education

6. What information should be provided to the patient to enhance adherence, ensure successful therapy, and minimize adverse effects?

## CLINICAL COURSE: ALTERNATIVE THERAPY

Mrs Flowers understands that she must stop the St. John's wort she has been taking because of an interaction with her prescribed mirtazapine, but she wonders if it would have been helpful if she had started it when she first began feeling depressed. See Section 19 in this casebook for questions about the use of St. John's wort for treatment of depression.

## SELF-STUDY ASSIGNMENTS

1. Because the SSRI antidepressants are commonly used and have the same reuptake pharmacology, contrast the agents in this class, considering relative side effects, dosing, and drug interactions.
2. Compare other antidepressants with SSRIs with regard to adverse effects and relative advantages and disadvantages.
3. Discuss the role of combination drug therapy in the treatment of depression, including the use of drugs not usually classified as antidepressants.
4. Review the medical literature and evaluate the scientific evidence for the efficacy of St. John's wort in the treatment of depression.

## CLINICAL PEARL

Although the selective serotonin reuptake inhibitors are a pharmacologic class, they are not a chemical class. Failure to respond to one SSRI does not reliably predict failure to respond to others.

## REFERENCES


1. Cuijpers P, Dekker J, Hollon SD, Anderson G. Adding psychotherapy to pharmacotherapy in the treatment of depressive disorders in adults: a meta-analysis. J Clin Psychiatry 2009;70:1219–1229.
2. Cipriani A, Furukawa TA, Salanti G, et al. Comparative efficacy and acceptability of 12 new-generation antidepressants: a multiple-treatments meta-analysis. Lancet 2009;373:746–758.
3. Cipriani A, La Ferla T, Furukawa TA, et al. Sertraline versus other antidepressive agents for depression. Cochrane Database Syst Rev 2010;4:CD006117.
4. Cassano P, Fava M. Tolerability issues during long-term treatment with antidepressants. Ann Clin Psychiatry 2004;16:15–25.
5. Preskorn SH, Shah R, Neff M, et al. The potential for clinically significant drug–drug interactions involving the CYP2D6 system: effects with fluoxetine and paroxetine versus sertraline. J Psychiatr Pract 2007;13:5–12.
6. Perry PJ. Pharmacotherapy for major depression with melancholic features: relative efficacy of tricyclic versus selective serotonin reuptake inhibitor antidepressants. J Affect Disord 1996;39:1–6.
7. Freeman MP, Mischoulon D, Tedeschini E, et al. Complementary and alternative medicine for major depressive disorder: a meta-analysis of patient characteristics, placebo-response rates, and treatment outcomes relative to standard antidepressants. J Clin Psychiatry 2010;71:682–688.


# 78

# BIPOLAR DISORDER

Don't Hate Me Because I'm Beautiful . . . . . . Level II

Lawrence J. Cohen, PharmD, BCPP, FASHP, FCCP

## LEARNING OBJECTIVES

After completing this case study, the reader should be able to:

- Outline a mental status examination and identify target symptoms of bipolar disorder when given patient interview information.
- Recommend appropriate pharmacotherapy for patients with acute mania.
- Generate parameters for monitoring anticonvulsant therapy for bipolar disorder.
- Identify the pharmacotherapeutic options for treating the subtypes of bipolar disorder.

## PATIENT PRESENTATION

### Chief Complaint

"There are hundreds of vampires in this city, and I have the documents to prove it."

### HPI

Michael Harrison is a 25-year-old man seen today in the Crisis Center triage by the ACT team. If he is detained, this is his third possible psychiatric admission. According to neighbors who called the police, the patient has been acting increasingly strange. The lights in the house are left on all night, and spiritual music is played at all hours. Last evening, he dug a trench around his front yard with an electric lawn edger and filled it with garlic cloves. This evening, he painted crosses on the front of the house and threw furniture into his yard and the street. When approached by neighbors, he apparently began screaming and preaching at them. When the police arrived, they found the patient standing naked on the dining room table in his front yard preaching. When the police approached, he began throwing garlic tablets at them and screaming, "Become naked in the eyes of the Lord and you will be saved." He became increasingly hostile during the arrest shouting, "Don't hate me because I'm beautiful." He then tried to bite one of the officers.

### PMH

Manic episodes first occurred while he was in college, leading to psychiatric admissions at ages 21 and 23 for acute mania. Patient was treated with haloperidol 5 mg po once daily and lithium 600 mg po Q AM and 900 mg po at bedtime, with adequate response and discharged on both occasions after about a month.
Medical problems include migraine headaches.

### Patient Interview

Patient is disheveled with pungent body odor. He is pacing the room, waving his hands in the air and preaching in an elated, loud, sing-songy voice. He is dressed flamboyantly in a brightly colored bathrobe and appears to be wearing a garlic necklace. He is carrying a Bible. When asked how he felt, he stated, "Playful, with intense clarity, sharp, spiffy, and clean." He then became angry, insisting that he be discharged before sunrise or he would "face the light of the right and mighty and burn in 'demonocratic' hell." He then asked for a priest to exorcise the homosexual demons from his body. He believes that vampires live in the city. He stated he has the documents to prove it and that the vampires are pursuing him to keep him from exposing their existence to Christians everywhere. He spoke in long run-on sentences with many political, religious, and sexual references. He was very difficult to interrupt. For example, at one point he stated, "Can't you see, or are you an idiot?! I am being persecuted by the right, 100 points of light, Republicans, redeeming the public, for the republic, under which I stand because I have no one to lean on, one gay man, bitten by the Democrat, the 'demoncrat,' doomed and miserable for loving the company I keep, and that's why misery loves company, and if you don't get that you're an idiot."

When asked about his sleep, he angrily replied, "Would you sleep at a time like this? If I sleep, America will fall, and it will all be on my shoulders. The towers in New York City have already fallen because I didn't get there in time." The patient stated that he has not been eating and has not taken his lithium in several days because, "Lithium is of the ground, the underworld. The Lord will sustain me."

Through his verbose conversation, it becomes apparent that a man he picked up in a gay bar last week bit him on the neck. He also seems to believe that he has been given a mission from God as penance for visiting this bar. Several times during the interview, he began crying and wailing loudly, begging to be saved and shouting, "I'm sorry." He appears distraught, tearful, irritable, and agitated. He said something about the trials of Job and that he would be the next to die. He then sang "Swing Low Sweet Chariot" in a very loud voice. When told that he might need to be in the hospital so we can help him with his problems, he screamed, "You can't help me! Only the Lord can help me! They have drunk from the fruit of the vine. I am that fruit."

### AIMS

Excessive eye blinking and mild grimacing; unclear whether abnormal (patient states this is the "demon blood trying to take over my body"). He is bothered by it in that to him it represents his "sinful nature."

### FH

Father has a history of depression; paternal grandmother was placed in an "asylum" for hysteria secondary to childbirth. Mother and brother have type 2 diabetes.

### SH

Recently fired from his job as a nurse at a local hospital. Patient is a single homosexual. Religious upbringing as a Southern Baptist. Smokes one ppd for 5 years. Patient states that he drinks "only occasionally," but he was noted to be intoxicated, with a BAC 0.14%, on a previous admission.

### Meds

Ergotamine and ibuprofen PRN for migraines

### All

NKDA

### ROS

Migraine headaches about twice a month, no aura, (+) nausea and photophobia. Occasional GI upset with no clear relationship to meals or time of day; frequent loose stools.

### Physical Examination

*VS*

BP 118/73, P 83, RR 16, T 37.1°C; Wt 94 kg, Ht 5′sy2″

*HEENT*

PERRLA; EOMI; fundi benign; throat and ears clear; TMs intact; rapid eye blinking and facial grimacing (may indicate early tardive dyskinesia)

*Skin*

Psoriasis evident on both elbows

*Neck*

Supple, bite mark, no nodes

*Lungs*

CTA & P

*CV*

RRR; $S_1$, $S_2$ normal; no MRG

*Abd*

(+) BS, nontender

*Ext*

Full ROM, pulses 2+ bilaterally

*Neuro*

A & O × 3; reflexes symmetric; toes downgoing; normal gait; normal strength; sensation intact; CNs II–XII intact

### Labs

See Table 78-1.

**TABLE 78-1 Lab Values**

| | | | | |
|---|---|---|---|---|
| Na 141 mEq/L | Hgb 14.6 g/dL | WBC 12.0 × $10^3$/mm$^3$ | AST 32 IU/L | Ca 9.7 mg/dL |
| K 3.8 mEq/L | Hct 45.7% | Neutros 67% | ALT 21 IU/L | Phos 5.3 mg/dL |
| Cl 103 mEq/L | RBC 4.73 × $10^6$/mm$^3$ | Lymphs 23% | Alk phos 87 IU/L | TSH 4.1 μIU/mL |
| $CO_2$ 24 mEq/L | MCV 90.2 μm$^3$ | Monos 7% | GGT 46 IU/L | RPR: neg |
| BUN 19 mg/dL | MCH 31 pg | Eos 2% | T. bili 0.9 mg/dL | Lithium 0.1 mEq/L |
| SCr 1.1 mg/dL | MCHC 34.4 g/dL | Basos 1% | Alb 3.7 g/dL | |
| Glu 89 mg/dL | Plt 256 × $10^3$/mm$^3$ | | T. chol 218 mg/dL | |

### UA

Color yellow; appearance slightly cloudy; glucose (–), bili (–), ketones trace; SG 1.025, blood (–), pH 6.0, protein (–), nitrites (–), leukocyte esterase (–)

### Assessment

Axis I: bipolar disorder, current episode mixed
Axis II: deferred
Axis III: migraine headache by history, obese, possible early tardive dyskinesia
Axis IV: recently fired from his job

# QUESTIONS

## Problem Identification

1.a. From the case information and patient interview, write a mental status examination for this patient.

1.b. Create a list of this patient's drug therapy problems.

1.c. What information (target symptoms, laboratory values) indicates the presence and severity of bipolar disorder, mixed episode?

## Desired Outcome

2. What are the goals of pharmacotherapy in this patient?

## Therapeutic Alternatives

3.a. What nondrug therapies might be useful for this patient?

3.b. What feasible pharmacotherapeutic alternatives are available for treatment of bipolar disorder?

## Optimal Plan

4.a. What drug, dosage form, dose, schedule, and duration of therapy are best for this patient?

4.b. What alternatives would be appropriate if the initial therapy fails or cannot be used?

## Outcome Evaluation

5. Which clinical and laboratory parameters are necessary to evaluate response to therapy and to detect or prevent adverse effects?

## Patient Education

6. What information should be provided to the patient to enhance adherence, ensure successful therapy, and minimize adverse effects?

# SELF-STUDY ASSIGNMENTS

1. Perform a literature search and explore the role of the newer anticonvulsants (lamotrigine, oxcarbazepine, and topiramate) in the treatment of bipolar disorder. Also, identify the current FDA-approved mood disorder indications for each of the atypical antipsychotics.
2. Determine which of the mood stabilizers can be administered once daily in order to improve adherence. How would you go about changing a patient's dosing regimen to improve adherence? Based on the literature, which patients are most suitable for conversion to once- or twice-daily dosing with lithium, carbamazepine, or valproate? Can regular-release products be used, or must the patient be converted to extended-release products?
3. Design an algorithm for the treatment of bipolar disorder including treatment strategies for acute mania, rapid cycling, bipolar depression, and mixed states.

# CLINICAL PEARL

When a patient admitted with acute mania is taking an antidepressant, the antidepressant should be tapered and withdrawn. In some patients, antidepressants may activate mania or increase the rate of cycling, and potentially delay response to antimanic/mood stabilizers. Antidepressants can always be added back, if needed, to the regimen after the patient is more stable.

# REFERENCES


1. Swann AC, Bowden CL, Morris D, et al. Depression during mania: treatment response to lithium or divalproex. Arch Gen Psychiatry 1997;54:37–42.
2. Freeman TW, Clothier JL, Pazzaglia P, Lesem MD, Swann AC. A double-blind comparison of valproate and lithium in the treatment of acute mania. Am J Psychiatry 1992;149:108–111.
3. Allen MH, Hirschfeld RM, Wozniak PJ, Baker JD, Bowden CL. Linear relationship of valproate serum concentration to response and optimal serum levels for acute mania. Am J Psychiatry 2006;163:272–275.
4. Tohen M, Jacobs TG, Grundy SL, et al. Efficacy of olanzapine in acute bipolar mania: a double-blind, placebo-controlled study. The Olanzapine HGGW Study Group. Arch Gen Psychiatry 2000;57:841–849.
5. Tohen M, Sanger TM, McElroy SL, et al. Olanzapine versus placebo in the treatment of acute mania. Olanzapine HGEH Study Group Trial. Am J Psychiatry 1999;156:702–709.
6. Calabrese J, Keck PE, Mcfadden W, et al. A randomized, double-blind, placebo-controlled trial of quetiapine in the treatment of bipolar I or II depression. Am J Psychiatry 2005;162:1351–1360.
7. Bowden CL, Calabrese JR, Sachs G, et al. A placebo-controlled 18-month trial of lamotrigine and lithium maintenance treatment in recently manic or hypomanic patients with bipolar disorder I. Arch Gen Psychiatry 2003;60:392–400.
8. Goldsmith DR, Wagstaff AJ, Ibbotson T, Perry CM. Spotlight on lamotrigine in bipolar disorder. CNS Drugs 2004;18:63–67.

9. Gerner RH, Stanton A. Algorithm for patient management of acute manic states: lithium, valproate, or carbamazepine? J Clin Psychopharmacol 1992;12:57S–63S.
10. Hartong EG, Moleman P, Hoogduin CA, Broekman TG, Nolen WA. Prophylactic efficacy of lithium versus carbamazepine in treatment-naive bipolar patients. J Clin Psychiatry 2003;64:144–151.
11. McElroy SL, Keck PE, Tugrul KC, et al. Valproate as a loading treatment in acute mania. Neuropsychobiology 1993;27:146–149.
12. Citrome L. Asenapine for schizophrenia and bipolar disorder: a review of the efficacy and safety profile for the newly approved sub-lingually absorbed second-generation antipsychotic. Int J Clin Pract 2009;63(12):1762–1784.
13. Sachs GS, Printz DJ, Kahn DA, Carpenter D, Docherty JP. The expert consensus guideline series: medication treatment of bipolar disorder 2000. Postgrad Med 2000;Spec No:1–104.
14. Ghaemi SN. New treatments for bipolar disorder: the role of atypical neuroleptic agents. J Clin Psychiatry 2000;61(Suppl 14):33–42.
15. Calabrese JR, Vieta E, Sheldon MD. Latest maintenance data on lamotrigine in bipolar disorder. Eur Neuropsychopharmacol 2003;13 (Suppl 2):S57–S66.

## ADDITIONAL RESOURCES

1. Systematic Treatment Enhancement Program for Bipolar Disorder (STEP-BD). Available at: *http://www.stepbd.org/referencelist.html.*
2. Texas Medication Algorithm Project (TMAP). Available at: *http://www.dshs.state.tx.us/mhprograms/disclaimer.shtm.*
3. Canadian Network for Mood and Anxiety Treatments (CANMAT) and International Society for Bipolar Disorders (ISBD) collaborative update of CANMAT guidelines for the management of patients with bipolar disorder: update 2009. Bipolar Disord 2009;11:225–255.
4. Practice Guidelines for the Treatment of Patients with Bipolar Disorder, 2nd ed. American Psychiatric Association, 2005. Available at: *http://www.psychiatryonline.com/pracGuide/pracGuideTopic_8.aspx.* (*Note*: 3rd edition was being developed as of the time of writing of this casebook chapter.) Accessed February 5, 2011.

# 79

# GENERALIZED ANXIETY DISORDER

Nervous Neddie . . . . . . . . . . . . . . . . . . . . . . . . Level I

**Sarah T. Melton, PharmD, BCPP, CGP**
**Cynthia K. Kirkwood, PharmD, BCPP**

## LEARNING OBJECTIVES

After completing this case study, the reader should be able to:

- Identify target symptoms associated with GAD.
- Construct treatment goals of pharmacotherapy for GAD.
- Recommend appropriate pharmacotherapy and duration of treatment for the acute, continuation, and maintenance phases of GAD.
- Develop a plan to counsel patients and consult with providers about the pharmacotherapy used in the treatment of GAD.
- Develop a monitoring plan for a patient treated for GAD based on the treatment regimen.

## PATIENT PRESENTATION

### Chief Complaint

"I am so worried all the time that I can't do anything else. I need some serious help."

### HPI

Ned Johnson is a 55-year-old man who presents to his family physician with complaints of severe irritability, feelings of "being on edge," and inability to fall asleep at night. He states that he always feels tense and exhausted with constant muscle tension and body aches. He was laid off from his job as a manager at a building supply store 9 months ago. Over the past year, he has had difficulty concentrating when filling out job application forms, and his mind often "goes blank" when talking with people. His irritability has impacted his relationship with his wife, and he is worried that she will leave him. He has developed frequent abdominal pain and daily episodes of diarrhea. He constantly worries about the lack of financial resources, his wife losing her job, and his relationship with his wife. He is afraid that he and his wife will lose their house and cars. He states that he cannot control his constant worry and that his anxiety has increased in intensity over the past 6 months. He denies having obsessive–compulsive thoughts or behaviors or symptoms of panic disorder. He recently went to the emergency department because he was so worried about multiple issues in his life that he could not eat or sleep for 2 days. He was given an IM injection of hydroxyzine and sent home with a prescription for hydroxyzine 25-mg capsules orally four times daily as needed for anxiety. He stopped this medication last week secondary to constipation and decreased urinary flow. He tried kava kava from a herbal store a few months ago. It was not effective, and he discontinued it after 2 weeks because of severe abdominal pain.

### PMH

Records from the family physician indicate frequent visits over the past 9 months for insomnia, headaches, abdominal pain, and diarrhea. He has been treated with buspirone for anxiety for the past 6 months.

After a recent visit to the ED, he was prescribed hydroxyzine to be taken up four times daily as needed for anxiety.

Past psychiatric history is significant for episode of depression and alcohol abuse when he was 33 years old that was treated with fluoxetine. He took the fluoxetine for 2 weeks and discontinued it secondary to insomnia.

### FH

Father, 80 years old, on "nerve medication" for several years. Mother deceased at age 73 from breast cancer with history of major depression and alcohol abuse. Patient has one sister who has been treated with multiple medications in the past for anxiety and depression and was treated for benzodiazepine abuse 5 years ago.

### SH

Married for 25 years; no children; high school graduate; past tobacco user (quit 5 years ago with 40 pack-year history); past alcohol abuse (has been sober for 10 years and attends Alcoholics Anonymous on a weekly basis); little exercise because of time constraints; drinks four to five cups of coffee per day, and three to four Mountain Dew soft drinks throughout the day. He admits to occasional marijuana use when his anxiety is "out of control." He does not have any prescription drug coverage at this time.

## CHAPTER 79

■ Meds

Buspirone 30 mg po BID for anxiety
Sudafed PE 10 mg po QID PRN nasal congestion
Loperamide 2 mg po Q 6 h PRN diarrhea

■ All

Sulfa (hives); codeine (nausea)

■ ROS

Positive only for paresthesias and mild diaphoresis; negative for dizziness, palpitations, SOB, chest pain

■ Physical Examination

*Gen*

Nervous, well-groomed man sitting on examination table; cooperative; oriented × 3

*VS*

BP 125/85, P 90, RR 18, T 36.5°C; Wt 90 kg, Ht 5′11″

*Skin*

Clammy; no rashes, lesions, or track marks

*HEENT*

EOMI; PERRLA; fundi benign; ear and nose clear; dentition intact; tonsils 1+

*Neck/Lymph Nodes*

Supple, no lymphadenopathy; thyroid symmetric and of normal size

*Lungs/Chest*

Symmetric chest wall movement; BS equal bilaterally; no rub; clear to A & P

*CV*

RRR, normal $S_1$ and $S_2$, no MRG

*Abd*

Symmetric; NTND; normal BS; no organomegaly or masses

*Genit/Rect*

Deferred

*MS/Ext*

Average frame; normal bones, joints, and muscles

*Neuro*

CNs II–XII intact; motor and sensory grossly normal; coordination intact

*MSE*

*Appearance and behavior:* well groomed, fair eye contact, wringing hands, and bouncing legs
*Speech:* well spoken and coherent with normal rate and rhythm
*Mood:* anxious, worried about everything in his life, and concerned that he is very sick
*Affect:* full
*Thought processes:* linear, logical, and goal-directed
*Thought content:* negative for suicidal or homicidal ideations, obsessions/compulsions, delusions, or hallucinations
*Memory:* 3/3 at 0 minutes, 2/3 at 5 minutes; spelled "world" backwards
*Abstractions:* good
*Judgment:* good by testing
*Insight:* fair
Score on Hamilton Anxiety Scale = 34 points (see Appendix A)

■ Labs

| | |
|---|---|
| Na 142 mEq/L | Hgb 14.0 g/dL |
| K 4.3 mEq/L | Hct 38% |
| Cl 105 mEq/L | TSH 3 mIU/L |
| $CO_2$ 28 mEq/L | AST 23 IU/L |
| BUN 15 mg/dL | ALT 20 IU/L |
| SCr 0.9 mg/dL | Alk phos 23 IU/L |
| Glu 80 mg/dL | Vit D 25-OH 51 ng/mL |

■ ECG

NSR; rate 88 bpm

■ Urine Toxicology Screen

Positive for 9-carboxy-THC

■ Assessment

GAD

# QUESTIONS

## Problem Identification

1.a. Create a list of the patient's drug therapy problems.

1.b. Is there anything in the patient's medication history that could cause or worsen anxiety?

1.c. What information (signs, symptoms, laboratory values) indicates the presence or severity of GAD?

## Desired Outcome

2. What are the goals of pharmacotherapy in this case?

## Therapeutic Alternatives

3.a. What nondrug therapies might be useful for this patient?

3.b. What feasible pharmacotherapeutic alternatives are available for the treatment of GAD?

## Optimal Plan

4.a. What drug, dosage form, dose, schedule, and duration of therapy are best for this patient?

4.b. What pharmacotherapeutic alternatives would be appropriate if the optimal plan fails or cannot be used?

## Outcome Evaluation

5. What clinical and laboratory parameters are necessary to evaluate the therapy for achievement of the desired therapeutic outcome and to detect or prevent adverse effects?

## Patient Education

6. What information should be provided to the patient to enhance adherence, ensure successful therapy, and minimize adverse effects?

## CLINICAL COURSE: ALTERNATIVE THERAPY

Mr. Johnson is still worried about both the side effects of prescription drugs to treat his anxiety and whether he will be able to afford them. He states that he has read a lot of information about kava, that "it really works for anxiety." Mr. Johnson says, "Maybe I was just using a bad product last time I tried it and that's why it didn't help much and hurt my stomach. Should I get a better product and try it again?" Please see Section 19 of this Casebook for questions about the use of kava kava for the treatment of GAD.

## SELF-STUDY ASSIGNMENTS

1. Perform a literature search to review the role of atypical antipsychotics in the treatment of GAD. Write a summary of the controlled trials that evaluated the use of atypical antipsychotics in GAD as adjunctive agents or monotherapy.
2. Individuals with GAD may misuse alcohol, cannabis, or other substances in an effort to ameliorate their anxiety. Review and summarize the recommendations put forth by the International Psychopharmacology Algorithm Project on treating patients with GAD and a history of or current substance abuse.
3. Many patients with mental illness do not have prescription drug insurance coverage and this impacts the choice of pharmacotherapy. Using this case example, go to a Web-based patient assistance program and document how you would go about helping this patient obtain a first-line agent that he otherwise would not be able to afford (e.g., escitalopram, duloxetine, venlafaxine extended-release capsules).

## CLINICAL PEARL

With effective pharmacotherapy available for the acute and long-term therapy of GAD, the treatment goal for anxiety is remission. Many patients exhibit treatment response but still have anxiety symptoms and social and functional impairment. Remission is a more rigorous treatment goal that requires a HAM-A score of ≤7 or reduction of at least 70% in baseline levels of symptoms.

## REFERENCES


1. Hamilton M. Hamilton Anxiety Scale. In: Guy W, ed. ECDEU Assessment Manual for Psychopharmacology. Rockville, MD, US Department of Health, Education, Welfare, 1976:193–198.
2. Bandelow B, Zohar J, Hollander E, Kasper S, Moller H, WFSBP Task Force on Treatment Guidelines for Anxiety, Obsessive–Compulsive and Post-Traumatic Stress Disorders. World Federation of Societies of Biological Psychiatry (WFSBP) guidelines for the pharmacological treatment of anxiety, obsessive–compulsive and post-traumatic stress disorders—first revision. World J Biol Psychiatry 2008;9(4):248–312.
3. McIntosh A, Cohen A, Turnbull N, et al. Clinical guidelines and evidence review for panic disorder and generalised anxiety disorder. 2004. Sheffield/London, University of Sheffield/National Collaborating Centre for Primary Care. Available at: *http://www.nice.org.uk/nicemedia/pdf/cg022fullguideline.pdf*. Accessed May 1, 2010.
4. International Psychopharmacology Algorithm Project (IPAP). GAD Algorithm Notes & References and Flowchart. 2006. Available at: *http://www.ipap.org/gad/index.php*. Accessed May 1, 2010.
5. Baldwin DS, Anderson IM, Nutt DJ, et al. Evidence-based guidelines for the pharmacological treatment of anxiety disorders: recommendations from the British Association for Psychopharmacology. J Psychopharm 2005;19:567–596.
6. Bech P. Dose–response relationship of pregabalin in patients with generalized anxiety disorder. A pooled analysis of four placebo-controlled trials. Pharmacopsychiatry 2007;40(4):163–168.
7. Bandelow B, Chouinard G, Bobes J, et al. Extended-release quetiapine fumarate (quetiapine XR): a once-daily monotherapy effective in generalized anxiety disorder. Data from a randomized, double-blind, placebo- and active-controlled study. Int J Neuropsychopharmacol 2010;13(3):305–320.
8. Connor KM, Payne V, Davidson JR. Kava in generalized anxiety disorder: three placebo-controlled trials. Int Clin Psychopharmacol 2006;21:249–253.
9. Katzman MA. Current considerations in the treatment of generalized anxiety disorder. CNS Drugs 2009;23(2):103–120.

## APPENDIX A

## The results of the HAM-A Scale (ECDEU version)[1] for this patient:

Mark and score as follows: 0, not present; 1, mild; 2, moderate; 3, severe; 4, very severe

**Anxious mood**

__4__ Worries, anticipation of the worst, fearful anticipation, irritability

**Tension**

__3__ Feelings of tension, fatigability, startle response, moved to tears easily, trembling, feelings of restlessness, inability to relax

**Fears**

__1__ Of dark, of strangers, of being left alone, of animals, of traffic, of crowds

**Insomnia**

__4__ Difficulty in falling asleep, broken sleep, unsatisfying sleep and fatigue on waking, dreams, nightmares, night terrors

**Intellectual**

__3__ Difficulty in concentration, poor memory

**Depressed mood**

__1__ Loss of interest, lack of pleasure in hobbies, depression, early waking, diurnal swing

**Somatic (muscular)**

__3__ Pains and aches, twitchings, stiffness, myoclonic jerks, grinding of teeth, unsteady voice, increased muscular tone

**Somatic (sensory)**

__1__ Tinnitus, blurring of vision, hot and cold flushes, feelings of weakness, pricking sensation

**Cardiovascular symptoms**

__2__ Tachycardia, palpitations, pain in chest, throbbing of vessels, fainting feelings, sighing, dyspnea

**Respiratory symptoms**

__1__ Pressure or constriction in chest, choking feelings, sighing, dyspnea

**Gastrointestinal symptoms**

__3__ Difficulty in swallowing, wind, abdominal pain, burning sensations, abdominal fullness, nausea, vomiting, borborygmi, looseness of bowels, loss of weight, constipation

**Genitourinary symptoms**

__2__ Frequency of micturition, urgency of micturition, amenorrhea, menorrhagia, development of frigidity, premature ejaculation, loss of libido, impotence

**Autonomic symptoms**

__3__ Dry mouth, flushing, pallor, tendency to sweat, giddiness, tension, headache, raising of hair

**Behavior at interview**

__3__ Fidgeting, restlessness or pacing, tremor of hands, furrowed brow, strained face, sighing or rapid respiration, facial pallor, swallowing, etc.

**Total score:** __34__

# 80

# OBSESSIVE–COMPULSIVE DISORDER

Five Is the Magic Number . . . . . . . . . . . . . . . . . Level I

**Sarah T. Melton, PharmD, BCPP, CGP**

**Cynthia K. Kirkwood, PharmD, BCPP**

## LEARNING OBJECTIVES

After completing this case study, the reader should be able to:

- Identify target symptoms associated with obsessive–compulsive disorder (OCD).
- Construct goals of pharmacotherapy for OCD.
- Recommend nonpharmacologic therapies for OCD.
- Develop an appropriate pharmacotherapy plan and duration of therapy for the management of OCD.
- Counsel patients and consult with providers about the pharmacotherapy used for OCD.
- Develop a monitoring plan for a patient treated for OCD based on the treatment regimen.

## PATIENT PRESENTATION

### Chief Complaint

"I am so afraid that I'm going to hurt my child."

### HPI

Sonya Reed is a 30-year-old woman presenting to her family physician accompanied by her mother after threatening to overdose on Benadryl. The patient has complaints of anxiety and feelings of unease that were increasing in severity over the past 2 weeks to the point that she had thoughts of killing herself. She reports having intrusive thoughts of throwing her 2-year-old child down the stairs. Because these thoughts are becoming more frequent, she feels she is a bad mother and may actually harm her child. She recently started checking all appliances in the house multiple times during the day to make sure they are turned off because she fears starting a fire that will injure the child. At first, she incessantly checked on the toddler but now is beginning to avoid the child because of her fears. She states that she knows that these thoughts are irrational. She is concerned because the checking behavior consumes 2–3 hours each day. She stopped going out with the child last week because she has to check and recheck the car seat safety belts so often that she usually does not make it to her destination. She also reports rubbing her arm in multiples of 5 to feel some relief from the overwhelming anxiety that develops throughout the day from the intrusive thoughts. She states that she has tried to hide this behavior from her parents, but it has become so time-consuming and distressful that she felt the only way out was to overdose. She now regrets ever thinking about killing herself.

### PMH

$G_2P_1A_1$—normal spontaneous vaginal delivery
Obesity
Kidney stone at age 25 years
Dental surgery 2 months ago

### PPH

No hospitalizations or outpatient psychiatric treatment, but she recalls from childhood doing strange counting rituals while lying in bed or watching TV. She has always felt a need to "control things."

### FH

Father, 68 years old, with history of major depression. Mother, 65 years old, with multiple sclerosis. Older brother is a "perfectionist" and has to have everything "just right."

### SH

Divorced for 7 years and recently broke up with boyfriend of 2 years about a month ago; degree in hotel restaurant management and works part-time at a local hotel; denies tobacco use but admits to occasional alcohol use. After her son was born she had excessive worrying that the baby was starving because he was not getting enough breast milk. She does not have prescription coverage.

### Meds

Multivitamin, one po daily.
Acetaminophen 500 mg po PRN headaches (patient uses one to two times per month).
Diphenhydramine 25 mg po PRN insomnia (patient uses three to four times per month).

### All

Sulfa (hives), adhesive bandages

### ROS

Unremarkable except patient reports that she feels she is "going insane" and has guilt over her obsessions. Patient denies fatigue, change in appetite, sleep pattern, difficulty concentrating, and crying spells. No palpitations or dyspnea.

### Physical Examination

*Gen*

Anxious, obese woman sitting on examination table rubbing her arm up and down, cooperative, oriented × 3

*VS*

BP 120/75, P 90, RR 19, T 36.5°C; Wt 80.3 kg, Ht 5′4″

*Skin*

Left arm red and slightly inflamed from elbow to wrist; no rashes, lesions, or track marks. Warm to touch.

*HEENT*

EOMI; PEERLA; fundi benign; ear and nose clear; dentition intact; tonsils 1+

*Neck/Lymph Nodes*

Supple, no lymphadenopathy; thyroid symmetric and of normal size

*Lungs/Chest*

Symmetric chest wall movement, BS equal bilaterally, no rub; clear to A & P

*Breasts*

Normal, expecting menstruation

*CV*

RRR, normal $S_1$ and $S_2$, no MRG

*Abd*

Symmetric; NTND; normal BS; no organomegaly or masses

*Gyn*

Normal hair distribution and external genitalia; normal urethra; parous cervix with no lesions or discharge; uterus normal; no adnexal masses or tenderness

*MS/Ext*

Small frame; normal bones, joints, muscles

*Neuro*

CNs II–XII intact; motor and sensory grossly normal; coordination intact; no tremor

*MSE*

*Appearance and behavior:* well groomed, poor eye contact, rubbing arm up and down in a slow methodical manner
*Speech:* well spoken, coherent with normal rate and rhythm
*Mood:* anxious, worried that she is a "bad mother"
*Affect:* anxious, frightened
*Thought processes:* linear, logical, and goal-directed
*Thought content:* negative for suicidal or homicidal ideations; positive for obsessions about harming her child; compulsions including checking and rubbing arm in multiples of 5; denies delusions and hallucinations
*Memory:* 3/3 at 0 minutes, 3/3 at 5 minutes (ball, pencil, chair); spelled "world" backwards
*Abstractions:* fair
*Judgment:* good by testing
*Insight:* good
Score on Yale–Brown Obsessive Compulsive Scale = 30 points

### Labs

| | |
|---|---|
| Na 140 mEq/L | Hgb 15.0 g/dL |
| K 3.7 mEq/L | Hct 40% |
| Cl 107 mEq/L | TSH 2.8 mIU/L |
| $CO_2$ 28 mEq/L | AST 28 IU/L |
| BUN 14 mg/dL | ALT 25 IU/L |
| SCr 0.8 mg/dL | Alk phos 42 IU/L |
| Glu 75 mg/dL | HCG negative |

### ECG

NSR; rate 88 bpm

### Urine Toxicology Screen

Negative

### Drug Levels

Acetaminophen 10 mcg/mL

### Assessment

OCD

### Plan

Start paroxetine 20 mg po daily.

## QUESTIONS

### Problem Identification

1.a. Create a list of the patient's drug therapy problems.

1.b. What information (signs, symptoms, laboratory values) indicates the presence or severity of OCD?

### Desired Outcome

2. What are the goals of pharmacotherapy for OCD in this case?

### Therapeutic Alternatives

3.a. What are the most appropriate nonpharmacologic therapies for this patient?

3.b. What pharmacotherapeutic alternatives are available for the treatment of OCD?

### Optimal Plan

4.a. What drug, dosage form, dose, schedule, and duration of therapy are best for this patient?

4.b. What pharmacotherapeutic alternatives would be appropriate if the optimal plan fails?

4.c. When is a patient with OCD considered to be "treatment-refractory?" What other pharmacologic alternatives are available if this patient is determined to be refractory to standard pharmacotherapy?

### Outcome Evaluation

5. Which clinical and laboratory parameters are necessary to evaluate the therapy for achievement of the desired therapeutic outcomes and to detect or prevent adverse effects?

### Patient Education

6. What information should be provided to the patient to enhance adherence, ensure successful therapy, and minimize adverse effects?

## FOLLOW-UP QUESTIONS

1. When is a decrease in the Y-BOCS score considered clinically significant?
2. If this patient had presented to the physician desiring to become pregnant after 6 months of pharmacotherapy, what would your recommendations be regarding pharmacotherapy?

## SELF-STUDY ASSIGNMENTS

1. Prepare a grid contrasting the pros and cons of each SSRI in the management of OCD.
2. Perform a literature search and write a short paper describing the symptoms of trichotillomania and the association with OCD. How is this disorder treated?

3. Discuss the pharmacotherapeutic agents used to augment antidepressant monotherapy in the treatment of OCD in patients who have a partial response.
4. Visit the Web site for the International OCD Foundation and review the patient brochure "What You Need to Know about Obsessive–Compulsive Disorder," especially the section on children and teens with OCD.

## CLINICAL PEARL

Higher dosages of antidepressant medication than those typically used for depression are often required to obtain antiobsessional effects. A response to pharmacotherapy may not occur until a therapeutic dose has been maintained for at least 10–12 weeks.

## REFERENCES

1. Goodman WK, Price LH, Rasmussen SA, et al. The Yale–Brown Obsessive Compulsive Scale I. Development, use, and reliability. Arch Gen Psychiatry 1989;46:1006–1011.
2. Kamath, P, Reddy YC, Kandavel T. Suicidal behavior in obsessive–compulsive disorder. J Clin Psychiatry 2007;68:1741–1750.
3. Jenike MA. Obsessive–compulsive disorder. N Engl J Med 2004;350: 259–265.
4. American Psychiatric Association. Practice Guideline for the Treatment of Patients with Obsessive–Compulsive Disorder. Arlington, VA, American Psychiatric Association, 2007. Available at: *http//www.psych.org/psych_pract/treatg/pg/prac_guide.cfm*. Accessed August 19, 2010.
5. Denys D. Pharmacotherapy of obsessive–compulsive disorder and obsessive–compulsive spectrum disorders. Psychiatr Clin North Am 2006;29:553–584.
6. Maina G, Albert U, Salvi V, Bogetto F. Weight gain during long-term treatment of obsessive–compulsive disorder: a prospective comparison between serotonin reuptake inhibitors. J Clin Psychiatry 2004;65: 1365–1371.
7. Hollander E, Allen A, Steiner M, Wheadon DE, Oakes R, Burnham DB. Acute and long-term treatment of prevention of relapse of obsessive–compulsive disorder with paroxetine. J Clin Psychiatry 2003;64: 1113–1121.
8. Phelps NJ, Cates ME. The role of venlafaxine in the treatment of obsessive–compulsive disorder. Ann Pharmacother 2005;39:136–140.

# 81

# INSOMNIA

Poor Adherence and Poor Sleep. . . . . . . . . . . Level II

**Mollie Ashe Scott, PharmD, BCPS, CPP**

**Amy M. Lugo, PharmD, BCPS, BC-ADM**

## LEARNING OBJECTIVES

After completing this case study, the reader should be able to:

- Identify the psychosocial, disease-related, and drug-induced causes of insomnia.
- Explain the impact of poor medication adherence on chronic illnesses.
- Educate a patient regarding nonpharmacologic treatments for insomnia.
- Design a therapeutic plan for treatment of insomnia.

## PATIENT PRESENTATION

### Chief Complaint

"I can't sleep."

### HPI

Jenny Moore is a 48-year-old woman who is referred by her family medicine physician to a Pharmacotherapy Clinic for medication therapy management for insomnia. She receives help paying for her medications from medication assistance programs. She reports that she is unable to sleep at all during the week and then sleeps all day on Sunday. Ms Moore is currently taking temazepam 30 mg daily at bedtime that was recently increased from 15 mg. She is also experiencing depression due to an abusive relationship with her boyfriend as well as lack of current employment. Her most recent Patient Heath Questionnaire-9 (PHQ-9) result was 20. She admits to being nonadherent to her medication regimen.

### PMH

Insomnia for many years
COPD
Depression
Migraine headaches
GERD
Allergic rhinitis

### FH

Mother is alive and well and lives nearby.

### SH

Single, lives with her abusive boyfriend. Unemployed, but receives some money from her mother. She smokes approximately five cigarettes per day, but has smoked up to two ppd in the past. She denies alcohol use. She sees a deacon at her church to discuss depressive issues. She receives medication assistance for several of her medications from a local agency.

### Medications

Temazepam 30 mg po QHS PRN sleep
Fluticasone/salmeterol DPI 250/50, one inhalation BID
Albuterol MDI, two puffs Q 6 hours PRN SOB
Tiotropium DPI, one inhalation daily
Citalopram 20 mg po Q AM
Olanzapine 3 mg/fluoxetine 25 mg po Q PM
Sumatriptan 100 mg po PRN migraine
Atenolol 25 mg po Q AM for migraine prophylaxis
Dexlansoprazole 60 mg po Q AM
Ibuprofen 200–400 mg po Q 6 hours PRN pain
Tramadol 50 mg po Q 6 hours PRN pain
Pseudoephedrine 30 mg po Q 6 hours PRN allergies

### Allergies

NKDA

### ROS

Patient reports that she does not sleep during the week and only sleeps on Sunday. She reports poor sleep hygiene, because she reads and watches television in bed. She drinks a great deal of caffeine throughout the day and really does not pay attention to how late she eats or exercises. Patient reports difficulty going to sleep and staying asleep, and she reports having had this problem for several years. Additionally, the temazepam does not seem to help much. She has a long history of depression but has never been hospitalized. She currently denies a "blue mood" or any thoughts of suicide, and her PHQ-9 score today is 20. She currently takes citalopram and the combination olanzapine/fluoxetine to help with her depressive symptoms. Her COPD is secondary to a long history of smoking but is currently controlled on tiotropium, fluticasone/salmeterol, and albuterol PRN. She has experienced migraine headaches for several years and uses sumatriptan and ibuprofen PRN and atenolol daily for prophylaxis. Her GERD, which she experiences when she is supine, is currently controlled on dexlansoprazole. She has runny nose, congestion, and itchy eyes in the spring.

### Physical Examination (From the Last Visit With Her PCP)

*Gen*

Obese woman in NAD who looks her stated age

*VS*

BP 125/80, P 76, RR 16, T 37°C; Wt 105 kg; Ht 5′6″

*Skin*

Normal skin color and turgor, no lesions noted

*HEENT*

Normocephalic, PERRLA, EOMI

*Neck/Lymph Nodes*

Supple with normal size thyroid, (–) adenopathy

*Lungs*

CTA bilaterally

*CV*

Normal $S_1$, $S_2$; no MRG

*Abd*

NTND, no HSM

*Genit/Rect*

Deferred

*Ext*

No C/C/E; normal muscle bulk and tone; muscle strength 5/5 and equal in all extremities; normal pulses

*Neuro*

Oriented to person, place, and time; CN II–XII intact; Mini-Mental State Examination results: 30/30

### Labs

| | | | |
|---|---|---|---|
| Na 140 mEq/L | Hgb 14 g/dL | AST 34 IU/L | *Lipid panel:* |
| K 4.2 mEq/L | Hct 43% | ALT 32 IU/L | TC 212 mg/dL |
| Cl 105 mEq/L | RBC 4.7 × $10^6$/mm$^3$ | LDH 112 IU/L | LDL 135 mg/dL |
| $CO_2$ 28 mEq/L | Plt 262 × $10^3$/mm$^3$ | GGT 47 IU/L | HDL 45 mg/dL |
| BUN 11 mg/dL | WBC 6.2 × $10^3$/mm$^3$ | T. bili 0.3 mg/dL | TG 160 mg/dL |
| SCr 0.8 mg/dL | TSH 3.9 mIU/L | T. prot 7.1 g/dL | |
| Glu 82 mg/dL | Free $T_4$ 4.1 ng/dL | Alb 4.0 g/dL | |

### Assessment

1. Insomnia uncontrolled with temazepam, poor sleep hygiene
2. Depression
3. Migraine headaches
4. COPD, currently controlled
5. GERD, current controlled
6. Nonadherence
7. Allergic rhinitis
8. Health maintenance issues

## QUESTIONS

### Problem Identification

1.a. Create a drug-related problem list for the patient.

1.b. Which information (signs, symptoms, laboratory values) indicates the presence or severity of insomnia?

1.c. Could any of the patient's problems have been caused by drug therapy?

1.d. What additional information is needed to satisfactorily assess this patient's insomnia?

### Desired Outcome

2. What are the goals of pharmacotherapy in this case?

### Therapeutic Alternatives

3.a. What nonpharmacologic therapies might be useful for this patient's insomnia?

3.b. What feasible pharmacotherapeutic alternatives are available for treatment of insomnia?

### Optimal Plan

4.a. What drug, dosage form, dose, schedule, and duration of therapy are best for this patient's insomnia?

4.b. What alternatives would be appropriate if the initial therapy fails or cannot be used?

### Outcome Evaluation

5. Which clinical and laboratory parameters are necessary to evaluate the therapy for achievement of the desired therapeutic outcome and to detect or prevent adverse effects?

### Patient Education

6. What information should be provided to the patient to enhance adherence, ensure successful therapy, and minimize adverse effects?

## FOLLOW-UP QUESTION

1. What other medication adjustments should be made at this time?

## SELF-STUDY ASSIGNMENTS

1. Discuss clinical pharmacy interventions that can improve medication adherence.
2. Explain important monitoring parameters for patients receiving atypical antipsychotics.

## CLINICAL PEARL

Patients with underlying depression frequently have insomnia, and poor medication adherence to antidepressants can exacerbate sleep disorders.

## ACKNOWLEDGMENT

Special thanks to Rachel Selinger, PharmD, for her contribution in the initial development of this case.

## REFERENCES

1. Morin A, Jarvis C, Lynch A. Therapeutic options for sleep-maintenance and sleep-onset insomnia. Pharmacotherapy 2007;27:89–110.
2. National Sleep Foundation. Available at: *http://www.sleepfoundation.org/article/sleep-topics/healthy-sleep-tips*. Accessed April 14, 2010.
3. Ramakrishnan K, Scheid D. Treatment options for insomnia. Am Fam Physician 2007;76:517–526.
4. Fick DM, Cooper JW, Wade WE, et al. Updating the Beers' Criteria for potentially inappropriate medication use in older adults. Results of a U.S. consensus panel of experts. Arch Intern Med 2003;163:2716–2724.
5. Montplaisir J, Hawa R, Moller C, et al. Zopiclone and zaleplon vs benzodiazepines in the treatment of insomnia. Canadian consensus statement. Hum Psychopharmacol 2003;18:29–38.
6. US Food and Drug Administration Center for Drug Evaluation and Research. Sleep Disorder (Sedative–Hypnotic) Drug Information. Available at: *http://www.fda.gov/Drugs/DrugSafety/PostmarketDrugSafetyInformationforPatientsandProviders/ucm101557.htm*. Accessed April 14, 2010.
7. ADA, American Psychiatric Association, American Association of Clinical Endocrinologists, North American Association for the Study of Obesity. Consensus development conference on antipsychotic drugs and obesity and diabetes. Diabetes Care 2004;27:596–601.
8. Trivedi MH, Fava M, Wisniewski SR, et al. Medication augmentation after the failure of SSRIs for depression. N Engl J Med 2006;354:1243–1252.

# SECTION 8
# ENDOCRINOLOGIC DISORDERS

## 82

## TYPE 1 DIABETES MELLITUS AND KETOACIDOSIS

Disconnected . . . . . . . . . . . . . . . . . . . . . . . . . . Level II

Holly S. Divine, PharmD, CGP, CDE

Carrie L. Johnson, PharmD, CDE

## LEARNING OBJECTIVES

After completing this case study, the reader should be able to:

- Recognize signs and symptoms of diabetic ketoacidosis (DKA).
- Determine laboratory parameters for the diagnosis and monitoring of DKA.
- Identify anticipated fluid and electrolyte abnormalities associated with DKA and their treatment.
- Recommend appropriate insulin therapy for treating DKA.
- Identify therapeutic decision points in DKA treatment and provide parameters for altering therapy at those points.

## PATIENT PRESENTATION

### Chief Complaint

"I felt weak and nauseated during softball practice. I checked my blood glucose and it read 'HI.'"

### HPI

Mary McGee is a 21-year-old woman with a history of type 1 diabetes, diagnosed 3 years ago. She is a college senior at the local university where she also plays softball. She started using an insulin pump approximately 6 months ago.

She noticed she was unusually tired and short of breath at the beginning of her practice and then began feeling weak and nauseated. She was also very thirsty during practice. Her softball coach said she seemed "a little confused." He advised her to check her blood glucose and it read HI. She checked her insulin pump and noticed the pump had become disconnected. She is unsure how long she has been without insulin. She vomited × 2 since shortly thereafter and was transported via emergency medical services to the emergency department.

### PMH

Type 1 DM diagnosed 3 years ago

### FH

Parents are alive and healthy. One twin sister who also has type 1 diabetes.

### SH

College student; no tobacco, alcohol, or illicit drug use

### Meds

NovoLog 100 U/mL, per insulin pump  
*Basal rates:*  
0.6 U/h 0000–0300  
0.9 U/h 0300–0700  
0.8 U/h 0700–1100  
0.7 U/h 1100–1730  
0.8 U/h 1730–0000  
Correction factor: 1 U:40 mg/dL >120 mg/dL  
*Insulin:carbohydrate ratios:*  
1:10 insulin:carbohydrate before breakfast  
1:15 insulin:carbohydrate before lunch and dinner  
Glucagon injection kit, as needed

### Allergies

NKDA

### ROS

Complains of blurry vision, lethargy, shortness of breath, nausea, polyuria, and polydipsia. Denies constipation, diarrhea, and headache.

### Physical Examination

#### *Gen*

WDWN Caucasian female appearing her stated age, with deep respirations, ketones on her breath, and slurred speech; slightly confused, but responds appropriately to questions

#### *VS*

BP 101/72, P 123, RR 32, T 37.0°C; Wt 56 kg, Ht 5′6″

#### *Skin*

Unremarkable

#### *HEENT*

PERRLA, EOMI; mucous membranes are dry

#### *Neck/Lymph Nodes*

Supple without lymphadenopathy or thyromegaly

#### *Lungs*

CTA, Kussmaul respirations

#### *CV*

$S_1$ and $S_2$ are normal without $S_3$, $S_4$, murmur or rub; RRR

**TABLE 82-1 Lab Values**

| | |
|---|---|
| 136 mEq/L | $16.0 \times 10^3/mm^3$ |
| 4.8 Eq/L | $4.61 \times 10^6/mm^3$ |
| 101 mEq/L | 14.2 g/dL |
| 10 mEq/L | 40.7% |
| 23 mg/dL | $239 \times 10^3/mm^3$ |
| 1.4 mg/dL | Positive |
| 479 mg/dL | |

*Abd*

NT/ND

*Genit/Rect*

Deferred

*MS/Ext*

No edema, pulses 2+ throughout, mild calluses

*Neuro*

A & O × 3; DTRs 2+ throughout; feet with normal sensation and vibration

■ Labs

| | |
|---|---|
| Na | WBC |
| K | RBC |
| Cl | Hgb |
| $CO_2$ | Hct |
| BUN | Platelets |
| SCr | Ketones |
| Glu | |

■ ABG

pH 7.26; $pCO_2$ 21 mm Hg; $pO_2$ 128 mm Hg; $HCO_3$ 7.1 mEq/L; oxygen sat 97%

■ UA

(+) Ketones; (+) glucose

■ Chest X-Ray

Normal

■ ECG

Sinus tachycardia

■ Assessment

DKA precipitated by insulin deficiency

## QUESTIONS

### Problem Identification

1.a. What signs, symptoms, and laboratory findings indicate the presence and severity of DKA in this patient?

1.b. What are the precipitating risk factors for DKA, and which of those risk factors are present in this patient?

1.c. What are the diagnostic criteria for DKA?

1.d. What problems need to be addressed in DKA besides hyperglycemia?

### Desired Outcome

2. What are the goals of therapy for this patient?

### Therapeutic Alternatives

3. What therapies are available to correct the metabolic derangements of DKA?

### Optimal Plan

4. Design a pharmacotherapeutic plan to resolve this patient's DKA.

### Outcome Evaluation

5.a. What monitoring is necessary for the therapeutic plan that you developed for the patient?

5.b. What if glucose does not fall by at least 10% in the first hour? Provide the rationale for your answer. What changes in the therapeutic regimen should be considered when the blood glucose drops below 200 mg/dL?

5.c. At what point is the DKA considered to be resolved, and when can IV insulin therapy be converted to subcutaneous therapy?

5.d. Outline a plan for converting the patient from IV to subcutaneous insulin after resolution of the DKA.

### Patient Education

6. What additional counseling or interventions should occur with this patient regarding prevention of future DKA?

## ■ SELF-STUDY ASSIGNMENTS

1. What does the American Diabetes Association state about DKA and hyperosmolar hyperglycemic nonketotic syndrome (HHS) in patients with type 2 diabetes? Compare these two disorders with respect to prevention, precipitating causes, signs and symptoms, pathophysiology, and treatment.
2. Investigate other causes of DKA, such as illness, and write a sick day management plan for this patient.

## CLINICAL PEARL

DKA is the second most common complication seen with insulin pump therapy. Young persons who have recurrent DKA should be evaluated for psychological problems, including eating disorders, as a potential contributing factor.

## REFERENCES

1. Kitabchi AE, Umpierrez GE, Miles JM, Fisher JN. Hyperglycemic crises in adult patients with diabetes. Diabetes Care 2009;32:1335–1343.
2. Wilson JF. In clinic. Diabetic ketoacidosis. Ann Intern Med 2010;152(January):ITC 1-1–ITC 1-16.
3. American Diabetes Association clinical practice recommendations. Diabetes Care 2010;33:S11–S61.
4. American College of Endocrinology consensus statement on guidelines for glycemic control. Endocr Pract 2002;8(Suppl 1):January/February.
5. Umpierriez GE, Cuervo R, Karabell A, Latif K, Freire AX, Kitabchi AE. Treatment of diabetic ketoacidosis with subcutaneous insulin aspart. Diabetes Care 2004;27:1873–1878.
6. Potti LG, Haines ST. Continuous subcutaneous insulin infusion therapy: a primer on insulin pumps. J Am Pharm Assoc 2009;49:e1–e17.

# 83

# TYPE 2 DIABETES MELLITUS: NEW ONSET

The Candy Man . . . . . . . . . . . . . . . . . . . . . . . . Level II

**Scott R. Drab, PharmD, CDE, BC-ADM**

**Deanne L. Hall, PharmD, CDE**

## LEARNING OBJECTIVES

After completing this case study, the reader should be able to:

- Recognize the signs, symptoms, and risk factors associated with type 2 diabetes mellitus (DM).
- Identify the comorbidities in type 2 DM associated with insulin resistance (metabolic syndrome).
- Compare the pharmacotherapeutic options in the management of type 2 DM including mechanism of action, contraindications, and side effects.
- Describe the role of self-monitoring of blood glucose (SMBG) and identify factors to enhance patient adherence.
- Develop a patient-specific pharmacotherapeutic plan for the treatment and monitoring of type 2 DM.

## PATIENT PRESENTATION

### Chief Complaint

"My vision has been blurred lately and it seems to be getting worse."

### HPI

Alfonso Giuliani is a 68-year-old man who presents to his family physician's office complaining of periodic blurred vision for the past month. He further complains of fatigue and lack of energy that prohibits him from working in his garden.

### PMH

HTN × 18 years
Dyslipidemia × 8 years
Gouty arthritis × 16 years with complicated course of uric acid urolithiasis
Hypothyroidism × 15 years
Obesity × 25 years

### FH

Diabetes present in mother. A.G. immigrated to the United States with his mother and sister after their father died suddenly for unknown reasons at age 45. One younger sibling died of breast cancer at age 48.

### SH

Retired candy salesman, married × 46 years with three children. No tobacco use. Drinks one to two glasses of homemade wine with meals. He reports compliance with his medications.

### Meds

Lisinopril 20 mg po once daily
Allopurinol 300 mg po once daily
Levothyroxine 0.088 mg po once daily

### All

NKDA

### ROS

Occasional polydipsia, polyphagia, fatigue, weakness, and blurred vision. Denies chest pain, dyspnea, tachycardia, dizziness or lightheadedness on standing, tingling or numbness in extremities, leg cramps, peripheral edema, changes in bowel movements, GI bloating or pain, nausea or vomiting, urinary incontinence, or presence of skin lesions.

### Physical Examination

*Gen*

The patient is a centrally obese, Caucasian man who appears to be restless and in mild distress.

*VS*

BP 124/76 without orthostasis; P 80; RR 18; T 37.2°C; Wt 77 kg; Ht 66″; BMI 27.4 kg/m$^2$

*Skin*

Dry with poor skin turgor; no ulcers or rash

*HEENT*

PERRLA; EOMI; TMs intact; no hemorrhages or exudates on funduscopic examination; mucous membranes normal; nose and throat clear w/o exudates or lesions

*Neck/LN*

Supple; without lymphadenopathy, thyromegaly, or JVD

*CV*

RRR; normal $S_1$ and $S_2$; no $S_3$, $S_4$, rubs, murmurs, or bruits

*Lungs*

CTA

*Abd*

Soft, NT, central obesity; normal BS; no organomegaly or distention

*GU/Rect*

Normal external male genitalia

*Ext*

Normal ROM and sensation; peripheral pulses 2+ throughout; no lesions, ulcers, or edema

*Neuro*

A & O × 3, CN II–XII intact; DTRs 2+ throughout; feet with normal vibratory and pinprick sensation (5.07/10 g monofilament)

### Labs

| | | |
|---|---|---|
| Na 141 mEq/L | Ca 9.9 mg/dL | A1C 7.8% |
| K 4.0 mEq/L | Phos 3.2 mg/dL | *Fasting lipid profile* |
| Cl 96 mEq/L | AST 21 IU/L | T. chol 280 mg/dL |

| | | |
|---|---|---|
| $CO_2$ 22 mEq/L | ALT 15 IU/L | HDL 27 mg/dL |
| BUN 24 mg/dL | Alk phos 45 IU/L | LDL 193 mg/dL |
| SCr 1.1 mg/dL | T. bili 0.9 mg/dL | Trig 302 mg/dL |
| Random Glu 202 mg/dL | | |

### UA

(–) Ketones, (–) protein, (–) microalbuminuria

### Assessment

1. Elevated random glucose and A1C, diagnostic for type 2 DM, new onset
2. Dyslipidemia requiring treatment
3. Hypertension apparently well controlled
4. Obesity
5. Gouty arthritis; patient claims not to have had an acute attack in over 3 years; will obtain a uric acid level to evaluate
6. Hypothyroidism; will obtain a thyroid panel to evaluate

## CLINICAL COURSE

The patient returned to clinic 3 days later for lab work, which revealed: TSH 1.8 mIU/L, free $T_4$ 1.2 ng/dL, UA 1.2 mg/dL, and FBG 157 mg/dL.

## QUESTIONS

### Problem Identification

1.a. What risk factors for type 2 DM are present in this patient?

1.b. What information (signs, symptoms, laboratory values) supports the diagnosis of type 2 DM?

1.c. What information indicates the presence of insulin resistance?

1.d. Create a list of this patient's drug therapy problems.

### Desired Outcome

2.a. What are the desired goals for the treatment of this patient's diabetes?

2.b. Considering his other medical problems, what other treatment goals should be established?

### Therapeutic Alternatives

3.a. What nonpharmacologic therapies might be useful in the management of this patient?

3.b. What feasible pharmacotherapeutic alternatives are available for the treatment of this patient's DM? Identify the factors that will influence your choice of initial therapy.

### Optimal Plan

4.a. Outline a complete pharmacotherapeutic plan to manage this patient's current problems including drug, dosage form, dose, schedule, and rationale for your selections.

4.b. What changes in therapy would you recommend if your initial plan fails to achieve adequate glycemic control?

### Outcome Evaluation

5.a. What clinical and laboratory parameters will you monitor to evaluate glycemic efficacy and to detect or prevent adverse effects?

5.b. The patient's physician suggested that he obtain a blood glucose meter for self-testing. What are the health care provider's responsibilities with respect to patients and SMBG?

5.c. Identify at least four potential situations in which the information provided by SMBG would be useful to patients and health care providers.

5.d. What factors should be considered in the selection of an appropriate blood glucose meter?

### Patient Education

6.a. What information should be provided to the patient about diabetes and its treatment to enhance adherence, ensure successful therapy, minimize adverse effects, and prevent future complications?

6.b. How would you educate the patient regarding how and when to check his blood glucose?

## FOLLOW-UP QUESTIONS

1. Which nonprescription products could be recommended for patients to use in treating hypoglycemic episodes?
2. List several potential sources of error in SMBG.
3. When starting patients on insulin, the use of combination oral antihyperglycemic agents and insulin offers several advantages over switching entirely to insulin:
   (a) What are the advantages of adding insulin to existing therapies with oral agents?
   (b) List an appropriate method of starting insulin therapy to adequately control fasting hyperglycemia in patients on combination oral agents.

## SELF-STUDY ASSIGNMENTS

1. Describe how you would evaluate and monitor this patient's quality of life.
2. Characterize the relationship between insulin resistance and the risk for atherosclerotic vascular disease.
3. Prepare a list of medications that have been associated with increasing blood glucose. Provide literature evidence on the strength of the association with each medication.
4. Review the literature and conduct a comparative review of the efficacy of inhaled insulin therapy relative to the insulin products commercially available for subcutaneous injection.

## CLINICAL PEARL

Approximately 24 million Americans have diabetes, and approximately one fourth are undiagnosed. From 1990 to 2003, the CDC reported that the number of Americans with diabetes rose 94%, providing further evidence that diabetes is a major public health threat of epidemic proportions. Excess caloric intake, low physical activity, and increasing levels of obesity are the main contributors to the increased incidence.

## REFERENCES

1. American Diabetes Association. Standards of medical care in diabetes—2007. Diabetes Care 2007;30(Suppl 1):S4–S41.
2. American Diabetes Association. Diagnosis and classification of diabetes mellitus. Diabetes Care 2007;30(Suppl 1):S42–S47.

3. Frohlich M, Imhof A, Berg G, et al. Association between C-reactive protein and features of the metabolic syndrome: a population-based study. Diabetes Care 2000;23:1835–1839.
4. Bloomgarden ZT. Insulin resistance: current concepts. Clin Ther 1998;20:216–231.
5. American College of Endocrinology, American Association of Clinical Endocrinologists. Medical guidelines for the management of diabetes mellitus: the AACE system of intensive diabetes self-management. Endocr Pract 2002;8(Suppl 1).
6. Grundy SM, Cleeman JI, Merz CN, et al. Implications of recent clinical trials for the National Cholesterol Education Program Adult Treatment Panel III guidelines. Circulation 2004;110:227–239.
7. American Diabetes Association. Evidence-based nutrition principles and recommendations for the treatment and prevention of diabetes and related complications. Diabetes Care 2003;26(Suppl 1): S51–S61.
8. Byetta Prescribing Information. San Diego, CA, Amylin Pharmaceuticals, February 2007.
9. Januvia Prescribing Information. Whitehouse Station, NJ, Merck & Co, 2006.
10. Oki J, Isley WL. Diabetes mellitus. In: Dipiro JT, et al, eds. Pharmacotherapy: A Pathophysiologic Approach, 6th ed. New York, McGraw-Hill, 2004.
11. American Diabetes Association. The pharmacological treatment of hyperglycemia in NIDDM. Diabetes Care 1996;19(Suppl 1):S54–S61.
12. Lanham MSM, Lebovic DI, Domino SE. Contemporary medical therapy for polycystic ovary syndrome. J Gynecol Obstet 2006;95: 236–241.
13. American Diabetes Association. Hypertension management in adults with diabetes. Diabetes Care 2004;27(Suppl 1):S65–S67.
14. National Cholesterol Education Program (NCEP) Expert Panel. Executive summary of the third report of the NCEP Expert Panel on Detection, Evaluation, and Treatment of High Blood Cholesterol in Adults (Adults Treatment Panel III). JAMA 2001;285;2486–2497.
15. Garg A. Dyslipoproteinemia and diabetes. Endocrinol Metab Clin North Am 1998;27:613–625.
16. American Diabetes Association. Influenza and pneumococcal immunization in diabetes. Diabetes Care 2004;27(Suppl 1):S111–S113.
17. American Diabetes Association. Aspirin therapy in diabetes. Diabetes Care 2004;27(Suppl 1):S72–S73.

# 84

# TYPE 2 DIABETES MELLITUS (EXISTING DISEASE)

Establishing Optimal Control . . . . . . . . . . . . . . Level II

**Antoinette B. Coe, PharmD**

**Sharon B.S. Gatewood, PharmD**

## LEARNING OBJECTIVES

After completing this case study, the reader should be able to:

- Identify the goals of therapy for the treatment of type 2 diabetes mellitus (DM).
- Discuss the risk factors and comorbidities associated with type 2 DM.
- Compare options for drug therapy management of type 2 DM including mechanisms of action, combination therapies, comorbidities, and patient-friendly treatment plans.
- Develop an individualized drug therapy management plan including dosage regimens, therapeutic endpoints, and monitoring parameters.
- Provide patient education regarding medications and the importance of adhering to the treatment plan, monitoring the disease state, maintaining blood glucose control, and seeking advice from health care providers when necessary.

## PATIENT PRESENTATION

### Chief Complaint

"I have had diabetes for about six months and would like to have my blood sugar tested. I think that my blood sugar is running low because I have a terrible headache."

### HPI

Sarah Martin is a 45 yo woman who comes to the pharmacy for a diabetes education class taught by the pharmacist. She would like for the pharmacist to check her blood sugar before the class begins. She was diagnosed with type 2 DM about 6 months ago. She had been attempting to control her disease with diet and exercise, but had no success. Her physician started her on metformin 1,000 mg twice daily with food about 3 months ago. She has gained 10 lb over the past year. She monitors her blood sugar once a day, and her results have ranged from 215 to 280 mg/dL. Her fasting blood sugars have averaged 200 mg/dL.

### PMH

Type 2 DM × 6 months
HTN × 17 years
Bipolar disorder × 25 years
Dyslipidemia × 12 years
Morbid obesity × 20 years

### FH

Father has history of HTN, dyslipidemia, and bipolar disorder. Mother has a history of dyslipidemia and hypothyroidism. Brother has DM thought to be secondary to alcoholism.

### SH

S.M. has been married for 23 years. She has two children who are teenagers and one child in college. She works as a sales associate in the electronics department of a local mass merchandiser. She denies any use of tobacco products after stopping smoking 10 years ago, but does drink alcohol occasionally (three beers or glasses of wine per week).

### Meds

Metformin 1,000 mg po BID with food
Lisinopril 20 mg po once daily
Zyprexa 5 mg po QHS
Carbamazepine ER 200 mg po BID
Lorazepam 1 mg po TID PRN
Fluoxetine 20 mg po Q AM
EC ASA 81 mg po once daily
Pravastatin 40 mg PO once daily

### All

Penicillin—hives

### ROS

S.M. complains of nocturia, polyuria, and polydipsia on a daily basis. Denies nausea, constipation, diarrhea, signs or symptoms of hypoglycemia, paresthesias, and dyspnea.

### Physical Examination

*Gen*

WDWN severely obese, white woman in NAD

*VS*

BP 154/90, P 98, RR 18, T 37.0°C; Wt 109 kg, Ht 5′8″, waist circ 38 in

*HEENT*

PERRLA, EOMI, R & L fundus exam without retinopathy

*Neck/Lymph Nodes*

No LAN

*Lungs*

Clear to A & P

*CV*

RRR, no m/r/g

*Abd*

NT/ND

*Genit/Rect*

Deferred

*MS/Ext*

Carotids, femorals, popliteals, and right dorsalis pedis pulses 2+ throughout; left dorsalis pedis 1+; feet show mild calluses on MTPs

*Neuro*

DTRs 2+ throughout, feet with normal sensation (5.07 monofilament) and vibration

### Labs

| | | *Fasting lipid profile* |
|---|---|---|
| Na 138 mEq/L | Ca 9.4 mg/dL | T. chol 244 mg/dL |
| K 3.7 mEq/L | Phos 3.3 mg/dL | LDL 141 mg/dL |
| Cl 103 mEq/L | AST 16 IU/L | HDL 58 mg/dL |
| $CO_2$ 31 mEq/L | ALT 19 IU/L | Trig 225 mg/dL |
| BUN 16 mg/dL | Alk phos 62 IU/L | TC/HDL ratio 4.2 |
| SCr 0.9 mg/dL | T. bili 0.4 mg/dL | |
| Gluc (random) 243 mg/dL | A1C 10.0% | |

### UA

1+ protein, (+) microalbuminuria

### Assessment

The patient reports that she exercises at most once a week and her diet is difficult to maintain due to being busy with her children's schedules and having an erratic eating schedule at both work and home. Her glycemic control has worsened from an A1C of 8.9% 6 months ago. She has had a moderate weight gain of 10 lb over the past year. Her blood pressure and cholesterol are not at goal on the current drug therapy. Her bipolar disorder is controlled on the current drug therapy. When the patient is in a depression or manic phase, she tends to use food to "treat" the symptoms.

## QUESTIONS

### Problem Identification

1.a. What are this patient's drug therapy problems?

1.b. What findings indicate poorly controlled diabetes in this patient?

### Desired Outcome

2.a. What are the goals of treatment for type 2 diabetes in this patient?

2.b. What individual patient characteristics should be considered in determining the treatment goals?

### Therapeutic Alternatives

3.a. What nonpharmacologic interventions should be recommended for this patient's drug therapy problems?

3.b. What pharmacologic interventions could be considered for this patient's drug therapy problems?

### Optimal Plan

4. What pharmacotherapeutic regimen would you recommend for each of the patient's drug therapy problems?

### Outcome Evaluation

5. What parameters should be monitored to evaluate the efficacy and possible adverse effects associated with the optimal regimens you selected?

### Patient Education

6. What information should be given to the patient regarding DM, hypertension, dyslipidemia, bipolar disorder, obesity, and her treatment plan to increase adherence, minimize adverse effects, and improve outcomes?

## FOLLOW-UP QUESTION

1. What alternative therapies might be appropriate if the initial plan for diabetes treatment fails?

## SELF-STUDY ASSIGNMENTS

1. Discuss the phenomenon known as the metabolic syndrome and the role that insulin resistance is postulated to play in its sequelae.
2. Explore and discuss the importance of monitoring postprandial blood glucose levels and its impact on overall glucose control, A1C levels, and progression of diabetes complications.
3. Research the various blood glucose monitors available, and compare among available monitors the features that meet the needs of individual patients and improve adherence to testing regimens.
4. Research new therapies for diabetes and discuss their potential role in the management of patients with type 2 DM.
5. Keep a food diary, including carbohydrate counting for each meal, and exercise log for 1 week. Evaluate and discuss your experience from the viewpoint of a patient with type 2 DM.

6. Investigate continuous blood glucose monitoring systems (CGMS) technology and discuss the role of CGMS in a patient with type 2 DM.
7. Research and compare current insulin pumps in the market. Discuss the role of insulin pump therapy in a patient with type 2 DM and what patient characteristics make or eliminate the patient as an insulin pump candidate.

## CLINICAL PEARL

Although metformin is now considered the first-line therapy for a patient with type 2 diabetes, not all patients with type 2 diabetes are appropriate candidates for metformin. Metformin has several contraindications, and patients generally must have good renal, hepatic, cardiac, and respiratory function to be considered a candidate for metformin therapy. Thus, a thorough assessment of the patient's comorbid conditions must be made. Early initiation of insulin therapy in patients who do not meet target goals is recommended.

## REFERENCES


1. American Diabetes Association. Standards of medical care in diabetes. Diabetes Care 2010;33(Suppl 1):S11–S61.
2. Grundy SM, Cleeman JI, Merz CN, et al. Implications of recent clinical trials for the National Cholesterol Education Program Adult Treatment Panel III guidelines. Circulation 2004;110:227–239.
3. Expert Panel on Detection, Evaluation, Treatment of High Blood Cholesterol in Adults. Executive summary of the third report of the National Cholesterol Education Program (NCEP) Expert Panel on Detection, Evaluation, and Treatment of High Blood Cholesterol in Adults (Adult Treatment Panel III). JAMA 2001;285:2486–2497.
4. Joint National Committee on Prevention, Detection, Evaluation, Treatment of High Blood Pressure. The seventh report of the Joint National Committee on Prevention, Detection, Evaluation, Treatment of High Blood Pressure. Arch Intern Med 2003;42:1206–1252.
5. NHLBI Obesity Education Initiative Expert Panel on the Identification, Evaluation, and Treatment of Overweight and Obesity in Adults. NIH Publication No. 98-4083. National Institutes of Health, September 1998.
6. Haupt DW. Differential metabolic effects of antipsychotic treatments. Eur Neuropsychopharmacol 2006;16:S149–S155.
7. Koski RR. Practical review of oral antihyperglycemic agents for type 2 diabetes mellitus. Diabetes Educ 2006;32(2):869–876.
8. American Diabetes Association. Medical management of hyperglycemia in type 2 diabetes: a consensus algorithm for the initiation and adjustment of therapy. Diabetes Care 2009;32(1):193–203.
9. Pepine CJ, Handberg EM, Cooper-DeHoff RM. A calcium antagonist vs a noncalcium antagonist hypertension treatment strategy for patients with coronary artery disease: the International Verapamil–Trandolapril Study (INVEST): a randomized control trial. JAMA 2003;290: 2805–2816.
10. Colhoun HM, Betteridge DJ, Durrington PN, et al. Primary prevention of cardiovascular disease with atorvastatin in type 2 diabetes in the Collaborative Atorvastatin Diabetes Study (CARDS): multicentre randomised placebo-controlled trial. Lancet 2004;364: 685–696.
11. Collins R, Armitage J. Heart Protection Study Collaborative Group: MRC/BHF Heart Protection Study of cholesterol-lowering with simvastatin in 5963 people with diabetes: a randomised placebo-controlled trial. Lancet 2003;361:2005–2016.
12. Edwards SJ, Smith CJ. Tolerability of atypical antipsychotics in the treatment of adults with schizophrenia or bipolar disorder: a mixed treatment comparison of randomized controlled trials. Clin Ther 2009;31:1345–1359.


# 85

# HYPERTHYROIDISM: GRAVES' DISEASE

Gland Central . . . . . . . . . . . . . . . . . . . . . . . . . Level II

**Kristine S. Schonder, PharmD**

## LEARNING OBJECTIVES

After completing this case study, the reader should be able to:

- Describe the signs, symptoms, and laboratory parameters associated with hyperthyroidism and relate them to the pathophysiology of the disease.
- Select and justify appropriate patient-specific initial and follow-up pharmacotherapy for patients with hyperthyroidism.
- Develop a plan for monitoring the pharmacotherapy for hyperthyroidism.
- Provide appropriate education to patients receiving drug therapy for hyperthyroidism.

## PATIENT PRESENTATION

### Chief Complaint

"My heart feels like it is racing, and I feel jittery."

### HPI

Carrie Gibson is a 23-year-old woman who presents to her PCP with complaints of palpitations and a fine tremor. The palpitations started a few months ago and would come and go until the past week when they began occurring more frequently, almost daily. She denies CP. She reports that she began noticing a fine tremor approximately 3 weeks ago. She also reports loose stools and a 5-kg weight loss over the past 6 months, despite a good appetite and food intake. She feels hot all of the time and sweats a lot. She further states that she has been losing her hair recently and that she is more irritable than usual.

### PMH

She has been healthy up to this point with no medical conditions. She reports having had "the flu" last November, but states that she did not seek medical attention at that time.

### FH

Father has HTN; mother had a history of Graves' disease and passed away 1 year ago from breast CA at age 53. Her oldest sister is 32 years of age and has breast CA; she has two other sisters, ages 29 and 25, and one brother, age 27, all of whom are healthy. Her aunt (mother's sister) and grandmother both had Graves' disease.

### SH

She smokes 1.5 ppd × 5 years and drinks alcohol socially on the weekends ("a few drinks on Fridays and Saturdays").

**TABLE 85-1 Lab Values**

| | | | | |
|---|---|---|---|---|
| Na 140 mEq/L | Hgb 12.8 g/dL | RDW 10.2% | AST 14 IU/L | Total $T_4$ 24 mcg/dL |
| K 4.1 mEq/L | Hct 38.4% | WBC 4.8 × $10^3$/mm$^3$ | ALT 16 IU/L | Free $T_4$ 4 ng/dL |
| Cl 98 mEq/L | RBC 3.08 × $10^6$/mm$^3$ | Polys 72% | T. bili 0.2 mg/dL | TSH 0.02 mIU/L |
| $CO_2$ 23 mEq/L | Plt 298 × $10^3$/mm$^3$ | Lymphs 27% | Amylase <30 IU/L | $T_3$ resin uptake 35% |
| BUN 9 mg/dL | MCV 86.4 μm$^3$ | Monos 1% | Ca 9.5 mg/dL | Total $T_3$ 550 ng/dL |
| SCr 0.6 mg/dL | MCH 27.1 pg | Basos 2% | Mg 2.0 mEq/L | Free thyroxine index 28.7 |
| Glu 78 mg/dL | MCHC 31.8 g/dL | | Phos 3.7 mg/dL | |

■ **Meds**

Drospirenone/ethinyl estradiol daily

■ **All**

None

■ **ROS**

She reports no visual changes, CP, or dyspnea. She has occasional N/V/D.

■ **Physical Examination**

*Gen*

Patient is a thin, tanned WF in NAD. She appears anxious and has a fine motor tremor in her hands.

*VS*

BP 136/80, P 120, RR 18, T 38.1°C; Wt 48 kg, Ht 5′6″

*Skin*

Hair is fine and sparse in the temporal area.

*HEENT*

PERRL, EOMI, (+) lid lag, no proptosis (no ophthalmoplegia) or periorbital edema

*Neck/Lymph Nodes*

Supple, (+) smooth, symmetrically enlarged thyroid (approximately twice the normal size), prominent pulsations in neck vessels

*Lungs*

CTA bilaterally, no wheezes or rales

*CV*

Regular rhythm, tachycardic without murmurs; (−) bruits

*Abd*

Soft, NT/ND; (+) hyperactive BS; no HSM or masses. Aortic pulsations palpable.

*Rect*

Guaiac (−) stool

*Ext*

Normal pulses bilaterally, no calf tenderness. No cyanosis. Fingernails and toenails are flaking. Thumbnails have prominent ridges.

*Neuro*

A & O ×3; fine tremor with outstretched hands; hyperreflexia at knees; no proximal muscle weakness

■ **Labs**

See Table 85-1.

■ **ECG**

NSR, with heart rate of 120 bpm

■ **Assessment**

A 23-year-old woman with goiter, probable hyperthyroidism. Most likely cause is Graves' disease.

## QUESTIONS

### Problem Identification

1.a. Create a list of the patient's drug therapy problems.

1.b. What signs, symptoms, and laboratory values indicate the presence or severity of hyperthyroidism?

### Desired Outcome

2. What are the goals of pharmacotherapy for this patient?

### Therapeutic Alternatives

3.a. What nondrug therapies might be useful for this patient?

3.b. What feasible pharmacotherapeutic alternatives are available for the treatment of Graves' disease?

### Optimal Plan

4. What drug, dosage form, dose, schedule, and duration of therapy are best for this patient?

### Outcome Evaluation

5. What clinical and laboratory parameters are necessary to evaluate thyroid replacement therapy to achieve euthyroidism and prevent adverse effects?

### Patient Education

6. What information should be provided to the patient to enhance adherence, ensure successful therapy, and minimize adverse effects?

## ■ CLINICAL COURSE

The patient is started on the treatment you recommended and returns for a 6-month follow-up visit. She reports that she has noticed marked improvement in her symptoms. The palpitations and tremor have both resolved. She states that she missed her last menses and is concerned that she may be pregnant. The following information is obtained:

VS: BP 124/70, P 88, RR 16, T 37.2°C

| | | |
|---|---|---|
| Hgb 12.5 g/dL | WBC 5.8 ×10$^3$/mm$^3$ | AST 18 IU/L |
| Hct 37.5% | Polys 65% | ALT 16 IU/L |
| MCV 85.6 μm$^3$ | Lymphs 30% | T. bili 0.2 mg/dL |
| MCH 26.5 pg | Monos 2% | Total $T_4$ 14.2 mcg/dL |
| MCHC 30.9 g/dL | Basos 2% | TSH <0.17 mIU/L |
| RDW 9.4% | Basos 1% | hCG 2637 mIU/mL |

## Follow-Up Questions

1. What changes to the patient's treatment for Graves' disease, if any, would you suggest at this point?
2. What other interventions would you recommend for this patient?

## ■ SELF-STUDY ASSIGNMENTS

1. Develop a monitoring protocol for the pharmacotherapy of hyperthyroidism.
2. Design a systematic approach for a patient counseling technique for the drug therapy of hyperthyroidism.

## CLINICAL PEARL

Ophthalmopathy associated with Graves' disease can produce significant morbidity in patients and can cause blindness in severe cases that affect the optic nerve or cornea. Graves' ophthalmopathy is thought to be an autoimmune disorder mediated by autoreactive T lymphocytes and cytokine release. The most common symptoms include diplopia, photophobia, tearing, and pain. Correction of the underlying hyperthyroidism can improve symptoms of Graves' ophthalmopathy in most cases. However, symptoms can temporarily worsen with radioactive iodine treatment, until the hyperthyroidism is corrected. Severe cases of Graves' ophthalmopathy should be treated with systemic or intraocular glucocorticoids. Alternative therapies include orbital radiotherapy and other immunomodulating drugs, such as cyclosporine and rituximab. Surgery is reserved for the most severe cases or those refractory to steroids.

## REFERENCES


1. Brent GA. Graves' disease. N Engl J Med 2009;358(24):2594–2605 [correction: N Engl J Med 2008;359;1407–1409].
2. Bahn RS, Burch HS, Cooper DS, et al. The role of propylthiouracil in the management of Graves' disease in adults: report of a meeting jointly sponsored by the American Thyroid Association and the Food and Drug Administration. Thyroid 2009;19(7):673–674.
3. Metso S, Auvinen A, Huhtala H, Salmi J, Oksala H, Jaatinen P. Increased cancer incidence after radioiodine treatment for hyperthyroidism. Cancer 2007;109:1972–1979 [erratum: Cancer 2007;110:1875].
4. Glinoer D, de Nayer P, Bex M. Effects of L-thyroxine administration, TSH-receptor antibodies and smoking on the risk of recurrence in Graves' hyperthyroidism treated with antithyroid drugs: a double-blind prospective randomized study. Eur J Endocrinol 2001;144:475–483.
5. Chan GW, Mandel SJ. Therapy insight: management of Graves' disease during pregnancy. Nat Clin Pract Endocrinol Metab 2007;3(6):470–478.
6. Bartalena L, Tanda ML. Graves' ophthalmopathy. N Engl J Med 2009;360(10):994–1001.


# 86

# HYPOTHYROIDISM

Trying to Have a Baby is Making Me Tired! . . . . Level II

**Michael D. Katz, PharmD**

## LEARNING OBJECTIVES

After completing this case study, the reader should be able to:

- Recognize the signs, symptoms, and associated complications of mild and overt hypothyroidism.
- Identify the goals of therapy for hypothyroidism.
- Develop an appropriate treatment and monitoring plan for thyroid replacement based on individual patient characteristics.
- Select an appropriate product for thyroid replacement therapy.
- Properly educate a patient taking thyroid replacement therapy.

## PATIENT PRESENTATION

### ■ Chief Complaint

"We are trying so hard to have a baby. Maybe that's why I'm so tired all the time … too much pressure."

### ■ HPI

Vickie Greene is a 31-year-old African-American woman who presents with her husband Eric (age 33) to the Endocrinology Clinic after being referred by her OB-GYN based on the results of some recent blood work. The Greenes have been trying to have a baby for almost 2 years, without Vickie becoming pregnant. The infertility workup done by the OB-GYN showed that Eric had a normal sperm count and sperm motility, and that Vickie had no anatomical abnormalities of her reproductive tract and no evidence of endometriosis. Vickie's serum sex hormone and gonadotropin levels were all normal. The couple is contemplating in vitro fertilization, but wants to make sure there are no hormone-related causes of her infertility. Vickie says that for the past few months she has felt increasingly fatigued, which she attributes to the stress of her unsuccessful attempts to become pregnant. She wonders if she is becoming depressed. She also notes that for the past few months, she has had more difficulty concentrating at work, and she has "gained a few pounds." Over the past 6 months, Vickie has noticed that her periods are a little heavier than normal and are somewhat more irregular. She notes that 2 years ago, she attended a local health fair that provided a variety of laboratory tests. The result of her TSH at that time was 4.2 mIU/L. Her PCP at that time felt that the TSH value was within the normal range and required no follow-up.

### ■ PMH

Infertility × 2 years
Iron deficiency anemia as a teenager

### ■ FH

Father, age 55, has mild COPD; mother, age 54, has type 2 DM, HTN; she has one sister, age 32, who has hypothyroidism. No history of sickle cell trait or disease.

■ SH

Married × 6 years, first marriage for both. No history of STDs. Works as an immigration attorney for a private firm. Social drinker in past but has not used alcohol since attempting to become pregnant; (−) tobacco or illicit drug use.

■ Meds

MiraLAX po daily PRN constipation
Seasonale one po daily (stopped 2 years ago)
$FeSO_4$ 300 mg po daily
Calcium carbonate 500 mg po twice daily
Acetaminophen 325–650 mg po PRN headache, body aches

■ All

Skin rash from sulfa drug

■ ROS

(+) Fatigue that she attributes to stress, (+) occasional insomnia, (+) constipation relieved with MiraLAX; (+) occasional headaches relieved with non-aspirin pain reliever; (−) tinnitus, vertigo, or infections; (−) urinary symptoms; (+) dry skin

■ Physical Examination

*Gen*

Well-appearing African-American woman in NAD

*VS*

BP 112/74, P 64, RR 12, T 36.8°C; Wt 62 kg, Ht 5′7″

*Skin*

Slightly dry-appearing skin; (−) rashes or lesions

*HEENT*

PERRLA, EOMI; (−) sinus tenderness; TMs appear normal

*Neck/Lymph Nodes*

(−) Thyroid nodules, possible slight thyroid enlargement; (−) lymphadenopathy, (−) carotid bruits

*Lungs/Thorax*

CTA

*Breasts*

(−) Lumps/masses

*CV*

RRR, normal $S_1$, $S_2$; (−) $S_3$ or $S_4$

*Abd*

NT/ND, (−) organomegaly

*Neuro*

A & O ×3; CN II–XII intact; DTRs 2+, symmetric

*GU*

Deferred given recent extensive w/u by OB-GYN

■ Labs (Fasting)

Na 138 mEq/L
K 4.2 mEq/L
Cl 98 mEq/L
$CO_2$ 25 mEq/L
BUN 8 mg/dL
SCr 0.7 mg/dL
Glu 98 mg/dL

Hgb 13.1 g/dL
Hct 39.2%
WBC 6.8 ×$10^3$/mm$^3$
MCV 89 μm$^3$
Ca 9.6 mg/dL
Mg 2.0 mEq/L
$PO_4$ 3.8 mg/dL
Albumin 4.0 g/dL
AST 22 IU/L
ALT 19 IU/L
T. bili 0.4 mg/dL
Alk phos 54 IU/L

Anti-TPO antibody +
TSH 9.8 mIU/L
Free $T_4$ 0.72 ng/dL
T. chol 212 mg/dL
LDL chol 142 mg/dL
HDL chol 45 mg/dL
TG 125 mg/dL

■ Assessment

A 31-year-old woman with infertility, fatigue, other nonspecific symptoms, and an elevated TSH level, suggestive of hypothyroidism

## QUESTIONS

### Problem Identification

1.a. Identify this patient's drug therapy problems.

1.b. What information (signs, symptoms, laboratory values) indicates the presence of hypothyroidism?

1.c. Could hypothyroidism be a cause of her infertility?

1.d. List examples of medications that are known to cause hypothyroidism. Could any of the patient's complaints have been caused by drug therapy?

1.e. What was the significance, if any, of her previous TSH of 4.2 mIU/L?

### Desired Outcome

2. What are the goals of pharmacotherapy in this case?

### Therapeutic Alternatives

3.a. What nondrug therapies might be useful for this patient?

3.b. What feasible pharmacotherapeutic alternatives (including complementary/alternative medicine products) are available for treatment of hypothyroidism?

### Optimal Plan

4. What drug, dosage form, dose, schedule, and duration of therapy are best for this patient?

### Outcome Evaluation

5. Which clinical and laboratory parameters are necessary to evaluate the therapy for achievement of the desired therapeutic outcome and to detect or prevent adverse effects?

### Patient Education

6. What information should be provided to the patient to enhance adherence, ensure successful therapy, and minimize adverse effects?

## ■ FOLLOW-UP QUESTIONS

1. How should this patient's elevated LDL cholesterol be managed now? What if her cholesterol continues to be elevated after she becomes euthyroid?
2. What changes in her thyroid therapy might be necessary if she does become pregnant?

3. Evaluate this patient's continued need for iron and calcium. Should they be discontinued? If not, what potential problems (if any) might be expected once thyroid replacement therapy is started?

## SELF-STUDY ASSIGNMENTS

1. Review the effects of untreated hypothyroidism during pregnancy on both mother and baby.
2. Research information on the US bioequivalence testing of levothyroxine ($LT_4$) products. How does US bioequivalence testing of $LT_4$ products differ from that of other oral products? Does $LT_4$ bioequivalence ensure therapeutic equivalence? Is there a consensus regarding the substitution of $LT_4$ product?
3. Review the factors that may alter $LT_4$ dose requirements, including drug interactions

## CLINICAL PEARL

Pregnant women who are receiving $LT_4$ replacement must undergo monthly monitoring of the TSH level to assure adequate replacement. The majority of such women will require an increase of their $LT_4$ dose during pregnancy to assure adequate replacement for both mother and fetus.

## REFERENCES


1. Aoki Y, Belin RM, Clickner R, Jeffries R, Phillips L, Mhafey KR. Serum TSH and total $T_4$ in the United States population and their association with participant characteristics. National Health and Nutrition Examination Survey (NHANES 1999–2002). Thyroid 2007;17:1211–1223.
2. Canaris GJ, Manowitz NR, Mayor G, Ridgway EC. The Colorado thyroid disease prevalence study. Arch Intern Med 2000;160:526–534.
3. Trokoudes KM, Skordis N, Picolos MK. Infertility and thyroid disorders. Curr Opin Obstet Gynecol 2006;18:446–451.
4. Poppe K, Velkeniers B, Glinoer D. The role of thyroid autoimmunity in fertility and pregnancy. Nat Clin Pract Endocrinol Metab 2008;4:394–405.
5. Wartofsky L, Dickey RA. The evidence for a narrower thyrotropin reference range is compelling. J Clin Endocrinol Metab 2005;90: 5483–5488.
6. Vaidya B, Pearce SHS. Management of hypothyroidism in adults. BMJ 2008;337:284–289.
7. Blakesley V, Awni W, Locke C, Ludden T, Granneman GR, Braverman LE. Are bioequivalence studies of levothyroxine sodium formulations in euthyroid volunteers reliable? Thyroid 2004;14:191–200.
8. Carr D, McLeod DT, Parry G, Thornes HM. Fine adjustment of thyroxine replacement dosage: comparison of the thyrotropin releasing hormone test using a sensitive thyrotropin assay with measurement of free thyroid hormones and clinical assessment. Clin Endocrinol 1988;28:325–333.
9. Dong BJ, Hauck WW, Gambertoglio JG, et al. Bioequivalence of generic and brand-name levothyroxine products in the treatment of hypothyroidism. JAMA 1997;277:1205–1213.
10. Mayor GH, Orlando T, Kurtz NM. Limitations of levothyroxine bioequivalence evaluation: an analysis of an attempted study. Am J Ther 1995;2:417–432.
11. Grozinsky-Glasberg S, Fraser A, Nahashoni E, Weizman A, Leibovici L. Thyroxine triiodothyronine combination therapy versus thyroxine monotherapy for clinical hypothyroidism: a meta-analysis of randomized controlled trials. J Clin Endocrinol Metab 2006;91: 2592–2599.
12. Fatourechi V. Subclinical hypothyroidism: an update for primary care physicians. Mayo Clin Proc 2009;84:65–71.
13. Abalovich M, Amino N, Barbour LA, et al. Management of thyroid dysfunction during pregnancy and postpartum: an Endocrine Society clinical practice guideline. J Clin Endocrinol Metab 2007;92(Suppl):S1–S47.


# 87

# CUSHING'S SYNDROME

A Tale of Two Glands.................... Level II

**Steven M. Smith, PharmD**

**John G. Gums, PharmD, FCCP**

## LEARNING OBJECTIVES

After completing this case study, the reader should be able to:

- Recognize and differentiate the signs, symptoms, and laboratory changes associated with the various forms of Cushing's syndrome.
- Recognize the biochemical, anatomic, and emotional changes that can occur with Cushing's syndrome.
- Recommend appropriate treatment regimens for patients with Cushing's syndrome.
- Suggest appropriate adjunctive pharmacotherapy to other health care providers for patients with Cushing's disease.
- Provide patient counseling on proper dosing, administration, and adverse effects of treatment for Cushing's disease.

## PATIENT PRESENTATION

### Chief Complaint

"I have been tired and weak lately, and I've noticed some swelling in my legs recently."

### HPI

Susan Taylor is a 31-year-old woman who presents to her family physician complaining of fatigue, weakness, and edema. She also reports weight gain (50 lb over 2 years) and depression with insomnia.

### PMH

Patient has been healthy with no other major medical illnesses, except seasonal allergic rhinitis. She had two healthy children by uncomplicated vaginal deliveries.

### FH

Mother is alive at age 54 with type 2 DM; father is living at age 56 with HTN. She has two sisters: one is healthy and the other has depression.

### SH

Patient does not smoke, and drinks occasionally. She is a photographer. Children are ages 6 and 3.

### Meds

Triphasil-21 as directed
Nasonex two sprays in each nostril once daily PRN allergic symptoms
Unisom PRN sleep
Advil PRN headache

### All

Sulfa—rash

### ROS

(+) For fatigue, weakness, occasional back pain, and weight gain; also reports episodes of sadness, depressed mood, and insomnia; skin bruises easily; occasional headache, blurred vision, and heartburn; no CP, wheezing, or SOB. Normal menstruation with regular periods.

### Physical Examination

*Gen*

WDWN obese, cushingoid-appearing white woman in NAD

*VS*

BP 165/86, HR 85, RR 14, T 37.0°C; Wt 82.1 kg, Ht 5′3″

*Skin*

Thin skin with some bruising and scratches; purple striae visible on abdomen

*HEENT*

Rounded face; moderate facial hair; PERRLA; EOMI; funduscopic exam shows normal retinal background, optic cup-to-disk ratios 0.4; visual fields appear to be grossly intact; OP moist and pink

*Neck/Lymph Nodes*

Supple; (+) JVD at 30° (7 cm); (−) bruits, adenopathy, or thyromegaly

*Chest*

CTA bilaterally

*Breasts*

No lumps or masses

*CV*

RRR, no MRG

*Abd*

Obese, soft, NT, (−) masses or organomegaly

*Genit/Rect*

Guaiac (−); normal external genitalia; no masses

*MS/Ext*

Appears to have decreased strength bilaterally; DTR 1–2+ and symmetric throughout all four extremities; 2+ pitting pedal edema bilaterally; pedal pulses palpable with moderate intensity

*Neuro*

Oriented ×3; flat affect; CNs II–XII intact

### Labs

| | | | |
|---|---|---|---|
| Na 138 mEq/L | Hgb 13.4 g/dL | AST 9 IU/L | TSH 2.33 mIU/L |
| K 3.3 mEq/L | Hct 38.5% | ALT 7 IU/L | A1C 7.1% |
| Cl 105 mEq/L | RBC 4.0 $\times 10^6$/mm$^3$ | Alk phos 180 IU/L | *Fasting lipid profile* |
| $CO_2$ 25 mEq/L | Plt 264 $\times 10^3$/mm$^3$ | T. bili 0.5 mg/dL | T. chol 261 mg/dL |
| BUN 12 mg/dL | WBC 14.5 $\times 10^3$/mm$^3$ | Alb 4.5 g/dL | HDL 62 mg/dL |
| SCr 0.9 mg/dL | | UA 5.6 mg/dL | LDL 120 mg/dL |
| Glu 160 mg/dL | | | Trig 396 mg/dL |

### Assessment

Probable Cushing's syndrome of unknown etiology requiring further evaluation by an endocrinologist

## CLINICAL COURSE

The patient was seen by an endocrinologist for further evaluation. Baseline 24-hour UFC was 356 and 362 mcg on separate days. A midnight salivary cortisol level was 0.54 mcg/dL. An overnight 1-mg DST showed a plasma cortisol of 9.2 mcg/dL. Plasma ACTH levels on 2 consecutive days at 1:00 PM were 103 and 110 pg/mL. A CRH stimulation test revealed a baseline plasma cortisol of 10.4 mcg/dL and ACTH of 108 pg/mL, with an increase to a plasma cortisol of 13.5 mcg/dL and ACTH of 187 pg/mL following CRH administration. An MRI revealed an enlarged pituitary gland; the same finding was seen on a focused repeat MRI. There was no focal inhomogeneity that would suggest an isolated adenoma (i.e., the tumor cannot be localized).

The risks and benefits of all the treatments were explained to Ms Taylor. She preferred to undergo radiation treatments rather than exploratory-type surgery. She indicated that she would like to have more children and would prefer to try other treatments prior to surgery.

## QUESTIONS

### Problem Identification

1.a. Create a list of this patient's drug therapy problems.

1.b. What information (signs, symptoms, laboratory values) indicates the presence or severity of Cushing's syndrome?

1.c. What information (presentation, history, laboratory values, imaging) can be used to identify the most likely etiology of Cushing's syndrome?

### Desired Outcome

2. What are the goals of pharmacotherapy in this case?

### Therapeutic Alternatives

3.a. What nondrug therapies might be useful for this patient?

3.b. What feasible pharmacotherapeutic alternatives are available for the treatment of Cushing's disease?

### Optimal Plan

4.a. What drug, dosage form, dose, schedule, and duration of therapy are best for treating this patient's Cushing's disease?

4.b. What adjunctive pharmacotherapy may be required if the therapy identified above is successful?

### Outcome Evaluation

5. What clinical and laboratory parameters are necessary to evaluate the therapy for achievement of the desired therapeutic outcome and to detect or prevent adverse events?

## Patient Education

6. What information should be provided to the patient to enhance adherence, ensure successful therapy, and minimize adverse events?

## ■ FOLLOW-UP QUESTIONS

1. What advantages does measuring late-night salivary cortisol have over measuring late-night serum cortisol levels?
2. What changes, if any, should be made to the treatment of allergic rhinitis?

## ■ CLINICAL COURSE

The patient received radiation therapy with adjuvant pharmacotherapy to reduce cortisol levels. Given that it may take several months for therapy to normalize cortisol levels, several other interventions were initiated to ameliorate the complications of Cushing's disease. She received hydrochlorothiazide 25 mg daily for hypertension, pioglitazone 30 mg daily for elevated blood sugars, atorvastatin 10 mg daily for dyslipidemia, and citalopram 20 mg daily for depression. A DXA scan revealed a *Z*-score of –2.4 standard deviations at the hip and –2.6 vertebrally. Accordingly, she received a diagnosis of steroid-induced osteoporosis. One month following initiation of the above agents, she presented to her physician for follow-up. She reported increased weakness, leg cramps, and palpitations. Lab work revealed a serum potassium of 2.7 mEq/L.

3. What pharmacologic therapy would you recommend to reduce her risk of fracture?
4. What medication changes would you suggest at this time?

## ■ SELF-STUDY ASSIGNMENTS

1. Many of the tests used in the differential diagnosis of Cushing's syndrome require drug therapy (e.g., DST, CRH). Create a table to assist health care providers in performing these tests correctly (include possible adverse events, timing, critical values, and evaluation of the results).
2. Compare the retail costs in your area for each of the pharmacotherapeutic alternatives for the treatment of Cushing's syndrome. Write a brief summary of your findings, and describe whether this information would cause you to change your recommendation for the initial drug therapy for this patient.
3. Describe methods that may be used to minimize drug-induced Cushing's syndrome.

## CLINICAL PEARL

Most patients with Cushing's disease are treated with transsphenoidal surgery because of its high cure rate (80–90%). Pharmacotherapy is usually used as adjunctive therapy rather than primary therapy.

## REFERENCES


1. Newell-Price J, Bertagna X, Grossman AB, Nierman LK. Cushing's syndrome. Lancet 2006;367:1605–1617.
2. Nieman LK, Biller BMK, Findling JW, et al. The diagnosis of Cushing's syndrome: an Endocrine Society clinical practice guideline. J Clin Endocrinol Metab 2008;93:1527–1540.


# 88

# ADDISON'S DISEASE

Behavior Changes with a Tan . . . . . . . . . . . . . Level II


**Cynthia P. Koh-Knox, PharmD**

**Zachary Weber, PharmD, BCPS**


## LEARNING OBJECTIVES

After completing this case study, the reader should be able to:

- Recognize the clinical presentation, symptoms, and laboratory changes associated with Addison's disease.
- Optimize pharmacologic and nonpharmacologic therapy for patients with Addison's disease and comorbid conditions.
- Provide education and counseling to patients and family members about Addison's disease and the proper administration, side effects, and adverse effects of corticosteroids and mineralocorticoids, and the importance of adherence to therapy.
- Provide counseling and education about common side effects associated with high and low cortisol serum concentrations.
- Compare corticosteroids with respect to relative glucocorticoid and mineralocorticoid potencies.

## PATIENT PRESENTATION

### ■ Chief Complaint

"I've noticed that over the past six months, my son's skin is getting darker, and he has been more lethargic, somewhat withdrawn, and sleeping more. I have also noticed that he has been making some poor choices, in terms of friends and activities."

### ■ HPI

Gregory Waters is a 19 yo man who is brought to the emergency department by his mother after she finds him crying, confused, and disoriented. His mothers states that she has recently noticed that he has not had the same level of energy, and has been complaining about not being able to run and play basketball with his friends at the park. She has also noticed he has been hanging out with a different group of friends, and she is concerned he may be involved in some abhorrent activities and may not be taking his medications appropriately.

### ■ PMH

Type 1 diabetes mellitus × 7 years
Hypothyroidism × 3 years

### ■ FH

Mother, 52 years old, has hypertension; father, 54 years old, has hypothyroidism; sister, 24 years old, has both hypertension and type 1 diabetes mellitus.

### ■ SH

Denies use of alcohol, tobacco, or illicit drugs; lives with his mother

■ Meds

Lantus 24 units subcutaneously QHS
NovoLog 1:15 scale carb counting ratio subcutaneously with meals
Levothyroxine 100 mcg po daily

■ All

NKDA

■ ROS

Increased tanning of the skin noted over the past 6 months. Increased fatigue, nausea, and a 2.5-kg weight loss over the past month.

■ Physical Examination

*Gen*

Alert, somewhat disoriented and confused

*VS*

BP 84/47, HR 91, RR 16, T 36.2°C, Wt 62.5 kg, Ht 5′4″

*Skin*

Warm, dry, and intact. Slightly tanned color.

*HEENT*

Normocephalic; oral mucosa moist. Pupils equal, round, and reactive to light. EOMI.

*Neck*

No JVD. Nontender. No thyroid nodularity.

*Lungs*

Lungs are clear to auscultation. Respirations are nonlabored.

*CV*

Normal rate and rhythm. No murmurs. Normal perfusion. No edema.

*Abd*

Soft, nontender, and nondistended. Normal bowel sounds.

*MS/Ext*

No CCE; normal ROM.

*Neuro*

Alert, somewhat disoriented.

*Psych*

Somnolent, but cooperative.

■ Labs (Fasting, Drawn at 10:15 AM)

| | | | |
|---|---|---|---|
| Na 116 mEq/L | Hgb 14.2 g/dL | AST 111 IU/L | T. chol 168 mg/dL |
| K 4.9 mEq/L | Hct 43.8% | ALT 59 IU/L | Trig 120 mg/dL |
| Cl 99 mEq/L | RBC 4.88 × $10^6$/mm$^3$ | Alk phos 75 IU/L | Fe 93 mcg/dL |
| $CO_2$ 26 mEq/L | Plt 244 × $10^3$/mm$^3$ | GGT 63 IU/L | TSH 25.8 mIU/L |
| BUN 14 mg/dL | WBC 3.6 × $10^3$/mm$^3$ | LDH 173 IU/L | Free $T_4$ 0.41 ng/dL |
| SCr 0.9 mg/dL | Neutros 41% | T. bili 1.1 mg/dL | Cortisol 0.4 mcg/dL |
| Glu 140 mg/dL | Lymphos 43% | D. bili 0.5 mg/dL | β-HCG Qual neg |
| Ca 9.2 mg/dL | Monos 13% | T. prot 7.3 g/dL | ACTH 2003 pg/mL |
| Phos 5.1 mg/dL | Eos 2% | Alb 4.1 g/dL | A1C 8.2% |
| Uric acid 4.1 mg/dL | Basos 1% | | |

Reference range for cortisol: AM 8–25 mcg/dL, PM 4–20 mcg/dL; ACTH 0–130 pg/mL

■ UA

Clear, pale yellow, SG 1.020, pH 6.8

■ Other

CT scan and ECG both negative

■ Assessment

1. Primary adrenal insufficiency, most likely due to an autoimmune disease.
2. Hypothyroidism with an elevated TSH, likely secondary to nonadherence to prescribed levothyroxine regimen.
3. Type 1 diabetes mellitus with an elevated A1C, likely secondary to nonadherence to prescribed insulin regimen.

## QUESTIONS

### Problem Identification

1.a. Create a list of the patient's drug therapy problems.

1.b. What information (signs, symptoms, laboratory values) indicates the presence or severity of Addison's disease?

### Desired Outcome

2. What are the goals of pharmacotherapy in this case?

### Therapeutic Alternatives

3.a. What nondrug therapies might be useful for this patient?

3.b. What feasible pharmacotherapeutic alternatives are available for the treatment of Addison's disease?

3.c. What psychosocial considerations are applicable to this patient?

### Optimal Plan

4. What drug, dosage form, dose, schedule, and duration of therapy are best for this patient?

### Outcome Evaluation

5. Which clinical and laboratory parameters are necessary to evaluate the response to therapy and to detect or prevent adverse effects?

### Patient Education

6. What information should be provided to the patient to enhance adherence, ensure successful therapy, and minimize adverse effects?

## ■ SELF-STUDY ASSIGNMENTS

1. Review the signs and symptoms of an acute adrenal crisis, and describe the treatment.
2. Differentiate the glucocorticoids with respect to duration of activity, glucocorticoid potency, and mineralocorticoid potency.
3. Differentiate the biologic functions of cortisol and aldosterone.
4. Explain why the skin becomes pigmented in adrenal insufficiency.
5. Identify drugs that may precipitate acute adrenal insufficiency or adrenal crisis.

## CLINICAL PEARL

Primary adrenal insufficiency (autoimmune polyglandular syndrome [APS]) is seen in up to 2% of patients with type 1 diabetes mellitus due to antiadrenal autoantibodies.

## REFERENCES


1. Baker SJ, White K. Addison's Disease Owner Manual. Available at: *http://www.addisons.org.uk/info/manual/adshgguidelines.pdf.* Accessed April 25, 2010.
2. Kaushik ML, Sharma C. Addison's disease presenting as depression. Indian J Med Sci 2003;57(6):249–251. Available at: *http://www.indianjmedsci.org/article.asp?issn=0019-5359;year=2003;volume=57;issue=6;spage=249;epage=251;aulast=Kaushik.* Accessed April 21, 2010.
3. Kordonouri O, Maguire AM, Knip M, et al. Other complications and associated conditions with diabetes in children and adolescents. Pediatr Diab 2009:10(Suppl 12):204–210.
4. Vaidya B, Chakera AJ, Dick C. Easily missed? Addison's disease. BMJ 2009;339(July):104–107.
5. Chakera AJ, Vaidya B. Addison disease in adults: diagnosis and management. Am J Med 2010;123:409–413.
6. Reisch N, Arit W. Fine tuning for quality of life: 21st century approach to treatment of Addison's disease. Endocrinol Metab Clin North Am 2009;38:407–418.
7. Arit W. The approach to the adult with newly diagnosed adrenal insufficiency. J Clin Endocrinol Metab 2009;94(4):1059–1067.
8. Elbelt U, Hahner S, Allolio B. Altered insulin requirement in patient with type 1 diabetes and primary adrenal insufficiency receiving standard glucocorticoid replacement therapy. Eur J Endocrinol 2009;160:919–924.


# 89

# HYPERPROLACTINEMIA

The Missing Period. . . . . . . . . . . . . . . . . . . . . . Level I


**Amy Heck Sheehan, PharmD**

**Karim Anton Calis, PharmD, MPH, FASHP, FCCP**


## LEARNING OBJECTIVES

After completing this case study, the reader should be able to:

- Recognize the signs and symptoms of hyperprolactinemia.
- Recommend appropriate treatment options for hyperprolactinemia.
- Design a plan to monitor the response to the pharmacologic treatment of hyperprolactinemia.

## PATIENT PRESENTATION

### Chief Complaint

"I haven't had my period for almost a year."

### HPI

Susan Oliver is a 31-year-old woman with a history of oligomenorrhea (menstrual cycle every 2–6 months) since menarche at age 14. She presents to her gynecologist after 11 months of amenorrhea and a small amount of milky discharge from her left breast, which she first noticed 1–2 months ago. The patient and her husband would like to have a baby, but she is concerned that she may be unable to have children. The patient states that she and her husband have not used birth control for more than 1 year, and she has had several negative home pregnancy tests.

### PMH

GERD
Seasonal allergies
Depression

### FH

Father died at age 58 from an AMI; mother (age 62) has type 2 DM and HTN. Patient has two brothers (ages 33 and 35) who are alive and well.

### SH

The patient is employed as an administrative assistant. She does not smoke and has less than one drink of alcohol per month. She has been married for 5 years and lives with her husband and two stepdaughters (ages 7 and 9).

### Meds

Omeprazole 20 mg po daily
Desloratadine 5 mg po daily
Fluoxetine 20 mg po daily
Prenatal vitamins one tablet po daily
Acetaminophen 500 mg po PRN

### All

Codeine (hives)

### ROS

Galactorrhea of the left breast and amenorrhea for 11 months as described in the HPI. No visual defects. No active GERD or migraine symptoms.

### Physical Examination

*Gen*

The patient is a WDWN white woman in NAD.

*VS*

BP 124/71, P 72, RR 13, T 37.1°C; Wt 72 kg, Ht 5′8″

*Skin*

Normal, intact, warm, and dry

*HEENT*

PERRLA, EOMI, normal funduscopic exam, normal visual fields

*Neck/Lymph Nodes*

Normal thyroid, no lymphadenopathy

*Lungs/Chest*

Clear to A & P

*Breasts*

Galactorrhea of left breast, no masses

*CV*

RRR, $S_1$ and $S_2$ normal, no MRG

*Abd*

Soft, nontender, no organomegaly, (+) bowel sounds

*GU*

LMP 11 months ago, normal pelvic exam and Pap smear

*MS/Ext*

Normal range of motion, no edema, pulses 2+ throughout

*Neuro*

A & O ×3, bilateral reflexes intact, normal gait, CNs II–XII intact

### Labs

| | | |
|---|---|---|
| Na 138 mEq/L | AST 23 IU/L | TSH 2.1 mIU/L |
| K 4.0 mEq/L | ALT 31 IU/L | $T_3$ 111 ng/dL |
| Cl 101 mEq/L | Alk phos 110 IU/L | Total $T_4$ 7.5 mcg/dL |
| $CO_2$ 25 mEq/L | T. bili 0.5 mg/dL | Free $T_4$ 1.3 ng/dL |
| BUN 13 mg/dL | | Serum β-HCG negative |
| SCr 0.8 mg/dL | | |
| Glu 89 mg/dL | | |

FSH 12 IU/L

Serum prolactin on 3 separate days: 133, 159, and 142 mcg/L

### Other Test Results

DXA T-score −0.90 at the lumbar spine (no previous DXA results)

MRI of the pituitary gland revealed an 8-mm pituitary adenoma

### Assessment

Hyperprolactinemia due to a microprolactinoma

# QUESTIONS

## Problem Identification

1.a. List this patient's drug therapy problems.

1.b. What signs, symptoms, and laboratory values indicate the presence of hyperprolactinemia?

1.c. Could this patient's hyperprolactinemia be drug-induced?

## Desired Outcome

2. What are the goals of treatment for a woman with hyperprolactinemia?

## Therapeutic Alternatives

3.a. What nondrug therapies can be considered for the treatment of hyperprolactinemia?

3.b. What pharmacotherapeutic options are available for the treatment of hyperprolactinemia in this woman?

## Optimal Plan

4. What medication regimen would you recommend for this patient?

## Outcome Evaluation

5.a. What clinical and laboratory parameters are necessary to monitor the patient's response to therapy?

5.b. If the initial therapy you recommend is effective, how soon can the patient hope to become pregnant?

## Patient Education

6. What information should be provided to the patient to enhance adherence, ensure successful therapy, and minimize adverse effects?

# CLINICAL COURSE

The patient was started on the regimen you recommended, and she returned to the clinic 4 weeks later complaining of significant nausea and abdominal pain that was temporally associated with medication administration. Serum prolactin concentrations measured 10 minutes apart were 140, 151, and 137 mcg/L. Galactorrhea and amenorrhea were unchanged.

## Follow-Up Questions

1. Identify the possible reasons for the patient's poor initial response to therapy.
2. Given the new patient information, what alternative therapies should be considered?
3. How long will this patient require drug treatment for the prolactinoma?

# SELF-STUDY ASSIGNMENTS

1. Review the available information on the safety of dopamine agonist pharmacotherapy in pregnant women. If this patient eventually becomes pregnant, should a dopamine agonist be continued throughout the pregnancy?
2. Research information on the use of hormone replacement therapy in patients with hyperprolactinemia. Is this patient a candidate for hormone replacement therapy? Why or why not?
3. Describe the treatment of hyperprolactinemia in the presence of a macroadenoma. How would the management of hyperprolactinemia be different if the patient were diagnosed with a macroprolactinoma instead of a microprolactinoma?

# CLINICAL PEARL

Although dopamine agonists are the mainstay of therapy for hyperprolactinemia, approximately 5–10% of patients do not respond to these agents because of poor compliance, suboptimal dosing, or the presence of a treatment-resistant prolactinoma.

# REFERENCES


1. Gillam MP, Molitch ME, Lombardi P, Colao A. Advances in the treatment of prolactinomas. Endocr Rev 2006;27:485–534.
2. DiSarno A, Landi ML, Cappabianca P, et al. Resistance to cabergoline as compared with bromocriptine in hyperprolactinemia: prevalence, clinical definition, and therapeutic strategy. J Clin Endocrinol Metab 2001;86:5256–5261.
3. Casanueva FF, Molitch ME, Schlechte JA, et al. Guidelines of the Pituitary Society for the diagnosis and management of prolactinomas. Clin Endocrinol 2006;65:265–273.
4. Molitch ME. Medical management of prolactin-secreting pituitary adenomas. Pituitary 2002;5:55–65.
5. Mah PM, Webster J. Hyperprolactinemia: etiology, diagnosis, and management. Semin Reprod Med 2002;20:365–373.
6. Klibanski A. Prolactinomas. N Engl J Med 2010;362:1219–1226.

SECTION 9
# WOMEN'S HEALTH (GYNECOLOGIC DISORDERS)

# 90

## PREGNANCY AND LACTATION

Pregnant at This Age? .................... Level II

Lisa Biondo, PharmD

Kelsey Briggs, PharmD

## LEARNING OBJECTIVES

After completing this case study, the reader should be able to:

- Define each FDA pregnancy category using the US Food and Drug Administration Drug Classification System.
- Determine the factors (clinical vs. pharmacologic) that should be considered when treating a pregnant or lactating patient.
- List the risks and benefits associated with medication use during pregnancy for hypertension, depression, and mechanical heart valve requiring chronic anticoagulation for thromboembolism prophylaxis.
- Identify alternative therapies that are considered safe during pregnancy for the treatment of depression and hypertension, and for thromboembolism prophylaxis in a patient with a mechanical heart valve.
- Design a pharmacotherapeutic plan for a pregnant patient with depression, hypertension, and a mechanical heart valve including treatment options, appropriate monitoring, and therapeutic goals.
- Educate a patient on the treatment options, benefits, risks, and monitoring of antidepressants, antihypertensives, and anticoagulants during pregnancy.

## PATIENT PRESENTATION

### Chief Complaint

"I have been nauseated and vomiting for the past week. I took a pregnancy test yesterday, and it was positive! How am I going to handle a pregnancy at this age? Plus, I am taking a lot of different medications. Could I have harmed my baby?"

### HPI

Laurel Livingston is a 40 yo woman who reports experiencing two to three episodes of nausea per day with vomiting occasionally in the evenings. Her GI symptoms began about 2 weeks ago and have remained consistent, preventing her from going to work. Around the same time her GI symptoms began, she started having frequent, painful urination and was diagnosed with a UTI. She is on day 5 of 7 of antibiotic treatment with nitrofurantoin. She states that she feels "run down" all the time and needs to start feeling better soon, or she will lose her job. Also she is extremely concerned about her "blood thinner" medication, remembering that she could not take it with her previous three pregnancies. Due to the death of her brother 5 years ago, Laurel was prescribed an antidepressant and is currently stable (no depressive episodes for the last 3 years). She eats well, exercises, and admits stopping her birth control due to weight gain.

### PMH

Depression
Mechanical prosthetic heart valve
Hypothyroidism
Hypertension

### FH

Mother alive and well; father died of pancreatic cancer at age of 67. Patient has one sister, age 45, who is alive and well; brother died in car accident 5 years ago at the age of 32.

### SH

Married, mother of two daughters, ages 10 and 13 (both healthy), and one son, 6 years old with cerebral palsy. She is a physical therapist at the local community hospital. She runs three times a week and follows a strict low-fat diet. She was a smoker (one pack per day) but is currently tobacco-free and occasionally drinks a glass of wine or alcoholic beverage on the weekends. She has no prior history of thromboembolism.

### Medications

Paroxetine 20 mg po once daily
Levothyroxine 125 mcg po once daily
Warfarin 7.5 mg po once daily
Lisinopril 10 mg po once daily
Nitrofurantoin 100 mg po twice daily × 7 days

### Allergies

NKDA

### ROS

(+) Nausea/vomiting × 2 weeks; fatigue; weight loss

### Physical Examination

*Gen*

WDWN concerned female

*VS*

BP 160/90, P 76, RR 17, T 36.3°C; Wt 82 kg, Ht 5′8″

*Skin*

Warm, dry, no eruptions, boils, or lesions

*HEENT*

WNL

*Neck/Lymph Nodes*

No adenopathy, no thyromegaly, supple

*Lungs*

CTA bilaterally

*Breasts*

Tender to palpation; no masses

*CV*

Mechanical click systolic murmur, Grade 2/4

*ABD*

Soft, NT, (+) BS; no masses, no bruits

*Genit/Rect*

Pelvic exam confirms pregnancy; stool heme/guaiac (−)
Urine (−) for protein/glucose

*Ext*

(−) CCE; pulses intact

*Neuro*

Normal sensory and motor levels

### Labs

| | | |
|---|---|---|
| Na 138 mEq/L | Hgb 13 g/dL | Blood type: O− |
| K 4 mEq/L | Hct 40% | PT/INR 10.0 seconds/3.0 |
| Cl 102 mEq/L | WBC 8.0 × $10^3$/mm$^3$ | Random glucose 100 mg/dL |
| $CO_2$ 27 mEq/L | Plt 345 × $10^3$/mm$^3$ | |
| BUN 10 mg/dL | TSH 1.45 mIU/L | |
| SCr 0.9 mg/dL | | |

Urinalysis: culture negative (no growth)
Ultrasound: confirmed pregnancy

### Assessment

A 40-year old pregnant woman presenting with nausea, vomiting, and fatigue who is concerned about the safety of her medications during pregnancy

# QUESTIONS

## Problem Identification

1. Create a list of the patient's potential drug therapy problems (now that she is pregnant). Be sure to include the information that indicates the severity of this patient's problems: FDA pregnancy category with definition for the patient's medications and specific malformations and/or risks associated with each medication.

## Desired Outcome

2. What are the goals of therapy for this patient's preexisting disease states/conditions (hypertension, depression, mechanical heart valve requiring anticoagulation, hypothyroidism) during her pregnancy?

## Therapeutic Alternatives

3.a. What are the benefits and risks of treating this patient's depression and hypertension and in providing anticoagulation for thromboembolism prophylaxis in light of the patient's mechanical heart valve?

3.b. What pharmacotherapeutic alternatives may be used to manage the patient's depression, hypertension, and anticoagulation for her heart valve?

## Optimal Plan

4.a. The physician decided to prescribe methyldopa for the patient's hypertension and enoxaparin for anticoagulation. What dose, schedule, and duration are the best for this patient for each of these medications?

4.b. The patient has been asymptomatic for more than a year and has agreed to discontinue her antidepressant. What are your recommendations for stopping the medication?

## Outcome Evaluation

5. What clinical and laboratory parameters are necessary to evaluate the therapy for achievement of the desired therapeutic outcomes for the patient's hypertension and anticoagulation therapy and to detect or prevent medication-related adverse effects?

## Patient Education

6. What information should be provided to the patient to enhance adherence to the medication, ensure successful therapy, and minimize adverse effects?

# CLINICAL COURSE

The patient returns to your office 4 weeks after she delivers her healthy baby boy. She reports that her clinical symptoms of depression have intensified postpartum and would like to know if she should reinitiate her antidepressant, and if so, at what dose.

## Follow-Up Question

1. Based on the 2008 American College of Obstetrics and Gynecology (ACOG) guidelines, what would you recommend to the patient?

# ADDITIONAL QUESTIONS

1. What is the definition of a teratogen?
2. What factors are used to decide whether or not to treat a pregnant or breastfeeding patient (clinical vs. pharmacologic)?

# SELF-STUDY ASSIGNMENTS

1. Review the ACOG Practice Bulletin: Clinical Management Guidelines for Obstetrician–Gynecologists (see reference 3).
2. Research the use of antidepressants for treatment of depression during pregnancy and lactation. Discuss the general treatment concepts, and outline the clinical recommendations for depression.

## CLINICAL PEARLS

1. There is little information regarding the risk of most medications used in human pregnancy and lactation at the time they receive their FDA approval and are initially marketed. Although only few drugs are known or strongly suspected to be teratogens, the majority of all drugs marketed in the United States are classified category C; <1% are category A.[5] Out of 2,150 products in the physician desk reference (PDR) 2002, only 124 drugs are category X. Of those 124 drugs, the majority of the labels contain only a black box warning. Only 13 of the 124 drugs contain specific pregnancy prevention risk management strategies in the label, and only 3 drugs (isotretinoin, acitretin, and thalidomide) have formal pregnancy prevention risk management programs.[5]

   Very few studies have thoroughly investigated drug concentrations in the breast milk. Most data available are for the tricyclic antidepressants, the majority of these being case reports.[5]

   The bottom line is that we desperately need more research and studies regarding the risks associated with medication use during pregnancy and lactation, as the lack of information available today often poses an ethical dilemma.

2. Electronic resources for information related to fetal and neonatal effects in pregnancy and lactation include Reprotox (www.reprotox.org) and TERIS (http://depts.washington.edu/terisweb). There are also postmarketing pregnancy exposure registries available through the US Food and Drug Administration Pregnancy Labeling Task Force. Alternatively, there is General Practice Research Database (GPRD) that can be utilized as data sources for investigating drug exposure during pregnancy.

## REFERENCES


1. Gonsalves L, Schuermeyer I. Treating depression in pregnancy: practical suggestions. Clev Clin J Med 2006;73:1098–1104.
2. Tuccori M, Testi A, Antonioli L, et al. Safety concerns associated with the use of serotonin reuptake inhibitors and other serotonergic/noradrenergic antidepressants during pregnancy: a review. Clin Ther Theme Issue 2009;31:1426–1453.
3. American College of Obstetrics and Gynecology. ACOG practice bulletin clinical management guidelines for obstetrician–gynecologists: use of psychiatric medications during pregnancy and lactation. Obstet Gynecol 2008;111:1001–1020.
4. Buhimschi C, Weiner C. Medications in pregnancy and lactation: part 1. Teratology. Obstet Gynecol 2009;113:166–188.
5. Cooper WO, Hernandez-Diaz S, Arbogast PG, et al. Major congenital malformations after first trimester exposure to ACE inhibitors. N Engl J Med 2006;354:2443.
6. Sibai, B. Chronic hypertension in pregnancy. Am J Obstet Gynecol 2002;100:369–377.
7. Buhimschi C, Weiner C. Medications in pregnancy and lactation: part 2. Drugs with minimal or unknown human teratogenic effect. Obstet Gynecol 2009;113(2 Pt 1):417–432.
8. Bates S, Greer I, Pabinger I, Hirsch J. Venous thromboembolism, thrombophilia, antithrombotic therapy, and pregnancy: American College of Chest Physicians evidence-based clinical practice guidelines (8th edition). Chest 2008;133;844S–886S.
9. Bonow RO, Carabello BA, Chatterjee K, et al. 2008 focused update incorporated into the ACC/AHA 2006 guidelines for the management of patients with valvular heart disease: a report of the American College of Cardiology/American Heart Association Task Force on Practice Guidelines. J Am Coll Cardiol 2008;52:e1–e142.
10. McLintock C, McCowan LME, North RA. Maternal complications and pregnancy outcome in women with mechanical prosthetic heart valves treated with enoxaparin. BJOG 2009;116:1585–1592.
11. Larsen LA, Ito S, Koren G. Prediction of milk/plasma concentration ratio of drugs. Ann Pharmacother 2003;37:1299–1306.


# 91

# CONTRACEPTION

Babies Aren't Us Yet . . . . . . . . . . . . . . . . . . . . Level II

Julia M. Koehler, PharmD, FCCP

## LEARNING OBJECTIVES

After completing this case study, the reader should be able to:

- Discuss the absolute and relative contraindications to the use of hormonal contraceptives.
- Discuss the advantages and disadvantages of the various forms of hormonal contraceptives, including both oral and nonoral formulations.
- Compare and contrast the marketed OC combinations and be able to select the best product for an individual patient.
- Develop strategies for managing the possible side effects of OCs and prepare appropriate alternative treatment plans.
- Provide specific patient education on the administration and expected side effects of selected hormonal contraceptives.

## PATIENT PRESENTATION

### Chief Complaint

"My fiancé and I are getting married soon, and we're not ready for kids just yet."

### HPI

Macy Madison is a 25-year-old graduate student who presents to the women's health clinic for contraceptive counseling. She and her fiancé, Fritz, are planning to be married in approximately 4 months. Macy states that she and Fritz have been in a monogamous sexual relationship for the past 3 years, and that their primary method of contraception has been via the inconsistent use of male condoms. She is here today to be evaluated for the use of hormonal contraceptives. The patient states she began menses at age 14, with irregular cycles of 25–36 days in length. Her last menses was 2 weeks ago. The patient states she has heard about contraceptive options that "decrease your number of periods," and she wants to know more about those options, and if they would be okay for her to try.

### PMH

Migraine headaches without aura or focal neurologic symptoms; well controlled for the past 12 months on prophylactic therapy

### FH

Mother, age 56, has HTN and osteoporosis and is postmenopausal. Grandmother died from complications of breast cancer, which was diagnosed at age 60. Father, age 58, has osteoarthritis, hypothyroidism, HTN, and hyperlipidemia. Grandfather died at age 74 of MI.

### SH

Currently lives in a house on campus, which she rents with three other graduate students. Once she and Fritz are married, they plan to rent an apartment together until she finishes graduate school. She admits to occasional social use of tobacco and alcohol ("a few drinks and a couple of cigarettes at parties on the weekends"). Otherwise, she denies regular smoking or alcohol use during the week, and she denies illicit drug use.

### Meds

Propranolol LA 160 mg po once daily for migraine prophylaxis
Naproxen 220 mg, one to two tablets po Q 8 h PRN menstrual cramps

### All

NKDA

### ROS

Menstrual periods are the most irregular during mid-term and final exam times. Migraine headaches are not accompanied by aura or focal neurologic symptoms, and have been well controlled on prophylactic medication. (Patient states she has not had a migraine for more than 12 months; however, prior to being placed on propranolol for migraine prophylaxis, she reported experiencing menstrual-related headaches in addition to frequent migraines.)

### Physical Examination

*Gen*

Thin, well-developed female in NAD

*VS*

BP 112/70, P 66, RR 14, T 37°C; Wt 59 kg, Ht 5′7″, BMI 20.4 kg/m$^2$

*Skin*

Mild facial acne

*HEENT*

PERRLA; EOMI; TMs intact; oral mucosa clear

*Neck/Lymph Nodes*

Supple without lymphadenopathy or thyromegaly

*Lungs*

CTA, no wheezing

*CV*

RRR; no MRG

*Breasts*

Symmetric in size without nodularity or masses, nontender; nipples appear normal without discharge

*Abd*

Soft, NT, no masses or organomegaly

*Genit/Rect*

Normal-appearing external genitalia; normal cervical and vaginal exam w/o tenderness or masses; rectal exam not performed

*MS/Ext*

Normal ROM; normal muscle strength

*Neuro*

A & O × 3

### Labs

Negative Pap test and UPT

### Assessment

A young, generally healthy, sexually active female with history of migraine headache disorder that has been well controlled with prophylactic medication is requesting hormonal contraceptives for birth control.

## QUESTIONS

### Problem Identification

1.a. Create a list of the patient's potential drug therapy problems.

1.b. What medical problems are absolute contraindications to hormonal contraceptive use, and do any of those conditions apply to this patient?

1.c. What medical problems are relative contraindications to hormonal contraceptive use, and do any of these apply to this patient?

1.d. What other information should be obtained before creating a pharmacotherapeutic plan?

### Desired Outcome

2. What are the goals of pharmacotherapy in this case?

### Therapeutic Alternatives

3. What pharmacotherapeutic alternatives are available for prevention of pregnancy in this patient, and what are the advantages or disadvantages of each?

### Optimal Plan

4. What contraceptive method, dose, and schedule are best for this patient?

### Outcome Evaluation

5. What clinical and laboratory parameters are necessary to evaluate the therapy for efficacy and adverse effects?

### Patient Education

6. What information should be provided to the patient to enhance adherence, ensure successful therapy, and minimize adverse effects?

## CLINICAL COURSE

Macy returns to the clinic in 2 months complaining of worsening acne and breakthrough bleeding.

### Follow-Up Questions

1. What medical conditions can be the cause of breakthrough bleeding?
2. If breakthrough bleeding is not caused by an underlying medical condition, how can it be managed?

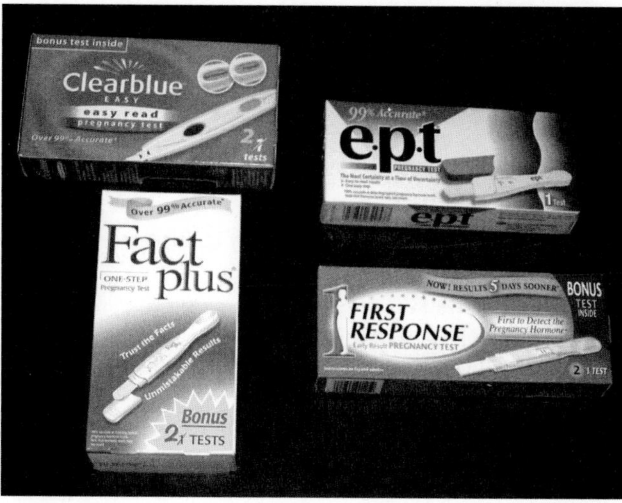


**FIGURE 91-1.** Several examples of home pregnancy test kits. *(Photo courtesy of R. Bowman.)*

3. What recommendations can be made to address this patient's complaint of worsening acne?

## ■ SELF-STUDY ASSIGNMENTS

1. Compare the costs of each method of birth control and prepare a report that contains your conclusions as to which method provides the best efficacy at the most reasonable cost.
2. Visit a pharmacy and review the various home pregnancy tests; determine how you would counsel a patient to use each one, and evaluate them for ease of use (Fig. 91-1).

## CLINICAL PEARL

Oral, transdermal, transvaginal, injectable, and implantable hormonal contraceptives, as well as intrauterine devices and most barrier contraceptives (with the exception of latex and synthetic condoms), do not protect against the acquisition of sexually transmitted infections. Thus, it is important to properly educate patients who are sexually active about the importance of taking necessary precautions to minimize their risk for acquiring a sexually transmitted infection, regardless of the type of hormonal contraceptive used.

## REFERENCES


1. Hatcher RA, Trussell J, Nelson AL, Cates W Jr, Stewart FH, Kowal D. Contraceptive Technology, 19th revised ed. New York, Ardent Media Inc, 2007.
2. Lewis MA, Spitzer WO, Heinemann LA, Thorogood M, MacRae KD. Third generation oral contraceptives and risk of myocardial infarction: an international case–control study. Transitional Research Group on Oral Contraceptives and the Health of Young Women. BMJ 1996;312:88–90.
3. Joint National Committee on Prevention, Detection, Evaluation, and Treatment of High Blood Pressure. The seventh report of the Joint National Committee on Prevention, Detection, Evaluation, and Treatment of High Blood Pressure. JAMA 2003;289:2560–2572.
4. Centers for Disease Control and Prevention. U.S. medical eligibility criteria for contraceptive use, 2010. Adapted from the World Health Organization medical eligibility criteria for contraceptive use, 4th ed. MMWR 2010;59:1–86 [early release].
5. Schoenen J, Sándor PS. Headache with focal neurological signs or symptoms: a complicated differential diagnosis. Lancet Neurol 2004;3:237–245.
6. Knopp RH, Broyles FE, Cheung M, Moore K, Marcovina S, Chandler WL. Comparison of lipoprotein, carbohydrate, and hemostatic effects of phasic oral contraceptives containing desogestrel or levonorgestrel. Contraception 2001;63:1–11.
7. Natazia—a new oral contraceptive. Med Lett Drugs Ther 2010;52(1346):71–72.
8. Vercellini P, Frontino G, De Giorgi O, Pietropaolo G, Pasin R, Crosignani PG. Continuous use of an oral contraceptive for endometriosis-associated recurrent dysmenorrhea that does not respond to a cyclic pill regimen. Fertil Steril 2003;80:560–563.
9. Product information for levonorgestrel 90 mcg and ethinyl estradiol 20 mcg (Lybrel). Philadelphia, PA, Wyeth Pharmaceuticals Inc, May 2007.
10. ACOG Committee on Practice Bulletins—Gynecology. ACOG practice bulletin. No. 73: use of hormonal contraception in women with co-existing medical conditions. Obstet Gynecol 2006;107:1453.
11. Audet M, Moreau M, Koltun WD, et al. Evaluation of contraceptive efficacy and cycle control of a transdermal contraceptive patch vs an oral contraceptive: a randomized controlled trial. JAMA 2001;285:2347–2354.
12. Bjarnadottir RI, Tuppurainen M, Killick SR. Comparison of cycle control with a combined contraceptive vaginal ring and oral levonorgestrel/ethinyl estradiol. Am J Obstet Gynecol 2002;186:389–395.
13. Choice of contraceptives. Treat Guidel Med Lett 2007;5(64):101–108.
14. Machado RB, Pereira AP, Coelho GP, Neri L, Martins L, Luminoso D. Epidemiological and clinical aspects of migraine in users of combined oral contraceptives. Contraception 2010;81:202–208.
15. Executive summary of the third report of the National Cholesterol Education Program (NCEP) Expert Panel on Detection, Evaluation, Treatment of High Blood Cholesterol in Adults (Adult Treatment Panel III). JAMA 2001;285:2486–2497.


# 92

# EMERGENCY CONTRACEPTION

Uh Oh . . . . . . . . . . . . . . . . . . . . . . . . . . . . . . . . Level II

**Emily C. Farthing-Papineau, PharmD, BCPS**

## LEARNING OBJECTIVES

After completing this case study, the reader should be able to:

- Describe the advantages and disadvantages of the various options for emergency contraception.
- Discuss the possible side effects and contraindications of the various forms of emergency contraceptives, including both oral and nonoral options.
- Provide patient education regarding the use of emergency contraception.

## PATIENT PRESENTATION

### ■ Chief Complaint

"I forgot to restart my birth control pill pack. I have gone 9 days without a 'real' pill. I'm not ready to be pregnant yet!"

#### HPI

Isabelle Furtel is a 23-year-old woman who presents to the Family Medicine Clinic in a panic. She states that she typically throws out the last week of pills in her pack, "since they are not 'real' pills anyway," and she forgot to start her new pill pack on time. She had intercourse with her husband 2 days ago and wants to know what she should do to avoid pregnancy.

#### PMH

Seasonal allergies

#### FH

Mother, age 47, with type 2 diabetes. Father, age 45, with hypertension. Maternal grandmother, age 69, with COPD.

#### SH

Denies smoking
Enjoys an occasional glass of wine
Married × 2 years—mutually monogamous relationship

#### Meds

Cetirizine 10 mg po once daily × 5 years
Aviane (ethinyl estradiol 20 mcg/levonorgestrel 0.1 mg) one tablet po once daily × 2 years

#### All

NKDA

#### ROS

I.F. is a nulligravida woman whose menstrual periods are regular with the use of the combined oral contraceptive pill. She denies any breakthrough bleeding or spotting with routine use. She is tolerating the contraceptive pill well.

#### Physical Examination

*Gen*

WDWN female appearing anxious

*VS*

BP 106/70, P 60, RR 13, T 37°C; Wt 53.5 kg, Ht 5′5″

*Skin*

Clear

*Exam*

Deferred; she had a complete examination 3 months ago that was normal.

#### Labs

3 months ago:
Negative Pap smear
2 years ago:
Tests negative for *Chlamydia*, gonorrhea, syphilis, and HIV

#### Assessment

I.F. is a healthy, sexually active female who missed two doses of her combined oral contraceptive pill, extending her pill-free interval >7 days. Emergency contraceptive options to prevent pregnancy should be discussed.

## QUESTIONS

### Problem Identification

1. Identify the patient's drug therapy problem.

### Desired Outcome

2. What are the goals of pharmacotherapy in this case?

### Therapeutic Alternatives

3.a. What pharmacotherapeutic options are available for emergency contraception for this patient, and what are the advantages or disadvantages of each?

3.b. What contraindications exist to the use of emergency contraception, and do they apply to this patient?

### Optimal Plan

4. Recommend an appropriate emergency contraceptive method and dose for this patient.

### Outcome Evaluation

5. What clinical and laboratory parameters are necessary to evaluate the efficacy of the therapy?

### Patient Education

6.a. Counsel the patient regarding how the emergency contraceptive regimen works, how to take it, and what side effects may occur.

6.b. Explain to the patient how she will know if the emergency contraception regimen was effective.

6.c. Instruct the patient on when emergency contraception may be warranted, should she need to use it in the future.

6.d. When should the patient reinitiate her combined oral contraceptive pill?

6.e. How can the patient minimize the need for emergency contraception in the future?

## CLINICAL COURSE

A few weeks later, Isabelle calls into the clinic to report that she started her period and is not pregnant. She states she is thankful for the advice provided to her.

## SELF-STUDY ASSIGNMENTS

1. For other forms of hormonal contraception, such as the patch, the ring, progestin-only pills, and injectables, create a table identifying when emergency contraception may be needed if these methods are not used appropriately.
2. Identify strategies to minimize the hormone-free interval with the use of hormonal contraception and thereby diminish the potential need for emergency contraception.
3. For patients not using hormonal contraception, identify additional scenarios for which emergency contraception may be utilized.

## CLINICAL PEARL

Although not FDA-approved for this purpose, a copper IUD may also be used as emergency contraception within the first 120 hours after unprotected intercourse.

## REFERENCES


1. Stewart F, Trussel J, Van Look PF. Emergency contraception. In: Hatcher RA, Trussell J, Nelson AL, et al, eds. Contraceptive Technology, 19th ed. New York, Ardent Media Inc, 2007:87–116.
2. American College of Obstetricians and Gynecologists. ACOG practice bulletin no. 112: emergency contraception. Obstet Gynecol 2010;115(5):1100–1109.
3. Bastianelli C, Farris M, Benagiano G. Emergency contraception: a review. Eur Soc Contracept 2008;13(1):9–16.
4. Fine P, Mathe H, Ginde S, Cullins V, Morfesis J, Gainer E. Ulipristal acetate taken 48–120 hours after intercourse for emergency contraception. Obstet Gynecol 2010;115:257–263.
5. Glasier AF, Cameron ST, Fine PM, et al. Ulipristal acetate versus levonorgestrel for emergency contraception: a randomised non-inferiority trial and meta-analysis. Lancet 2010;375:555–562.
6. Ulipristal [Package Insert]. Morristown, NJ, Watson Pharma Inc, 2010.
7. Grimes DA. Intrauterine devices (IUDs). In: Hatcher RA, Trussell J, Nelson AL, et al, eds. Contraceptive Technology, 19th ed. New York, Ardent Media Inc, 2007:117–143.
8. Baird DT. Emergency contraception: how does it work? Reprod Biomed Online 2009;18(1):32–36.
9. Centers for Disease Control and Prevention. U.S. medical eligibility criteria for contraceptive use, 2010. Adapted from the World Health Organization medical eligibility criteria for contraceptive use, 4th edition. MMWR 2010;59(May):1–86 [early release].


# 93

# PREMENSTRUAL DYSPHORIC DISORDER

A Gloomy Girl. . . . . . . . . . . . . . . . . . . . . . . . . . Level II

**Larissa N. Hall, PharmD, BCPS**

## LEARNING OBJECTIVES

After completing this case study, the reader should be able to:

- Differentiate between the clinical presentation and diagnosis of premenstrual syndrome (PMS) and premenstrual dysphoric disorder (PMDD).
- Identify the desired therapeutic outcomes for patients with PMDD.
- Design an appropriate therapeutic plan for a patient with PMDD.
- Design an appropriate monitoring plan for a patient with PMDD, taking into account patient-specific factors (Table 93-1).
- Educate patients and other health care professionals about PMDD and therapeutic options.

## PATIENT PRESENTATION

### Chief Complaint

"I think my boss may fire me if I don't get some help."

**TABLE 93-1 Item Content of the Daily Record of Severity of Problems (DRSP)**

| |
|---|
| 1.a. Felt depressed, sad, "down," or "blue" |
| 1.b. Felt hopeless |
| 1.c. Felt worthless or guilty |
| 2. Felt anxious, tense, "keyed up," or "on edge" |
| 3.a. Had mood swings (e.g., suddenly felt sad or tearful) |
| 3.b. Was more sensitive to rejection or my feelings were easily hurt |
| 4.a. Felt angry, irritable |
| 4.b. Had conflicts or problems with people |
| 5. Had less interest in usual activities (e.g., work, school, friends, hobbies) |
| 6. Had difficulty concentrating |
| 7. Felt lethargic, tired, fatigued, or had a lack of energy |
| 8.a. Had increased appetite or overate |
| 8.b. Had cravings for specific foods |
| 9.a. Slept more, took naps, found it hard to get up when intended |
| 9.b. Had trouble getting to sleep or staying asleep |
| 10.a. Felt overwhelmed or that I could not cope |
| 10.b. Felt out of control |
| 11.a. Had breast tenderness |
| 11.b. Had breast swelling, felt "bloated," or had weight gain |
| 11.c. Had headache |
| 11.d. Had joint or muscle pain |
| At work, at school, at home, or in daily routine, at least one of the problems noted above caused reduction of productivity or inefficiency |
| At least one of the problems noted above interfered with hobbies or social activities (e.g., avoid or do less) |
| At least one of the problems noted above interfered with relationships with others |

### HPI

Gloria Gray, a 29-year-old woman, is an established patient at the Family Physician clinic who returns with complaints of bloating, breast tenderness, angry outbursts, irritability, depression, and fatigue. She has kept a record of her symptoms over the past 3 months, and it appears that her symptoms occur during the last week of her menstrual cycle each month. During this time, she really has a difficult time at work in particular. She gets angry easily and yells at coworkers. She feels very fatigued during this time, which causes her to lose focus and fall behind on her work. She is really concerned that she may lose her job. In addition, even though her husband has been very patient with her during these episodes, she can tell that it is really negatively affecting their relationship because they argue more frequently. She has tried over-the-counter ibuprofen and Midol Teen Formula, but these agents helped only minimally. Her symptoms typically resolve within the first few days of her menses. She says that she is depressed about her current situation, and she would really like some help. On an additional note, she states that she and her husband are not ready to have children as they previously thought. She says that there has just been too much stress in their lives lately, so she is interested in taking birth control. She and her husband use condoms, but they want to take every precaution at this time to effectively prevent pregnancy.

### PMH

Migraines without aura
Irritable bowel syndrome

### FH

Mother has dyslipidemia. Father has irritable bowel syndrome.

## SH

Married for 4 years. No children. Previous smoker 10 years ago, but no current tobacco use. She drinks alcohol socially on the weekends. She works full-time as a professor at a small community college.

## Meds

Metamucil one teaspoonful of powder in 8 oz of water daily
Propranolol 20 mg Q 6 hours
Sumatriptan 100 mg PRN migraine headache, may repeat × one dose
Women's multivitamin daily

## All

NKDA

## Physical Examination

*Gen*

Tearful, petite female

*VS*

BP 108/66, P 55, RR 17, T 98.3°F; Wt 112 lb, Ht 5′6″

*Skin*

Normal; intact; warm and dry

*HEENT*

PERRLA; EOMI; moist mucous membranes; TMs intact

*Neck/Lymph Nodes*

Supple without evidence of JVD, lymphadenopathy, or thyromegaly

*Lungs/Thorax*

Clear to A & P

*Breasts*

Symmetric; no lumps or masses; nipples without discharge; tender to touch

*CV*

RRR without MRG

*Abd*

Soft, NT/ND; +BS; no masses

*Genit/Rect*

Normal pelvic exam and pap smear

*Ext*

Normal ROM; pulses 2+; No CCE

*Neuro*

A & O × 3; CN II–XII intact; DTRs 2+

## Labs

Na 141 mEq/L, K 3.5 mEq/L, Cl 104 mEq/L, $CO_2$ 27 mEq/L, Glu 81 mg/dL, BUN 14 mg/dL, SCr 0.9 mg/dL

Ca 9.2 mg/dL, AST 20 IU/L, ALT 17 IU/L, Alb 3.9 g/dL, TSH 0.74 mIU/L

TC 190 mg/dL (fasting), TG 120 mg/dL (fasting), LDL 95 mg/dL (fasting), HDL 71 mg/dL (fasting)

WBC 6 × $10^3$/mm$^3$, Hgb 13 g/dL, Hct 39%, MCV 92.8 μm$^3$, MCH 31.7 pg, MCHC 34.2 g/dL, Plt 249 × $10^3$/mm$^3$

## Assessment

1. PMDD
2. Desire for contraception
3. Migraines without aura, currently well controlled
4. Irritable bowel syndrome, currently well controlled

# QUESTIONS

## Problem Identification

1.a. Create a list of the patient's drug therapy problems.

1.b. What symptoms in the patient's clinical presentation indicate PMDD?

1.c. How does this patient's clinical presentation differ from that of a patient suffering from PMS? What are the diagnostic differences between PMS and PMDD?

## Desired Outcome

2. What are the desired therapeutic outcomes in this patient with regard to PMDD?

## Therapeutic Alternatives

3.a. What nondrug therapies might be useful for a patient with PMDD?

3.b. What feasible pharmacotherapeutic alternatives are available for treatment of PMDD?

## Optimal Plan

4. What drug(s), dosage form, dose, schedule, and duration of therapy is/are best for this patient?

## Outcome Evaluation

5. What clinical and laboratory parameters are necessary to evaluate the therapy for achievement of the desired therapeutic outcome and to detect or prevent adverse effects?

## Patient Education

6. What information should be provided to the patient to enhance adherence, ensure successful therapy, and minimize adverse effects?

## SELF-STUDY ASSIGNMENTS

1. Develop a patient educational handout that outlines the differences between PMS and PMDD and provides resources for patients to get more information on PMDD.
2. List diseases that mimic the symptoms of PMDD that must be ruled out before the diagnosis of PMDD can be confirmed in a patient.
3. Discuss how migraine headaches and irritable bowel syndrome may be affected by the menstrual cycle.

## CLINICAL PEARL

PMDD and PMS are similar in many ways, but they differ in diagnostic criteria and severity. While up to 80% of women experience PMS, only up to 8% of women suffer from PMDD. PMDD is classified as a psychiatric disease. Therefore, it is important to differentiate PMDD from PMS in order to appropriately treat patients who suffer from the disease.

## REFERENCES


1. American Psychiatric Association. Diagnostic and Statistical Manual of Mental Disorders, 4th ed. Washington, DC, American Psychiatric Press, 2000:771–774.
2. Futterman LA, Rapkin AJ. Diagnosis of premenstrual disorders. J Reprod Med 2006;51:349–358.
3. Endicott J, Nee J, Harrison W. Daily record of severity of problems (DRSP): reliability and validity. Arch Women Ment Health 2006;9:41–49.
4. Clinical Management Guidelines for Premenstrual Syndrome. ACOG Practice Bulletin. No. 15. Washington, DC, the American College of Obstetricians and Gynecologists, April 2000.
5. Kroll R, Rapkin AJ. Treatment of premenstrual disorders. J Reprod Med 2006;51:359–370.
6. Noncontraceptive Uses of Hormonal Contraceptives. ACOG Practice Bulletin. No. 110. Washington, DC, the American College of Obstetricians and Gynecologists, January 2010.


# 94

# ENDOMETRIOSIS

Persistent Pelvic Pain . . . . . . . . . . . . . . . . . . . . Level II

**Connie Kraus, PharmD, BCPS**

## LEARNING OBJECTIVES

After completing this case study, the reader should be able to:

- Identify the signs and symptoms associated with endometriosis.
- Compare and contrast the benefits and risks associated with various hormonal medications used for treatment of endometriosis-associated pelvic pain.
- Determine a treatment approach for this case taking into account other health issues and potential health benefits.
- Discuss possible side effects associated with treatment for endometriosis.

## PATIENT PRESENTATION

### Chief Complaint

"Although the pain associated with my menstrual period is better, the naproxen upsets my stomach, and I am still having pain in my lower abdomen at other times during the month."

### HPI

Lisbeth Anderson is a 30-year-old woman who was diagnosed with endometriosis 3 months ago based on a history of dysmenorrhea, intermittent pain with defecation, and past history of dyspareunia. She presents to the nurse practitioner today for evaluation and management of continued endometriosis-related pain despite treatment with naproxen.

### PMH

s/p deep vein thrombosis 4 years ago after a flight to Southeast Asia; treated for 6 months with warfarin; no recurrence

G1P1A0; one healthy male child aged 2 years

### FH

Mother (aged 57 years) has a history of endometriosis, no other health conditions; father (aged 58 years) has hypertension and elevated cholesterol; one female sibling (aged 25 years) is healthy.

### SH

Patient is a freelance photographer. She has one child. She is single; not currently sexually active. She does not smoke and consumes no more than two alcohol-containing beverages per week. She exercises 30 minutes most days of the week.

### Meds

Naproxen 250 mg three times daily with food at first sign of menses for 5–7 days was begun at previous visit.

Multivitamin one daily.

### All

NKDA

### ROS

(+) For moderate pain in pelvic region, (–) for constipation, menstrual periods occur at regular intervals of 29 days

### Physical Examination

*Gen*

WDWN female in NAD

*VS*

BP 115/70, P 65, RR 15, T 37°C; Wt 72 kg, Ht 5′11″; patient has maintained same weight pre-pregnancy and postpregnancy

*Skin*

No lesions

*HEENT*

WNL

*Neck/Lymph Nodes*

Supple, no bruits, no adenopathy, no thyromegaly

*Lungs/Thorax*

CTA bilaterally

*Breasts*

Supple; no masses

*CV*

RRR, normal $S_1$ and $S_2$

*Abd*

Soft; patient states at baseline she experiences pain that averages a "4" on a 0–10 pain scale (with 10 being the worst possible pain), (+) BS; no masses noted

*Genit/Rect*

Pelvic exam: (+) adnexal pain elicited and rated at "6" on a 10-point scale, no masses

*MS/Ext*

Pulses intact

*Neuro*

Normal sensory and motor levels

### Labs

Na 135 mEq/L
K 3.8 mEq/L
Cl 104 mEq/L
$CO_2$ 25 mEq/L
BUN 10 mg/dL
SCr 0.6 mg/dL
Random Glu 89 mg/dL

*Fasting lipid profile*
T. chol 140 mg/dL
LDL 55 mg/dL
HDL 65 mg/dL
Trig 100 mg/dL

### Other

PAP smear: Normal
Chlamydia/gonorrhea: Negative
Urine pregnancy test: Negative

### Assessment

A 30-year-old woman with recent diagnosis of endometriosis with chronic pelvic pain; partial relief from dysmenorrhea with naproxen. Because of naproxen-related side effects and pain at other times besides during menses, would like to consider hormonal treatment options.

# QUESTIONS

## Problem Identification

1.a. What are the patient's current medication-related problems?

1.b. What information indicates the severity of this patient's problems?

## Desired Outcome

2. What are the goals of therapy for this patient's endometriosis pain?

## Therapeutic Alternatives

3.a. What nondrug therapies might be useful for this patient?

3.b. What hormonal options are available for the treatment of endometriosis?

3.c. What are the potential risks and benefits of the various treatment options for this patient?

3.d. Are there any treatments contraindicated in this patient?

## Optimal Plan

4. What drug, dosage form, dose, schedule, and duration are best for this patient?

## Outcome Evaluation

5. What clinical and laboratory parameters are necessary to evaluate the therapy for achievement of the desired therapeutic outcome and to detect or prevent adverse effects?

## Patient Education

6. What information should be provided to the patient to enhance adherence to the medication, ensure successful therapy, and minimize adverse effects?

# CLINICAL COURSE

The patient returns to her nurse practitioner 6 months after starting medroxyprogesterone acetate 150 mg intramuscular injections every 3 months. She reports that her pelvic pain is better controlled with an overall average rating pain of "1" on the 10-point scale. She states that she had intermittent spotting initially, but now has no menstrual periods.

## Follow-Up Questions

1. What is the optimal length of time for a patient to continue on medroxyprogesterone acetate injections for treatment of endometriosis-related chronic pelvic pain?
2. Are there other options that this patient could select to achieve similar results with the same or better side-effect profile?
3. Would your recommendation change if this patient had risk factors for osteopenia or future osteoporosis?
4. Would your recommendation change if this patient had indicated an interest in having another child in the next 1–2 years?

# SELF-STUDY ASSIGNMENTS

1. Research complementary therapies that have been studied for the relief of endometriosis, and compare the evidence for their efficacy with standard treatments.
2. Review the contraindications of the various contraceptive agents used for treatment of endometriosis.

# CLINICAL PEARL

Pharmacologic treatment of endometriosis may be useful for decreasing pain. Pharmacotherapeutic agents that mimic pregnancy or menopause are the cornerstone of treatment. All of these agents have similar efficacy in treating pain, but have different side-effect profiles. Treatment with hormonal therapy does not improve fertility, which can also be a potential consequence of the disease.

# REFERENCES


1. Wieser F, Cohen M, Gaeddert A, et al. Evolution of medical treatment for endometriosis: back to the roots? Hum Reprod Update 2007;13(5):487–499.
2. Flower A, Liu JP, Chen S, Lewith G, Little P. Chinese herbal medicine for endometriosis. Cochrane Database Syst Rev 2009;(8):CD006568.
3. The Practice Committee of the American Society for Reproductive Medicine. Treatment of pelvic pain associated with endometriosis. Fertil Steril 2006;86(Suppl 4):S18–S27.
4. Ozkan S, Arici A. Advances in treatment options of endometriosis. Gynecol Obstet Invest 2009:67:81–91.
5. Garquhar C. Endometriosis. BMJ 2007;334:249–253.

6. Petta CA, Ferianni RA, Abrao MS, et al. Randomized clinical trial of a levonorgestrel-releasing intrauterine system and a depot GnRH analogue for the treatment of chronic pelvic pain in women with endometriosis. Hum Reprod 2005;7:1993–1998.
7. Walch K, Unfried G, Huber J, et al. Implanon® versus medroxyprogesterone acetate: effects on pain scores in patients with symptomatic endometriosis—a pilot study. Contraception 2009;70:29–34.
8. Selak V, Farquhar C, Prentice A, Singla A. Danazol for pelvic pain associated with endometriosis. Cochrane Database Syst Rev 2007;(4):CD000068.
9. Davis L, Kennedy SS, Moore J, Prentice A. Modern combined oral contraceptives for pain associated with endometriosis. Cochrane Database Syst Rev 2007;(3):CD001019.
10. Hatcher RA, Trussell J, Nelson AL, Cates W Jr, Stewart FH, Kowal D. Contraceptive Technology, 19th ed. Contraceptive Technology Communications Inc, 2007.
11. Department of Reproductive Health, World Health Organization. Medical eligibility criteria for contraceptive use. Available at: *http://www.who.int/reproductivehealth/publications/family_planning/9789241563888/en/index.html*. Accessed May 9, 2010.

# 95

# MANAGING MENOPAUSAL SYMPTOMS

A Hot Topic. . . . . . . . . . . . . . . . . . . . . . . . . . . . Level II

**Nicole S. Culhane, PharmD, FCCP, BCPS**

## LEARNING OBJECTIVES

After completing this case study, the reader should be able to:

- Identify the signs and symptoms associated with menopause.
- List the risks and benefits associated with hormone therapy (HT), and identify appropriate candidates for HT.
- Differentiate between topical and systemic forms of HT.
- Recommend nonpharmacologic therapy for menopausal symptoms.
- Identify alternative, nonhormonal therapies for women unable to take HT.
- Design a comprehensive pharmacotherapeutic plan for a patient on HT including treatment options and monitoring.
- Determine the desired therapeutic outcomes for a patient taking HT.
- Educate patients on the treatment options, benefits, risks, and monitoring of HT.

## PATIENT PRESENTATION

### Chief Complaint

"I have been having hot flashes for the past few months, and I just can't take it anymore."

### HPI

Emma Peterson is a 50 yo woman who reports experiencing two to three hot flashes per day, occasionally associated with insomnia. She also states she is awakened from sleep about two to three times per week needing to change her bed clothes and linens. Her symptoms began about 3 months ago, and over that time they have worsened to the point where they have become very bothersome. She states that her mother was prescribed a pill for this, but she is hesitant to take the same thing because she heard on the news and from friends that the medication may not be safe. She also does not want to "get her period back" if possible. Successfully treated for depression in the past, she is currently controlled on paroxetine therapy. She currently exercises three times a week and tries to follow a low-cholesterol diet.

### PMH

Depression
GERD
HTN
Hypothyroidism

### FH

Mother died of stroke at age 67; father died of lung cancer at age 62. Patient has one brother, 52, and one sister, 48, who are alive and well, but both with HTN.

### SH

Married, mother of two healthy daughters, ages 21 and 25. She is an RN in a neighboring physician's office. She walks on her treadmill three times a week and is trying to follow a dietitian-designed low-cholesterol diet. She does not smoke and occasionally drinks a glass of red wine with dinner.

### Meds

Hydrochlorothiazie 25 mg po once daily
Omeprazole 20 mg po once daily
Paroxetine 20 mg po once daily
Synthroid 0.75 mg po once daily

### All

NKDA

### ROS

(+) Hot flashes, occasional night sweats and insomnia, vaginal dyness. (−) For weight gain, constipation. LMP 12 months ago.

### Physical Examination

*Gen*

WDWN female in NAD

*VS*

BP 128/86, P 78, RR 15, T 36.4°C; Wt 76.2 kg, Ht 5′6″

*Skin*

Warm, dry, no lesions

*HEENT*

WNL

*Neck/LN*

Supple, no bruits, no adenopathy, no thyromegaly

*Lungs/Thorax*

CTA bilaterally

*Breasts*

Supple; no masses

*CV*

RRR, normal $S_1$ and $S_2$; no m/r/g

*Abd*

Soft, NT/ND, (+) BS; no masses

*Genit/Rect*

Pelvic exam normal except (+) mucosal atrophy; stool guaiac (−)

*Ext*

(−) CCE; pulses intact

*Neuro*

Normal sensory and motor levels

### Labs

| | | | |
|---|---|---|---|
| Na 136 mEq/L | Hgb 12.7 g/dL | Ca 9.3 mg/dL | *Fasting lipid profile* |
| K 3.9 mEq/L | Hct 39.3% | AST 32 IU/L | T. chol 190 mg/dL |
| Cl 104 mEq/L | WBC 6.5 × $10^3$/mm$^3$ | ALT 30 IU/L | LDL 132 mg/dL |
| $CO_2$ 25 mEq/L | Plt 208 × $10^3$/mm$^3$ | TSH 2.46 mIU/L | HDL 50 mg/dL |
| BUN 10 mg/dL | | FSH 87.8 mIU/mL | Trig 180 mg/dL |
| SCr 0.7 mg/dL | | UPT (−) | |
| Random Glu 98 mg/dL | | | |

### Other

Pap smear and mammogram: Normal

### Assessment

A 50 yo symptomatic postmenopausal woman considering HT versus other treatment options.

# QUESTIONS

## Problem Identification

1.a. Create a list of the patient's drug therapy problems.

1.b. What information (signs, symptoms, laboratory values) indicates the presence or severity of this patient's problems as she begins menopause?

## Desired Outcome

2. What are the goals of therapy for this patient's menopausal symptoms?

## Therapeutic Alternatives

3.a. What nondrug therapies might be useful for this patient?

3.b. What are the benefits and risks of HT for this patient?

3.c. What pharmacotherapeutic *hormonal* therapies are available for the treatment of menopause?

3.d. What *nonhormonal* alternatives may be used to manage menopausal symptoms?

## Optimal Plan

4. What drug, dosage form, dose, schedule, and duration are best for this patient?

## Outcome Evaluation

5. What clinical and laboratory parameters are necessary to evaluate the therapy for achievement of the desired therapeutic outcome and to detect or prevent adverse effects?

## Patient Education

6. What information should be provided to the patient to enhance adherence to the medication, ensure successful therapy, and minimize adverse effects?

## CLINICAL COURSE

The patient returns to her physician after taking HT for 1 year. She reports that her hot flashes, night sweats, and occsional insomnia have significantly decreased and would like to know if she should continue taking the HT regimen and if so, for how long.

## Follow-Up Questions

1. What is the optimal dose and length of time for a patient to continue on HT?
2. How should HT be discontinued after successful treatment?
3. Would your recommendation for HT change if the patient had been complaining of genital symptoms only? Why or why not?
4. Would your recommendation for HT change if this patient were to have had significant risk factors for coronary artery disease (CAD) or a personal history of breast cancer? Why or why not?
5. How would you responsd to the patient if she asked you about taking bioidentical HT?

## CLINICAL COURSE: ALTERNATIVE THERAPY

Because Mrs Peterson is considering stopping her HT because of her family history of breast cancer but still desires some relief from hot flushes, she asks for additional information on other alternatives. She has heard that black cohosh should not be used in women with breast cancer, but she has a friend who also has a family history of breast cancer who has been on black cohosh for about 9 months on the recommendation of her physician, although the friend must have a checkup with lab tests every 6 months. Mrs Peterson asks if black cohosh or soy would be an appropriate option to help keep her hot flushes under control. See Section 19 in this casebook for questions about the use of black cohosh for managing menopausal symptoms.

## SELF-STUDY ASSIGNMENTS

1. Research nonhormonal therapies that have been studied for the relief of menopausal symptoms and compare the scientific evidence of their efficacy to traditional hormonal medications.
2. Review the results of the Women's Health Initiative (WHI) study from 2002 as well as the 2007 reanalysis of the WHI results regarding the impact of HT on cardiovascular disease related to age and duration of HT use, and provide a summary of the overall findings regarding HT and cardiovascular risk and breast cancer risk.

## CLINICAL PEARL

Women should receive a thorough history and physical exam, including assessing CAD and breast cancer risk factors, before HT is considered. If a woman does not have any contraindications to HT, including CAD or significant CAD risk factors, and also does not have a personal history of breast cancer, HT would be an appropriate therapy option as it remains the most effective treatment for vasomotor symptoms and vulvovaginal atrophy.

## REFERENCES


1. Bolland MJ, Ames RW, Horne AM, Orr-Walker BJ, Gamble GD, Reid IR. The effect of treatment with a thiazide diuretic for 4 years on bone density in normal postmenopausal women. Osteoporos Int 2007;18:479–486.
2. Grady D. Management of menopausal symptoms. N Engl J Med 2006;355:2338–2347.
3. Hulley S, Grady D, Bush T, et al. Randomized trial of estrogen plus progestin for secondary prevention of coronary heart disease in postmenopausal women. Heart and Estrogen/Progestin Replacement Study (HERS) Research Group. JAMA 1998;280:605–613.
4. Rossouw JE, Anderson GL, Prentice RL, et al. Writing Group for the Women's Health Initiative Investigators. Risks and benefits of estrogen plus progestin in healthy postmenopausal women: principal results from the Women's Health Initiative randomized controlled trial. JAMA 2002;288:321–333.
5. Rossouw JE, Prentice RL, Manson JE, et al. Postmenopausal hormone therapy and risk of cardiovascular disease by age and years since menopause. JAMA 2007;297:1465–1477.
6. Anderson GL, Limacher M, Assaf AR, et al. Effects of conjugated equine estrogen in postmenopausal women with hysterectomy: the Women's Health Initiative randomized controlled trial. JAMA 2004;291:1701–1712.
7. Utian WH, Shoupe D, Backmann G, Pinkerton JV, Pickar JH. Relief of vasomotor symptoms and vaginal atrophy with lower doses of conjugated equine estrogens and medroxyprogesterone acetate. Fertil Steril 2001;75:1065–1079.
8. Fugate SE, Church CO. Nonestrogen treatment modalities for vasomotor symptoms associated with menopause. Ann Pharmacother 2004;38:1482–1499.
9. Speroff L, Gass M, Constantine G, Olivier S. Efficacy and tolerability of desvenlafaxine succinate treatment for menopausal vasomotor symptoms. Obstet Gynecol 2008;111:77–87.
10. Grady D. A 60-year-old woman trying to discontinue hormone replacement therapy. JAMA 2002;287(16):2130–2137.

SECTION 10
# UROLOGIC DISORDERS

## 96

# ERECTILE DYSFUNCTION

Where There's a Pill, There's a Way . . . . . . . . Level III

**Cara Liday, PharmD, BCPS, CDE**

## LEARNING OBJECTIVES

After completing this case study, students should be able to:

- Recognize risk factors associated with development of erectile dysfunction (ED).
- Provide brief descriptions of the advantages and disadvantages of the common therapies available for treating ED.
- Compare and contrast the available PDE-5 inhibitors.
- Recommend appropriate lifestyle changes and other therapy for ED in a specific patient.
- Provide patient education on administration and expected side effects of selected treatment modalities for ED.

## PATIENT PRESENTATION

### Chief Complaint

"My sex life just isn't what it used to be …."

### HPI

Peter Johnson is a 63-year-old man who presents to his PCP with the above complaint. On questioning, he states that for the last year he has been able to achieve only partial erections that are insufficient for intercourse. He does not notice nocturnal penile tumescence. He feels that the problem is leading to a strained relationship with his wife, and he is interested in trying an herbal product or "nutritional supplement" for help.

### PMH

Type 2 DM × 14 years

HTN

HF (NYHA class II)

Dyslipidemia

### FH

Father deceased at age 72 of cancer; mother alive with HTN

### SH

Married for 38 years; no history of marital problems; does not smoke or drink alcohol; walks for 30 minutes 5 days per week with slight SOB

### Meds

Insulin glargine 45 U SC at bedtime

Metformin 1,000 mg po BID

Sitagliptin 100 mg po once daily

Lisinopril 40 mg po once daily

Carvedilol 25 mg po BID

Furosemide 20 mg po every morning

Simvastatin 40 mg po once daily

ASA 81 mg po once daily

### All

NKDA

### ROS

Denies significant life stressors, fatigue, nocturia, urgency, or symptoms of prostatitis. Complains of occasional nocturia, numbness in his feet, and difficulty achieving and maintaining erections. Occasionally has transient edema in his ankles, and many of his toenails are brittle and yellowing.

### Physical Examination

*Gen*

Alert, well-developed, cooperative man in NAD

*VS*

BP 136/84, P 60, RR 18, T 37.2°C; Wt 120 kg, Ht 5′11″

*Skin*

Warm, dry; no lesions

*HEENT*

NC/AT; EOMI; PERRLA; funduscopic examination shows no arteriolar narrowing, hemorrhages, or exudates

*Neck/Lymph Nodes*

Supple without JVD, lymphadenopathy, masses, or goiter

*Lungs/Chest*

Clear to A & P bilaterally

*CV*

RRR; normal $S_1$ and $S_2$; no MRG

*Abd*

Soft, obese; NTND; normal bowel sounds; no masses or organomegaly

*Genit/Rect*

Normal scrotum, testes descended; NT w/o masses; penis without discharge or curvature; slightly enlarged prostate

*MS/Ext*

Muscle strength 5/5 throughout; full ROM in all extremities; pulses 2+ throughout; no edema present; multiple toenails with yellow discoloration and thickening

*Neuro*

CNs II–XII intact; DTRs 2+ and equal bilaterally. No sensory/motor deficits; reduced sensation in extremities bilaterally with vibratory and monofilament testing

■ Labs

| | | | |
|---|---|---|---|
| Na 139 mEq/L | Hgb 16.0 g/dL | Ca 9.5 mg/dL | *Fasting lipid profile* |
| K 3.9 mEq/L | Hct 50% | Mg 1.8 mEq/L | T. chol 192 mg/dL |
| Cl 102 mEq/L | AST 35 IU/L | A1C 8.5% | HDL 41 mg/dL |
| $CO_2$ 24 mEq/L | ALT 18 IU/L | Testosterone | LDL 94 mg/dL |
| BUN 12 mg/dL | | 700 ng/dL | TG 129 mg/dL |
| SCr 1.0 mg/dL | | TSH 1.54 mIU/L | VLDL 19 mg/dL |
| Glu (fasting) 166 mg/dL | | BNP 79 pg/mL | |

■ UA

SG 1.00; pH 5.1; leukocyte esterase (–); nitrite (–); protein 100 mg/dL; ketones (–); urobilinogen normal; bilirubin (–); blood (–)

Microalbumin/Cr ratio 18 mg/g

■ Assessment

A 63-year-old male with ED, poor long-term control of type 2 diabetes, hypertension, HF, dyslipidemia, and probable diagnosis of onychomycosis

## CLINICAL COURSE

Mr Johnson was referred to his cardiologist for exercise treadmill testing. It was determined that he may safely resume sexual activity at this time. He is to call immediately if he has significant SOB or chest pain during or after intercourse.

# QUESTIONS

## Problem Identification

1.a. Create a list of the patient's drug therapy problems.

1.b. What risk factors for ED are present in this patient?

1.c. What are the etiologies of ED, and what is this patient's most likely etiology?

1.d. Could any of the patient's problems have been caused by drug therapy?

## Desired Outcome

2. What are the goals of therapy in this case?

## Therapeutic Alternatives

3.a. What nondrug therapies are available for the treatment of ED?

3.b. What pharmacologic alternatives are available for the treatment of ED?

## Optimal Plan

4. What therapy is most appropriate and effective for initial treatment of this patient? If drug therapy is indicated, list the drug, dosage form, dose, schedule, and duration of therapy.

## Outcome Evaluation

5. What clinical parameters are necessary to evaluate the therapy for achievement of the desired therapeutic outcome and to detect or prevent adverse effects?

## Patient Education

6. What information should be provided to the patient to enhance compliance, ensure successful therapy, and minimize adverse effects?

## ■ SELF-STUDY ASSIGNMENTS

1. If therapy for onychomycosis is desired, what medication would be optimal, and how would the addition of this agent change your treatment of the patient's ED?
2. β-Blockers are typically associated with an increased incidence of ED. Determine why nebivolol may have a lower incidence of ED and may possibly improve erectile function.
3. Discuss the possible benefits of using a PDE-5 inhibitor in patients with symptomatic benign prostatic hyperplasia (BPH).
4. Evaluate the incidence of women's sexual dysfunction and options for therapy in this population.

## CLINICAL PEARL

Patients with cardiovascular (CV) disease have a greater risk of developing ED. In addition, the presence of ED in otherwise healthy individuals may indicate an increased risk of subsequent CV disease. The development of ED may precede the onset of CV symptoms by 3 years or more. Providers should use this opportunity to screen or treat CV disease appropriately.

## REFERENCES

1. McVary KT. Erectile dysfunction. N Engl J Med 2007;357;2472–2481.
2. Schwarz ER, Rastogi S, Kapur V, Sulemanjee N, Rodriguez JJ. Erectile dysfunction in heart failure patients. J Am Coll Cardiol 2006; 48:1111–1119.
3. Esposito K, Giugliano FR, DiPalo C, et al. Effect of lifestyle changes on erectile dysfunction in obese men. JAMA 2004;291:2978–2984.
4. Heidelbaugh JJ. Management of erectile dysfunction. Am Fam Physician 2010;81:305–312.
5. Tsertsvadze A, Fink HA, Yazdi F, et al. Oral phosphodiesterase-5 inhibitors and hormonal treatments for erectile dysfunction: a systematic review and meta-analysis. Ann Intern Med 2009;151:650–661.
6. Ellsworth P, Kirshenbaum EM. Current concepts in the evaluation and management of erectile dysfunction. Urol Nurs 2008;28: 357–369.

7. Consumer Updates. Hidden risks of erectile dysfunction "treatments" sold online. U.S. Food and Drug Administration. Available at: *www.fda.gov/ForConsumers/ConsumerUpdates/ucm048386.htm*. Accessed February 24, 2010.
8. Rosen RC, Jackson G, Kostis JB. Erectile dysfunction and cardiac disease: recommendations of the second Princeton consensus conference. Curr Urol Rep 2006;7:490–496.

# 97

# BENIGN PROSTATIC HYPERPLASIA

Long-Lasting Love. . . . . . . . . . . . . . . . . . . . . . . Level II

**Catherine A. Heyneman-Cashmore, PharmD, MS, ANP, FASCP**
**Kevin W. Cleveland, PharmD, ANP**

## LEARNING OBJECTIVES

After completing this case study, students should be able to:

- Recognize the clinical manifestations of BPH.
- Differentiate between obstructive and irritative symptoms in patients with BPH.
- Recommend appropriate pharmacotherapeutic treatment for BPH.
- Identify and manage drug interactions associated with BPH pharmacotherapy.
- Recognize when surgical therapies should be considered for patients with BPH.
- Understand how some drugs can exacerbate BPH symptoms.

## PATIENT PRESENTATION

### Chief Complaint

"I'm up four or five times a night feeling that I have to urinate, and then when I get to the bathroom all I do is dribble. I'm very lightheaded when I stand up, and sometimes I don't make it to the bathroom in time. I have a girlfriend now, but I am finding it difficult to be intimate with her. Also, going to the bathroom all night is really impacting my love life."

### HPI

Jimmy McCracken is a 62-year-old man with a long-standing history of UTIs. He has a history of urosepsis requiring hospitalization. He is being evaluated because of complaints of worsening urinary hesitancy, nocturia, and dribbling. He also has a new complaint of ED.

### PMH

HTN

Laminectomy 10 years ago

BPH with urge incontinence

Chronic UTIs

Type 2 DM (well controlled with glyburide/metformin)

Allergy to cat dander

ED

Obesity

Hx headaches

Osteoarthritis

### FH

Educated through the 12th grade. Father died of massive MI at age 78; mother died of natural causes at age 91.

### SH

Worked for 35 years in a grocery store; retired 7 years ago. Married once. Wife deceased 6 months ago (stroke); one daughter, two granddaughters. Lives alone but is socially active. Recently started dating a 59-year-old woman he met through his square-dancing group. Patient is emphatic about maximizing the use of natural products in his therapy, including continued use of saw palmetto. Used smokeless tobacco × 35 years; heavy ETOH in the past, occasional glass of wine now.

### ROS

In conversation, he is alert, friendly, and courteous. He has no c/o dyspepsia, dysphagia, abdominal pain, hematemesis, or visible blood in the stool.

### Meds

Glyburide/metformin 5/500 mg po BID

Amitriptyline 50 mg po at bedtime (HA prophylaxis)

Terazosin 10 mg po QD

Saw palmetto 200 mg po BID

Ibuprofen 800 mg po BID

Claritin-D 24-hour one tablet po daily (allergy to cats)

### All

NKDA; allergic to cat dander

### Physical Examination

*Gen*

White male in NAD; well-kept appearance; A & O × 3

*VS*

BP 110/60, P 85, RR 18, T 37°C; Wt 115.2 kg, Ht 6′0″

*Skin*

Vertical scars on neck and lower back from laminectomies

*HEENT*

PERRLA; EOMI; TMs WNL; nose and throat clear w/o exudate or lesions

*Neck/Lymph Nodes*

Supple w/o LAD or masses; thyroid in midline

*Lungs/Thorax*

CTA, distant sounds

*CV*

RRR w/o murmurs

*Abd*

Soft, NTND w/o masses or scars; (+) BS

*Genit/Rect*

Testes ↓↓, penis circumcised w/o DC; guaiac (+) stool

*MS/Ext*

Neurovascular intact; distal pulses 1–2+

*Neuro*

DTRs 2+; CNs II–XII grossly intact

### UA

Color straw; appearance clear; SG 1.010; pH 6.5; glucose (–); bilirubin (–); ketones (–); blood (–); urobilinogen 0.2 mg/dL; nitrite (–); leukocyte esterases (–); epithelial cells—occasional per hpf; WBC—occasional per hpf; RBC—none seen; bacteria—trace; amorphous—none seen; crystals—1+ calcium oxalate; mucus—none seen. Culture not indicated.

### GU Consult

Patient treated for UTI 2 weeks ago with Cipro 250 mg Q 12 h × 3 days. Urine clear; negative for glucose. Bladder examination with ultrasound revealed postvoid residual estimate of 200 mL. Prostate approximately 35 g, benign. AUA Symptom Score = 20. Uroflowmetry ($Q_{max}$) = 8 mL/s.

### Assessment

BPH with urge incontinence

ED

Symptomatic hypotension

Normocytic anemia possibly secondary to UGI bleed

### Labs

See Table 97-1.

## QUESTIONS

### Problem Identification

1.a. Create a list of the patient's drug therapy problems.

1.b. Describe the natural history and epidemiologic characteristics of BPH.

1.c. Which of this patient's complaints are consistent with obstructive symptoms of BPH? Which are consistent with irritative symptoms?

1.d. What steps are recommended in the initial evaluation of all patients presenting with BPH (Fig. 97-1)?

1.e. What other medical conditions should be ruled out before treating this patient for BPH?

### Desired Outcome

2. What are the goals of pharmacotherapy in this case?

### Therapeutic Alternatives

3. What are the treatment alternatives for BPH?

### Optimal Plan

4. What drug, dosage form, dose, schedule, and duration of therapy are best for this patient?

### Outcome Evaluation

5. What clinical and laboratory parameters are necessary to evaluate the therapy for achievement of the desired therapeutic outcome and to detect or prevent adverse effects?

### Patient Education

6. What information should be provided to the patient to enhance compliance, ensure successful therapy, and minimize adverse effects?

## CLINICAL COURSE: ALTERNATIVE THERAPY

As the pharmacist in the team, you perform a literature search on the use of saw palmetto for BPH. You discover that there are reports of the dietary supplement both improving and worsening symptoms of ED. Because the patient's ED symptoms began while he was taking saw palmetto, you decide that it is plausible that saw palmetto could be contributing to ED symptoms. In addition, your readings indicate that saw palmetto should really only be used by patients with mild to moderate BPH. Based on this information, your recommendation is to stop the saw palmetto. However, because the patient is emphatic about wanting to continue a natural product, you search for alternative dietary supplements that may provide some benefit for this patient's BPH without contributing to ED. Would *Pygeum africanum* be a reasonable option to consider? For questions related to the use of *P. africanum* for the treatment of BPH, please see Section 19 of this casebook.

## CLINICAL COURSE

Mr McCracken's blood pressure increased to 130/90, and the BPH and ED symptoms improved remarkably after your recommendations were implemented. Over the ensuing weeks, he continued to experience occasional urgency and hesitancy, so 6 months later he opted for laser prostatectomy. This procedure was successful in alleviating his symptoms.

**TABLE 97-1 Lab Values**

| | | | | |
|---|---|---|---|---|
| Na 136 mEq/L | Hgb 12.6 g/dL | WBC 5.6 × $10^3$/mm$^3$ | AST 12 IU/L | Ca 8.5 mg/dL |
| K 4.1 mEq/L | Hct 37.9% | Neutros 75% | ALT 16 IU/L | Phos 3.5 mg/dL |
| Cl 103 mEq/L | MCV 92.5 μm$^3$ | Lymphs 16% | Alk phos 55 IU/L | Uric acid 3.5 mg/dL |
| $CO_2$ 41 mEq/L | MCH 30.8 pg | Monos 5% | LDH 121 units/L | $T_4$ 7.3 mcg/dL |
| BUN 9 mg/dL | MCHC 33.3 g/dL | Eos 3% | T. bili 0.6 mg/dL | TSH 1.04 mIU/L |
| SCr 0.7 mg/dL | Plt 191 × $10^3$/mm$^3$ | Basos 1% | T. prot 6.1 g/dL | A1C 7.5% |
| Glu 120 mg/dL | | | T. chol 146 mg/dL | PSA 4.5 ng/mL |

Patient Name: ______________ DOB: __________ ID: ______________ Date of assessment: __________

Initial Assessment ( ) Monitor during: __________ Therapy ( ) after: ______________ Therapy/surgery ( ) __________

AUA BPH Symptom Score

| | Not at all | Less than 1 time in 5 | Less than half the time | About half the time | More than half the time | Almost always | |
|---|---|---|---|---|---|---|---|
| 1. Over the past month, how often have you had a sensation of not emptying your bladder completely after you finished urinating? | 0 | 1 | 2 | 3 | 4 | 5 | |
| 2. Over the past month, how often have you had to urinate again less than two hours after you finished urinating? | 0 | 1 | 2 | 3 | 4 | 5 | |
| 3. Over the past month, how often have you found you stopped and started again several times when you urinated? | 0 | 1 | 2 | 3 | 4 | 5 | |
| 4. Over the past month, how often have you found it difficult to postpone urination? | 0 | 1 | 2 | 3 | 4 | 5 | |
| 5. Over the past month, how often have you had a weak urinary stream? | 0 | 1 | 2 | 3 | 4 | 5 | |
| 6. Over the past month, how often have you had to push or strain to begin urination? | 0 | 1 | 2 | 3 | 4 | 5 | |
| | None | 1 time | 2 times | 3 times | 4 times | 5 or more times | |
| 7. Over the past month, how many times did you most typically get up to urinate from the time you went to bed at night until the time you got up in the morning? | 0 | 1 | 2 | 3 | 4 | 5 | |
| | | | | Total Symptom Score | | | |

**FIGURE 97-1.** The American Urologic Association (AUA) symptom index for benign prostatic hyperplasia (BPH). *(Reprinted with permission from BPH, Main Report: Roehrborn CG, McConnell JD, Barry MJ, et al. AUA Guideline on the Management of Benign Prostatic Hyperplasia. American Urological Association Education and Research Inc, © 2003.)*

## SELF-STUDY ASSIGNMENTS

1. Compare the efficacy of saw palmetto (*Serenoa repens*) to finasteride and $\alpha_1$-antagonists for the treatment of BPH.
2. Perform a literature search for evidence that supports the use of phosphodiesterase type 5 inhibitors and $\alpha_1$-antagonists as combination therapy for BPH/ED.
3. Identify the BPH patient subpopulation that would benefit the most from finasteride/dutasteride therapy.
4. Compare treatment options for ED in patients with BPH. Identify the risks and potential benefits of using $\alpha_1$-antagonists and 5$\alpha$-reductase inhibitors in treating comorbid ED and BPH.

## CLINICAL PEARL

Physiologic measurements such as postvoid residuals, uroflowmetry, and pressure–flow studies often do not correlate well with the patient's perception of BPH symptom severity.

## REFERENCES


1. Miner M, Rosenberg MT, Perelman MA. Treatment of lower urinary tract symptoms in benign prostatic hyperplasia and its impact on sexual function. Clin Ther 2006;28:13–25.
2. Kaminetsky JC. Comorbid LUTS and erectile dysfunction: optimizing their management. Curr Med Res Opin 2006;22:2497–2506.
3. AUA Practice Guidelines Committee. AUA guideline on management of benign prostatic hyperplasia (2003/2006 update). Available at: *www.auanet.org/guidelines/bph.cfm|http//www.auanet.org/guidelines/bph.cfm*. Accessed March 10, 2010.
4. Narayan P, Evans CP, Moon T. Long-term safety and efficacy of tamsulosin for the treatment of lower urinary tract symptoms associated with benign prostatic hyperplasia. J Urol 2003;170(Pt 1):498–502.
5. McConnell JD, Bruskewitz R, Walsh P, et al. The effect of finasteride on the risk of acute urinary retention and the need for surgical treatment among men with benign prostatic hyperplasia. N Engl J Med 1998;338:557–563.
6. Lowe FC, McConnell JD, Hudson PB, et al, Finasteride Study Group. Long-term 6-year experience with finasteride in patients with benign prostatic hyperplasia. Urology 2003;61:791–796.
7. Roehrborn CG, Boyle P, Nickel JC, et al. Efficacy and safety of a dual inhibitor of 5-alpha-reductase types 1 and 2 (dutasteride) in men with benign prostatic hyperplasia. Urology 2002;60:434–441.
8. McConnell JD, Roehrborn CG, Bautista OM, et al, Medical Therapy of Prostatic Symptoms (MTOPS) Research Group. The long-term effect of doxazosin, finasteride, and combination therapy on the clinical progression of benign prostatic hyperplasia. N Engl J Med 2003;349:2387–2398.
9. Bent S, Kane C, Shinohara K, et al. Saw palmetto for benign prostatic hyperplasia. N Engl J Med 2006;354:557–566.
10. Liguori G, Trombetta C, De Giorgi G, et al. Efficacy and safety of combined oral therapy with tadalafil and alfuzosin: an integrated approach to the management of patients with lower urinary tract symptoms and erectile dysfunction. Preliminary report. J Sex Med 2009;6:544–552.

# 98

# URINARY INCONTINENCE

Bladder Matters . . . . . . . . . . . . . . . . . . . . . . . Level II

**Mary Lee, PharmD, BCPS, FCCP**

**Roohollah R. Sharifi, MD, FACS**

## LEARNING OBJECTIVES

After completing this case study, students should be able to:

- Distinguish overactive bladder syndrome from stress urinary incontinence, overflow urinary incontinence, and functional urinary incontinence.
- Determine when anticholinergic drugs should be recommended for the management of overactive bladder syndrome.
- Compare and contrast muscarinic receptor selectivity, lipophilicity, and pharmacokinetic properties of commonly used antimuscarinic agents for management of overactive bladder and discuss the clinical implications of these properties.
- Discuss the potential advantages of extended-release oral and transdermal formulations of antimuscarinic agents in the elderly with overactive bladder syndrome.
- Identify concomitant drug therapy that may exacerbate overactive bladder syndrome.
- Recommend appropriate nondrug therapy for the management of overactive bladder syndrome.

## PATIENT PRESENTATION

### Chief Complaint

"I can't seem to control my urine. I feel like I have to urinate all the time. However, when I do go to the bathroom, I often pass only a small amount of urine. Sometimes I wet myself. I was started on a medication for my leaking a few weeks ago, but it doesn't seem to be working."

### HPI

Susan Jones is an 83-year-old woman with urinary urgency, frequency, and incontinence. She reports soiling her underwear at least one to three times during the day and night and has resorted to wearing panty liners or changing her underwear several times a day. The patient has curtailed much of her volunteer work and social activities because of this problem. Urinary leakage is not worsened by laughing, coughing, sneezing, carrying heavy objects, or walking up and down stairs. She does not report wetting herself without warning. She has been taking Detrol LA 2 mg po daily for the past month with no improvement in her voiding symptoms, and she complains of new-onset constipation, confusion, and difficulty remembering routine tasks.

### PMH

HTN for many years, treated with medications for 10 years. Dyslipidemia for 5 years, controlled with a low-cholesterol diet, weight control, regular exercise, and medication. Menopausal; stopped ovulating at age 52; no longer has hot flashes. Has difficulty falling asleep and often has sleepless nights. She has no history of spinal or pelvic surgery.

### FH

Noncontributory

### SH

Nonsmoker; social drinker; married

### Meds

Hydrochlorothiazide 25 mg po once daily with supper

Pravastatin 40 mg po at bedtime

Diovan® (valsartan) 160 mg po every morning

Detrol LA 2 mg po daily

Sominex® (diphenhydramine) 15 mg po at bedtime as needed

Amitriptyline 50 mg po at bedtime as needed

### All

NKDA

### ROS

Negative except for complaints noted above

### Physical Examination

*Gen*

WDWN female

*VS*

BP 135/84, P 90, RR 16, T 37°C; Wt 65 kg, Ht 5′2″

*Skin*

No rashes, wounds, or open sores

*HEENT*

PERRLA; EOMI; no AV nicking or hemorrhages

*Neck/Lymph Nodes*

No palpable thyroid masses; no lymphadenopathy

*Pulm*

Clear to A & P

*Breasts*

Normal; no lumps

*CV*

Regular $S_1$, $S_2$; (+) $S_4$; (−) $S_3$, murmurs, or rubs

*Abd*

Soft, NTND: (+) bowel sounds

*Genit/Rect*

Genital examination shows atrophic vaginitis consistent with menopausal status. Perineal sensation and anal sphincter tone are normal.

Pelvic examination shows no uterine prolapse and a mild degree of cystocele. Cervix is normal. No pelvic, adnexal, or uterine masses found.

External hemorrhoids; heme (−) stool.

*Ext*

Normal; equal motor strength in both arms and legs

*Neuro*

A & O × 3, CNs II–XII grossly intact; DTRs 3/5 bilaterally; negative Babinski. When asked to recall a series of five objects after 5 minutes, the patient had difficulty and could only recall one object.

### Labs

| | |
|---|---|
| Na 145 mEq/L | Hgb 12 g/dL |
| K 4.2 mEq/L | Hct 37% |
| Cl 105 mEq/L | Plt 400 × $10^3/mm^3$ |
| $CO_2$ 28 mEq/L | WBC 5.0 × $10^3/mm^3$ |
| BUN 15 mg/dL | |
| SCr 1.0 mg/dL | |
| Glu 100 mg/dL | |

### UA

No bacteria; no WBC

### Other

Using an ultrasonic bladder scan, a residual urine volume was measured after the patient voided. No residual urine was found. The bladder was then filled with 300 mL of saline. The patient felt the first desire to void at 100 mL. The catheter was removed. The patient was asked to cough in different positions. No stress urinary incontinence was demonstrated. The patient voided the entire volume of saline that was instilled.

### Assessment

Overactive bladder with symptoms of urinary urgency, frequency, and incontinence, which is not responding to Detrol LA 2 mg po daily. Patient is also having new-onset constipation and CNS problems that must be addressed. Will evaluate carefully and consider alternative medication options.

## QUESTIONS

### Problem Identification

1.a. Create a list of the patient's drug therapy problems.

1.b. What information (signs, symptoms, medical history, laboratory values, other test results) suggests the presence or severity of urge incontinence?

1.c. Differentiate urge incontinence from stress incontinence, overflow incontinence, and functional incontinence.

1.d. Define overactive bladder syndrome.

1.e. In addition to the medications the patient is currently taking, what other drugs could exacerbate the symptoms of overactive bladder syndrome?

### Desired Outcome

2. What are the goals of pharmacotherapy in this case?

### Therapeutic Alternatives

3.a. What nondrug therapies might be useful for this patient?

3.b. What pharmacotherapeutic alternatives are available for treatment of overactive bladder? Compare and contrast antimuscarinic agents for treatment of overactive bladder syndrome.

3.c. What are the possible consequences of persistent CNS adverse effects of anticholinergic agents in this patient?

### Optimal Plan

4. What drug, dosage form, dose, schedule, and duration of therapy are best for this patient?

### Outcome Evaluation

5. What clinical and laboratory parameters are necessary to evaluate the therapy for achievement of the desired therapeutic outcome and to detect or prevent adverse effects?

### Patient Education

6. What information should be provided to the patient to enhance compliance, ensure successful therapy, and minimize adverse effects?

## CLINICAL COURSE

After 3 weeks of the medication regimen you recommended, the patient returns to the clinic. Although her voiding symptoms have resolved, her confusion persists and constipation has worsened. She complains of feeling bloated all the time. She says that she cannot tolerate these problems and wants different drug treatment.

### Follow-Up Questions

1. Explain how these adverse effects could be attributed to the alternative antimuscarinic agent the patient is now taking.
2. What alternative medication would you recommend for this patient to manage her voiding symptoms with the lowest potential for adverse effects?
3. Why should medications with anticholinergic effects be used cautiously in elderly patients?

## SELF-STUDY ASSIGNMENTS

1. Patients have been classified as extensive versus poor metabolizers of tolterodine. Describe the characteristics of these patients and the clinical implications of this patient classification.
2. Botulinum toxin has been reported to be effective for relieving symptoms of overactive bladder. Explain how it is administered and the adverse effects associated with its use.
3. Duloxetine has been used in selected patients with overactive bladder. Identify the ideal patients for such treatment.

## CLINICAL PEARL

A uroselective antimuscarinic agent generally exerts systemic clinical effects. This is because $M_3$ receptors may predominate in a particular organ, but they are not organ specific. $M_3$ receptors are also located in the brain and GI tract. Therefore, antagonism of $M_3$ receptors may relieve symptoms of overactive bladder but may also produce dose-related undesirable anticholinergic adverse effects outside of the urinary bladder.

## REFERENCES


1. Cartwright R, Renganathan A, Cardozo L. Current management of overactive bladder. Curr Opin Obstet Gynecol 2008;20:489–495.
2. Kay GG, Ebinger U. Preserving cognitive function for patients with overactive bladder: evidence for a differential effect of darifenacin. Int J Clin Pract 2008;62:1792–1800.

3. Ellsworth PI, Brunton SA, Wein AJ, et al. Frequently asked questions in the evaluation and management of overactive bladder. J Fam Pract 2009;58:S1–S11.
4. Andersson KE, Chapple CR, Cardozo L, et al. Pharmacological treatment of overactive bladder: report from the International Consultation on Incontinence. Curr Opin Urol 2009;19:380–394.
5. Abrams P, Andersson KE. Muscarinic receptor antagonists for overactive bladder. BJU Int 2007:100:987–1006.
6. Shaw GL, Patel HRH. Transdermal oxybutynin: a review. Expert Opin Drug Metab Toxicol 2007;3:435–439.
7. Salvatore S, Serati M, Bolis P. Tolterodine for the treatment of overactive bladder. Expert Opin Pharmacother 2008;9:1249–1255.
8. Biastre K, Burnakis T. Trospium chloride treatment of overactive bladder. Ann Pharmacother 2009;43:283–295.
9. Chughtai B, Levin R, De E. Choice of antimuscarinic agents for overactive bladder in the older patient: focus on darifenacin. Clin Interv Aging 2008;3:503–509.
10. Hoffstetter S, Leong FC. Solifenacin succinate for the treatment of overactive bladder. Expert Opin Drug Metab Toxicol 2009;5:345–350.
11. Michel MC. Fesoterodine: a novel muscarinic receptor antagonist for the treatment of overactive bladder syndrome. Expert Opin Pharmacother 2008;9:1787–1796.

# SECTION 11
# IMMUNOLOGIC DISORDERS

# 99

## SYSTEMIC LUPUS ERYTHEMATOSUS

Tired to the Bone. . . . . . . . . . . . . . . . . . . . . . . Level II

**Nicole Paolini Albanese, PharmD, CDE**

**Mark J. Wrobel, PharmD**

## LEARNING OBJECTIVES

After completing this case study, students should be able to:

- Discuss the clinical presentation of SLE, including its complications.
- Design appropriate therapy for the treatment of SLE and the complications of APS and iron deficiency anemia.
- Construct a monitoring plan for SLE, including disease activity, drug efficacy, and drug toxicity.

## PATIENT PRESENTATION

### Chief Complaint

"My knees are killing me, I'm tired all the time, and I've got horrible pain in my stomach."

### HPI

Ann Baker is a 32-year-old woman who has been having knee pain on and off for about 2 years. She has been to the doctor a few times since then with the same complaint. Workups showed no radiologic changes to the knees, and the doctor settled on a diagnosis of early arthritis. She was not evaluated by a rheumatologist. Despite scheduled APAP and ibuprofen throughout the day, the pain has not decreased much. The pain seems to be cyclical; it is very bad for a period of weeks, and then it wanes over time. It is also worse in the summer. She thinks the rashes she gets now and then on her face and arms have something to do with the pain, since the rash happens around the same time of a bad flare-up. No matter how much sleep she gets, it does not seem to be enough; a couple of sleep medications later, she is no better than before she tried them. She has also noticed a darkening of her stool over the past couple of months.

### PMH

Knee pain × 2 years
HTN × 1 year
Depression × 3 years
Fatigue × 1 year

### FH

Father alive in his mid-60s; has HTN and dyslipidemia. Mother alive in her mid-60s; has asthma and seasonal allergies.

### SH

Employed as a travel agent; married 5 years; occasional EtOH use and no current or past tobacco use. On inquiry, Ms Baker states she and her husband are trying to conceive.

### Meds

Hydrochlorothiazide 12.5 mg po once daily
Amlodipine 5 mg po once daily
Fluoxetine 20 mg po once daily
Ibuprofen 800 mg po four times daily
Acetaminophen 500 mg po three times daily
*Past meds*: Zolpidem 10 mg po at bedtime and ramelteon 8 mg po at bedtime (stopped using both after inefficacy)

### All

NKDA

### ROS

(+) Fatigue, rash; (–) fever, chills, peripheral edema, or alopecia

### Physical Examination

*Gen*

Tired-looking woman in moderate pain.

Pain scale: Presently 6/10; per patient, her worst pain is 10/10; her best score is 0/10.

*VS*

BP 136/82, P 74, RR 17, T 38°C, Wt 59 kg, Ht 5′4″

*Skin*

Warm, moist to touch, slight red, scaly rash on forearms and across both cheekbones but sparing the nasolabial folds

*HEENT*

PERRLA; EOMI

*Neck/Lymph Nodes*

Supple without adenopathy

*Lungs/Thorax*

CTA; no rales/rhonchi

*CV*

RRR; $S_1$ and $S_2$ heard

*Abd*

Tender, nondistended; (+) bowel sounds; (+) stool guaiac

*Ext*

Peripheral pulses intact; no edema

*Joint examination:* (–) bony proliferation, synovitis, crepitus, muscle atrophy, or deformities; no limitations on range of motion

*Neuro*

A & O × 3; CN II–XII intact; Babinski negative

### Labs

| | | |
|---|---|---|
| Na 136 mEq/L | Hgb 10.0 g/dL | RF titer 1:40 |
| K 4.7 mEq/L | Hct 31% | Anti-CCP antibody (–) |
| Cl 105 mEq/L | WBC 7.2 × $10^3$/mm$^3$ | ANA titer 1:320 (rim pattern) |
| $CO_2$ 25 mEq/L | Plt 250 × $10^3$/mm$^3$ | C3 50 mg/dL |
| BUN 13 mg/dL | Fe 35 mcg/dL | C4 10 mg/dL |
| SCr 0.8 mg/dL | TIBC 455 mcg/dL | Lupus anticoagulant (+) |
| Uric acid 5.5 mg/dL | Ferritin 8 ng/mL | Anticardiolipin Ab (+) |
| Glucose 82 mg/dL | ESR 66 mm/h | dsDNA Ab (+) |

### UA

(–) WBC, RBC, RBC casts; (+) microalbuminuria; (–) protein

### Radiologic Joint Evaluation

(–) Patellar or tibial fracture, (–) displacement, (–) fragments, (–) ligament damage, no evident soft tissue damage

### Assessment

Mild-to-moderate SLE with biomarkers for APS; iron deficiency anemia possibly secondary to NSAID use; possible NSAID-associated gastropathy

## QUESTIONS

### Problem Identification

1.a. What information (signs, symptoms, laboratory values) indicates the development of SLE?

1.b. What information (signs, symptoms, laboratory values) indicates the development of iron deficiency anemia?

### Desired Outcome

2.a. What are the goals of pharmacotherapy for SLE in this patient?

2.b. What are the goals of pharmacotherapy for APS in this patient?

2.c. What are the goals of pharmacotherapy for iron deficiency anemia in this patient?

### Therapeutic Alternatives

3.a. What nondrug suggestions can you make to this patient for the treatment of SLE?

3.b. What pharmacotherapeutic options are available for the treatment of SLE in this patient?

3.c. What options are available for prophylaxis of thrombotic events due to APS?

### Optimal Plan

4.a. What is the optimal regimen for SLE in this patient, and are there any concerns with this regimen if she were to conceive?

4.b. What is your choice for prophylaxis against thrombotic events due to APS?

4.c. What are your recommendations for treating this patient's iron deficiency anemia and NSAID-associated gastropathy?

4.d. Should any changes be made in this patient's antihypertensive therapy?

### Outcome Evaluation

5. What clinical and laboratory parameters are necessary to evaluate the therapy for achievement of the desired therapeutic outcome and to detect or prevent adverse events?

### Patient Education

6. What information can be provided to the patient to minimize future relapses, ensure successful therapy, and minimize adverse events?

## FOLLOW-UP QUESTIONS

1. What can this patient do to increase the chances of having a successful pregnancy?
2. If your initial medication regimen does not work, what is the next step in treating this patient?

## SELF-STUDY ASSIGNMENTS

1. How do B lymphocyte stimulator antagonists work, and where do they fit in with the pharmacotherapeutic management of SLE?
2. Devise a comprehensive patient education plan for women with SLE who wish to start a family.

## CLINICAL PEARL

Because UV light exacerbates SLE, drugs that induce photosensitivity should be avoided in patients with the disease.

## REFERENCES


1. Giles I, Rahman A. How to manage patients with systemic lupus erythematosus who are also antiphospholipid antibody positive. Best Pract Res Clin Rheumatol 2009;23:525–537.
2. Ruiz-Irastorza G, Khamashta MA. Managing lupus patients during pregnancy. Best Pract Res Clin Rheumatol 2009;23:575–582.
3. ACR Committee on SLE Guidelines. Guidelines for referral and management of systemic lupus erythematosus in adults. American College of Rheumatology Ad Hoc Committee on Systemic Lupus Erythematosus Guidelines. Arthritis Rheum 1999;42:1785–1796.
4. Farquharson RG, Quenby S, Greaves M. Antiphospholipid syndrome in pregnancy: a randomized, controlled trial of treatment. Obstet Gynecol 2002;100:408–413.
5. Alarcon GS, McGwin G, Bertoli AM, et al. Effect of hydroxychloroquine on the survival of patients with systemic lupus erythematosus: data from LUMINA, a multiethnic US cohort (LUMINA L). Ann Rheum Dis 2007;66:1168–1172.
6. Fessler BJ, Alarcon GS, McGwin G Jr, et al. Systemic lupus erythematosus in three ethnic groups: XVI. Association of hydroxychloroquine use with reduced risk of damage accrual. Arthritis Rheum 2005;52:1473–1480.
7. Ostensen M, Khamashta M, Lockshin M, et al. Anti-inflammatory and immunosuppressive drugs and reproduction. Arthritis Res Ther 2006;8:209 [Epub May 11, 2006].
8. Levy RA, Vilela VS, Cataldo MJ, et al. Hydroxychloroquine (HCQ) in lupus pregnancy: double-blind and placebo-controlled study. Lupus 2001;10:401–404.

9. Yeomans ND, Tulassay Z, Juhasz L, et al. A comparison of omeprazole with ranitidine for ulcers associated with nonsteroidal antiinflammatory drugs. N Engl J Med 1998;338:719–726.
10. Duran-Barragan S, McGwin G Jr, Vila LM, Reveille JD, Alarcon GS. Angiotensin-converting enzyme inhibitors delay the occurrence of renal involvement and are associated with a decreased risk of disease activity in patients with systemic lupus erythematosus—results from LUMINA (LIX): a multiethnic US cohort. Rheumatology 2008;47:1093–1096.

# 100

# ALLERGIC DRUG REACTION

Return of the 3-Day Itch . . . . . . . . . . . . . . . . . Level II

**Lynne M. Sylvia, PharmD**

## LEARNING OBJECTIVES

After completing this case study, students should be able to:

- Interpret drug allergy information (e.g., timing of the reaction, signs, and symptoms) to identify the likelihood of an IgE-mediated reaction.
- Assess the potential for cross-sensitivity between penicillins and carbapenems.
- Differentiate desensitization from graded challenge dosing procedures and identify patients who are appropriate candidates for each procedure.
- Select appropriate antibiotic therapy for a patient with multiple antibiotic allergies.

## PATIENT PRESENTATION

### Chief Complaint

"My cough is back and I feel like I did when I was admitted two weeks ago."

### HPI

Alan Adams is a 55-year-old man with a history of COPD who presents today to the pulmonary clinic for a follow-up visit. Two weeks ago, he presented to the ER complaining of a 3-day history of tiredness and a cough productive of greenish sputum. Sputum cultures at that time revealed *Pseudomonas aeruginosa* sensitive to aztreonam and cefepime with intermediate sensitivity to piperacillin–tazobactam and tobramycin. Due to his multiple antibiotic allergies, the patient underwent desensitization to cefepime. He was subsequently treated for 7 days with IV cefepime without incident. He was discharged from the hospital to his home 2 weeks ago. He has had four admissions this year for COPD and pneumonia.

### PMH

COPD × 17 years
Chronic empyema secondary to bronchial pleural fistulae with chest tube placement 7 months ago
Right upper lobe abscess secondary to *Candida* and *Aspergillus*; S/P upper lobe lobectomy 11 years ago
HTN × 10 years
S/P MI 15 years ago

### SH

Lives with his mother; he is unemployed. He has a 40 pack-year smoking history. Admits to occasional alcohol use; denies use of recreational drugs.

### Meds

Albuterol MDI two puffs Q 6 h PRN
Ipratropium MDI two puffs Q 6 h
Aspirin 325 mg po once daily
Amlodipine 10 mg po once daily
Prednisone 20 mg po daily (initiated as 60 mg po daily during previous hospital admission; plan was to taper the dose and discontinue therapy within 2 weeks of hospital discharge)

### All

Ampicillin–sulbactam: facial edema, tongue swelling, periorbital edema
Ceftazidime: urticarial rash on chest and face with shortness of breath
Codeine: nausea, pruritus

### ROS

(+) Fatigue, fever, sore throat, shortness of breath, and cough with thick sputum; (–) nausea, vomiting, diarrhea, chills, or chest pain

### Physical Examination

*Gen*

A 55-year-old Caucasian man appearing older than his stated age in moderate respiratory distress. He is lethargic and hard of hearing.

*VS*

BP 100/60, P 85, RR 16, T 39°C; Wt 52 kg, Ht 5′5″

*Skin*

Dry scaly skin; no tenting

*HEENT*

PERRLA, EOM intact, dry mucous membranes

*Neck/Lymph Nodes*

(–) Bruits, (–) lymphadenopathy

*Lungs/Thorax*

(+) Diffuse crackles at the left base; wheezes throughout with poor breath sounds

*CV*

Normal $S_1$ and $S_2$, RRR, (–) MRG

*Abd*

Distended with (+) bowel sounds; (–) hepatosplenomegaly

*Genit/Rect*

Deferred

*Ext*

(+) Clubbing; (–) cyanosis or edema; poor muscle tone

## Labs

| | | |
|---|---|---|
| Na 137 mEq/L | Hgb 14.8 g/dL | WBC 17 × $10^3$/mm$^3$ |
| K 3.7 mEq/L | Hct 44.6% | Neutros 72% |
| Cl 96 mEq/L | RBC 5.36 × $10^6$/mm$^3$ | Bands 5% |
| $CO_2$ 29 mEq/L | Plt 244 × $10^3$/mm$^3$ | Eos 4% |
| BUN 22 mg/dL | MCV 83.2 μm$^3$ | Lymphs 11% |
| SCr 1.0 mg/dL | MCHC 33.2 g/dL | Monos 8% |
| Glu 119 mg/dL | | Basos 0% |

## ABG

pH 7.44, $pO_2$ 55 mm Hg, $pCO_2$ 38 mm Hg, $O_2$ sat 90%

## Chest X-Ray

Haziness in the left lower lobe S/P right upper lobe resection

## Sputum Gram Stain

Pending

## Sputum Cultures

Pending

## Blood Cultures

Pending

## Assessment

1. HCAP
2. Multiple allergies to antibiotics
3. COPD
4. HTN
5. S/P MI

# QUESTIONS

## Problem Identification

1.a. Based on the patient's allergy history, how should his allergies to ampicillin–sulbactam and ceftazidime be categorized—as minor, moderate, or severe?

1.b. What additional information would be helpful to fully assess the patient's risk of hypersensitivity reactions to β-lactam antibiotics?

1.c. What additional information would be helpful to assess whether the patient experiences true hypersensitivity versus pseudoallergy to codeine?

## Desired Outcome

2. What are the goals for the treatment of pneumonia in this case?

## CLINICAL COURSE

The patient is admitted to the hospital from the pulmonary clinic. He is started on albuterol 2.5 mg by nebulizer Q 2 h PRN, ipratropium 0.5 mg by nebulizer Q 2 h PRN, guaifenesin with codeine (100 mg/10 mg per 5 mL) po Q 4 h PRN, acetaminophen 325–650 mg po Q 4 h PRN, and prednisone 40 mg po once daily. While cultures are pending, the medical resident reviews this patient's recent hospital course, the cultures and sensitivities obtained 2 weeks ago, and the hospital's guidelines for treating HCAP. Consideration is given to initiating empiric therapy with meropenem 500 mg IV Q 6 h, ciprofloxacin 400 mg IV Q 12 h, and vancomycin 750 mg IV Q 24 h. Prior to writing these orders, the medical resident asks for your advice on the initiation of meropenem in this patient.

**TABLE 100-1 Initial Empiric Treatment for HCAP and HAP in Patients with Risk Factors for Drug-Resistant Pathogens[a]**

| **Combination antibiotic therapy** |
|---|
| Antipseudomonal cephalosporin (cefepime, ceftazidime) |
| *Or* |
| Antipseudomonal carbapenem (imipenem or meropenem) |
| *Or* |
| β-Lactam/β-lactamase inhibitor (piperacillin–tazobactam) |
| *Plus* |
| Antipseudomonal fluoroquinolone (ciprofloxacin or levofloxacin) |
| *Plus* |
| Linezolid or vancomycin |

[a]American Thoracic Society and the Infectious Diseases Society of America. Guidelines for the management of adults with hospital-acquired, ventilator-associated and health care-associated pneumonia. Am J Respir Crit Care Med 2005;171:388–416.

## Therapeutic Alternatives

3.a. The initial empiric regimens currently recommended for HCAP are summarized in Table 100-1. Both cefepime and aztreonam are alternatives to meropenem in these multidrug regimens. Based on this patient's history, are cefepime and aztreonam safe alternatives to meropenem for empiric therapy of HCAP? (See Fig. 100-1 for the chemical structures of cefepime and ceftazidime.)

3.b. If a multidrug regimen including cefepime was chosen for empiric therapy, would this patient require another course of desensitization prior to initiation of full-dose cefepime therapy?

## Optimal Plan

4. Assess the risk of a hypersensitivity cross-reaction to meropenem in this patient. Based on your review of the literature, determine which of the following courses of action is best: (a) initiation of full-dose meropenem therapy; (b) desensitization to meropenem prior to initiating full treatment doses; or (c) graded challenge dosing of meropenem prior to initiating full treatment doses. Substantiate your position on the most appropriate course of action based on evidence from the literature.

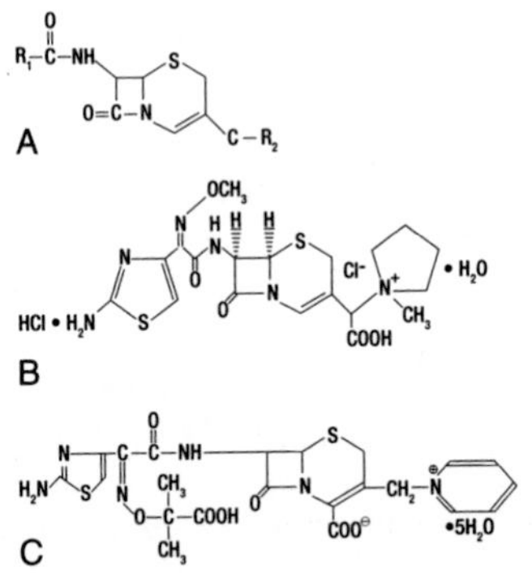

A

B

C

**FIGURE 100-1.** Chemical structures of cefepime and ceftazidime. ***A.*** Basic cephalosporin structure. ***B.*** Cefepime (*Maxipime [cefepime] product information, Bristol Myers Squibb Company, Princeton, NJ, 2003*). ***C.*** Ceftazidime (*Fortaz [ceftazidime] product information, GlaxoSmithKline, Research Triangle Park, NC, October 2005*).

## CHAPTER 101

## Outcome Evaluation

5. In patients who undergo desensitization and/or graded challenge dosing, what clinical and laboratory parameters should be evaluated during and after these procedures to detect or prevent allergic events?

## Patient Education

6. What information should be provided to the patient about his drug allergies to minimize allergic events in the future?

## SELF-STUDY ASSIGNMENTS

1. Define the following terms: CAP, HAP, HCAP, and VAP. Differentiate the initial empiric regimens for each of these types of pneumonia.
2. Develop a care map for patients allergic to penicillin for whom a carbapenem is ordered. Outline the process by which the clinician would determine the most appropriate course of action for these patients. Be specific to the type of allergy to the penicillin (i.e., maculopapular rash vs. Stevens–Johnson syndrome vs. anaphylactic reaction).
3. Apply the concepts of graded challenge dosing and desensitization (see the section "Clinical Pearl") to the issue of β-lactam hypersensitivity. Develop criteria describing those patients with history of β-lactam hypersensitivity who would be appropriate candidates for graded challenge dosing versus desensitization to structurally related antibiotics.

## CLINICAL PEARL

A graded challenge dose (test dosing) involves the cautious administration of a medication to a patient. Graded challenge doses of a medication are often recommended for patients who have history of hypersensitivity to a structurally related medication and the risk of a cross-reaction is deemed unlikely. Unlike desensitization, graded challenge dosing does not alter the body's immune response to an antigenic medication.

## REFERENCES


1. Sylvia LM. Drug allergy, pseudoallergy and cutaneous diseases. In: Tisdale JE, Miller DA, eds. Drug-Induced Diseases: Prevention, Detection and Management, 2nd ed. Bethesda, MD, ASHP Publications, 2010:51–97.
2. Solensky R. Drug hypersensitivity. Med Clin North Am 2006;90: 233–260.
3. Romano A, Di Fonso M, Viola M, et al. Selective hypersensitivity to piperacillin. Allergy 2000;55:787.
4. Pichichero ME. Cephalosporins can be prescribed safely for penicillin-allergic patients. J Fam Pract 2006;55:106–112.
5. Kelkar PS, Li JT. Cephalosporin allergy. N Engl J Med 2001;345:804–809.
6. Win PH, Brown H, Zankar A, et al. Rapid intravenous cephalosporin desensitization. J Allergy Clin Immunol 2005;116:225–228.
7. Solensky R. Drug desensitization. Immunol Allergy Clin North Am 2004;24:425–443.
8. Prescott WA, Kusmierski KA. Clinical importance of carbapenem hypersensitivity in patients with self-reported and documented penicillin allergy. Pharmacotherapy 2007;27(1):137–142.
9. Romano A, Viola M, Gueant-Rodriguez RM, et al. Imipenem in patients with immediate hypersensitivity to penicillins. N Engl J Med 2006;354:2835–2837.
10. Romano A, Viola M, Gueant-Rodriguez RM, et al. Brief communication: tolerability of meropenem in patients with IgE-mediated hypersensitivity to penicillins. Ann Intern Med 2007;146:266–269.
11. Atanaskovic-Markovic M, Gaeta F, Medjo B, et al. Tolerability of meropenem in children with IgE-mediated hypersensitivity to penicillins. Allergy 2008;63:237–240.
12. Wilson DL, Owens RC, Zuckerman JB. Successful meropenem desensitization in a patient with cystic fibrosis. Ann Pharmacother 2003;37:1424–1428.


# 101

# SOLID ORGAN TRANSPLANTATION

Kidney—Don't Fail Me Now! . . . . . . . . . . . . . . Level III

**Kristine S. Schonder, PharmD**

## LEARNING OBJECTIVES

After completing this case study, students should be able to:

- Develop a patient-specific therapeutic plan for acute cellular rejection following solid organ transplantation.
- Assess a transplant medication regimen for potential drug interactions and develop a plan to resolve any identified interactions.
- Describe possible adverse effects of immunosuppressive medications and prophylactic medications for solid organ transplant recipients and develop a plan to resolve these effects.
- Counsel a transplant recipient on the importance of medication adherence and implement mechanisms to enhance adherence.

## PATIENT PRESENTATION

### Chief Complaint

"I have pain over my kidney transplant, my legs are swollen, and my urine output is decreased."

### HPI

Brent Salston is a 42-year-old man who presents to the renal transplant clinic for evaluation of diarrhea and the above complaints.

### PMH

6 months S/P living kidney transplant from his wife
ESRD secondary to PCKD
HTN
Gout
Peripheral neuropathy, diagnosed 2 weeks ago by PCP

### FH

Mother is alive with hypertension; father deceased from kidney disease. Two aunts and sister also have kidney disease. He is married with two children, Sarah and Justin, who are alive and well.

### SH

He drinks beer occasionally with friends, but not since his transplant. He has no history of smoking or IVDA.

## ROS

He has pain over his kidney and bilateral edema in his lower extremities. He reports mild pain and tingling in lower extremities. Urine output has decreased from baseline.

## Meds

Tacrolimus 4 mg po BID (last dose taken last night at 8:00 PM)
Prednisone 5 mg po once daily
Mycophenolate mofetil 1,000 mg po BID
Dapsone 100 mg po daily
Valganciclovir 900 mg po daily
Aspirin 81 mg po once daily
Sodium bicarbonate 650 mg po BID
Ferrous sulfate 325 mg po TID
Metoprolol XL 100 mg po daily
Amlodipine 10 mg po daily
Famotidine 20 mg po BID
Fludrocortisone 0.1 mg po daily
Magnesium chloride 64 mg po BID
Allopurinol 100 mg po daily
Carbamazepine 200 mg po BID, started 2 weeks ago by PCP

## All

Sulfa (rash)

## Physical Examination

*Gen*

WDWN man in NAD

*VS*

BP 169/92, P 66 reg, RR 14, T 37.4°C; Wt 87 kg (previous Wt 85 kg 2 weeks ago), Ht 5′10″

*Skin*

Warm and dry

*HEENT*

PERRLA; EOMI

*Chest*

CTA & P

*CV*

Normal $S_1$ and $S_2$; no MRG

*Abd*

Tenderness over kidney allograft; incisional wound healed; liver size normal

*Ext*

3+ pitting edema in LE; 2+ DP pulses bilaterally. No cyanosis.

*Neuro*

A & O × 3; CN II–XII intact; DTRs 2+ throughout

## Labs

At 8:00 AM today (fasting):

Na 141 mEq/L
K 5.7 mEq/L
Cl 104 mEq/L
$CO_2$ 23 mEq/L
FBS 78 mg/dL
BUN 39 mg/dL (last was 20 mg/dL)
SCr 2.5 mg/dL (last was 1.1 mg/dL)

Hgb 12.2 g/dL
Hct 36.6%
RBC 5.1 × $10^6$/mm$^3$
Plt 289 × $10^3$/mm$^3$
WBC 1.9 × $10^3$/mm$^3$
 Polys 68%
 Lymphs 27%
 Monos 2%
 Eos 1%
 Basos 2%

Ca 8.9 mg/dL
Phos 2.3 mg/dL
Mg 1.4 mg/dL
Uric acid 6.8 mg/dL
FK <2 ng/mL[a]

[a]Tacrolimus whole blood concentration (therapeutic range, 5–20 ng/mL).

## Renal Biopsy

Moderate acute cellular rejection (Banff 2A)

## Assessment

Acute rejection of kidney allograft, hyperkalemia, leukopenia

# QUESTIONS

## Problem Identification

1.a. Create a list of the patient's drug therapy problems.

1.b. Which signs, symptoms, and laboratory values indicate rejection of the kidney allograft?

1.c. What are the potential causes of hyperkalemia in this patient?

1.d. What are the potential causes of leukopenia in this patient?

1.e. What are the potential causes of the other medical problems in this patient?

## Desired Outcome

2. What are the goals of pharmacotherapy in this case?

## Therapeutic Alternatives

3.a. What nonpharmacologic therapies and education might be useful for this patient?

3.b. What pharmacotherapeutic alternatives are available for the treatment of kidney allograft rejection?

3.c. What pharmacotherapeutic alternatives are available for treating hyperkalemia in this patient?

3.d. What pharmacotherapeutic alternatives are available for treating leukopenia in this patient?

## Optimal Plan

4.a. What drug, dosage form, dose, schedule, and duration of therapy are best to treat this patient's kidney allograft rejection?

4.b. What alternatives would be appropriate if the initial therapy fails or cannot be used?

4.c. Design a pharmacotherapeutic plan to treat this patient's hyperkalemia, leukopenia, and other medical problems.

## Outcome Evaluation

5. What clinical and laboratory parameters are necessary to evaluate the response to therapy and to detect or prevent adverse effects?

## Patient Education

6. What information should be provided to the patient to enhance adherence, ensure successful therapy, and minimize adverse effects?

## CLINICAL COURSE

The patient receives the treatment you recommended for acute cellular rejection. The rejection episode resolves and renal function returns to baseline levels. He is now presenting 3 months later for a routine follow-up appointment.

### Meds

Tacrolimus 7 mg po BID (last dose taken last night at 8:00 PM)
Prednisone 15 mg po once daily
Mycophenolate mofetil 1,000 mg po BID
Dapsone 100 mg po daily
Valganciclovir 900 mg po daily
Aspirin 81 mg po daily
Sodium bicarbonate 650 mg po BID
Ferrous sulfate 325 mg po TID
Metoprolol XL 100 mg po daily
Amlodipine 10 mg po daily
Famotidine 20 mg po BID
Fludrocortisone 0.1 mg po BID
Magnesium chloride 128 mg po BID
Allopurinol 100 mg po daily
The patient's PCP decided to discontinue the carbamazepine and begin gabapentin 100 mg po at bedtime and titrate the dose upward slowly over the next several months based on the patient's response. The patient began this treatment 1 day ago.

### Labs (at 8:00 AM Today)

| | | |
|---|---|---|
| Na 139 mEq/L | Hgb 12.1 g/dL | Ca 9.1 mg/dL |
| K 3.8 mEq/L | Hct 36.3% | Phos 3.5 mg/dL |
| Cl 109 mEq/L | RBC 5.2 × $10^6$/mm$^3$ | Mg 2.2 mg/dL |
| $CO_2$ 31 mEq/L | Plt 278 × $10^3$/mm$^3$ | FK 5.4 ng/mL |
| FBS 82 mg/dL | WBC 3.7 × $10^3$/mm$^3$ | |
| BUN 19 mg/dL | | |
| SCr 1.1 mg/dL | | |

## FOLLOW-UP QUESTION

1. What changes, if any, should be made to the patient's drug regimen?

## SELF-STUDY ASSIGNMENTS

1. Develop a pharmacotherapeutic plan for the different strategies to treat acute cellular rejection of the allograft in solid organ transplant recipients.
2. Design a systematic approach for patient education for a new solid organ transplant recipient focusing on immunosuppressive therapies, adverse effects and drug interactions, and strategies to manage patient compliance with a complicated regimen.
3. Formulate a pharmacotherapeutic plan for the management of hyperkalemia that identifies different strategies based on the onset and magnitude of hyperkalemia.

## CLINICAL PEARL

Acute rejection can occur in up to 20% of kidney transplant recipients within the first 6 months after transplant. Although an abrupt rise in serum creatinine ≥30% over baseline can signal an acute rejection episode, a renal biopsy must be performed for a definitive diagnosis. The greatest risk factor for acute cellular rejection is a decrease in the level of immunosuppression. Treatment of acute rejection is typically based on the severity of the rejection episode.

## REFERENCES


1. KDOQI clinical practice guidelines on hypertension and antihypertensive agents in chronic kidney disease. Available at: *http://www.kidney.org/professionals/KDOQI/guidelines_bp/index.htm*. Accessed March 3, 2010.
2. Tylicki L, Habicht A, Watschinger B, Hörl WH. Treatment of hypertension in renal transplant recipients. Curr Opin Urol 2003;13:91–98.
3. Webster AC, Pankhurst T, Rinaldi F, Chapman RJ, Craig JC. Monoclonal and polyclonal antibody therapy for treating acute rejection in kidney transplant recipients: a systematic review of randomized trial data. Transplantation 2006;81:953–965.
4. Ghanekar H, Welch BJ, Moe OW, Sakhaee K. Post-renal transplantation hypophosphatemia: a review and novel insights. Curr Opin Nephrol Hypertens 2006;15:97–104.

SECTION 12
# BONE AND JOINT DISORDERS

# 102

## OSTEOPOROSIS

Bona fide Treatment. . . . . . . . . . . . . . . . . . . . . Level II

Emily C. Farthing-Papineau, PharmD, BCPS

### LEARNING OBJECTIVES

After completing this case study, students should be able to:

- Identify the risk factors for the development of osteoporosis and utilize the FRAX tool to assess risk of an osteoporotic fracture.
- Recommend appropriate nonpharmacologic measures for the prevention and treatment of osteoporosis.
- Recommend the correct amount and form of calcium supplementation required for the prevention and treatment of osteoporosis.
- Design an appropriate pharmacologic treatment regimen for the treatment of osteoporosis in postmenopausal women.
- Provide appropriate patient education regarding osteoporosis and its therapy.

### PATIENT PRESENTATION

#### Chief Complaint

"I've taken alendronate twice, and I can't stand the heartburn and stomach pain that it is causing me. I am not going to take this medication anymore. Why can't I just take my calcium and vitamin D?"

#### HPI

Evelyn Smith is a 66-year-old woman with a history of HTN, dyslipidemia, COPD, hypothyroidism, GERD, and recently diagnosed osteoporosis. She presents to the family medicine clinic for a follow-up visit for her HTN, dyslipidemia, and osteoporosis.

#### PMH

HTN first diagnosed at age 50
S/P MI 12 years ago
Dyslipidemia × 13 years
Hypothyroidism × 27 years
Osteoporosis diagnosed by DXA scan 2 months ago
COPD (Stage II) diagnosed 3 years ago and currently stable. Had one exacerbation 9 months ago, which was her only exacerbation in the past 3 years.
Breast cancer with mastectomy of left breast and radiation therapy at age 40
Menopause at age 51
GERD

#### FH

Paternal history (+) for CAD; father died at age 60 of "heart trouble"
Maternal history (+) for stroke and vascular disorders; hip fracture

#### SH

Widowed; $G_2P_3$; one ppd smoker; drinks occasionally

#### ROS

Worsened heartburn with alendronate therapy; reports vaginal dryness; has noticed that her height has decreased by 2 in since she was 35 years old; denies shortness of breath or chest pain

#### Meds

Advair 250/50 one puff BID × 9 months
Albuterol MDI two puffs Q 6 h PRN shortness of breath
Alendronate 70 mg po once monthly × 2 months
Aspirin 81 mg po once daily × 12 years
Atenolol 50 mg po once daily × 10 years
Lovastatin 20 mg po once daily × 3 months
Omeprazole 20 mg po once daily × 1 year
Os-Cal 500 po BID × 2 months
Ramipril 10 mg po BID × 2 years
Synthroid 100 mcg po once daily × 20 years

#### All

NKDA

#### Physical Examination

*Gen*

WDWN Caucasian woman in NAD

*VS*

BP 148/92, P 64, RR 18, T 37°C; Wt 53.5 kg, Ht 5′3″

*Skin*

Fair complexion, color good, no lesions

*HEENT*

PERRLA; EOMI; eyes and throat clear; funduscopic exam reveals mild arteriolar narrowing, with AV ratio 1:3; no hemorrhages, exudates, or papilledema

*Neck/Lymph Nodes*

Supple, without obvious nodes; no JVD

*Chest*

Decreased breath sounds bilaterally; air movement decreased; no rales or rhonchi

*Breasts*

Mastectomy scar left breast; right breast normal

*CV*

RRR; no murmurs, rubs, or gallops

*Abd*

Soft, NT/ND, (+) BS

*Genit/Rect*

Deferred

*MS/Ext*

Good pulses bilaterally

*Neuro*

CN II–XII intact; DTRs 2+; sensory and motor levels intact

### Labs

| | | *Current fasting lipid profile* | *Three months ago* |
|---|---|---|---|
| Na 144 mEq/L | Ca 9.1 mg/dL | | T. chol 211 mg/dL |
| K 4.0 mEq/L | TSH 3.492 mIU/L | T. chol 177 mg/dL | TG 165 mg/dL |
| Cl 104 mEq/L | AST 32 IU/L | TG 148 mg/dL | HDL 38 mg/dL |
| $CO_2$ 25 mEq/L | ALT 27 IU/L | HDL 41 mg/dL | LDL 140 mg/dL |
| BUN 18 mg/dL | | LDL 106 mg/dL | AST 20 IU/L |
| SCr 1.0 mg/dL | | | ALT 17 IU/L |
| Glu 97 mg/dL | | | |

### Other

*DXA scan results from Hologic machine:*

Lumbar spine 2 months ago reveals: L2–4 = 0.780 g/cm$^2$ (T score: –3.2 SD); right femoral neck = 0.52 g/cm$^2$ (T score: –2.8 SD).

X-ray of the spine 2 months ago shows a compression fracture on L3.

### Assessment

1. Severe osteoporosis requiring alteration in therapy due to medication intolerance
2. Hypertension not adequately controlled
3. Hyperlipidemia responding to therapy, but not at goal
4. Stable Stage II COPD
5. Hypothyroidism well controlled on current regimen

## QUESTIONS

### Problem Identification

1.a. Create a list of the patient's drug therapy problems.

1.b. What information (signs, symptoms, laboratory values, FRAX score) indicates the presence or severity of the patient's osteoporosis? What are the patient's risk factors for developing osteoporosis?

### Desired Outcome

2. What are the goals of pharmacotherapy for osteoporosis in this case?

### Therapeutic Alternatives

3.a. What nondrug therapies might be useful for this patient's osteoporosis?

3.b. What feasible pharmacotherapeutic alternatives are available for treatment of the osteoporosis?

### Optimal Plan

4.a. What drug, dosage form, dose, schedule, and duration of therapy are best for treating this patient's osteoporosis?

4.b. What alternatives would be appropriate if the initial therapy fails or cannot be used?

### Outcome Evaluation

5. Which clinical and laboratory parameters are necessary to evaluate the therapy for achievement of the desired therapeutic outcome and to detect or prevent adverse effects?

### Patient Counseling

6. What information should be provided to the patient to enhance adherence, ensure successful therapy, and minimize adverse effects?

## SELF-STUDY ASSIGNMENTS

1. Create a list of medications associated with an increased risk for developing osteoporosis.
2. Investigate the new drugs and drug classes under development for the treatment of osteoporosis.
3. Develop an exercise plan to prevent osteoporosis.

## CLINICAL PEARL

In elderly patients or those on acid-suppressive therapy, recommend calcium citrate instead of calcium carbonate, as this salt form does not require an acidic gastric pH for dissolution.

## REFERENCES

1. Yang YX, Lewis JD, Epstein S, Metz DC. Long-term proton pump inhibitor therapy and risk of hip fracture. JAMA 2006;296:2947–2953.
2. National Institutes of Health. JNC 7 express; seventh report of the Joint National Committee on Prevention, Detection, Evaluation, and Treatment of High Blood Pressure. Bethesda, MD, National Heart, Lung, and Blood Institute; 2003. NIH Publication No. 03-5233.
3. Feskanich D, Willett WC, Stampfer MJ, Colditz GA. A prospective study of thiazide use and fractures in women. Osteoporos Int 1997;7:79–84.
4. National Cholesterol Education Program Expert Panel. Final report of the third report of the National Cholesterol Education Program (NCEP) Expert Panel on Detection, Evaluation, and Treatment of High Blood Cholesterol in Adults (Adult Treatment Panel III). Bethesda, MD, National Heart, Lung, and Blood Institute. National Institutes of Health; 2002. NIH Publication No. 02-5215.
5. Grundy SM, Cleeman JI, Merz CN, et al, for the Coordinating Committee of the National Cholesterol Education Program. Implications of recent clinical trials for the National Cholesterol Education Program Adult Treatment Panel III guidelines. Circulation 2004;110:227–239.
6. Global strategy for diagnosis, management and prevention of COPD (updated 2009). The Global Initiative for Chronic Obstructive Lung Disease Web site. Available at: *http://www.goldcopd.org/Guidelineitem.asp?l1=2&l2=1&intId=2003*. Updated December 2009. Accessed April 20, 2010.

7. The North American Menopause Society. Management of osteoporosis in postmenopausal women: 2010 position statement of the North American Menopause Society. Menopause 2010;17(1):25–54.
8. American Association of Clinical Endocrinologists Osteoporosis Task Force. AACE medical guidelines for clinical practice for the prevention and treatment of postmenopausal osteoporosis: 2001 edition, with selected updates for 2003. Endocr Pract 2003;9:544–564.
9. National Osteoporosis Foundation. Clinician's guide to prevention and treatment of osteoporosis. National Osteoporosis Foundation Web site. Available at: *http://www.nof.org/professionals/Clinicians_Guide.htm*. Updated January 2010. Accessed April 20, 2010.
10. Treating tobacco use and dependence: 2008 update. U.S. Department of Health and Human Services Web site. Available at: *http://www.surgeongeneral.gov/tobacco/index.html*. Published May 2008. Accessed April 20, 2010.
11. Tucker KL, Morita K, Qiao N, Hannan MT, Cupples A, Kiel DP. Colas, but not other carbonated beverages, are associated with low bone mineral density in older women: the Framingham Osteoporosis Study. Am J Clin Nutr 2006;84:936–942.
12. Levenson DI, Bockman RS. A review of calcium preparations. Nutr Rev 1994;52:221–232.
13. American College of Rheumatology Ad Hoc Committee on Glucocorticoid-Induced Osteoporosis. Recommendations for the prevention and treatment of glucocorticoid-induced osteoporosis, 2001 update. Arthritis Rheum 2001;44:1496–1503.
14. Houghton LA, Veith R. The case against ergocalciferol (vitamin $D_2$) as a vitamin supplement. Am J Clin Nutr 2006;84:694–697.
15. Update of safety review follow-up to the October 1, 2007, early communication about the ongoing safety review of bisphosphonates. Food and Drug Administration Web site. Available at: *http://www.fda.gov/Drugs/DrugSafety/PostmarketDrugSafetyInformationforPatientsandProviders/DrugSafetyInformationforHeathcareProfessionals/ucm136201.htm*. Published November 11, 2008. Accessed April 20, 2010.
16. U.S. Preventive Services Task Force. Hormone therapy for the prevention of chronic conditions in postmenopausal women: recommendations from the U.S. Preventive Services Task Force. Ann Intern Med 2005;142:855–860.
17. FDA drug safety communication: ongoing safety review of oral bisphosphonates and atypical subtrochanteric femur fractures. Food and Drug Administration Web site. Available at: *http://www.fda.gov/Drugs/DrugSafety/PostmarketDrugSafetyInformationforPatientsandProviders/ucm203891.htm*. Published March 10, 2010. Accessed April 20, 2010.
18. Cummings SR, San Martin J, McClung MR, et al. Denosumab for prevention of fractures in postmenopausal women with osteoporosis. N Engl J Med 2009;361:756–765.


# 103

# RHEUMATOID ARTHRITIS

Joint Project . . . . . . . . . . . . . . . . . . . . . . . . . . . Level II

**Amy W. Rudenko, PharmD**

## LEARNING OBJECTIVES

After completing this case study, the reader should be able to:

- Identify the signs and symptoms of RA.
- Recommend appropriate drug therapy for the management of RA.
- Recognize alternative therapies for the treatment of pain and inflammation in patients with RA.
- Recommend appropriate nonpharmacologic options for managing patients with RA.
- Counsel patients about the drug therapy used to treat RA.

## PATIENT PRESENTATION

### Chief Complaint

"I ache all over, I feel exhausted, and I am having a hard time getting going in the morning. I want to have a baby, but I don't think I can do it feeling like this."

### HPI

Irene Schwartz is a 33-year-old woman who presents to her rheumatologist with generalized arthralgias, fatigue, and morning stiffness. She presented with similar symptoms 3 months ago, at which time she was started on a regimen of methotrexate and prednisone. She reports slight improvement in her symptoms relative to her visit 3 months ago.

### PMH

RA × 3 months

### FH

Father is alive and is being treated for hypertension and hypercholesterolemia. Mother is alive and suffers with severe RA and osteoporosis. Two siblings—no health concerns.

### SH

Executive secretary; married for 3 years; wants to start a family within the next year. Denies tobacco use. Drinks one to two glasses of wine per week.

### Meds

Prednisone 5 mg, one tablet po Q AM
Methotrexate 2.5 mg, six tablets po once a week
Folic acid 1 mg, one tablet po once daily
Patient receives medications at a local community pharmacy. Medication profile indicates that she refills her medications on time the first of each month.

### All

None

### ROS

Eighteen tender joints and 16 swollen joints bilaterally; decreased ROM in hands and wrists; morning stiffness every day for about 2 hours; fatigue experienced daily during afternoon hours; swelling in hands, knees, and feet; denies HA, chest pain, SOB, bleeding episodes, or syncopal attacks; denies nausea, vomiting, diarrhea, loss of appetite, or weight loss.

### Physical Examination

*Gen*

Caucasian woman in moderate distress because of pain, swelling, and fatigue related to arthritis

*VS*

BP 118/76, P 82, RR 14, T 37.1°C; Wt 65 kg, Ht 5′6″

*Skin*

No rashes; normal turgor; no breakdown or ulcers

*HEENT*

Atraumatic; moon facies; moist mucous membranes; PERRLA; EOMI; pale conjunctiva bilaterally; TMs intact

*Neck/Lymph Nodes*

Supple, no JVD or thyromegaly; no bruits; palpable lymph nodes

*Chest*

CTA

*Breasts*

Normal; no lumps

*CV*

RRR; normal $S_1$, $S_2$; no MRG

*Abd*

Soft, NT/ND; (+) BS

*Genit/Rect*

Deferred

*MS/Ext*

Hands: mild RA changes; swelling of the second, third, fourth, and fifth PIP joints bilaterally; pain in the third and fourth MCP joints bilaterally; decreased grip strength, L > R (patient is left-handed)

Wrists: decreased ROM

Elbows: good ROM

Shoulders: decreased ROM (especially abduction) bilaterally

Hips: good ROM

Knees: good ROM, pain bilaterally

Feet: 1+ edema bilaterally; full plantar flexion; reduced dorsiflexion; 3+ pedal pulses

*Neuro*

CN II–XII grossly intact; muscle strength 5/5 UE, 5/5 LE, DTRs 4/4 biceps and triceps, 2/4 patella

■ Labs

See Table 103-1.

■ UA

Normal

■ Chest X-Ray

No fluid, masses, or infection; no cardiomegaly

■ Hand X-Ray

Multiple erosions of MCP and PIP joints bilaterally; measurable joint space narrowing from previous x-ray 3 months ago

■ DXA Scan of Hip/Spine

T score reported as –0.9

■ DAS 28

7.59 reported 3 months ago

6.97 reported today

■ Assessment

A 33-year-old woman in moderate distress with RA not adequately controlled with current therapy. DAS exhibits high disease activity although patient reports slight improvement in symptoms over 3 months ago. Patient is adherent with current medication regimen. Patient expresses desire to start a family within the next year.

## QUESTIONS

### Problem Identification

1.a. List the patient's drug therapy problems.

1.b. What information (signs, symptoms, laboratory values) indicates the presence and severity of RA?

1.c. What additional information is needed to assess the patient?

### Desired Outcome

2. What are the goals of pharmacotherapy in this case?

### Therapeutic Alternatives

3.a. What nonpharmacologic modalities may be beneficial for this patient?

3.b. What pharmacologic alternatives are available for the treatment of RA?

3.c. What economic and psychosocial considerations are applicable to this patient?

### Optimal Plan

4. What drug, dosage form, dose, schedule, and duration of therapy are best for this patient?

### Outcome Evaluation

5. What clinical and laboratory parameters are necessary to evaluate the patient's drug therapy?

**TABLE 103-1 Lab Values**

| | | | | |
|---|---|---|---|---|
| Na 135 mEq/L | Hgb 10.8 g/dL | AST 15 IU/L | CK <20 IU/L | *Fasting lipid profile* |
| K 4.1 mEq/L | Hct 31% | ALT 12 IU/L | ANA negative | T. chol 186 mg/dL |
| Cl 101 mEq/L | WBC 13.0 × $10^3$/mm$^3$ | Alk phos 56 IU/L | Wes ESR 55 mm/h | LDL 106 mg/dL |
| $CO_2$ 22 mEq/L | Plt 356 × $10^3$/mm$^3$ | T. bili 0.8 mg/dL | RF (+) 1:1,280 | HDL 50 mg/dL |
| BUN 12 mg/dL | Ca 9.1 mg/dL | Alb 4.2 g/dL | Anti-CCP (+) | TG 150 mg/dL |
| SCr 0.8 mg/dL | Urate 5.1 mg/dL | HbsAg (–) | aPTT 31 sec | |
| Glu 103 mg/dL | TSH 0.74 mIU/L | Anti-HCV (–) | INR 1.0 | |

## Patient Education

6. What information should be provided to the patient to enhance adherence, ensure successful therapy, and minimize adverse effects?

## SELF-STUDY ASSIGNMENTS

1. Perform a literature search and assess the risk of various treatments for RA during pregnancy and lactation.
2. Perform a literature search and assess the risk of cardiovascular events associated with NSAID use.
3. Create a list of the clinically significant drug interactions for NSAIDs and DMARDs, including methotrexate.
4. Compare the biologic agents used to treat RA with respect to class of agent, route of administration, efficacy, and incidence of side effects.

## CLINICAL PEARL

Teratogenicity of various agents used to treat RA needs to be considered for female patients of childbearing age. The American College of Rheumatology contraindicates the use of leflunomide, methotrexate, and minocycline in women who are pregnant or trying to become pregnant. Safety data with other agents are limited but the TNF-α agents are generally considered safe for use prior to pregnancy.

## REFERENCES


1. Fransen J, van Riel PLCM. The disease activity score and the EULAR response criteria. Rheum Dis Clin North Am 2009;35:745–757.
2. American College of Rheumatology Subcommittee on Rheumatoid Arthritis Guidelines. Guidelines for the management of rheumatoid arthritis: 2002, update. Arthritis Rheum 2002;46:328–346.
3. Saag KG, Teng GG, Patkar NM, et al. American College of Rheumatology 2008 recommendations for the use of nonbiologic and biologic disease-modifying antirheumatic drugs in rheumatoid arthritis. Arthritis Rheum 2008;59:762–784.
4. Singh JA, Christensen R, Wells GA, et al. Biologics for rheumatoid arthritis: an overview of Cochrane reviews. Cochrane Database Syst Rev 2009;(4). Art. no.: CD007848.
5. Statkute L, Ruderman EM. Novel TNF antagonists for the treatment of rheumatoid arthritis. Expert Opin Investig Drugs 2010;19:105–115.
6. Oldfield V, Dhillon S, Plosker GL. Tocilizumab: a review of its use in the management of rheumatoid arthritis. Drugs 2009;69:609–632.
7. Keeling SO, Oswald AE. Pregnancy and rheumatic disease: "by the book" or "by the doc". Clin Rheumatol 2009;28:1–9.


# 104

# OSTEOARTHRITIS

The Tolls of Labor. . . . . . . . . . . . . . . . . . . . . . . Level II

**Christopher M. Degenkolb, PharmD, BCPS**

## LEARNING OBJECTIVES

After completing this case study, the reader should be able to:

- Recognize the most common signs and symptoms of osteoarthritis.
- Design an appropriate pharmacotherapeutic regimen for treating osteoarthritis, taking into account a patient's other medical problems and drug therapy.
- Incorporate potential adjunctive therapies (pharmacologic, nonpharmacologic, and alternative) into the regimen of a patient with osteoarthritis.
- Assess and evaluate the efficacy of an analgesic regimen for a patient with osteoarthritis, and formulate an alternative plan if the regimen is inadequate or causes unacceptable toxicity.

## PATIENT PRESENTATION

### Chief Complaint

"What can I take to help this pain? This new medication I am taking is only taking the edge off!"

### HPI

Ray Kansella is a 74-year-old man who comes in to see his primary care physician today complaining of right knee and right hip pain for the last 10 years since he retired from an assembly plant. He often did very heavy lifting in his job and put a lot of strain on his back and legs; now the patient feels he is paying the price for all of his hard work. Mr Kansella wakes up every morning very stiff, and his right knee cracks when he gets up out of bed. The cracking in the joint goes away after he finishes his breakfast, but the aching in his knee and hip persists and chronically bothers him. He has been taking Vicodin®-ES for the past several months on a scheduled basis with only minimal benefit. He reports not being sure of what medications he has tried in the past; all he knows is that whatever he is taking is not really helping. He reports adherence to all medications prescribed to him. His primary care physician is now asking for your recommendation on a pain management regimen for this patient given his past medical and medication history.

### PMH

OA × 10 years
HTN × 20 years
Obesity × 15 years
Seizure disorder × 12 years (last seizure was 5 years ago)
CKD ×5 years

### PSH

Appendectomy 35 years ago

### FH

Father died at age 68 due to myocardial infarction
Mother died at age 81 of CVA
One brother (still living) with whom patient is not close

### SH

Retired and has good insurance plan and a steady pension from his company
Denies tobacco use
Occasional EtOH (two to three beers on weekends)

### Meds

Amlodipine 10 mg po daily in AM
Lisinopril 10 mg po daily in AM
Metoprolol 50 mg po BID
Hydrocodone/APAP 7.5 mg/750 mg two tablets po Q 6 h PRN pain
Levetiracetam 1,000 mg po BID

### All

NKDA; reports allergy to egg products

### ROS

Positive for pain and stiffness in the right knee and right hip; has low back pain with occasional shooting and aching pains radiating to the buttocks and groin area. Negative for headache, neck stiffness, joint swelling, or erythema. No SOB or palpitations. Has not had a bowel movement in the past 5 days.

### Physical Examination

*Gen*

Well-developed, obese, Caucasian male with moderate pain, but otherwise in NAD

*VS*

BP 148/89, P 68, RR 18, T 37.1°C; Ht 5′9″, Wt 225 lb, pain 6/10. No orthostatic changes.

*Skin*

Warm, dry, intact

*HEENT*

NC/AT; PERRLA; funduscopic exam reveals sharp disks; mild A-V nicking, but no hemorrhages or exudates; no scleral icterus; TMs intact; mucous membranes moist; poor dentition with gingival erythema; no lateral deviation of tongue; no pharyngeal edema or erythema

*Neck/Lymph Nodes*

Supple; no thyromegaly or lymphadenopathy; no carotid bruits

*Lungs*

CTA

*CV*

Distant heart sounds, normal $S_1$ and $S_2$; PMI at fifth ICS/MCL; RRR; no m/r/g; no JVD or HJR

*Abd*

Obese, soft, nontender; no guarding; diminished BS; unable to assess liver size on palpation

*Genit/Rect*

Prostate gland normal; normal sphincter tone; guaiac (−) stool in rectal vault

*MS/Ext*

Back pain radiating to right buttock with straight leg raising at 60°; right hip pain with flexion >90° and with internal and external rotation >45°; right hip tender to palpation; right knee (+) crepitus; no swelling or edema; good pedal pulses

*Neuro*

Oriented × 3; normal affect; appears at times to alternate between apathy and anger/frustration; CN II–XII intact; DTRs equal bilaterally except for slightly diminished Achilles reflexes bilaterally; no focal deficits; gait impaired secondary to hip and knee pain. Babinski's downgoing.

### Labs

| | | |
|---|---|---|
| Na 135 mEq/L | Hgb 11.8 g/dL | AST 38 IU/L |
| K 4.7 mEq/L | Hct 34.5% | Alk phos 96 IU/L |
| Cl 98 mEq/L | WBC 6.5 × $10^3$/mm$^3$ | T. prot 7.4 g/dL |
| $CO_2$ 26 mEq/L | Plt 286 × $10^3$/mm$^3$ | Alb 4.2 g/dL |
| BUN 18 mg/dL | MCV 85.3 μm$^3$ | Phos 4.5 mg/dL |
| SCr 1.9 mg/dL | MCH 28.4 pg | ESR 18 mm/h |
| Glu 99 mg/dL | MCHC 34.5 g/dL | Ca 11.2 mg/dL |

### UA

SG 1.011; pH 6.5; WBC (−), RBC (−), leukocyte esterase (−), nitrite (−), 2+ protein. Microscopic examination reveals two to five epithelial cells/hpf and no bacteria.

### X-Rays

Lumbar spine: advanced degenerative changes at L3–4 and at L4–5.

Right hip: moderate degenerative changes with some spurring of the femoral head and slight decrease in joint space.

Right knee: moderate degenerative changes. No effusion.

### Assessment

1. Pain secondary to moderate to severe OA of the lumbar spine, right hip, and right knee
2. Obesity (150% of IBW, BMI =33.2 kg/m$^2$)
3. HTN
4. CKD
5. Seizure disorder

# QUESTIONS

## Problem Identification

1.a. Create a list of the patient's drug therapy problems.

1.b. What information (symptoms, signs, laboratory values) indicates the presence or severity of the primary problem (osteoarthritis)?

1.c. What additional information is needed to satisfactorily assess this patient's major medical problems?

## Desired Outcome

2. What are the goals of pharmacotherapy for each of this patient's drug-related problems?

## Therapeutic Alternatives

3.a. What nondrug therapies might be useful for this patient?

3.b. What feasible pharmacotherapeutic alternatives are available for treatment of this patient's osteoarthritis?

## Optimal Plan

4.a. What drug, dosage form, schedule, and duration of therapy are best for treating this patient's osteoarthritis?

4.b. What alternatives would be appropriate if the initial therapy fails or cannot be used?

## Outcome Evaluation

5. What clinical and laboratory parameters are necessary to evaluate the therapy for achievement of the desired therapeutic outcome and to detect or prevent adverse effects?

## Patient Education

6. What information should be provided to the patient to enhance adherence, ensure successful therapy, and minimize adverse effects?

## FOLLOW-UP QUESTIONS

1. Evaluate the acetaminophen dosing given what the patient reports taking on a daily basis. What are the risks of the current regimen and how can these risks be minimized?
2. The patient tells you that he wants his physician to inject a drug into his knee in order to alleviate the pain. What are the therapeutic options for injection into joints to treat osteoarthritis, and when would you consider recommending this route of administration?
3. The physician is unsure of the dosing of this patient's levetiracetam for treating a seizure disorder. Is this current dose appropriate, and are there any considerations you should emphasize to the physician regarding monitoring of this medication?
4. Clinicians often rely on equianalgesic charts to convert from one opioid to another. What are some of the risks of relying too much on these dosing parameters, and how should you account for differences among the opioid medications?

## SELF-STUDY ASSIGNMENTS

1. Many patients who deal with pain and osteoarthritis often turn to unproven methods to control their pain. Research some of these unproven methods online and try to find active ingredients to determine if these are unsafe to recommend for patients with complex medication regimens.
2. Evaluate this patient's chronic kidney disease. What stage of chronic renal insufficiency does this patient have, and what is the most likely etiology of his renal disease? Prepare a paper describing some of the complications of long-standing kidney disease and how such complications should be managed.

## CLINICAL PEARL

Over 21 million Americans have osteoarthritis. It is a chronic debilitating condition associated with pain that affects activities of daily living. Managing patient's pain can maintain mobility and improve quality of life. Although use of long-acting opioids for osteoarthritis is not a first-line option, it may be a necessary therapy in certain circumstances. Therefore, it is important to dose cautiously with the lowest effective dose and monitor patient closely for side effects. Adjunctive therapies may always be considered to limit dose escalation of opioid analgesics.

## REFERENCES


1. Recommendations for the medical management of osteoarthritis of the hip and knee: 2000 update. American College of Rheumatology Subcommittee on Osteoarthritis guidelines. Arthritis Rheum 2000;43:1905–1915.
2. Felson DT. Osteoarthritis of the knee. N Engl J Med 2006;354:841–848.
3. Simon LS, Lipman AG, Jacox AK, et al. Pain in Osteoarthritis, Rheumatoid Arthritis and Juvenile Chronic Arthritis, 2nd ed. Glenview, IL, American Pain Society, 2002:1–179 (Clinical Practice Guideline, no. 2). Available at: *www.guideline.gov*. Accessed July 16, 2007.
4. Schilling A, Corey R, Leonard M, Eghtesad B. Acetaminophen: old drug, new warnings. Cleve Clin J Med 2010;77:19–27.
5. McPherson ML. Demystifying Opioid Conversion Calculations, 1st ed. Bethesda, MD, American Society of Health-System Pharmacists, 2010.
6. Neustadt DH. Intra-articular injections for osteoarthritis of the knee. Cleve Clin J Med 2006;73:897–911.
7. Lozada CJ. Glucosamine in osteoarthritis: questions remain. Cleve Clin J Med 2007;74:65–71.
8. Clegg DO, Reda DJ, Harris CL, et al. Glucosamine, chondroitin sulfate, and the two in combination for painful knee osteoarthritis. N Engl J Med 2006;354:795–808.


# 105

# GOUT AND HYPERURICEMIA

The King of Oktoberfest. . . . . . . . . . . . . . . . . . Level II

**Erik D. Maki, PharmD, BCPS**

## LEARNING OBJECTIVES

After completing this case study, the reader should be able to:

- Recognize major risk factors for developing gout in a given patient, including drugs that may contribute to or cause this disorder.
- Develop a pharmacotherapeutic plan for a patient with acute gouty arthritis that includes individualized drug selection and assessment of the treatment for efficacy or toxicity.
- Identify patients in whom maintenance therapy for gout and hyperuricemia is warranted.
- Identify medications not used primarily for gout that may have a beneficial effect on SUA levels.

## PATIENT PRESENTATION

### Chief Complaint

"My toe is on fire."

### HPI

Roy Huff is a 78-year-old man who presents to the emergency department complaining of significant toe pain. Mr Huff states, "I think I'm paying the price for my fun at Oktoberfest." He reports having spent the weekend indulging on beer and sausage at the local Oktoberfest festival. In the early hours of Monday morning (approximately 3 hours ago), he awoke to sudden excruciating pain in his right big toe. Over the last hour, this toe has become red, swollen, and so painful that he cannot walk. He has not experienced any trauma or injuries. He also denies having experienced these symptoms previously.

### PMH

HTN
PUD
Obesity

### SH

The patient typically drinks "a can of beer or two" daily but drank significantly on Friday, Saturday, and Sunday. He does not smoke or use illicit drugs.

## Meds

Chlorthalidone 25 mg po daily, started 1 month ago
Omeprazole 20 mg po daily

## All

NKDA

## ROS

Other than feeling somewhat dehydrated from all of his drinking, the patient has no major complaints prior to this ED visit. No chest pain, nausea/vomiting, or respiratory symptoms. Bowel habits are normal. He has no prior history of arthritic symptoms or joint problems.

## Physical Examination

*Gen*

A healthy-appearing, obese, white man in acute distress

*VS*

BP 120/60, P 110, RR 19, T 37.5°C; Wt 88 kg, Ht 5′6″

*Skin*

Poor skin turgor. No rashes or other dermatologic abnormalities

*HEENT*

PERRLA, dry mucous membranes, throat/ears clear of redness or inflammation

*Neck/Lymph Nodes*

Negative for lymph node swelling or masses

*Lungs/Thorax*

Clear to auscultation bilaterally, symmetric movement with inspiration

*CV*

Tachycardic, normal rhythm, normal $S_1$ and $S_2$

*Abd*

Obese, but soft, nontender. Positive bowel sounds in all quadrants

*Genit/Rect*

Deferred

*MS/Ext*

Erythematous, edematous right first metatarsophalangeal joint, which is very warm to touch. Joint is exquisitely painful with patient relating the pain as currently a 10/10 (on a 1–10 scale with "0" being no pain and "10" being the worse pain the patient has ever suffered). No swelling of any other joints. No signs of tophi present.

*Neuro*

A & O × 3. CN II–XII grossly intact, no focal neurologic deficits.

## Labs

| | | | |
|---|---|---|---|
| Na 145 mEq/L | Hgb 15.1 g/dL | WBC 12.8 × $10^3$/mm$^3$ | *Lipid panel (fasting)* |
| K 3.5 mEq/L | Hct 45% | Neutros 88% | HDL 50 mg/dL |
| Cl 101 mEq/L | RBC 4.9 × $10^6$/mm$^3$ | Bands 0% | Trig 190 mg/dL |
| $CO_2$ 23 mEq/L | Plt 210 × $10^3$/mm$^3$ | Eos 1% | LDL 92 mg/dL |
| BUN 40 mg/dL | MCV 81 μm$^3$ | Lymphs 10% | T. chol 180 mg/dL |
| SCr 3.0 mg/dL | MCHC 35 g/dL | | |
| Glu 105 mg/dL | ESR 45 mm/h | Monos 1% | |
| SUA 11.6 mg/dL | | RF negative | |

*Ankle and foot radiographs*: negative for break or damage
*Aspirated fluid from first metatarsophalangeal joint tap*: >50 WBC/HPF, containing negatively birefringent monosodium urate crystals

## Assessment

1. Primary presentation of acute gouty arthritis
2. Acute renal failure secondary to dehydration and diuretic use
3. Probable adverse drug reaction: drug-induced gout
4. Hypertension; currently well controlled
5. History of duodenal ulcer; on maintenance antisecretory therapy

# QUESTIONS

## Problem Identification

1.a. Create a list of the patient's drug therapy problems.

1.b. What patient information (symptoms, signs, laboratory values) indicates the presence or severity of acute gouty arthritis?

1.c. What risk factors in this case could contribute to or cause gouty arthritis?

## Desired Outcome

2. What are the goals of pharmacotherapy in this case?

## Therapeutic Alternatives

3.a. What nondrug therapies may be useful for this patient?

3.b. What pharmacotherapeutic modalities are available for the treatment of acute gouty arthritis?

3.c. Should chronic treatment to decrease the patient's serum uric acid level be initiated at this time? Why or why not?

## Optimal Plan

4.a. Considering the patient's information, what drug, dosage form, schedule, and duration of therapy are best in this case?

4.b. What agent would be best to treat the patient's hypertension assuming his renal function normalizes?

## Outcome Evaluation

5. Which clinical and laboratory parameters should be monitored to assess the efficacy of the pharmacotherapeutic plan and to prevent adverse effects?

## Patient Education

6. What information should be provided to the patient to enhance adherence, ensure successful therapy, and avoid adverse effects?

## CLINICAL COURSE

The patient responded to the therapy you recommended, and within 96 hours his pain has subsided significantly. Toe redness and swelling have decreased to near normal. Additionally, with fluids, his SCr has returned to baseline (0.8 mg/dL). After consultation with you, the patient's physician decides against maintenance therapy to decrease serum uric acid levels. The patient, remembering the severe pain this episode caused, follows your recommended lifestyle changes and is adherent to the new medication you recommended for his hypertension. At his 6-month follow-up appointment, he reports no more attacks of gout. He has lost 20 lb and no longer drinks ethanol. His serum uric acid level has decreased to 6.9 mg/dL, and his BP is 130/80 mm Hg.

## FOLLOW-UP QUESTIONS

1. At what point should maintenance therapy to decrease serum uric acid levels be considered?
2. If at some point maintenance therapy to decrease serum uric acid is begun, what additional therapy is needed to prevent acute flares?

## SELF-STUDY ASSIGNMENTS

1. List antihyperuricemic agents that are available in the United States and their relative advantages and disadvantages. Describe new agents that are being studied for this indication and what clinical data support their use.
2. List medications that can either raise or lower serum uric acid concentrations.

## CLINICAL PEARL

Historically, colchicine was used for treatment of acute gout flares at doses of 0.6 mg Q 1–2 h until symptoms resolved or adverse GI symptoms developed (6 mg maximum). GI side effects were employed as a clinical endpoint for discontinuing the drug because these side effects tended to occur prior to the more severe adverse effects of colchicine-induced myopathy and myelosuppression. However, current recommendations are to use low-dose colchicine at a dose of 1.2 mg, followed in 1 hour with a single dose of 0.6 mg. For patients receiving prophylactic colchicine prior to the flare, it is recommended to wait 12 hours after treatment dosing before resuming prophylactic dosing.

## REFERENCES


1. Richette P, Bardin T. Gout. Lancet 2010;375(9711):318–328.
2. Zhang W, Doherty M, Bardin T, et al. EULAR evidence based recommendations for gout. Part II: management. Report of a task force of the EULAR Standing Committee for International Clinical Studies Including Therapeutics (ESCISIT). Ann Rheum Dis 2006;65:1312–1324.
3. Jordan KM, Cameron JS, Snaith M, et al. British Society for Rheumatology and British Health Professionals in Rheumatology guideline for the management of gout. Rheumatology 2007;46:1372–1374.
4. Choi HK. A prescription for lifestyle change in patients with hyperuricemia and gout. Curr Opin Rheumatol 2010;22:166–172.
5. Hoskison KT, Wortmann RL. Management of gout in older adults: barriers to optimal control. Drugs Aging 2007:24(1):21–36.

SECTION 13

# DISORDERS OF THE EYES, EARS, NOSE, AND THROAT

# 106

## GLAUCOMA

Another Silent Disease. . . . . . . . . . . . . . . . . . . Level III

**Tien T. Kiat-Winarko, PharmD, BSc**

## LEARNING OBJECTIVES

After completing this case study, students should be able to:

- Recognize the importance of regular eye examinations and the difference between glaucoma and ocular hypertension.
- List the risk factors for developing open-angle glaucoma.
- Select and recommend agents from different pharmacologic classes when indicated and provide the rationale for drug selection.
- Recommend conventional glaucoma therapy as well as other options in glaucoma management when indicated.
- Implement the basic ophthalmologic monitoring parameters used in glaucoma therapy.
- Counsel patients on their medication regimen and proper ophthalmic administration technique.
- Explain and discuss possible adverse drug reactions with patients to increase therapy adherence.

## PATIENT PRESENTATION

### Chief Complaint

"My left eye is foggy, and I get blurred vision and headaches."

### HPI

Lee Angeles is a pleasant 48-year-old man with a history of advanced open-angle glaucoma who presents to his ophthalmologist with complaints of fogging and distortion of vision in the left eye lasting 6–12 hours. This occasionally progresses to tunnel vision, with chronic sensitivity to fluorescent lights and throbbing bandlike squeezing headaches lasting for hours. He also complains of periodic distortion in the left eye for the past 3 months, sometimes associated with central area visual blurring. Despite his condition, he continues to maintain self-independence. He often drives from Los Angeles to his weekend home in Palm Springs.

He was in his usual state of health until he had a skydiving accident 23 years ago and fractured his thoracic spine at the level of T9–10. During that hospitalization, he complained of blurred vision. Ophthalmology consult was sought, and he was ultimately diagnosed with advanced open-angle glaucoma (Fig. 106-1). He was managed by a general ophthalmologist for several years, who prescribed Timoptic 0.5% in both eyes BID, Propine 0.1% in both eyes BID, and Ocusert Pilo-40 in right eye and Ocusert Pilo-20 in left eye once every week. He was subsequently referred to a glaucoma specialist because of worsening of his condition. He had undergone laser trabeculoplasty in both eyes prior to his referral. The glaucoma specialist examined the patient, and a complete workup was done on the initial visit.

Bilateral laser trabeculoplasty was performed 18 years ago with an initial decrease in IOP; however, IOP subsequently increased several months later. Filtering surgery was performed in Boston on both eyes 17 years ago. Multiple prior brain MRIs revealed no abnormal findings. Other ocular history includes severe myopia since childhood, history of dry eyes, and history of contact lens wear.

### PMH

Childhood asthma that resolved at puberty
Depression as a consequence of chronic open-angle glaucoma and worsening of vision after completion of his PhD program
S/P ultrasonic renal lithotripsy secondary to nephrolithiasis associated with acetazolamide use
S/P tonsillectomy as a child

### FH

Father, mother, and sister have glaucoma. Father has HTN.

### SH

PhD in molecular biology from Harvard. Single. No history of smoking. Drank four cans of beer per day for 3 years during postgraduate study. Currently drinks two to three cans of beer per week.

### ROS

Negative except for occasional episodes of erectile dysfunction

### Meds

Betoptic 0.5% in both eyes BID
Iopidine 0.5% in left eye TID
Trusopt 2% in left eye TID
FML 0.1% in both eyes TID
Bion Tears in both eyes BID
Nifedipine 10 mg po TID
Trental 400 mg po TID
Paxil 20 mg po once daily
Also performs eye massage on both eyes QID
Past medications include pilocarpine 4%, Timoptic 0.5%, Propine, Diamox sequels 500 mg, and Pred-Forte 1%

### All

NKDA

### Physical Examination

*VS*

BP 126/88, P 78, R 19, T 36.4°C

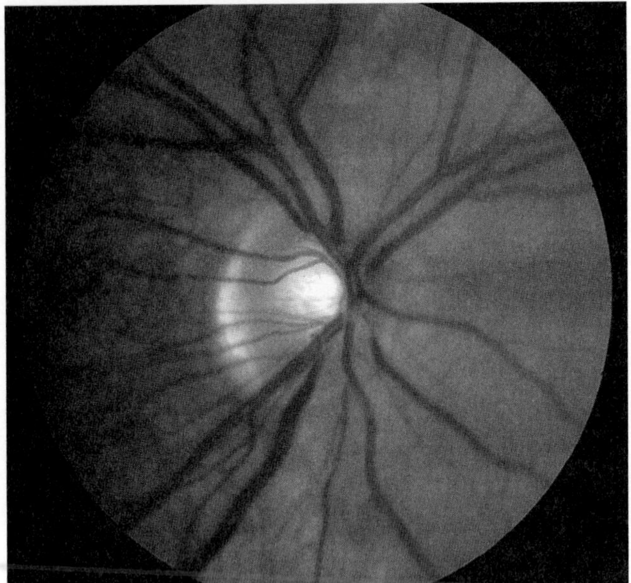
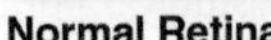
Normal Retina

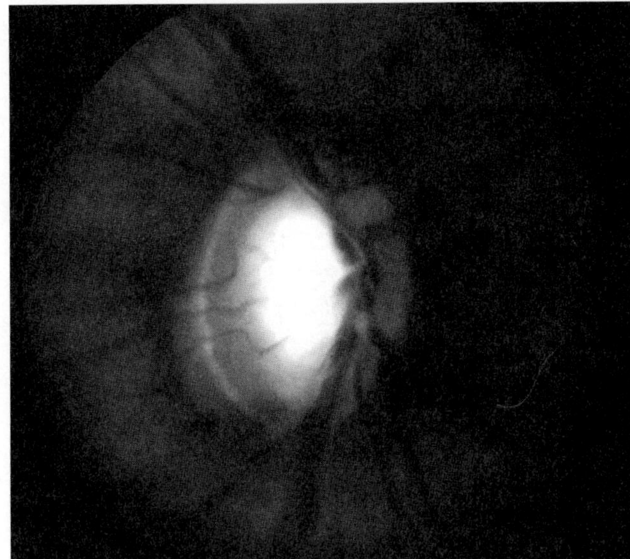
Retina with Glaucoma

**FIGURE 106-1.** Comparison of the retina in a patient with a healthy optic nerve *(left)* and in a patient with glaucoma and a large cup with a disc hemorrhage, typical of chronic open-angle glaucoma *(right)*. *(Photo courtesy of Dr Donald Minckler, University of California, Irvine.)*

*Eyes*

*Visual acuity:* OD—hand motion at 3 in with correction spectacles; OS—20/30.

*Slit-lamp exam:* Lid margins were without inflammation in both eyes; conjunctiva without injection; normal tear breakup, did not stain with fluorescein; cornea clear and smooth; anterior chamber deep and quiet; lenses—clear in both eyes; iris round without neovascularization or abnormality; no mass/nodules; filtering bleb is visible at 11 o'clock meridian.

*Intraocular pressure:* OD—14 mm Hg; OS—20 mm Hg.

*Vitreous examination:* Clear in both eyes.

*Disks:* OD—the disc appeared whitish, fully cupped and showed marked pallor; C/D ratio = 1.0; OS—C/D ratio = 0.99 with only a narrow rim present (normal C/D ratio ≤0.33).

*Color vision:* OD—unable to see; OS—WNL.

*Visual fields:* OD—unable to see the Amsler grid; can only see hand motion at 3 in away; OS—several paracentral scotomata with the Amsler grid; 20/30. Diurnal curve of IOP revealed pressures between 10 and 21 mm Hg.

*CV*

RRR without MRG; carotid pulses are brisk and equal bilaterally without bruits

*Neuro*

Smell and corneal sensation are intact bilaterally. Facial symmetry, tone, and sensation are intact bilaterally. Cranial nerves VIII–XII were intact. Gait was intact. Finger-to-nose and rapid alternating movement tests were normal. Reflexes were symmetric and normal. Sensation was intact and symmetric to pinprick, proprioception, and light touch. Motor strength of all extremities was 5/5.

### Labs

| | |
|---|---|
| Na 141 mEq/L | BUN 10 mg/dL |
| K 4.4 mEq/L | Scr 0.7 mg/dL |
| Cl 109 mEq/L | FBG 95 mg/dL |
| $CO_2$ 29 mEq/L | Vitamin $D_3$ 34 ng/mL |

### Assessment

1. High myopia with advanced chronic juvenile open-angle glaucoma
2. No evidence of macular edema
3. No cataracts
4. S/P filtering procedure in both eyes
5. Depression associated with chronic open-angle glaucoma

### Plan

Increase eye massage to eight times per day.

Follow up in 6 weeks.

Repeat filtering surgery/trabeculectomy with mitomycin C to further lower IOP.

Switch nifedipine to nimodipine for better CNS/ophthalmic absorption to increase blood flow.

Counsel with neuro-ophthalmologist, retina ophthalmologist, and neurologist.

# QUESTIONS

## Problem Identification

1.a. Identify this patient's drug therapy problems.

1.b. What risk factors for POAG are present in this patient?

1.c. What information (signs, symptoms) indicates the presence or severity of this patient's glaucoma?

1.d. This patient was diagnosed with advanced open-angle glaucoma during his hospital stay after a skydiving accident. Would earlier therapy have prevented the deterioration of POAG?

1.e. The patient reports occasional episodes of erectile dysfunction. Are phosphodiesterase-5 inhibitors such as sildenafil safe for patients with high intraocular pressure?

## Desired Outcome

2. What are the goals of pharmacotherapy in this case?

## Therapeutic Alternatives

3.a. What nondrug therapies might be useful for this patient?

3.b. What feasible pharmacotherapeutic alternatives are available for treating this patient's glaucoma?

3.c. Is antioxidant supplementation beneficial in maintaining eye health?

3.d. Discuss the possible benefit of neuroprotective agents such as memantine in patients with glaucoma.

## Optimal Plan

4.a. Devise an optimal pharmacotherapeutic regimen for treating this patient's glaucoma.

4.b. What alternatives would be appropriate if the initial therapy fails or cannot be used?

## Outcome Evaluation

5. What clinical and laboratory parameters are necessary to evaluate the therapy for achievement of the desired therapeutic outcome and to detect or prevent adverse effects?

## Patient Education

6. What information should the patient receive about the disease of glaucoma, proper medication administration technique, and possible side effects of treatment?

## SELF-STUDY ASSIGNMENTS

1. Perform a literature search on the reason why antimetabolites such as mitomycin C and 5-FU are used in glaucoma surgery. What is the mechanism of action of these antimetabolites in trabeculectomy pressure-lowering surgery?
2. Perform a literature search and explain the rationale for using nimodipine and pentoxifylline in advanced open-angle glaucoma. How do these agents work to increase blood flow to the eye and retard the progression of nerve damage?
3. Under what circumstances should the product Ocusert Pilo be used? Compare the advantages and disadvantages of using this long-acting ocular insert.

## REFERENCES

1. Schwartz GF. Compliance and persistency in glaucoma follow-up treatment. Curr Opin Ophthalmol 2005;16:114–121.
2. Kass MA, Gordon MO, Gao F, et al. Delaying treatment of ocular hypertension: the ocular hypertension treatment study. Arch Ophthalmol 2010;128:276–287.
3. Kane H, Gaasterland DE, Monsour M. Response of filtered eyes to digital ocular pressure. Ophthalmology 1997;104:202–206.
4. Liu JH. Circadian rhythm of intraocular pressure. J Glaucoma 1998;7:141–147.
5. Brandt JD, VanDenburgh AM, Chen K, et al. Comparison of once- or twice-daily bimatoprost with twice-daily timolol in patients with elevated IOP: a 3-month clinical trial. Ophthalmology 2001;108:1023–1031.
6. Aung T, Chew PT, Yip CC, et al. A randomized double-masked crossover study comparing latanoprost 0.005% with unoprostone 0.12% in patients with primary open-angle glaucoma and ocular hypertension. Am J Ophthalmol 2001;131:636–642.
7. Varma R, Winarko J, Winarko TK. Concentration of latanoprost ophthalmic solution after 4 to 6 weeks' use in an eye clinic setting. Invest Ophthalmol Vis Sci 2006;47:222–225.
8. Mundorf T, Williams R, Whitcup S, et al. A 3-month comparison of efficacy and safety of brimonidine-purite 0.15% and brimonidine 0.2% in patients with glaucoma or ocular hypertension. J Ocul Pharmacol Ther 2003;19:37–44.
9. Glaucoma Research Foundation. Alternative medicine. Available at: *www.glaucoma.org/treating/alternative_med.html* accessed February 11, 2011.
10. Doshi M, Edward DP, Osmanovic S. Clinical course of bimatoprost-induced periocular skin changes in Caucasians. Ophthalmology 2006;113:1961–1967.

# 107

# ALLERGIC RHINITIS

To Play or Not to Play . . . . . . . . . . . . . . . . . . . . Level I

**Brice Labruzzo Mohundro, PharmD**

**W. Greg Leader, PharmD**

## LEARNING OBJECTIVES

After completing this case study, students should be able to:

- Classify a patient's allergic rhinitis based on the signs and symptoms of the disease.
- Educate patients on appropriate measures to limit or avoid exposure to specific antigens.
- Compare and contrast available agents used to treat allergic rhinitis with respect to efficacy and safety.
- Develop a safe and effective therapeutic regimen for the management of allergic rhinitis based on disease severity.
- Educate patients with allergic rhinitis on appropriate medication use.

## PATIENT PRESENTATION

### Chief Complaint

"My nose is stopped up and I can't smell anything. During football practice, I sometimes start sneezing and can't stop. When I finally stop sneezing, my nose starts running and then gets stopped up again. I am having trouble at practice because I am so tired, and now my eyes are red and watery all the time and my ears and roof of my mouth are itchy. This happened last football season and playing wasn't as fun as it used to be so I am thinking about quitting the team."

### HPI

Caleb Thibodeaux is a 14-year-old boy presenting to a multidisciplinary family medicine clinic with complaints of upper respiratory symptoms. The symptoms have been occurring since the beginning of football practice and have worsened over the past month. He reports that it started with occasional sneezing spells but now includes congestion, red, watery eyes, and itchy nose and throat. He has not run a fever and does not have throat pain. He occasionally wakes up with a dry mouth in the mornings.

■ PMH

Atopic dermatitis
Recurrent otitis media
Tympanostomy tubes and adenoidectomy at age 4

■ FH

Father, age 44, with a history of asthma. Mother, age 38, with a history of migraine headaches. Brother, age 10, with severe persistent asthma, and sister, age 6, with perennial allergic rhinitis.

■ SH

Lives in a three-bedroom house built on a concrete slab with his parents. He has been living there for approximately 9 months. Neither parents nor siblings smoke. Family has a dog that lives indoors but sleeps in the laundry room. Caleb is in the seventh grade and is on both the football and baseball team.

■ Meds

Benadryl 25 mg po BID × 7 days
Oxymetazoline (Afrin) two sprays in each nostril BID × 7 days
Creatine 5 g po QID

■ All

Penicillin (anaphylaxis)

■ ROS

Admits to occasional headaches but denies shortness of breath, wheezing, chest pain, or abdominal discomfort

■ Physical Examination

*Gen*

The patient is a young boy who looks his stated age. He appears tired and sounds congested. He is continually wiping his nose upward with the palm of his hand and rubbing his eyes.

*VS*

BP 112/74, P 68, RR 18, T 36.9°C; Wt 105 lb, Ht 5′3″

*HEENT*

NC/AT; PERRLA; EOMI. Conjunctivae are injected. Periorbital edema and discoloration. TMs are intact. Swollen nasal mucous membranes and nasal turbinates with a pale, bluish hue and clear discharge. No tenderness over frontal and maxillary sinuses. There are no oropharyngeal lesions, and the throat is nonerythematous.

*Neck*

No lymphadenopathy or thyromegaly

*Chest*

CTA bilaterally; no wheezes

*Heart*

RRR without murmur or rub

*Abdomen*

Soft, nontender, (+) BS

*Genit/Rect*

Deferred

*Extremities*

No CCE, pulses 2+ throughout

*Neuro*

A & O × 3; DTRs 2+ throughout; 5/5 strength; CN I–XII intact

■ Other

Skin prick allergen skin test: Positive for ragweed allergy

■ Assessment

This is a 14-year-old boy with sneezing, nasal congestion, pruritus of the nose and palate, chemosis, and conjunctival injection most likely due to seasonal allergies.

■ Plan

Seasonal rhinitis: Develop a treatment regimen that effectively reliever the patient's symptoms with minimal side effects and reasonable coat.

# QUESTIONS

## Problem Identification

1.a. Create a list of the patient's drug therapy problems.

1.b. What information (signs, symptoms, laboratory values) indicates the presence or severity of allergic rhinitis?

1.c. Could any of the patient's problems have been caused by drug therapy?

1.d. What additional information from the patient history is needed to satisfactorily assess this patient?

## Desired Outcome

2. What are the goals of pharmacotherapy in this case?

## Therapeutic Alternatives

3.a. What nondrug therapies might be useful for this patient?

3.b. What feasible pharmacotherapeutic alternatives are available for treatment of allergic rhinitis?

## Optimal Plan

4.a. What drug, dosage form, dose, schedule, and duration of therapy are best for this patient?

4.b. What alternatives would be appropriate if the initial therapy fails?

## Outcome Evaluation

5. What clinical and laboratory parameters are necessary to evaluate the therapy for achievement of the desired therapeutic outcome and to detect or prevent adverse effects?

## Patient Education

6.a. What information should be provided to a patient receiving an intranasal corticosteroid to enhance compliance, ensure successful therapy, and minimize adverse effects?

6.b. What information should be provided to a patient receiving an ophthalmic antihistamine?

## CLINICAL COURSE: ALTERNATIVE THERAPY

Caleb's mother is quite concerned about drowsiness associated with prescription treatments for his symptoms because he has a tendency to nap when he is supposed to be doing homework. Mrs Thibodeaux uses butterbur extract for migraine prophylaxis and has heard that it is effective for allergy symptoms; she asks about using the same product for Caleb. For questions related to the use of butterbur extract for the treatment of allergic rhinitis, please see Section 19 of this casebook.

## SELF-STUDY ASSIGNMENTS

1. Recommend a treatment plan for an 80-year-old man in a nursing home who has moderate persistent allergic rhinitis. Discuss any age-related concerns that may be encountered.
2. Make recommendations for a single first-generation antihistamine, second-generation antihistamine, and intranasal corticosteroid to include on a hospital or HMO formulary. Support your recommendations with efficacy, safety, and economic data.
3. Search the literature on the use of complementary or alternative therapies for treatment of allergic rhinitis and prepare a table summarizing the results of controlled clinical trials.
4. Outline a treatment plan for a pregnant patient with allergic rhinitis. Justify your selection of pharmacologic agents based on their efficacy and safety profiles.

## CLINICAL PEARL

Immunotherapy is the only treatment for allergic rhinitis that has been demonstrated to alter the natural course of the disease.

## REFERENCES

1. Wallace DV, Dykewicz MS, Bernstein DI, et al, Joint Task Force on Practice, American Academy of Allergy, Asthma & Immunology, American College of Allergy, Asthma and Immunology, Joint Council of Allergy, Asthma and Immunology. The diagnosis and management of rhinitis: an updated practice parameter. J Allergy Clin Immunol 2008;122(2 Suppl):S1–S84.
2. Bousquet J, Khaltaev N, Cruz AA, et al. Allergic Rhinitis and its Impact on Asthma (ARIA) 2008 update (in collaboration with the World Health Organization, GA(2)LEN and AllerGen). Allergy 2008;63(Suppl 86): 8–160.
3. Casale TB, Blaiss MS, Gelfard E, et al. First do no harm: managing antihistamine impairment in patients with allergic rhinitis. J Allergy Clin Immunol 2003;111:S835–S842.
4. Horak F, Zieglmayer P, Zieglmayer R, et al. A placebo-controlled study of the nasal decongestant effect of phenylephrine and pseudoephedrine in the Vienna Challenge Chamber. Ann Allergy Asthma Immunol 2009;102:116–120.
5. Scadding GK. Corticosteroids in the treatment of pediatric allergic rhinitis. J Allergy Clin Immunol 2001;108(1 Suppl):S59–S64.
6. Rodrigo GJ, Yanez A. The role of antileukotriene therapy in seasonal allergic rhinitis: a systematic review of randomized trials. Ann Allergy Asthma Immunol 2006;96:779–786.
7. Wilson AM, O'Byrne PM, Parameswaran K. Leukotriene receptor antagonists for allergic rhinitis: a systematic review and meta-analysis. Am J Med 2004;116:338–344.
8. Schapowal A. Petasites Study Group. Butterbur Ze339 for the treatment of intermittent allergic rhinitis: dose-dependent efficacy in a prospective, randomized, double-blind, placebo-controlled study. Arch Otolaryngol Head Neck Surg 2004;130:1381–1386.
9. Casale TB, Busse WW, Kline JN, et al, Immune Tolerance Network Group. Omalizumab pretreatment decreases acute reactions after rush immunotherapy for ragweed-induced seasonal allergic rhinitis. J Allergy Clin Immunol 2006;117:134–140.

SECTION 14
# DERMATOLOGIC DISORDERS

## 108

## CUTANEOUS REACTION TO DRUGS

A Case of TEN . . . . . . . . . . . . . . . . . . . . . . . . Level III

Rebecca M.T. Law, BS Pharm, PharmD

## LEARNING OBJECTIVES

After completing this case study, students should be able to:

- Understand the approach to identifying or ruling out a suspected drug-induced skin reaction.
- Recognize the signs and symptoms of drug-induced Stevens Johnson syndrome (SJS) and toxic epidermal necrolysis (TEN).
- Name the drugs most commonly implicated in causing SJS and TEN.
- Determine an appropriate course of action for a patient with a suspected drug-induced skin reaction.
- Understand the treatment approach for a patient with TEN, including nonpharmacologic and pharmacologic therapies.
- Counsel patients with suspected drug-induced SJS or TEN about the nature of the reaction and necessary precautions, including which medications to avoid in the future.
- Identify patients with potentially serious skin reactions who should be referred for further medical evaluation and treatment.

## PATIENT PRESENTATION

### Chief Complaint

"My child has a blistering rash all over her body and is really sick!"

### HPI

April Rayne is a 14-year-old Caucasian girl who presented to the ED with a high fever, vomiting, diarrhea, and a 3-day history of a skin rash. The rash is maculopapular with blisters and has spread to involve 75% of her body surface area. She had a UTI about 1.5 weeks ago and was prescribed a 7-day course of TMP/SMX. She adhered to the regimen; her urinary tract symptoms of dysuria and frequency and her abdominal discomfort resolved within 2–3 days. This was her first UTI. She continued to take the TMP/SMX as directed. Seven days after starting therapy, she noticed red spots on her arms and legs that began to spread over the whole body. The rash began to blister. She became febrile, and last night she began vomiting and had two bouts of diarrhea. This morning her mother brought her to the ED and she was admitted to the ICU, where she was immediately intubated to protect her airway patency.

### PMH

Unremarkable

### FH

Parents A & W, no siblings

### SH

April is a student who just began taking jazz classes about 2 months ago, which she really enjoys.tr She is not sexually active, does not smoke, and does not use alcohol. There have been no recent changes in diet or in her living environment.

### Meds

Just completed a 7-day course of TMP/SMX. No additional drugs taken including OTCs, vitamins, herbals, or drugs of abuse. Not on oral contraceptives.

### Meds in Hospital

For intubation: Ketamine 40 mg IV × 1, midazolam 1 mg IV × 1, propofol 120 mg IV × 1

For BP support: Dopamine IV infusion at 12 mcg/kg/min

### All

NKDA

### ROS

Skin is tender to the touch, with rash and blisters. Continues to have loose BM. Vomited × 1 in ED. Otherwise negative except for complaints noted above.

### Physical Examination

*Gen*

Fairly anxious 14-year-old Caucasian girl looking acutely ill

*VS*

BP 90/50, HR 90, RR 25, T 40.1°C

*Skin*

Extensive maculopapular rash over 75% of BSA. Blisters involve over 30% of BSA and appear to still be spreading. Small blisters on discrete dark red purpuric macules symmetrically over face, hands, feet, limbs, and trunk with widespread erythema. Blisters and intensely red oozing erosions over lips (especially vermilion border), oral mucosa, and vaginal area. Some ruptured blisters on skin and some with necrotic centers. Positive Nikolsky's sign. Skin is tender to the touch.

*HEENT*

PERRLA, EOMI, fundi benign, TMs intact. Corneal abrasions but no blisters. Conjunctivitis with some debris collecting under eyelids. External nares clear. Blisters in oral cavity and ulceration on lower lip. Pharynx erythematous and blistering.

*Chest*

Upper airway congestion; debris and ulceration in mouth, throat, and epiglottis. (She was immediately intubated to protect airway patency.)

*Cor*

RRR without murmurs, rubs, or gallops; $S_1$ and $S_2$ normal

*Abd*

(+) BS, soft, nontender, no masses

*Genitourinary*

Blistering in vaginal area. Foley catheter inserted—urine output approximately 40–50 mL/h.

*Rectal*

Deferred

*MS/Ext*

Maculopapular rash and some blisters on arms and legs. Bilateral arthralgias and myalgias. Peripheral pulses present.

*Neuro*

Oriented × 3. No signs of confusion.

■ Labs

| | | | |
|---|---|---|---|
| Na 140 mEq/L | Glucose 95 mg/dL | WBC 11 × $10^3$/mm$^3$ | Hgb 12 g/dL |
| K 4.0 mEq/L | BUN 9 mg/dL | PMNs 65% | Hct 31% |
| Cl 101 mEq/L | SCr 0.7 mg/dL | Bands 5% | Plt 239 × $10^3$/mm$^3$ |
| $CO_2$ 32 mEq/L | AST 15 IU/L | Eos 8% | INR 1.24 |
| $PO_4$ 2.2 mg/dL | ALT 22 IU/L | Monos 1% | aPTT 32.4 sec |
| T. protein 6.5 g/dL | LDH 120 IU/L | Basos 1% | ESR 35 mm/h |
| Albumin 3.1 g/dL | | Lymphs 20% | RF negative |

Urinalysis: No protein, ketones, blood, WBC, or bacteria

■ Chest X-Ray

WNL

■ Clinical Course

*Day 2 of Admission*

Urine output still approximately 40–50 mL/h; 1,050 mL/previous 24 hours

*Day 3 of Admission*

Histopathology of biopsy specimen from lesion on lip: Epidermal degeneration with intraepidermal vesiculation and subepidermal bullae. Mild perivascular lymphocytic infiltrate.

Direct immunofluorescence of biopsy specimen from lip lesion: Negative.

Swab from blisters on arm: Coagulase-negative *Staphylococcus*, *Pseudomonas aeruginosa*.

Blood cultures: Coagulase-negative *Staphylococcus*, sensitive to vancomycin.

Urine culture (mid-stream urine): No growth.

■ Assessment

This is a 14-year-old girl with TEN, likely drug-induced, who has probably developed secondary *Staphylococcus epidermidis* bacteremia.

## QUESTIONS

### Problem Identification

1.a. Create a drug therapy problem list for this patient.

1.b. What signs and symptoms of TEN does this patient demonstrate?

1.c. Could the patient's signs and symptoms be caused by a drug?

1.d. What findings correlate with disease severity of TEN and a worse prognosis?

### Desired Outcome

2. What are the treatment goals for this patient?

### Therapeutic Alternatives

3.a. What nonpharmacologic alternatives are available for managing TEN in this patient?

3.b. What pharmacotherapeutic alternatives are available for managing this patient's TEN?

### Optimal Plan

4. Design an optimal pharmacotherapeutic plan for TEN in this patient.

### Outcome Evaluation

5. What efficacy and adverse effects monitoring is needed for the management strategies you recommended?

### Patient Education

6. How would you inform this patient (and her caregivers) about her drug therapies?

## ■ SELF-STUDY ASSIGNMENTS

1. Differentiate among the various types, terminology, and manifestations of cutaneous drug reactions, including irritant drug reactions, fixed drug reactions, maculopapular skin reactions, photoallergic and phototoxic reactions, bullous reactions, morbilliform and urticarial reactions, pigmentation, lichenoid eruptions, SJS, TEN, drug hypersensitivity syndrome, and vasculitis.
2. If this patient had SJS, how would the clinical presentation, disease course, and treatment differ from those of TEN?
3. Obtain information on the anticonvulsants and NSAIDs in the oxicam class that have been most commonly implicated in causing SJS/TEN.
4. Investigate the genetics of drug hypersensitivity, including associations with specific genetic markers (e.g., HLA-B*5701 and HLA-B*1502 alleles).

## CLINICAL PEARL

Aggressive and vigilant nondrug supportive therapies are vital to the effective management of TEN.

## REFERENCES

1. Cohen V, Jellinek SP, Schwartz RA. Toxic epidermal necrolysis. eMedicine updated February 12, 2009. Available at: *http://emedicine.medscape.com/article/229698-overview*. Accessed March 28, 2010.
2. Levi N, Bastuji-Garin S, Mockenhaupt M, et al. Medications as risk factors of Stevens–Johnson syndrome and toxic epidermal necrolysis in children: a pooled analysis. Pediatrics 2009;123;e297–e304 [originally published online January 19, 2009; DOI: 10.1542/peds.2008–1923].
3. Mittmann N, Chan BC, Knowles S, et al. IVIG for the treatment of toxic epidermal necrolysis. Skin Therapy Lett 2007;12:7–9. ©2007 SkinCareGuide.com. Posted by Medscape April 10, 2007. Available at: *www.medscape.com/viewarticle/554693*. Accessed May 21, 2010.
4. Playe S, Murphy G. Recognizing adverse reactions to antibiotics. Emerg Med 2006;38(6):11–20. Available at: *www.emedmag.com/html/pre/fea/features/061506.asp*. Accessed May 21, 2010.
5. Tilles SA. Practical issues in the management of hypersensitivity reactions: sulfonamides. South Med J 2001;94:817–824.
6. Roujeau JC, Kelly JP, Naldi L, et al. Medication use and the risk of Stevens–Johnson syndrome or toxic epidermal necrolysis. N Engl J Med 1995;333:1600–1607.
7. Mockenhaupt M, Viboud C, Dunant A, et al. Stevens–Johnson syndrome and toxic epidermal necrolysis: assessment of medication risks with emphasis on recently marketed drugs. The EuroSCAR-Study. J Invest Dermatol 2008;128:35–44.
8. Johnson KK, Green DL, Rife JP, et al. Sulfonamide cross-reactivity: fact or fiction? Ann Pharmacother 2005;39:290–301.
9. Strom BL, Schinnar R, Apter AJ, et al. Absence of cross-reactivity between sulfonamide antibiotics and sulfonamide nonantibiotics. N Engl J Med 2003;349:1628–1635.
10. Klein PA. Stevens–Johnson syndrome and toxic epidermal necrolysis. eMedicine updated February 20, 2009. Available at: *http://emedicine.medscape.com/article/1124127-overview*. Accessed May 25, 2010.
11. deShazo RD, Kemp SF. Allergic reactions to drugs and biologic agents. JAMA 1997;278:1895–1906.

# 109

# ACNE VULGARIS

The Graduate . . . . . . . . . . . . . . . . . . . . . . . . . . Level II

**Rebecca M.T. Law, BS Pharm, PharmD**

**Wayne P. Gulliver, MD, FRCPC**

## LEARNING OBJECTIVES

After completing this case study, students should be able to:

- Understand risk factors and aggravating factors in the pathogenesis of acne vulgaris.
- Understand the treatment strategies for acne, including appropriate situations for using nonprescription and prescription medications and use of topical and systemic therapies.
- Educate patients with acne on systemic therapies.
- Monitor the safety and efficacy of selected systemic therapies.

## PATIENT PRESENTATION

### Chief Complaint

"I can't stand this acne!"

### HPI

Elaine Morgan is an 18-year-old woman with a history of facial acne since age 15. One month ago, she completed a 3-month course of minocycline in combination with Differin (adapalene). Her acne has flared up again, and she has again presented to her family physician for treatment.

### PMH

Has irregular menses as a result of polycystic ovary syndrome diagnosed 3 years ago, which has not required medical treatment. However, it has resulted in an acne condition that was initially quite mild; she responded well to nonprescription topical products. In the past 2 years, the number of facial lesions has increased despite OTC, and, later, prescription drug treatments. Initially, Benzamycin Gel was beneficial, but this had to be discontinued because of excessive drying. Differin was used next, and it controlled her condition for about 6 months; then the acne worsened and oral antibiotics were added. Most recently, she has received two 3-month courses of minocycline over the past year. She has also noted some scarring and cysts in the past few months.

### FH

Parents alive and well; two older brothers (ages 21 and 25). Father had acne with residual scarring.

### SH

The patient is under some stress because she is graduating in a few weeks. She wants to do well in school so she will qualify for the best colleges. Both of her brothers graduated with honors. She is sexually active, and her boyfriend uses condoms.

### Meds

None currently

### All

NKDA

### ROS

In addition to the complaints noted above, the patient has irregular menstrual periods and mild hirsutism.

### Physical Examination

*Gen*

Alert, moderately anxious teenager in NAD

*VS*

BP 110/70, RR 15, T 37°C; Wt 45 kg, Ht 5′2″

*Skin*

Comedones on forehead, nose, and chin. Papules and pustules on the nose and malar area. A few cysts on the chin. Scars on malar area. Increased facial hair.

*HEENT*

PERRLA, EOMI, fundi benign, TMs intact

*Chest*

CTA bilaterally

*Cor*

RRR without MRG, $S_1$ and $S_2$ normal

*Abd*

(+) BS, soft, nontender, no masses

*MS/Ext*

No joint aches or pains; peripheral pulses present

*Neuro*

CN II–XII intact

### Labs

| | | | |
|---|---|---|---|
| Na 140 mEq/L | Hgb 13.0 g/dL | AST 21 IU/L | T. chol 170 mg/dL |
| K 3.7 mEq/L | Hct 38% | ALT 39 IU/L | LDL-C 90 mg/dL |
| Cl 100 mEq/L | Plt 300 × $10^3$/mm$^3$ | LDH 105 IU/L | Trig 90 mg/dL |
| $CO_2$ 25 mEq/L | WBC 7.0 × $10^3$/mm$^3$ | Alk phos 89 IU/L | HDL 45 mg/dL |
| BUN 12 mg/dL | | T. bili 1.0 mg/dL | DHEAS 221 mcg/dL (6 µmol/L) |
| SCr 1.0 mg/dL | | Alb 3.9 g/dL | Testosterone (free) 2.3 ng/mL |
| Glu 100 mg/dL | | FSH 30 mIU/mL | Prolactin 15 ng/mL |
| BUN 12 mg/dL | | LH 150 mIU/mL | |
| SCr 1.0 mg/dL | | | |

# QUESTIONS

## Problem Identification

1.a. Create a drug therapy problem list for this patient.

1.b. What signs and symptoms consistent with acne does this patient have?

1.c. How does polycystic ovary syndrome contribute to this patient's acne and other physical findings?

## Desired Outcome

2. What are the treatment goals for this patient?

## Therapeutic Alternatives

3. What feasible therapeutic alternatives are available for management of this patient's acne and hyperandrogenism?

## Optimal Plan

4. What treatment regimen is best suited for this patient?

## Outcome Evaluation

5. How would you monitor the therapy you recommended for efficacy and adverse effects?

## Patient Education

6. How would you educate the patient about this treatment regimen to enhance compliance and ensure successful therapy?

# CLINICAL COURSE

Two months later, the patient has developed bloating, weight gain, and increased appetite, likely related to the therapy prescribed. She also reveals that her maternal grandmother and aunt both died of melanoma, and a friend told her that she should not be using her new therapy.

## Follow-Up Question

1. What is the most appropriate course of action?

# SELF-STUDY ASSIGNMENTS

1. Review the dysmorphic syndrome associated with acne.
2. Review the nonpharmacologic management of acne, including stress reduction and dietary changes.

# CLINICAL PEARL

In females with acne, scarring + cysts + two courses of oral antibiotics means hormonal therapy and "consider isotretinoin."

# REFERENCES


1. Thielitz A, Gollnick H. Overview of new therapeutic developments for acne. Expert Rev Dermatol 2009;4(1):55–65.
2. Costello M, Shrestha B, Eden J, et al. Insulin-sensitising drugs versus the combined oral contraceptive pill for hirsutism, acne and risk of diabetes, cardiovascular disease, and endometrial cancer in polycystic ovary syndrome. Cochrane Database Syst Rev 2007;(1) [intervention review]. Art. no.: CD005552. DOI: 10.1002/14651858.CD005552.pub2 [edited, published in Cochrane Libr 2009;(1)].
3. Cheung AP, Chang RJ. Polycystic ovary syndrome. Clin Obstet Gynecol 1990;33:655–667.
4. Gollnick H, Cunliffe W, Berson D, et al. Management of acne: a report from a Global Alliance to Improve Outcomes in Acne. J Am Acad Dermatol 2003;49(1 Suppl):S1–S37 (Hormonal Therapy—pp. S20–S25, General Management Strategies—pp. S30–S31).
5. Law RM. The pharmacist's role in the treatment of acne. Am Pharm 2003;125:35–42.
6. Zaenglein AL, Thiboutot DM. Expert committee recommendations for acne management. Pediatrics 2006;118:1188–1199.
7. Strauss JS, Krowchuk DP, Leyden JJ, et al, American Academy of Dermatology/American Academy of Dermatology. Guidelines of care for acne vulgaris management. J Am Acad Dermatol 2007;56:651–663. Available at National Guidelines Clearinghouse at: *http://www.guidelines.gov/summary/summary.aspx?doc_id=10797*. Accessed May 2010.
8. Agency for Healthcare Research and Quality, September 2001. Evidence report/technology assessment number 17: management of acne. Available at: *www.ahcpr.gov/clinic/epcsums/acnesum.htm*. Accessed May 13, 2010. For a summary of this review, see Lehmann HP, Robinson KA, Andrews JS, et al. Acne therapy: a methodologic review. J Am Acad Dermatol 2002;47:231–240.
9. Stein-Gold L. Adapalene–benzoyl peroxide combination gel improves symptoms of acne vulgaris. In: American Academy of Dermatology (AAD) 68th Annual Meeting. Abstract P711. Presented March 6, 2010.
10. Wooltorton E. Diane-35 (cyproterone acetate): safety concerns. CMAJ 2003;168:455–456.
11. Seaman HE, deVries CS, Farmer RDT. The risk of venous thromboembolism in women prescribed cyproterone acetate in combination with ethinyl estradiol: a nested cohort analysis and case–control study. Hum Reprod 2003;18:522–526.
12. Karagas MR, Stukel TA, Dykes J, et al. A pooled analysis of 10 case–control studies of melanoma and oral contraceptive use. Br J Cancer 2002;86:1085–1092.

# 110

# PSORIASIS

The Harried School Teacher .............. Level II

Rebecca M.T. Law, BS Pharm, PharmD

Wayne P. Gulliver, MD, FRCPC

## LEARNING OBJECTIVES

After completing this case study, students should be able to:

- Describe the pathophysiology and clinical presentation of plaque psoriasis.
- Discuss the appropriate use of topical, photochemical, and systemic treatment modalities including BRMs for psoriasis, based on disease severity.
- Compare the efficacy and adverse effects of systemic therapies for psoriasis, including first-line standard therapies (methotrexate, acitretin, cyclosporine), second-line therapies (azathioprine, hydroxyurea, sulfasalazine), and the BRMs (alefacept, adalimumab, etanercept, infliximab, and ustekinumab).
- Select appropriate therapeutic regimens for patients with plaque psoriasis based on disease severity and patient-specific considerations such as organ dysfunction.
- Educate patients with psoriasis about proper use of pharmacotherapeutic treatments, potential adverse effects, and necessary precautions.

## PATIENT PRESENTATION

### Chief Complaint

"Nothing is helping my psoriasis."

### HPI

Gerald Kent is a 50-year-old man with a >25-year history of psoriasis who presented to the outpatient dermatology clinic 2 days ago with another flare-up of his psoriasis. He was admitted to the inpatient dermatology service for a severe flare-up of plaque psoriasis involving his arms, legs, elbows, knees, palms, abdomen, back, and scalp (Fig. 110-1).

He was diagnosed with plaque psoriasis at age 23. He initially responded to topical therapy with medium-potency topical corticosteroids, later to calcipotriol. He subsequently required photochemotherapy using PUVA to control his condition. PUVA eventually became ineffective, and 10 years ago he was started on oral methotrexate 5 mg once weekly. Dosage escalations kept his condition under fairly good control for about 5 years. Flare-ups during that period were initially managed with SCAT, but they eventually became more frequent and lesions were more widespread despite increasing the methotrexate dose. A liver biopsy performed about 5 years ago showed no evidence of fibrosis, hepatitis, or cirrhosis.

After requiring two SCAT treatments in a 4-month period, along with methotrexate 25 mg once weekly po (given as two doses of 12.5 mg 12 hours apart), a change in therapy was considered necessary at that time. Because he was receiving maximum recommended methotrexate doses and had already reached a lifetime cumulative methotrexate dose of 2.2 g, he was changed to his current cyclic regimen of cyclosporine microemulsion (Neoral) 75 mg twice daily for 3 months, followed by acitretin (Soriatane) 25 mg once daily with dinner for 3 months, and repeat. Flare-ups became infrequent and were again successfully managed by SCAT. However, in the last 6 months, he has already required two SCAT treatments for flare-ups. This is his third flare-up this year.

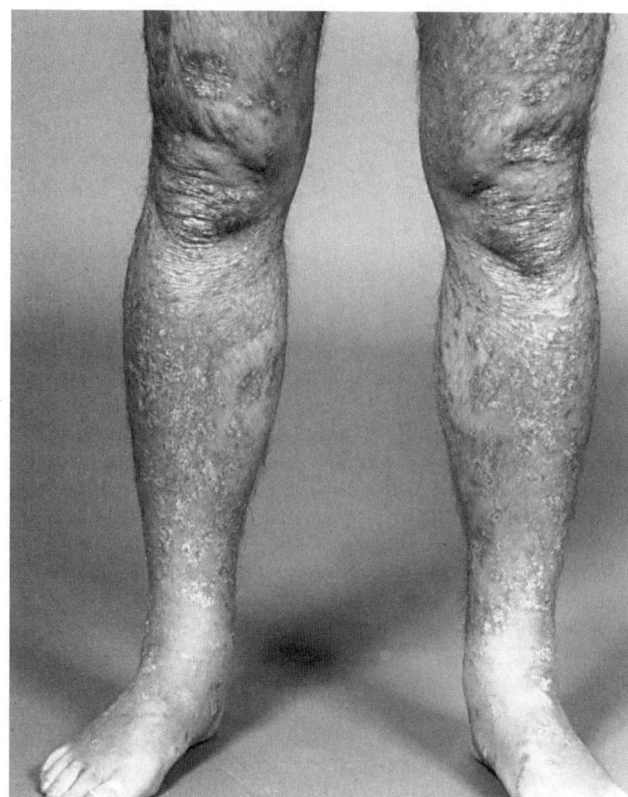

**FIGURE 110-1.** Example of severe plaque psoriasis involving the lower extremities in a male patient. *(Photo courtesy of Wayne P. Gulliver, MD.)*

### PMH

One episode of major depressive illness triggered by the death of his first wife, which occurred 16 years ago (age 34). He was treated by his family physician who prescribed fluoxetine for 6 months. He has had no recurrences. He has no other chronic medical conditions and no other acute or recent illnesses.

### FH

Parents alive and well. Father has HTN and type 2 diabetes. Two older sisters and a younger brother. Younger brother was diagnosed with psoriasis about 5 years ago. No history of other immune disorders or malignancy.

### SH

Patient is an elementary school teacher. He is currently a nonsmoker but used to be a heavy smoker in his younger years (20s and 30s); social use of alcohol (glass of wine with dinner). He is married and has two children ages 10 and 12 with his second wife. There has been an increased workload for the past year because of layoffs at his school board.

## Meds

Neoral 75 mg twice daily po; in 1 month, he is scheduled to change to acitretin 25 mg once daily for the following 3 months (cyclic therapy).

Acetaminophen for occasional headaches.

## All

NKDA

## ROS

Skin feels very itchy despite using a nonmedicated moisturizer TID. No joint aches or pains. No complaints of shortness of breath. Occasional nausea associated with a cyclosporine dose. Has been feeling jumpy and stressed because of tensions at work but does not feel depressed.

## Physical Examination

*Gen*

Alert, mildly anxious 50-year-old Caucasian man in NAD

*VS*

BP 139/86, P 88, T 37°C; Wt 75 kg, Ht 5′9″

*Skin*

Confluent plaque psoriasis with extensive lesions on abdomen, arms, legs, back, and scalp. Thick crusted lesions on elbows, knees, palms, and soles. Lesions are red to violet in color, with sharply demarcated borders except where confluent, and are loosely covered with silvery white scales. There are no pustules or vesicles. There are excoriations on trunk and extremities consistent with scratching.

*HEENT*

PERRLA, EOMI, fundi benign, TMs intact; extensive scaly lesions on scalp as noted

*Neck/Lymph Nodes*

No lymphadenopathy; thyroid nonpalpable

*Chest*

CTA bilaterally

*CV*

RRR without MRG; $S_1$ and $S_2$ normal

*Abd*

(+) BS, soft, nontender, no masses; extensive scaly lesions and excoriations on skin as noted in the section "Skin"

*Genit*

WNL

*Rect*

Deferred

*MS/Ext*

No joint swelling, increased warmth, or tenderness; skin lesions as noted in the section "Skin"; no nail involvement; peripheral pulses 2+ throughout

*Neuro*

A & O × 3; CN II–XII intact; DTRs 2+ toes downgoing

## Labs

| | | |
|---|---|---|
| Na 139 mEq/L | Hgb 13.5 g/dL | AST 22 IU/L |
| K 4.0 mEq/L | Hct 35.0% | ALT 38 IU/L |
| Cl 102 mEq/L | Plt 255 × $10^3$/mm$^3$ | LDH 107 IU/L |
| $CO_2$ 25 mEq/L | WBC 6.0 × $10^3$/mm$^3$ | Alk phos 98 IU/L |
| BUN 14 mg/dL | | T. bili 1.0 mg/dL |
| SCr 1.0 mg/dL | | Alb 3.7 g/dL |
| Glu 98 mg/dL | | Uric acid 4 mg/dL |
| | | T. chol 180 mg/dL |

# QUESTIONS

## Problem Identification

1.a. Create a list of this patient's drug therapy problems.

1.b. What signs and symptoms consistent with plaque psoriasis does this patient demonstrate?

1.c. What risk factors for developing psoriasis or experiencing a disease flare-up are present in this patient?

1.d. What comorbidities does this patient have?

1.e. Could the signs and symptoms be caused by any drug therapy he is receiving?

## Desired Outcome

2. What are the goals of pharmacotherapy for this patient's plaque psoriasis?

## Therapeutic Alternatives

3.a. What nonpharmacologic alternatives are available for managing the patient's psoriasis and its related symptoms?

3.b. What feasible pharmacotherapeutic alternatives are available for controlling the patient's disease and its related symptoms at this point?

## Optimal Plan

4. What drug regimen is best suited for treating this flare-up of the patient's psoriasis and its related symptoms?

## Outcome Evaluation

5. How should you monitor the therapy you recommended for efficacy and adverse effects?

## Patient Education

6. What information should be provided to the patient to enhance compliance and ensure successful therapy?

## CLINICAL COURSE: ALTERNATIVE THERAPY

Because of Mr Kent's frustration with his increased psoriasis flare-ups despite his prescription treatments, he is very interested in trying anything to help decrease his symptoms. A friend who takes fish oil for eczema told him it might help the psoriasis, so he asks about the possibility of adding fish oil on a daily basis. For questions related to the use of fish oil/omega-3 fatty acids for the treatment of psoriasis, please see Section 19 of this casebook.

## SELF-STUDY ASSIGNMENTS

1. Perform a literature search to identify potential future therapies for psoriasis: topical therapies such as NSAIDs, protein kinase

C inhibitors, methotrexate gel, and implantable 5-fluorouracil formulation; systemic therapies such as glucosamine, monoclonal antibodies, and cytokines.

2. Perform a literature search to review the current guidelines, opinions, and evidence regarding liver biopsies and long-term methotrexate use for patients with psoriasis.

## CLINICAL PEARL

Provide patient-specific therapies and always consider any psychosocial effects, debilities, and comorbidities related to the patient's psoriasis.

## REFERENCES


1. Law RMT. Psoriasis. In: Chisholm MA, Schwinghammer TL, Wells BG, et al, eds. Pharmacotherapy Principles and Practice, 2nd ed. New York, McGraw-Hill, 2010:1079–1091.
2. Schon MP, Boehncke WH. Psoriasis. N Engl J Med 2005;352: 1899–1912.
3. Menter A, Gottlieb A, Feldman SR, et al. Guidelines of care for the management of psoriasis and psoriatic arthritis. Section 1. Overview of psoriasis and guidelines of care for the treatment of psoriasis with biologics. J Am Acad Dermatol 2008;58:826–850.
4. Papp KA, Gulliver W, Lynde CW, Poulin Y (Steering Committee). Canadian Guidelines for the Management of Plaque Psoriasis, 1st ed. June 2009. Endorsed by the Canadian Dermatology Association. Available at: *http://www.dermatology.ca/guidelines/cdnpsoriasisguidelines.pdf*. Accessed January 7, 2010.
5. Rahman P, Elder JT. Genetic epidemiology of psoriasis and psoriatic arthritis. Ann Rheum Dis 2005;64(Suppl 2):ii37–ii39.
6. Smith N, Weymann A, Tausk FA, et al. Complementary and alternative medicine for psoriasis: a qualitative review of the clinical trial literature. J Am Acad Dermatol 2009;61:841–856.
7. Menter A, Korman NJ, Elmets CA, et al. 2009 guidelines of care for the management of psoriasis and psoriatic arthritis—Section 3. Guidelines of care for the management and treatment of psoriasis with topical therapies. J Am Acad Dermatol 2009;60:643–659.
8. Menter A, Korman NJ, Elmets CA, et al. 2009 guidelines of care for the management of psoriasis and psoriatic arthritis—Section 4. Guidelines of care for the management and treatment of psoriasis with traditional systemic agents. J Am Acad Dermatol 2009;61:451–485.
9. Menter A, Korman NJ, Elmets CA, et al. 2009 guidelines of care for the management of psoriasis and psoriatic arthritis—Section 5. Guidelines of care for the treatment of psoriasis with phototherapy and photochemotherapy. J Am Acad Dermatol 2010;62:114–135.
10. Rosmarin DM, Lebwohl M, Elewski BE, et al. Cyclosporine and psoriasis: 2008 National Psoriasis Foundation Consensus Conference. J Am Acad Dermatol 2010;62:838–853.
11. Kalb RE, Strober B, Weinstein G, Lebwohl M. Methotrexate and psoriasis: 2009 National Psoriasis Foundation Consensus Conference. J Am Acad Dermatol 2009;60:824–837.
12. Poulin Y, Langley RD, Teixeira HD, et al. Biologics in the treatment of psoriasis: clinical and economic overview. J Cutan Med Surg 2009:13(Suppl 2):S49–S57.
13. Leonardi CL, Kimball AB, Papp KA, et al. Efficacy and safety of ustekinumab, a human interleukin-12/23 monoclonal antibody, in patients with psoriasis: 76-week results from a randomised, double-blind, placebo-controlled trial (PHOENIX 1). Lancet 2008;371: 1665–1674.
14. Papp KA, Langley R, Lebwohl M, et al. Efficacy and safety of ustekinumab, a human interleukin-12/23 monoclonal antibody, in patients with psoriasis: 52-week results from a randomised, double-blind, placebo-controlled trial (PHOENIX 2). Lancet 2008;371: 1675–1684.


# 111

# ATOPIC DERMATITIS

The Itch that Erupts when Scratched . . . . . . . . Level I


**Rebecca M.T. Law, BS Pharm, PharmD**

**Poh Gin Kwa, MD, FRCPC**




## LEARNING OBJECTIVES

After completing this case study, students should be able to:

- Understand risk factors and aggravating factors in the pathophysiology of atopic dermatitis.
- Understand the treatment strategies for atopic dermatitis, including nonpharmacologic management.
- Educate patients and/or their caregivers about management of atopic dermatitis.
- Monitor the safety and efficacy of selected pharmacologic therapies.

## PATIENT PRESENTATION

### Chief Complaint

As stated by the patient's mother, "My child constantly wants to scratch her skin, and she can't sleep well during the night."

### HPI

Julia Chan is a 3.5-year-old girl who just started attending daycare about 1 month ago. She did not want to go and still exhibits a lot of clinging behavior when her mother tries to leave; she still cries when her mother eventually does manage to leave. Her mother says that Julia's atopic dermatitis has flared up again. Julia has had atopic dermatitis since she was about 6 months old. It had been well controlled by topical corticosteroids and liberal use of moisturizers. Her recent flare-up began about 2–3 weeks ago. She has not been sleeping well and is constantly trying to scratch her skin at night. Her mother has been using 100% cotton sheets for her bed since she was an infant. She has sewn mittens on Julia's 100% cotton pajamas to prevent her from scratching, because she had previously caused excoriations from scratching, which then became infected. During the day, Julia constantly wants to scratch her skin but has been told to just "pat" the itchy area. The caregivers at the daycare center keep an eye on her scratching behavior as well but are not always able to prevent her from scratching herself. They also inform her mother that Julia likes to eat food shared by other children.

### PMH

Julia was breastfed from birth for a total of 8 weeks, when her mother decided to return to work. Julia was then cared for at home by a babysitter and fed cow's milk, with oatmeal cereal being introduced as the first solid food. She was fed some lemon meringue pie (made with egg white) once, and developed generalized hives, which led to the recognition that Julia has an egg allergy. This was confirmed by allergic skin testing. Julia's atopic dermatitis presented at 6 months of age. The parents have recently become aware that the babysitter left Julia alone a lot (sitting on the floor/carpet to play by herself). That was the major reason for sending Julia to a daycare center.

## SH

Julia is the only child of a professional couple. Her father is an engineer and her mother is a litigation lawyer who often works long hours. The couple has a stressful lifestyle, and it appears that the stress is reflected in Julia's care. Sometimes Julia would be driven to one or another babysitter's homes at the last minute, when something urgent arises that the couple must attend to. There is very little family time. Unfortunately, their relatives do not live in the same city, and there is little social support for Julia on a day-to-day basis. The parents were hoping that the daycare center would be helpful, but so far that has proven to be another issue for Julia. She does not want to participate in activities there and has lots of temper tantrums. She does not play well with other children. Julia had been toilet trained but has now lost her toilet training and is using diapers again. Julia's mother started smoking again due to the recent stress; Julia keeps her up at night, and she is having difficulty dealing with Julia's multiple issues at home and at the daycare center.

## FH

There is a strong family history of atopy. Julia's father has a severe allergy to shellfish, and her mother has a history of hay fever. Her father's sister has multiple food allergies. Her maternal grandmother had asthma. Her paternal first cousin had infantile eczema. Her maternal first cousin has a severe peanut allergy (generalized hives).

## Meds

Hydrocortisone 1% cream applied to affected areas two to four times a day; although twice daily is her usual maintenance dose, she is currently using it three to four times a day.

Vaseline ad lib.

Diphenhydramine 0.5 teaspoonful at bedtime as needed (when skin is excessively itchy, to allow Julia to sleep).

## Allergies

NKDA. Multiple food allergies: egg (hives, developed allergy as an infant), strawberries, raspberries, and tomatoes.

## ROS

Not obtained

## Physical Examination

### *Gen*

Unhappy, cranky, thin, clinging girl who keeps sucking her thumb

### *VS*

BP 98/50, HR 96, RR 18, T 37°C; Wt 12.2 kg (10th percentile), Ht 98 cm (38.6″; 50th percentile), head circumference 49.5 cm (19.5″; 50th percentile)

### *Skin*

Generally dry. Eczematous skin lesions in flexure areas (behind ears, wrist joints, elbows, knees). Likely pruritic papules in flexure areas. Excoriations from scratching. Some bleeding seen but does not appear infected. Some cracking skin lesions seen behind the ears and knees. There are no lesions on the extensor parts of her body, no lesions on top of her nose, and no lesions in the diaper area.

The remainder of the physical exam was normal.

## Labs

| | | | |
|---|---|---|---|
| Na 135 mEq/L | Hgb 12.0 g/dL | WBC differential | AST 20 IU/L |
| K 4.0 mEq/L | Hct 35% | Neutros 50% | ALT 7 IU/L |
| Cl 102 mEq/L | Plt 230 × $10^3$/mm$^3$ | Bands 3% | IgE 300 IU/mL |
| $CO_2$ 26 mEq/L | WBC 5.0 × $10^3$/mm$^3$ | Eosinophils 18% | D-dimer 90 ng/mL |
| BUN 8 mg/dL | | Lymphs 27% | RAST elevated |
| SCr 0.2 mg/dL | | Basophils 1% | INR 1.1 |
| | | Monos 1% | aPTT 30 s |

*Note:* Reference ranges at age 3.5—BUN 8–20 mg/dL, SCr 0.2–0.8 mg/dL, AST 20–60 IU/L, ALT 0–37 IU/L, and IgE 0–25 IU/mL; WBC differential—neutros 20–65%, eos 0–15%, basos 0–2%, lymphs 20–60%, and monos 0–10%.

Swab of skin lesion where there is bleeding: No growth

## Assessment

This is a 3.5-year-old child with an exacerbation of atopic dermatitis, likely stress-induced.

# QUESTIONS

## Problem Identification

1.a. Create a drug therapy problem list for this patient.

1.b. What signs and symptoms of atopic dermatitis does this patient demonstrate?

1.c. What risk factors or aggravating factors may have contributed to the patient's atopic dermatitis flare?

1.d. Could the patient's signs and symptoms be caused by a drug?

## Desired Outcome

2. What are the treatment goals for this patient?

## Therapeutic Alternatives

3. What feasible nonpharmacologic and pharmacologic alternatives are available to manage this patient's pruritus and atopic dermatitis?

## Optimal Plan

4. What treatment regimen is best suited for this patient?

## Outcome Evaluation

5. What efficacy and adverse effects monitoring is needed for the management strategies you recommended?

## Patient Education

6. How would you inform the patient's caregiver about the treatment regimen to enhance compliance and ensure successful therapy?

## SELF-STUDY ASSIGNMENTS

1. Review the use of phototherapy for atopic dermatitis.
2. Discuss how an 8-month-old infant with atopic dermatitis might differ from a 3.5-year-old child (with respect to clinical presentation and treatment strategies).

## CLINICAL PEARL

In atopic dermatitis, minimizing preventable risk factors such as stress, eliminating triggers, providing appropriate skin care, and controlling the itch are as important as pharmacologic treatment.

## REFERENCES


1. National Institute of Arthritis and Musculoskeletal and Skin Diseases. Handout on Health: Atopic Dermatitis. US Department of Health and Human Services, May 2009. NIH Publication No. 09-4272. Available at: *www.niams.nih.gov/Health_Info/Atopic_Dermatitis/default.asp*. Accessed July 10, 2010.
2. Lynde C, Barber K, Claveau J, et al. Canadian practical guide for the treatment and management of atopic dermatitis. J Cutan Med Surg (incorporating Medical and Surgical Dermatology), published online June 28, 2005. Available at: *http://www.springerlink.com/content/r5432000056r2748/fulltext.html*. Accessed July 10, 2010.
3. Krafchik BR. Atopic Dermatitis. eMedicine updated January 19, 2010. Available at: *emedicine.medscape.com* (eMedicine Specialties → Dermatology → Allergy & Immunology). *http://emedicine.medscape.com/article/1049085-overview*. Accessed July 10, 2010.
4. Beltrani VS, Boguneiwicz M. Atopic dermatitis. Dermatol Online J 2003;9(2):1. Available at: *http://dermatology.cdlib.org/92/reviews/atopy/beltrani.html*. Accessed July10, 2010.
5. Bieber T. Mechanisms of disease: atopic dermatitis. N Engl J Med 2008;358:1483–1494.
6. Akdis CA. New insights into mechanisms of immunoregulation in 2007. J Allergy Clin Immunol 2008;122:700–709.
7. Koblenzer CS. Itching and the atopic skin. J Allergy Clin Immunol 1999;104(3 Pt 2):S109–S113.
8. Hanifin JM, Cooper KD, Ho VC, et al. Guidelines of care for atopic dermatitis. J Am Acad Dermatol 2004;50:391–404.
9. Burks AW, Laubach S, Jones SM. Oral tolerance, food allergy, and immunotherapy: implications for future treatment. J Allergy Clin Immunol 2008;121:1344–1350.
10. Hengge UR, Ruzicka T, Schwartz RA, et al. Adverse effects of topical glucocorticosteroids. J Am Acad Dermatol 2006;54:1–15.
11. Murch SH. Probiotics as mainstream allergy therapy? Arch Dis Child 2005;90:881–882.
12. Wickens K, Black PN, Stanley TV, et al. A differential effect of 2 probiotics in the prevention of eczema and atopy: a double-blind, randomized, placebo-controlled trial. J Allergy Clin Immunol 2008;122:788–794.

SECTION 15
# HEMATOLOGIC DISORDERS

## 112

# IRON DEFICIENCY ANEMIA

Wilbur is Tired and His Stomach Hurts . . . . . . Level I

**William J. Spruill, PharmD, FASHP, FCCP**
**William E. Wade, PharmD, FASHP, FCCP**

## LEARNING OBJECTIVES

After completing this case study, the student should be able to:

- Recognize that certain drugs such as NSAIDs can cause chronic blood loss and iron deficiency anemia (IDA).
- Identify the signs, symptoms, and laboratory manifestations of IDA.
- Select appropriate iron therapies for the treatment of IDA.
- Understand the monitoring parameters for both short- and long-term treatment of IDA.
- Inform patients of the potential adverse effects of iron therapy.
- Educate patients about the importance of adherence to their iron therapy regimen.

## PATIENT PRESENTATION

### Chief Complaint

"I have belly pain and feel tired all the time."

### HPI

Wilbur Cox is a 67 yo man who presents to your pharmacy with the above complaint. With further questioning, he relates the onset of his GI complaints shortly after he started self-medicating with ibuprofen 200 mg four tablets four times a day about 6 months ago for pain associated with "arthritis" in his right knee and ankle. His stomach pain has gotten progressively worse over the past few months. He describes this pain as a burning sensation that usually begins 30 minutes to 1 hour after meals and may or may not be relieved by antacid administration. Use of omeprazole as needed has likewise not provided much acute pain relief. Further questioning reveals a history of PUD approximately 5 years ago. You suggest he stop taking ibuprofen and all other OTC NSAIDs and recommend that he use acetaminophen not more than 2 g per day if needed. Additionally, you contact his primary care physician to make an appointment for Wilbur for further evaluation, and you let Wilbur know you will fax a brief note to his physician detailing the nature of your referral.

## CLINICAL COURSE

Three days later, he is evaluated by his family physician, which provides the following additional information.

### PMH

OA of the knees and ankles
PUD 5 years ago
GI bleed—approximately 7 years ago
COPD × 10 years
HTN × 10 years

### FH

Mother died in childbirth; father died of cancer at age 93.

### SH

Cigarette smoker—two ppd × 42 years. No alcohol; quit in 1990. He is married.

### ROS

No fever or chills; (+) burning pain in stomach after meals; (–) heartburn; (+) melena; good appetite; has one daily BM; no significant weight changes over past 5 years; (+) dry mouth; (+) fatigue, tires easily; (–) paralysis, fainting, numbness, paresthesia, or tremor; headache only occasionally; has myopic vision; (–) tinnitus or vertigo; has hay fever in spring; (+) cough, sputum production (about one cup per day); (+) wheezing; denies chest pain, edema; (+) dyspnea and orthopnea; denies nocturia, hematuria, dysuria, or Hx of stones; (+) bilateral joint pain in both knees and ankles, worse on the right side, for over 5 years

### Meds

Lisinopril 10 mg po daily
Tiotropium 18 mcg inhaled once daily
Formoterol 12 mcg inhaled Q 12 h
Ibuprofen 200 mg po three or four tablets three or four times a day for knee and ankle pain
Antacids po PRN for stomach pain
Prilosec OTC 20 mg PRN stomach pain

### All

Codeine (upset stomach)
Aspirin (upset stomach)

### Physical Examination

*Gen*

WM in acute distress who appears his stated age

*VS*

BP 118/51, P 121, RR 22, T 36.2°C, pulse oximetry 90% in room air; Wt 78 kg, Ht 6′1″

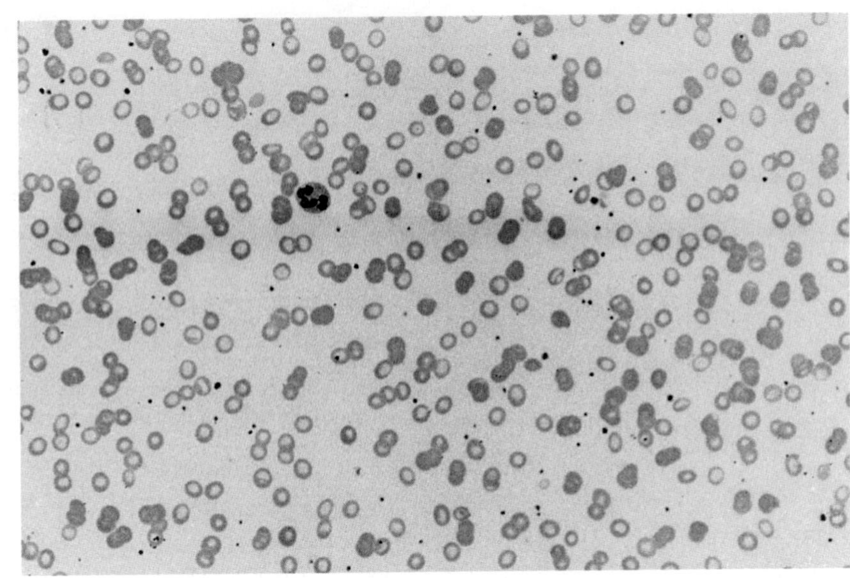

**FIGURE 112-1.** Blood smear with hypochromic, microcytic red blood cells (Wright–Giemsa ×330). *(Photo courtesy of Lydia C. Contis, MD.)*

*Skin*

Age- and sun-related lentigines and seborrheic keratoses noted

*HEENT*

PERRL; EOMI; conjunctivae are pale; mucous membranes pale and dry; normal funduscopic examination with no retinopathy noted; deviated nasal septum; no sinus tenderness; oropharynx clear

*Neck/Lymph Nodes*

Neck supple without masses; trachea midline; no thyromegaly, no JVD

*Thorax*

Breath sounds decreased bilaterally, increased anterior–posterior diameter, (+) rhonchi, pursed-lip breathing

*CV*

Tachycardia with a soft systolic murmur; PMI at fifth ICS, MCL; (–) bruits

*Abd*

Soft, tender to palpation; no masses or organomegaly; normal peristalsis

*Genit/Rect*

Normal external male genitalia; rectal examination (+) stool guaiac

*MS/Ext*

Slight knee joint enlargement, with pain and tenderness noted, and limited ROM of both knees and ankles, worse on right side; crepitation noted at the talus–tibia junction on dorsiflexion of the right foot; changes consistent with OA; strong pedal pulses bilaterally; no peripheral edema; pallor of the nail beds

*Neuro*

A & O × 3; DTR 2+; normal gait

*Other*

Peripheral blood smear: hypochromic, microcytic red blood cells (Fig. 112-1)

## Labs

See Table 112-1.

## Assessment

1. Severe IDA probably of GI origin, possibly secondary to NSAID-induced gastropathy
2. OA of both knees and ankles, worse on right side
3. COPD
4. HTN
5. FULL CODE status but patient does not wish to be left on a machine if there is no hope of recovery

**TABLE 112-1** Lab Values

| | | | | |
|---|---|---|---|---|
| Na 138 mEq/L | Hgb 7.2 g/dL | WBC 10.7 × $10^3$/mm$^3$ | AST 10 IU/L | Ca 8.7 mg/dL |
| K 3.7 mEq/L | Hct 25% | Segs 61% | ALT 23 IU/L | Iron 4 mcg/dL |
| Cl 104 mEq/L | RBC 3.77 × $10^6$/mm$^3$ | Bands 2% | T. bili 0.3 mg/dL | TIBC 465 mcg/dL |
| $CO_2$ 27 mEq/L | MCV 66.2 μm$^3$ | Lymphs 23% | LDH 85 IU/L | Transferrin sat 1% |
| BUN 12 mg/dL | MCH 19 pg | Monos 10% | T. prot 6.3 g/dL | Ferritin 5 ng/mL |
| SCr 0.8 mg/dL | MCHC 28.7 g/dL | Eos 3% | Alb 3.7 g/dL | $B_{12}$ 680 pg/mL |
| Glucose 90 mg/dL | RDW 20.9% | Basos 1% | Folic acid 8.2 ng/mL | |
| | MPV 8.1 fL | | | |
| | Microcytosis 2+ | | | |
| | Anisocytosis 1+ | | | |

■ Plan

Admit to hospital for further evaluation.
NPO.
Infuse 4 units PRBCs.
Begin D5% NS at 82 mL/h continuous.
Begin esomeprazole 40 mg po daily.
Consult GI service for suspected GI bleed.

## CLINICAL COURSE

The same day, the patient is seen by a gastroenterologist and undergoes both EGD and colonoscopy. Findings included severe gastritis with multiple bleeding lesions. Colonoscopy results were normal.

Final assessment: chronic, severe IDA secondary to bleeding gastric ulcer most likely secondary to NSAID therapy.

## QUESTIONS

### Problem Identification

1.a. What potential drug therapy problems does this patient have?

1.b. What signs, symptoms, and laboratory findings are consistent with the finding of IDA secondary to blood loss?

### Desired Outcome

2. What are the goals of pharmacotherapy for this patient's anemia?

### Therapeutic Alternatives

3.a. What nondrug therapy may be effective for managing this anemia?

3.b. Discuss all of the oral and parenteral pharmacotherapeutic alternatives that could be used to treat this patient's anemia.

### Optimal Plan

4. Outline an optimal pharmacotherapy plan for this patient.

### Outcome Evaluation

5. What clinical and laboratory parameters are necessary to evaluate the therapy for achievement of the desired therapeutic outcome and to detect and prevent adverse effects?

### Patient Education

6. What information should be provided to the patient to enhance compliance, ensure successful therapy, and minimize adverse effects?

## ■ CLINICAL COURSE

Mr Cox's hemoglobin and hematocrit increased after PRBCs to 12.6 g/dL and 40.8% by the second day of hospitalization. At that time, he was discharged on the treatment you recommended. For his OA, it is recommended that Wilbur be given a therapeutic trial of a nonacetylated salicylate such as choline magnesium trisalicylate along with acetaminophen up to two per day, if needed. A therapeutic trial of glucosamine can also be considered. Wilbur should be advised that NSAIDs, including those available over-the-counter, should be avoided because he is at high risk of a recurrent GI bleed that is related to both dose and length of NSAID therapy.

On his return to the clinic 1 month later for evaluation, he has no complaints of adverse effects from his medications. He indicates that he is fairly compliant with his iron therapy and is not experiencing any dose-limiting side effects. Stool exam for occult blood is negative. At that time, he is instructed to return in 2 more months. At that 3-month follow-up visit, his laboratory values continue to improve, and his next follow-up visit is scheduled in 3 more months. Laboratory values at 1, 3, and 6 months into therapy are shown in Table 112-2.

**TABLE 112-2** Laboratory Test Values at 1, 3, and 6 Months

| Test (Units) | 1 Month | 3 Months | 6 Months |
|---|---|---|---|
| RBC count ($\times 10^6$/mm$^3$) | 4.1 | 4.2 | 4.8 |
| Hgb (g/dL) | 11.1 | 13.0 | 14.9 |
| Hct (%) | 36 | 40 | 47 |
| MCV (μm$^3$) | 86 | 90 | 92 |
| MCH (pg) | 25 | 30 | 33 |
| MCHC (g/dL) | 31 | 34 | 36 |
| RDW (%) | 15.8 | 13.2 | 11.3 |
| Serum iron (mcg/dL) | 45 | 80 | 105 |
| TIBC (mcg/dL) | 489 | 491 | 500 |
| Transferrin saturated (%) | 9.0 | 19.0 | 21.0 |
| Ferritin (ng/mL) | 69 | 120 | 163 |
| Stool guaiac | Negative | Negative | Negative |

## ■ SELF-STUDY ASSIGNMENTS

1. Make a list of oral medications that should not be taken close to the time of iron administration; note the medications for which ferrous salts may interfere with their absorption.
2. Perform a literature search to determine the evidence supporting use of various sustained-release iron preparations, and determine the incremental cost of such products.
3. What monitoring steps should be incorporated into your pharmaceutical care plan to:
   (a) Check for recurrence of signs/symptoms of iron deficiency due to his chronic GI bleed?
   (b) Educate the patient concerning his risk of GI bleed associated with NSAID therapy and how he can minimize this risk?
   (c) Monitor for recurrence of signs and symptoms of gastropathy?
   (d) Monitor for efficacy of new treatments (such as acetaminophen or glucosamine) for his osteoarthritis?
4. Calculate the correct total dose of parenteral iron dextran (i.e., total dose iron dextran) for this patient, and write a comprehensive order for its administration.

## CLINICAL PEARL

In otherwise healthy patients, a transient increase in the reticulocyte count 3–10 days after beginning therapy can be used to confirm the correct diagnosis and treatment and to rule out other causes of anemia.

Therapeutic doses of iron must be given for 3–6 months to ensure repletion of all iron stores; the serum ferritin is the best parameter for monitoring iron stores after correction of the hemoglobin and hematocrit.

## REFERENCES

1. Alleyne M, Horne MK, Miller JL. Individualized treatment for iron-deficiency anemia in adults. Am J Med 2008;121:943–948.
2. Auerbach M, Rodgers GM. Intravenous iron. N Engl J Med 2007; 357:93–94.
3. Auerbach M, Goodnough LT, Picard D, Maniatis A. The role of intravenous iron in anemia management and transfusion avoidance. Transfusion 2008;48:988–1000.
4. Miller HJ, Hu J, Valentine JK, Gable PS. Efficacy and tolerability of intravenous ferric gluconate in the treatment of iron deficiency anemia in patients without kidney disease. Arch Intern Med 2007; 167:1327–1328.
5. Auerbach M, Ballard H, Glaspy J. Clinical update: intravenous iron for anemia. Lancet 2007;369:1502–1504.
6. Akarsu S, Taskin E, Yilmaz E, et al. Treatment of iron deficiency anemia with intravenous iron preparations. Acta Haematol 2006;116:51–57.
7. Gotloib L, Silverberg D, Fudin R, et al. Iron deficiency is a common cause of anemia in chronic kidney disease and can often be corrected with intravenous iron. J Nephrol 2006;19:161–167.
8. Marignani M, Angeletti S, Filippi L, et al. Occult and obscure bleeding, iron deficiency anemia and other gastrointestinal stories. Int J Mol Med 2005;15:129–135 [review].

# 113

# VITAMIN $B_{12}$ DEFICIENCY

Tongue Twister . . . . . . . . . . . . . . . . . . . . . . . Level II

**Jon P. Wietholter, PharmD, BCPS**

## LEARNING OBJECTIVES

After completing this case study, students should be able to:

- Recognize the signs, symptoms, and laboratory abnormalities associated with vitamin $B_{12}$ deficiency anemia.
- Select an appropriate dosage regimen for treatment of anemia resulting from vitamin $B_{12}$ deficiency.
- Describe monitoring parameters for the initial and subsequent evaluations of patients with anemia caused by vitamin $B_{12}$ deficiency.
- Educate patients about appropriate vitamin $B_{12}$ therapy.

## PATIENT PRESENTATION

### Chief Complaint

"I feel like I'm constantly tired and fatigued and my tongue is sore and swollen, making it extremely difficult for me to eat or drink anything."

### HPI

Caleb Chalk is a 65-year-old man who presents to your outpatient clinic with his wife. He claims that his fatigue and lethargy have been going on for years but have been worsening over the last 4–5 months to the point that he is constantly tired. Additionally, he claims that over the last 2–3 weeks his tongue has become extremely painful and swollen and that he struggles while eating food. His appetite has diminished as he tries to avoid eating anything that could worsen his pain and the fact that he feels "fuller" much quicker than he used to. On questioning, he also mentions a slight tingling and numbness in his feet that seems to worsen on finishing any physical activity. The patient has lost about 10 lb over the last 3 months and also states that he feels like he is running a constant low-grade fever. His wife adds that she feels that he is becoming more confused, and this has been worsening over the last several years.

### PMH

COPD
Type 2 diabetes mellitus
Gout

### FH

Father alive (85 years old) with CAD, HTN, glaucoma, and type 2 DM
Mother deceased at age 75; had HTN, dementia, and CKD

### SH

Married for 42 years, lives with his wife; has two children (one son and one daughter) who are both healthy and live in the area; (+) tobacco, 1.5 ppd since age 24; (–) alcohol, (–) illicit drugs; is a retired pharmacist with good health insurance

### Meds

Docusate sodium 100 mg po Q 12 h
Albuterol MDI two puffs Q 6 h PRN
Fluticasone/salmeterol 250/50 one puff Q 12 h
Tiotropium 18 mcg one puff daily
Metformin 1,000 mg po Q 12 h
Glyburide 5 mg po daily
Colchicine 0.6 mg po daily
Allopurinol 300 mg po daily

### All

Penicillin (hives)
Levofloxacin (anaphylaxis)

### ROS

Complains of tongue pain and tingling sensation in his toes; (–) SOB, headache, chest pain, psychiatric abnormalities, polyuria, or polydipsia; denies any visual changes, constipation, diarrhea, or urinary retention

### Physical Examination

*Gen*

Elderly Caucasian male; moderately overweight in no acute distress with normal affect and speech; seems slightly irritated and exceptionally fatigued

*VS*

BP 123/87, P 106, RR 16, T 38.0°C; Wt 92 kg, Ht 6′0″, BMI 27.4

*Skin*

Pale, turgor normal, no rashes or lesions

*HEENT*

PERRLA; EOMI; (–) photophobia; (+) red, smooth, swollen, sore tongue with loss of papillae; TMs appear normal

*Neck*

Supple; no masses, lymphadenopathy, or thyromegaly

*Chest*

Bilateral breath sounds; minor wheezing and rhonchi present on auscultation; (–) rales or orthopnea

*CV*

No discernible rhythm abnormality by auscultation; no murmurs or gallops; (+) tachycardia

*Abd*

Soft, nontender; mild splenomegaly; no masses; normal bowel sounds present

*Rect*

Deferred

*Ext*

No erythema, pain, or edema; normal pulses; (+) paresthesias; no joint redness or swelling; no limb weakness; reflexes intact

*Neuro*

A & O × 3; CN: visual fields and hearing intact; coordination intact; decreased pinprick in both lower extremities; decreased vibratory sensation in both lower extremities; decreased temperature sensation in both lower extremities; (–) ataxia, lightheadedness

### Labs (All Fasting)

| | | | |
|---|---|---|---|
| Na 136 mEq/L | Hgb 8.4 g/dL | AST 30 IU/L | Iron 124 mcg/dL |
| K 3.5 mEq/L | Hct 25.3% | ALT 24 IU/L | Ferritin 100 ng/mL |
| Cl 108 mEq/L | RBC 2.09 × $10^6$/$mm^3$ | Alk phos 79 IU/L | Transferrin 229 mg/dL |
| $CO_2$ 28 mEq/L | Plt 91 × $10^3$/$mm^3$ | T. bili 0.8 mg/dL | Antiparietal cell antibodies (–) |
| BUN 13 mg/dL | WBC 3.5 × $10^3$/$mm^3$ | D. bili 0.4 mg/dL | LDH 140 IU/L |
| SCr 1.0 mg/dL | MCV 121 $\mu m^3$ | T. chol 153 mg/dL | $B_{12}$ 101 pg/mL |
| Glu 134 mg/dL | MCH 40 pg | | Folate 12.3 ng/mL |
| A1C 6.8% | MCHC 33.2 g/dL | | |
| TSH 3.4 mIU/L | Reticulocyte (corr) 0.7% | | |

### Peripheral Blood Smear Morphology

Macro-ovalocytosis, hypersegmented granulocytes, large platelets, macrocytic red blood cells with megaloblastic changes (Fig. 113-1)

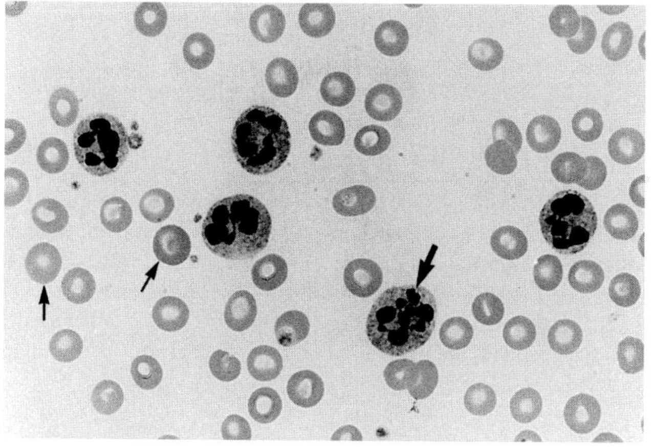

**FIGURE 113-1.** Blood smear with enlarged hypersegmented neutrophils, one with eight nuclear lobes (*large arrow*) and macrocytes (*small arrows*) (Wright–Giemsa ×1,650). (*Photo courtesy of Lydia C. Contis, MD.*)

### Assessment

1. Macrocytic anemia consistent with vitamin $B_{12}$ deficiency of unknown origin
2. Atrophic glossitis possibly associated with vitamin $B_{12}$ deficiency
3. Peripheral sensory neuropathy possibly associated with vitamin $B_{12}$ deficiency

## QUESTIONS

### Problem Identification

1.a. Create a drug therapy problem list for this patient.

1.b. What information indicates the presence or severity of vitamin $B_{12}$ deficiency?

1.c. Could the vitamin $B_{12}$ deficiency have been caused by drug therapy? If so, should any changes be made to the patient's current drug regimen to aid in the treatment of his vitamin $B_{12}$ deficiency?

### Desired Outcome

2. What are the pharmacotherapeutic goals in this case?

### Therapeutic Alternatives

3.a. What nondrug therapies for vitamin $B_{12}$ deficiency might be useful for this patient?

3.b. What pharmacotherapeutic options are available for treating this patient's vitamin $B_{12}$ deficiency?

### Optimal Plan

4. What drug, dosage form, dose, schedule, and duration of therapy are best for this patient?

### Outcome Evaluation

5. What clinical and laboratory parameters are necessary to evaluate the therapy for achievement of the desired therapeutic outcome and to detect or prevent adverse effects?

### Patient Education

6. What information should be provided to the patient to enhance compliance, ensure successful therapy, and minimize adverse effects?

## FOLLOW-UP QUESTION

1. Mr Chalk returns to your clinic 3 months later reporting that he is feeling much less fatigued and is able to eat a more consistent diet but is still suffering from the tingling in his toes and a milder form of tongue soreness. What information can you give him regarding these remaining maladies?

## CLINICAL PEARL

Pernicious anemia is a chronic illness arising from impaired absorption of vitamin $B_{12}$ due to a lack of intrinsic factor in gastric secretions. It garnered its name because it was universally fatal (pernicious is from the Latin word for violent death or destruction) due to a lack of available treatment options in the early stages of disease recognition. It can now be simply treated as any other vitamin $B_{12}$ deficiency and is a rather benign disease process if detected early.

## SELF-STUDY ASSIGNMENTS

1. A serum vitamin $B_{12}$ level is no longer the most reliable laboratory test for evaluation of vitamin $B_{12}$ deficiency. Review the diagnostic tests that are becoming more common and provide a rationale for their increased use.
2. The anemia resulting from vitamin $B_{12}$ deficiency can be corrected by giving patients folic acid. Why then must we differentiate between the two common causes of macrocytic anemia (folic acid deficiency and vitamin $B_{12}$ deficiency) instead of simply treating all patients with folic acid?
3. Describe the rationale for using tetracycline to normalize vitamin $B_{12}$ levels in patients diagnosed with blind loop syndrome.

## REFERENCES

1. Ting RZ, Szeto CC, Chan MH, Ma KK, Chow KM. Risk factors of vitamin $B_{12}$ deficiency in patients receiving metformin. Arch Intern Med 2006;166:1975–1979.
2. Dharmarajan TS, Adiga GU, Norkus EP. Vitamin $B_{12}$ deficiency. Recognizing subtle symptoms in older adults. Geriatrics 2003;58:30–38.
3. Herrmann W, Schorr H, Obeid R, Geisel J. Vitamin $B_{12}$ status, particularly holotranscobalamin II and methylmalonic acid concentrations, and hyperhomocysteinemia in vegetarians. Am J Clin Nutr 2003;78:131–136.
4. Dali-Youcef N, Andres E. An update on cobalamin deficiency in adults. QJM 2009;102:17–28.
5. Kaferle J, Strzoda CE. Evaluation of macrocytosis. Am Fam Physician 2009;79(3):203–208.
6. Andres E, Loukili NH, Noel E, et al. Vitamin $B_{12}$ (cobalamin) deficiency in elderly patients. CMAJ 2004;171:251–259.
7. Butler CC, Vidal-Alaball J, Cannings-John R, et al. Oral vitamin $B_{12}$ versus intramuscular vitamin $B_{12}$ for vitamin $B_{12}$ deficiency. Fam Pract 2006;23:279–285.
8. Hvas AM, Nexo E. Diagnosis and treatment of vitamin $B_{12}$ deficiency—an update. Haematologica 2006;91:1506–1512.
9. Smith AD, Refsum H. Vitamin $B_{12}$ and cognition in the elderly. Am J Clin Nutr 2009;89(Suppl):707S–711S.
10. Eussen SJ, de Groot LC, Joosten LW, et al. Effect of oral vitamin $B_{12}$ with or without folic acid on cognitive function in older people with mild vitamin $B_{12}$ deficiency: a randomized, placebo-controlled trial. Am J Clin Nutr 2006;84:361–370.

# 114

# FOLIC ACID DEFICIENCY

More Wine, Anyone? . . . . . . . . . . . . . . . . . . . Level I

**Jonathan Kline, PharmD, CACP, BCPS**

**Amber Chiplinski, PharmD, BCPS**

## LEARNING OBJECTIVES

After completing this case study, students should be able to:

- Recognize the signs, symptoms, and laboratory abnormalities associated with folic acid deficiency.
- Identify the confounding factors that may contribute to the development of folic acid deficiency (e.g., medications, concurrent disease states, dietary habits).
- Recommend an appropriate treatment regimen to correct anemia resulting from folic acid deficiency.
- Educate patients with folic acid deficiency regarding pharmacologic and nonpharmacologic interventions used to correct folic acid deficiency.
- Describe appropriate monitoring parameters for initial and subsequent monitoring of folic acid deficiency.

## PATIENT PRESENTATION

### Chief Complaint

"My stomach hurts and I have been throwing up today."

### HPI

Laura Jones is a 43-year-old woman with a 1-day history of vomiting and mild abdominal pain. The pain radiates down to the lower abdominal quadrants bilaterally. She presents to the ED after experiencing some chest discomfort late in the day. She denies any fevers, chills, or similar pains in the past. She also complains of loose stools and chronic fatigue for the past 2–3 months.

### PMH

Fibromyalgia
Celiac disease
Hypothyroidism
Osteopenia
History of endometriosis
Placenta previa—s/p TAH–BSO

### FH

Mother positive for lupus; sister with Crohn's disease; negative for DM, CAD, CVA, CA

### SH

Married; (+) alcohol—three to four glasses of wine per day, increased recently from one to two glasses after her mother-in-law moved in; (+) smoking tobacco 0.5 ppd × 25 years, (–) recreational drug use; unemployed

### Meds

Levothyroxine 100 mcg po daily
Estradiol 0.05 mg/24 h transdermal patch (Estraderm); replace twice weekly

### All

Doxycycline—rash

### ROS

(+) Generalized weakness; (–) dizziness; (–) weight gain or loss; (–) fever; (–) vision or hearing changes; (–) cough, chest pain, palpitations; (–) shortness of breath; (+) nausea/vomiting, abdominal pain, loose stools; (–) rectal bleeding; (–) nocturia or dysuria; (+) bilateral lower extremity weakness; (–) edema, rashes, or petechiae; (–) symptoms of depression or anxiety; (–) history of bleeding problems or VTE

### Physical Examination

*Gen*

Caucasian female who appears generally ill, but nontoxic

*VS*

BP 135/90, P 82, RR 40, T 35.5°C

*Skin*

No petechiae, rashes, ecchymoses, or active lesions; decreased skin turgor

*HEENT*

Atraumatic/normocephalic; PERRLA, EOMI; conjunctivae pink, sclera white; TMs intact and reactive; nose is patent; tongue is large and erythematous; dry mucous membranes

*Neck/Lymph Nodes*

Normal ROM; no JVD, adenopathy, thyromegaly, or bruits

*Lung/Thorax*

Lungs CTA bilaterally

*CV*

RRR; no murmurs, gallops, or rubs

*Abd*

Soft, nondistended, with midepigastric and right flank and right lower quadrant tenderness; (+) bowel sounds

*Genit/Rect*

Deferred

*MS/Ext*

Lower extremities warm with 2+ bipedal pulses; no clubbing, cyanosis, or edema

*Neuro*

CN II–XII grossly intact; decreased muscle strength 3/5 bilaterally in upper and lower extremities; DTRs throughout

### Labs

| | | | |
|---|---|---|---|
| Na 138 mEq/L | Hgb 12.6 g/dL | AST 128 IU/L | Folate 2.8 ng/mL |
| K 4.2 mEq/L | Hct 37.2% | ALT 52 IU/L | $B_{12}$ 242 pg/mL |
| Cl 102 mEq/L | RBC 3.78 × $10^6$/mm$^3$ | Alk phos 142 IU/L | |
| $CO_2$ 21 mEq/L | Plt 217 × $10^3$/mm$^3$ | GGT 288 IU/L | |
| BUN 7 mg/dL | WBC 6.3 × $10^3$/mm$^3$ | T. bili 2.1 mg/dL | |
| SCr 0.52 mg/dL | MCV 120.4 μm$^3$ | Alb 3.4 g/dL | |
| Glu 89 mg/dL | MCH 40.5 pg | TSH 2.06 mIU/L | |
| Amylase 404 IU/L | MCHC 33.6 g/dL | $T_4$, free 1.2 ng/dL | |
| Lipase 679 IU/L | RDW 12.1% | | |

### Assessment

Acute pancreatitis secondary to alcohol use
Dehydration
Macrocytic anemia secondary to folate deficiency

# QUESTIONS

## Problem Identification

1.a. Create a drug therapy problem list for this patient.

1.b. What signs, symptoms, and laboratory values indicate that this patient has anemia secondary to folate deficiency?

1.c. Could the patient's folate deficiency have been caused by drug therapy or comorbidity?

1.d. What additional information can be used to assess this patient's folate deficiency?

1.e. Why is it important to differentiate folate deficiency from vitamin $B_{12}$ deficiency, and how is this accomplished?

## Desired Outcome

2. What are the goals of pharmacotherapy for this patient's anemia?

## Therapeutic Alternatives

3.a. What nondrug therapies may be used to correct this patient's folic acid deficiency?

3.b. What pharmacotherapeutic alternatives are available for treating this patient's anemia?

## Optimal Plan

4. What are the most appropriate drug, dosage form, dose, schedule, and duration of therapy for resolving this patient's anemia?

## Outcome Evaluation

5. What parameters should be used to evaluate the efficacy and adverse effects of folic acid replacement therapy in this patient?

## Patient Education

6. What information would you provide to this patient about her folic acid replacement therapy?

# SELF-STUDY ASSIGNMENTS

1. What are the advantages and disadvantages of folinic acid (leucovorin calcium) over standard folic acid, and why is this preferred folate supplement in patients receiving high-dose methotrexate?
2. List and compare the mechanism for how the following drugs can lead to folic acid deficiency: azathioprine, trimethoprim, and phenytoin.
3. What is the role of folic acid in the management of methanol ingestion?

# CLINICAL PEARL

Unlike dietary folate, supplemented folic acid (pteroylglutamic acid) is absorbed even with abnormal function of GI mucosal cells. Likewise, persistent alcohol ingestion or the use of drugs affecting folic acid absorption, folate transport, or dihydrofolate reductase will not prevent a sufficient therapeutic response to oral supplementation.

# REFERENCES


1. Arafah BM. Increased need for thyroxine in women with hypothyroidism during estrogen therapy. N Engl J Med 2001;344:1743–1749.
2. Coppen A, Bolander-Gouaille C. Treatment of depression: time to consider folic acid and vitamin $B_{12}$. J Psychopharmacol 2005;19:59–65.
3. Snow CF. Laboratory diagnosis of vitamin $B_{12}$ and folate deficiency: a guide for the primary care physician. Arch Intern Med 1999;159:1289–1298.
4. Presutti RJ, Cangemi JR, Cassidy HD, Hill DA. Celiac disease. Am Fam Physician 2007;76:1795–1802.
5. Seppa K, Sillanaukee P, Saarni M. Blood count and hematologic morphology in nonanemic macrocytosis: differences between alcohol abuse and pernicious anemia. Alcohol 1993;10:343–347.

6. Kipps TJ, Kaushansky K. Hematopoietic agents: growth factors, minerals, and vitamins. In: Brunton LL, Lazo JS, Parker KL, eds. Goodman & Gilman's The Pharmacological Basis of Therapeutics, 11th ed. New York, NY, McGraw-Hill, 2005:1433–1466.
7. Rampersaud GC, Kauwell GP, Bailey LB. Folate: a key to optimizing health and reducing disease risk in the elderly. J Am Coll Nutr 2003;22:1–8.
8. Selhub J, Morris MS, Jacques PF. In vitamin $B_{12}$ deficiency, higher serum folate is associated with increased total homocysteine and methylmalonic acid concentrations. Proc Natl Acad Sci USA 2007;104:19995–20000.
9. Dhar M, Bellevue R, Carmel R. Pernicious anemia with neuropsychiatric dysfunction in a patient with sickle cell anemia treated with folate supplementation. N Engl J Med 2003;348:2204–2207.
10. Carmel R. Treatment of severe pernicious anemia: no association with sudden death. Am J Clin Nutr 1988;48:1443–1444.

# 115

# SICKLE CELL ANEMIA

Engineering a Crisis . . . . . . . . . . . . . . . . . . . . . . . . Level I

**Christine M. Walko, PharmD, BCOP**

## LEARNING OBJECTIVES

After completing this case study, students should be able to:

- Recognize the clinical characteristics associated with an acute sickle cell crisis.
- Discuss the presentation of acute chest syndrome and treatment options.
- Recommend optimal analgesic therapy based on patient-specific information.
- Identify optimal endpoints of pharmacotherapy in sickle cell anemia patients.
- Recommend treatment that may reduce the frequency of sickle cell crises.

## PATIENT PRESENTATION

### Chief Complaint

"I can't breathe and my chest hurts."

### HPI

Todd Jefferson is a 38-year-old African-American man with a history of sickle cell anemia who presents to the local community hospital ED with pain. On waking up yesterday morning, he experienced a sudden onset of pain in his right elbow, shoulder, and lower back. He began taking oxycodone 20 mg every 4 hours at that time with minor pain relief. This morning he experienced a fever of 102°F, progressive shortness of breath, and priapism, which caused him to see treatment at the ED.

### PMH

Sickle cell anemia (SS disease) diagnosed before the age of 1 with approximately three to four crises per year requiring hospitalization
Acute chest syndrome 2 years ago that required intubation
Plasma exchange (most recently during the intubation admission)
Several episodes of priapism, usually associated with sickle cell pain crisis

### FH

Mother and father alive and well, both with sickle cell trait. Patient has one sister with sickle cell trait.

### SH

Lives locally with his wife; currently works as chemical engineer

### ROS

Denies nausea, vomiting, or diarrhea. Cannot remember his last bowel movement but believes he has not had one in the last 3 days. Has had fever with some chills and sweats; no cough, nasal discharge, rashes, or skin lesions. Reports stuttering priapism with recurring episodes each lasting approximately 1 hour.

### Meds

Folic acid 1 mg po daily
Hydroxyurea 1,000 mg po BID
Oxycodone 20 mg po Q 4 h PRN pain

### All

Sulfa (reported rash when very young)
Codeine (nausea and dysphoria)

### Physical Examination

*Gen*

Thin, well-developed, diaphoretic African-American man in acute distress

*VS*

BP 115/72, P 110, RR 20, T 38.5°C; 72 kg; $O_2$ sat is 84% in room air improving to 97% on 4 L $O_2$, and then 89% on 40% face mask

*HEENT*

PERRL; EOMI; oral mucosa soft and moist; normal sclerae and funduscopic examination; no sinus tenderness

*Skin*

Normal turgor; no rashes or lesions

*Neck*

Supple; nontender, no lymphadenopathy or thyromegaly

*CV*

RRR; II/VI SEM; no rubs or gallops

*Lungs*

Crackles in both bases on auscultation; dullness to percussion

*Abd*

Voluntary guarding, mild distention, hypoactive bowel sounds, mild splenomegaly; no hepatomegaly or masses

*Genitourinary*

Priapism evident

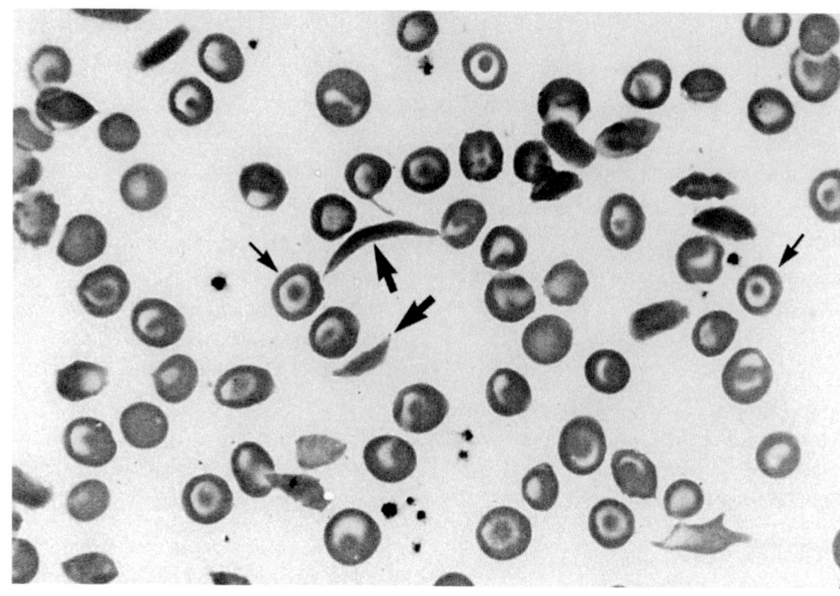

**FIGURE 115-1.** Peripheral blood with sickle cells (*large arrows*) and target cells (*small arrows*) (Wright–Giemsa ×1,650). (*Photo courtesy of Lydia C. Contis, MD.*)

*Ext*

No edema; notable tenderness in right shoulder and elbow; mild erythema and inflammation is present.

*Neuro*

A & O × 3; normal strength, reflexes intact

## Labs

| | | | |
|---|---|---|---|
| Na 143 mEq/L | Hgb 7.7 g/dL | AST 40 IU/L | Ca 8.8 mg/dL |
| K 4.2 mEq/L | Hct 20.8% | ALT 28 IU/L | Mg 1.9 mEq/L |
| Cl 112 mEq/L | Plt 480 × $10^3$/mm$^3$ | Alk phos 77 IU/L | Phos 3.9 mg/dL |
| $CO_2$ 28 mEq/L | MCV 110 μm$^3$ | T. bili 5.0 mg/dL | (+) Anti-E red cell antibody |
| BUN 50 mg/dL | Retic 18.2% | D. bili 0.8 mg/dL | |
| SCr 1.4 mg/dL | WBC 18.2 × $10^3$/mm$^3$ | I. bili 4.2 mg/dL | |
| Glu 92 mg/dL | Segs 74% | Alb 3.4 g/dL | |
| | Bands 7.5% | | |
| | Eos 1.5% | | |
| | Lymphs 14% | | |
| | Monos 3% | | |

## Other

Arterial blood gas: pH 7.49, $Pco_2$ 38, $pO_2$ 72, bicarb 30, $O_2$ sat 96% on oxygen

Hgb electrophoresis: Hgb $A_2$ 3%; Hgb F 8%; Hgb S 89%

Peripheral blood smear: Sickle forms and target cells present (Fig. 115-1).

## Chest X-Ray

This is a portable chest x-ray remarkable for diffuse interstitial infiltrates in both lung fields consistent with acute chest syndrome (Fig. 115-2). Cardiomegaly is also notable.

## ECG

Normal sinus rhythm

## Echocardiogram

Normal LV function

## Assessment

A 38-year-old, African-American man in sickle cell crisis with probable acute chest syndrome, priapism, and constipation

# QUESTIONS

## Problem Identification

1.a. Create a list of the patient's drug therapy problems.

1.b. What signs, symptoms, and laboratory values are consistent with an acute sickle cell crisis in this patient?

1.c. What signs, symptoms, and laboratory values support a diagnosis of acute chest syndrome in this patient?

1.d. What additional information is needed to satisfactorily assess this patient?

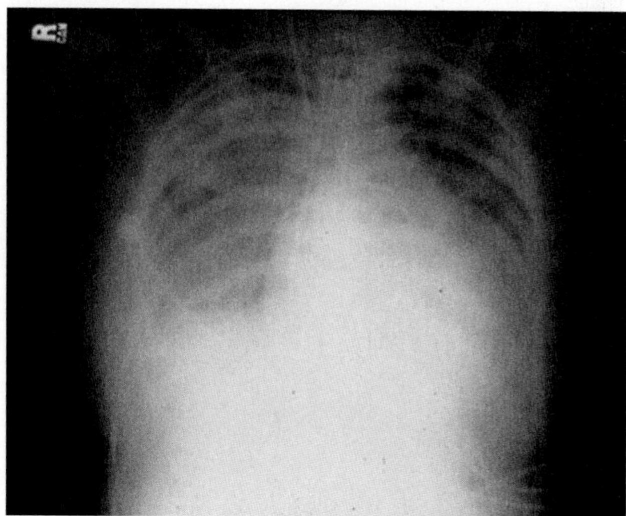

**FIGURE 115-2.** Lung radiograph of patient with acute chest syndrome secondary to sickle cell anemia. (*Photo courtesy of Kenneth I. Ataga, MD.*)

## Desired Outcome

2. What are the goals of pharmacotherapy in this case?

## Therapeutic Alternatives

3.a. What nondrug therapies might be useful for this patient?

3.b. What feasible pharmacotherapeutic alternatives are available for treatment of the patient's pain?

3.c. What feasible pharmacotherapeutic alternatives are available for treating opioid-induced constipation?

## Optimal Plan

4. Outline a detailed therapeutic plan to treat all facets of this patient's acute sickle cell crisis, acute chest syndrome, priapism, and constipation. For all drug therapies, include the dosage form, dose, schedule, and duration of therapy.

## Outcome Evaluation

5.a. What clinical and laboratory parameters are necessary to evaluate therapy for achievement of the desired therapeutic outcome and to detect or prevent adverse effects?

## CLINICAL COURSE

The plans you recommended have been initiated, and on the fourth day of hospitalization the patient's pain is markedly improved, oxygen saturation improved to 98% on room air, he is afebrile, and his priapism has resolved. He has had two bowel movements but still feels his bowel habits have not yet returned to normal. He is only using two to three demands on his PCA per day and is asking to switch back to oral medication.

5.b. Considering this information, what changes (if any) in the pharmacotherapeutic plan are warranted while the patient is hospitalized?

5.c. What evidence exists to suggest that the patient is adherent with hydroxyurea therapy, and how should this therapy continue to be monitored?

## Patient Education

6. What information should be provided to the patient to enhance compliance, ensure successful therapy, and minimize adverse effects?

## SELF-STUDY ASSIGNMENTS

1. Determine the likelihood of the patient's offspring having sickle cell trait and/or disease if the father has:
   (a) Normal hemoglobin
   (b) Sickle cell trait
   (c) Sickle cell disease
2. Describe the complications associated with frequent crises in each organ system.
3. Discuss the differences between sickle cell anemia and β-thalassemia in terms of etiologies, laboratory abnormalities, and disease complications.

## CLINICAL PEARL

Allogeneic bone marrow transplantation has proved curative in pediatric sickle cell anemia patients. Approximately 20% of patients have a matched sibling donor, and matches may also be found through the National Marrow Donor Program.

## REFERENCES


1. Vichinsky EP, Neumayr LD, Earles AN, et al. Causes and outcomes of the acute chest syndrome in sickle cell disease. National Acute Chest Syndrome Study Group. N Engl J Med 2000;342:1855–1865.
2. Vichinsky EP, Styles LA, Colangelo LH, et al. Acute chest syndrome in sickle cell disease: clinical presentation and course. Cooperative Study of Sickle Cell Disease. Blood 1997;89:1787–1792.
3. Steinberg MH. Management of sickle cell disease. N Engl J Med 1999;340:1021–1030.
4. Morris CR, Singer ST, Walters MC. Clinical hemoglobinopathies: iron, lungs and new blood. Curr Opin Hematol 2006;13:407–418.
5. Bellet PS, Kalinyak KA, Shukla R, et al. Incentive spirometry to prevent acute pulmonary complications in sickle cell diseases. N Engl J Med 1995;333:699–703.
6. Herndon CM, Jackson KC, Hallin PA. Management of opioid-induced gastrointestinal effects in patients receiving palliative care. Pharmacotherapy 2002;22:240–250.
7. Steinberg MH, Barton F, Castro O, et al. Effect of hydroxyurea on mortality and morbidity in adult sickle cell anemia: risks and benefits up to 9 years of treatment. JAMA 2003;289:1645–1651.

SECTION 16
# INFECTIOUS DISEASES

# 116

## USING LABORATORY TESTS IN INFECTIOUS DISEASES

Catheter-Related Bloodstream Infection. . . . . Level III

**Dustin Zeigler, PharmD, BCPS**

### LEARNING OBJECTIVES

After completing this case study, the reader should be able to:

- Discuss the appropriate procedure for drawing blood cultures.
- Discuss the use of new laboratory tests that help differentiate coagulase-negative staphylococci from *Staphylococcus aureus*.
- Design a therapeutic plan to treat a catheter-related bloodstream infection.
- Evaluate culture and sensitivity results, and determine the clinical significance of the MIC for *S. aureus*.
- Recommend a plan for monitoring efficacy and adverse effects of antimicrobial therapy.

### PATIENT PRESENTATION

#### Chief Complaint

Wife states her husband, "cannot catch his breath, and I am unable to wake him up. He just has not been acting himself the last several days."

#### HPI

Joe Johnson is a 67-year-old man arriving in the ED via ambulance. The patient's history is obtained from his wife. She describes a change in mental status and lethargy, and she has noted her husband having difficulty breathing. The symptoms started 2 days ago and have progressively worsened. Over the past 24 hours, he has become unarousable and developed a fever (38.9°C). She states Mr Johnson is currently undergoing chemotherapy for advanced lung cancer that was diagnosed approximately 1 month ago. His chemotherapy was last administered 3 days ago.

#### PMH

Stage IV non-small cell lung carcinoma status post thoracotomy undergoing chemotherapy
Diabetes mellitus
Hypertension
Depression
Pulmonary embolus diagnosed 3 months ago

#### FH

Both parents are deceased (mother, aged 88, of natural causes; father, aged 71, of stroke). He is married without any children.

#### SH

Retired welder, no tobacco or alcohol

#### Meds

Bevacizumab 1,200 mg IV every 3 weeks
Carboplatin 390 mg IV over 3 hours every 3 weeks
Carboplatin 750 mg IV every 3 weeks
Coumadin 1 mg po daily
Pioglitazone 30 mg po daily
Metformin 1,000 mg po BID
Amlodipine 10 mg po daily
Paroxetine 10 mg po daily
Megestrol ES 625 mg po daily
Prochlorperazine 10 mg Q 4 h po PRN nausea
Lorazepam 0.5 mg po Q 8 h PRN
Temazepam 15 mg po QHS
Oxycodone 5 mg po Q 4 h PRN pain

#### All

PCN—hives when he was a child
Lisinopril—lip swelling

#### ROS

Unable to obtain due to patient's condition

#### Physical Examination

*Gen*

The patient is frail, well groomed, appearing in respiratory distress.

*VS*

BP 86/63, P 155, RR 48, T 38.9°C; Wt 77.3 kg, Ht 71 in

*Skin*

Warm and diaphoretic; tunneled intravenous catheter present in left upper chest, no drainage or pus at insertion site, presence of erythema and warmth surrounding exit site noted

*HEENT*

NC/AT; PERRLA; conjunctivae pink; sclerae clear; EOMI; disk margins sharp; no arteriolar narrowing, AV nicking, hemorrhages, or exudates; ear canals clear and drums negative; nares normal; teeth intact, tonsils intact and normal; pharynx negative

*Neck/Lymph Nodes*

Trachea midline; thyroid palpable; no nodules; no evidence of jugular venous distention

*Chest*

Severe respiratory distress with marked respiratory effort and use of accessory muscles; generalized rhonchi

*CV*

Tachycardic; normal $S_1$ and $S_2$; no heaves, thrills, or bruits

*Abd*

Soft, nondistended; no palpable masses or tenderness; no hepatosplenomegaly

*Genit/Rect*

Not performed

*MS/Ext*

Deferred

*Neuro*

Does not respond to voice; responds to pain with withdrawal

### Labs

| | | |
|---|---|---|
| Na 133 mEq/L | Hgb 9.9 g/dL | WBC 3.1 × $10^3$/mm$^3$ |
| K 4.4 mEq/L | Hct 28.8% | Segs 90% |
| Cl 96 mEq/L | RBC 3.34 × $10^6$/mm$^3$ | Bands 2% |
| $CO_2$ 23 mEq/L | Plt 95 × $10^3$/mm$^3$ | Lymphs 6% |
| BUN 55 mg/dL | MCV 86.1 μm$^3$ | Monos 2% |
| SCr 2.11 mg/dL | MCH 29.7 pg | PT 39 sec |
| Glu 287 mg/dL | MCHC 34.5 g/dL | INR 4.12 |
| Lactate 2.5 mmol/L | RDW 16.6% | BNP 805 pg/mL |
| | D-dimer 17.3 μg/mL | |

Baseline ABG: pH 7.43; $pO_2$ 52 mm Hg; $pCO_2$ 35 mm Hg; $HCO_3$ 23 mEq/L; $O_2$ saturation 86%

Urinalysis obtained from foley: color, yellow; specific gravity, 1.170; pH 5; +1 protein; negative nitrites; negative LE; 15–20 RBC; few bacteria; 0–3/HPF WBC; moderate uric acid crystals

### Chest X-Ray

Mass in right lower lobe

### CT Angiography of Chest

Right pneumothorax, pulmonary emboli, pneumonia, and metastatic bone lesions in thoracic spine

### Assessment

1. Respiratory failure with differential diagnosis of lung cancer, pneumonia, or pulmonary embolus
2. Sepsis syndrome with unknown source of infection, pending workup

### Plan

1. Emergent intubation performed for impending respiratory failure.
2. STAT CT angiography of chest (done).
3. Collect two sets of blood cultures, one peripheral and one from the vascular catheter. Urine sample for urinalysis and culture via foley also collected. Once intubated, collect a respiratory culture via endotracheal aspirate.
4. Fluid resuscitation for hypotension; start norepinephrine drip if hypotension resistant to fluids.

## QUESTIONS

### Problem Identification

1.a. Create a list of this patient's drug therapy problems.

1.b. What subjective and objective data indicate the presence of infection?

1.c. What indicates a possible urinary tract infection on urinalysis? Does Mr Johnson's urinalysis represent the presence of an infection?

1.d. What are the criteria for SIRS? Does Mr Johnson meet these criteria?

1.e. Define sepsis.

### Desired Outcome

2.a. What are the desired treatment goals for Mr Johnson's current medical problems?

2.b. When should Mr Johnson's blood cultures be drawn in relation to antibiotic administration?

2.c. Why are a minimum of two sets of blood cultures obtained, including one from the lumen of intravascular catheter, when present?

## CLINICAL COURSE

After transferring to the ICU, the patient's blood pressure improved with 4 L of normal saline. Shortly after the patient arrived at the ICU, the microbiology lab calls the ICU physician and tells her that Mr Johnson's Gram stains from both blood cultures reveal gram-positive cocci in clusters, and the PNA FISH results indicate the presence of *S. aureus*. All cultures are plated and incubated to evaluate for bacterial growth. The Gram stain from the endotracheal suction shows <10 polys and <10 epithelial cells.

### Therapeutic Alternatives

3.a. Create a list of appropriate antibiotics to empirically treat Mr Johnson's infection pending final culture and sensitivity results.

3.b. In addition to antibiotic therapy, what nonpharmacologic interventions are required for this patient?

### Optimal Plan

4.a. What is the clinical advantage of using a rapid identification test, such as PNA FISH, to help determine the staphylococcal species?

4.b. How is a catheter-related bloodstream infection diagnosed?

4.c. What is the preferred antibiotic for this patient, including dose, route, frequency, and duration of therapy?

4.d. Develop a plan for monitoring for the occurrence of adverse drug events with the chosen antibiotic.

**TABLE 116-1** *S. aureus* Susceptibility Report

| Antibiotic | MIC/Interpretation |
|---|---|
| Clindamycin | ≤0.25/sensitive[a] |
| Erythromycin | ≥8/resistant |
| Gentamicin | ≤0.5/sensitive |
| Levofloxacin | 0.25/sensitive |
| Oxacillin | ≥4/resistant |
| Penicillin | ≥0.5/resistant |
| Rifampin | ≤0.5/sensitive |
| Trimethoprim/sulfamethoxazole | ≤10/sensitive |
| Vancomycin | 2/sensitive |
| Tetracycline | ≤1/sensitive |

[a]Positive for inducible clindamycin resistance.

## CLINICAL COURSE

Cardiology is consulted on the second day of admission for placement of an inferior vena cava filter. On the third day, the blood culture and sensitivity results are available (see Table 116-1). Urine culture final results revealed no growth. Surgery is consulted to remove the tunneled vascular catheter.

### Outcome Evaluation

5.a. What effect does the MIC of the organism have on the current treatment plan?

5.b. When are serum vancomycin concentrations collected to determine the appropriateness of drug dosing? How often are serum vancomycin concentrations checked? What is the goal trough serum concentration in this patient?

5.c. Outline a follow-up plan for monitoring the efficacy of this therapeutic regimen.

## SELF-STUDY ASSIGNMENTS

1. What role does antibiotic lock therapy have in the treatment of catheter-related infections?
2. If the patient were neutropenic (ANC <500), how would empiric antibiotic therapy change? What organism(s) would you empirically treat?
3. How do you interpret BAL cultures versus induced sputum cultures?
4. What organisms most frequently represent contaminants (or false-positives) in blood cultures?
5. When evaluating growth of cultures, how can differential time to positivity be useful in diagnosing catheter-related bloodstream infections?

## CLINICAL PEARL

The blood is a sterile body fluid; thus, when a blood culture grows pathogenic bacteria, the source of the bacteria must always be investigated. The infectious source must be identified to assist in determining the appropriate antimicrobial selection and duration of therapy to increase the likelihood of bacterial eradication.

## REFERENCES


1. Sobel JD, Kaye D. In: Mandell GL, Bennett JE, Dolin R, eds. Principles and Practices of Infectious Diseases, 6th ed. Philadelphia, PA, Elsevier Churchill Livingston, 2005:875–905.
2. Mermel LA, Allon M, Bouza E, et al. Clinical practice guidelines for the diagnosis and management of intravascular catheter-related infection: 2009 update by the Infectious Diseases Society of America. Clin Infect Dis 2009;49:1–45.
3. Ly T, Gulia J, Pyrgos V, Waga M, Shoham S. Impact upon clinical outcomes of translation of PNA FISH-generated laboratory data from the clinical microbiology bench to bedside in real time. Ther Clin Risk Manag 2008;4:637–640.
4. Hensley DM, Encina TR. An evaluation of the AvanDx *Staphylococcus aureus*/CNS PNA FISH assay. Clin Lab Sci 2009;22:30–33.
5. Rybak M, Lomaestro B, Rotschafer JC, et al. Therapeutic monitoring of vancomycin in adult patients: a consensus review of the American Society of Health-System Pharmacists, the Infectious Diseases Society of America, and the Society of Infectious Diseases Pharmacists. Am J Health Syst Pharm 2009;66:82–98.
6. Tenover FC, Moellering RC Jr. The rationale for revising the Clinical and Laboratory Standards Institute vancomycin minimal inhibitory concentration interpretive criteria for *Staphylococcus aureus*. Clin Infect Dis 2007;44:1208–1215.
7. Soriano A, Marco F, Martinez JA, et al. Influence of vancomycin minimum inhibitory concentration on the treatment of methicillin-resistant *Staphylococcus aureus* bacteremia. Clin Infect Dis 2008;46:193–200.


# 117

# BACTERIAL MENINGITIS

Space Invaders: The Cerebral Kind. . . . . . . . . Level II

**Sherry A. Luedtke, PharmD**

## LEARNING OBJECTIVES

After completing this case study, the reader should be able to:

- Identify risk factors and common presenting signs and symptoms of bacterial meningitis in infants and children.
- Differentiate common bacterial pathogens associated with meningitis in children of different ages.
- Recommend appropriate empiric and definitive antimicrobial therapy for bacterial meningitis.
- Identify appropriate parameters for monitoring antimicrobial therapy of bacterial meningitis.

## PATIENT PRESENTATION

### Chief Complaint

From mom: "Please help my baby, he won't wake up!"

### HPI

Jamie Hernandez is an 18-month-old, 11.9-kg, male infant who presents to the emergency department in the arms of his mother. She reports that she received a call from his daycare reporting a fever ($T_{max}$ 103°F/39.4°C) the previous day. She assumed he must have another ear infection and started him on some Tylenol and some "left over" amoxicillin that seemed to bring down the fever somewhat. She indicates that he had a restless night, waking up numerous times with irritability and was inconsolable. This morning, she had difficulty arousing him. She immediately called her pediatrician, who instructed her to take him directly to the emergency department.

## PMH

Jamie was a term infant who was born via an uncomplicated vaginal delivery. He has been relatively healthy to date, except for ear infections, the most recent of which was 1 month ago.

## FH

Paternal grandfather and mother diagnosed with diabetes mellitus

## SH

Lives with mother, father, and two siblings (4 and 7 years old). The eldest sibling attends first grade; the youngest two children attend daycare.

## Meds

None; immunizations up to date

## All

NKDA

## Physical Examination

*Gen*

Lethargic, ill-appearing infant

*VS*

BP 80/48, HR 156, RR 47, T 39.7°C; Wt 11.9 kg

*HEENT*

PERRL, tympanic membranes erythematous bilaterally

*Chest*

Lungs clear bilaterally

*CV*

Sinus tachycardia, regular rhythm, no murmurs

*Abd*

Soft, distended, (+) BS

*Extremities*

Capillary refill 3–4 seconds, extremities are somewhat mottled in appearance and cool to touch.

*Neuro*

Lethargic but arousable, (–) Kernig's and Brudzinski's sign

## Labs

| | | |
|---|---|---|
| Na 143 mEq/L | Hgb 15.4 g/dL | *CBG* |
| K 4.3 mEq/L | Hct 46.2% | pH 7.35 |
| Cl 105 mEq/L | Plt 297 × $10^3$/mm$^3$ | $pO_2$ 45 mm Hg |
| $CO_2$ 15 mEq/L | WBC 21.0 × $10^3$/mm$^3$ | $pCO_2$ 50 mm Hg |
| SCr 1.2mg/dL | Neutros 40% | $HCO_3$ 15 mEq/L |
| Glu 145 mg/dL | Bands 24% | BE –8 mEq/L |
| Ca 9.2 mg/dL | Lymphs 34% | Procalcitonin 40.8 ng/mL |
| Mg 1.6 mEq/L | Eos 1% | |
| $PO_4$ 4.5 mg/dL | Basos 1% | |
| TP 6.5 g/dL | | |
| Alb 4.2 g/dL | | |
| Bili 0.8mg/dL | | |
| AST 87 IU/L | | |
| ALT 22 IU/L | | |
| ALP 305 IU/L | | |

Urine and CSF serology: *Haemophilus influenzae* type B (–), *Streptococcus pneumoniae* (+), Group B *Streptococcus* (–), *Neisseria meningitidis* (–), *N. meningitidis B*/*Escherichia coli* (–)

CSF chemistry/cell count: Color/appearance hazy, glucose 45 mg/dL, protein 295 mg/dL, WBC 210/mm$^3$ (5% lymphs, 52% monos, 43% neutros), RBC 10,000/mm$^3$

Gram stain (CSF): Gram-positive cocci in pairs

Cultures: Blood, urine, CSF pending

## Chest X-Ray

Unremarkable

## Assessment

1. Suspected pneumococcal meningitis
2. Hypotension

# QUESTIONS

## Problem Identification

1.a. What drug therapy problems does this infant have?

1.b. What risk factors does this patient have for bacterial meningitis?

1.c. What clinical and laboratory findings indicate the presence of meningitis and its severity?

## Desired Outcome

2. What are the goals of drug therapy in this situation?

## Therapeutic Alternatives

3.a. What nondrug therapies might be useful for managing this patient?

3.b. Describe the empiric antimicrobial regimen that should be used in this patient.

3.c. Discuss adjuvant drug therapy options for the management of infants and children with meningitis.

3.d. What supportive therapies may be used to manage the patient's hypotension and resulting metabolic acidosis?

## CLINICAL COURSE

Blood cultures returned positive for *S. pneumoniae.* CSF cultures (drawn after antibiotics were initiated) and urine cultures were negative. Sensitivity studies revealed intermediate sensitivity to penicillin (MIC >0.01 mcg/mL) and cefotaxime/ceftriaxone (MIC >2.0 mcg/mL).

Repeat procalcitonin in 24 hours was 10.6 ng/mL, and the repeat CBC at that time revealed: Hgb 14.5 g/dL, Hct 43.5%, Plt 150 × $10^3$/mm$^3$, and WBC 19 × $10^3$/mm$^3$ (30% segs, 16% bands, 53% lymphs, 1% basos).

## Optimal Plan

4. Interpret the sensitivity report. Given this new information, are there any changes in drug therapy that you would recommend? What duration of therapy do you recommend?

## Outcome Evaluation

5. Describe the monitoring parameters necessary to evaluate the efficacy and safety of the therapy.

## CLINICAL COURSE

Over the next 48 hours, the infant was treated with the regimen you recommended and blood pressure and neurologic status improved. A repeat lumbar puncture was performed at that time and was clear. The patient was discharged on day 10 of therapy. Audiometry testing performed after completion of antibiotic therapy was normal. The child had no evidence of neurologic impairment as a consequence of the infection at follow-up evaluations.

## SELF-STUDY ASSIGNMENTS

1. Discuss the impact of universal pneumococcal immunization of infants with the conjugated pneumococcal polysaccharide vaccine on the incidence of pneumococcal meningitis in children and the rates of meningitis caused by non-PCV7 serotypes.
2. Describe the penetration of antimicrobials into the CNS and the properties that influence their penetration.
3. Discuss the use of alternative agents (i.e., meropenem and/or quinolones) in the management of resistant pneumococcal meningitis.
4. Review the sensitivity and specificity of other markers of serious infections in infants and young children (IL-6, CRP, TNF-α).

## CLINICAL PEARL

Resistant pneumococcal infections remain a serious cause of morbidity and mortality despite the implementation of universal vaccination with the conjugated pneumococcal vaccine (Prevnar).

## REFERENCES


1. Chavez-Bueno S, McCracken GH. Bacterial meningitis in children. Pediatr Clin North Am 2005;52:795–810.
2. Tunkel AR, Hartman BJ, Kaplan SL, et al. Practice guidelines for the management of bacterial meningitis. Clin Infect Dis 2004;39:1267–1284.
3. Chae YN, Chui NC, Huang FY. Clinical features and prognostic factors in childhood pneumococcal meningitis. J Microbiol Immunol Infect 2008;41(1):48–53.
4. Wasier AP, Chevret L, Essouri S, Durand P, Chevret S, Devictor D. Pneumococcal meningitis in a pediatric intensive care unit: prognostic factors in a series of 49 children. Pediatr Crit Care Med 2005;6(5):568–572.
5. Hsiao AL, Baker MD. Fever in the new millennium: a review of recent studies of markers of serious bacterial infection in febrile children. Curr Opin Pediatr 2005;17:56–61.
6. Saez-Llorens X, McCracken GH. Bacterial meningitis in children. Lancet 2003;361:2139–2148.
7. Kaplan SL. Management of pneumococcal meningitis. Pediatr Infect Dis J 2002;21:589–591.
8. Mongelluzzo J, Mohamad Z, Ten Have TR, Shah SS. Corticosteroids and mortality in children with bacterial meningitis. JAMA 2008;299(7):2048–2055.
9. Peltola H, Roine I, Fernandez J, et al. Hearing impairment in childhood bacterial meningitis is little relieved by dexamethasone or glycerol. Pediatrics 2010;125:e1–e8.
10. Von de Beck D, de Gans J, McIntyre P, Prasad K. Corticosteroids for acute bacterial meningitis. Cochrane Database Syst Rev 2007;(1). Art. no.: CD004405.


# 118

# ACUTE BRONCHITIS

The Collegiate Cough. . . . . . . . . . . . . . . . . . . . Level II

**Jessica Helmer Brady, PharmD, BCPS**

**Justin J. Sherman, MCS, PharmD**

## LEARNING OBJECTIVES

After completing this case study, the reader should be able to:

- Identify signs and symptoms of acute bronchitis and their duration, and evaluate relevant laboratory values in order to rule out more serious illness such as pneumonia.
- Discuss why obtaining sputum cultures and Gram stains is not relevant in evaluation and treatment of patients with uncomplicated acute bronchitis.
- Discuss why antibiotic treatment is not indicated for uncomplicated acute bronchitis.
- Select nonpharmacologic and pharmacologic treatment alternatives for supportive care, incorporating new data regarding efficacy.

## PATIENT PRESENTATION

### Chief Complaint

"I can't seem to stop coughing! It's keeping me and my roommate awake at night, not to mention totally disrupting my classes. And now my throat is also really sore. I even tried my roommate's asthma inhaler in hopes that my cough would stop, but it didn't. I just want an antibiotic to make this all go away!"

### HPI

Allie Comeaux, a 21-year-old college student, is being seen at her university's Student Health Center for complaints of a productive, purulent cough and sore throat for the past 5 days. On questioning, Allie denies that she has had any fever, chills, or myalgias. She does express concern that a dorm mate was recently hospitalized with pneumonia. She admits to using her roommate's asthma inhaler, which she recalls was albuterol, with no relief. While her throat is still sore, she is most concerned with her disruptive cough. "My history professor even asked me to leave the class when I couldn't stop coughing!"

### PMH

Mild acne × 5 years

Irregular menstrual cycle, ranging from 25 to 40 days in length

Current with age-appropriate vaccinations, with the exception of influenza and human papillomavirus

### FH

Father, 51, has been diagnosed with hypertension and hyperlipidemia and has a distant history of alcohol abuse. Mother, 50, is menopausal. The patient also has two younger brothers, ages 16 and 18, with no health issues.

### SH

Allie lives at University Dorm with a suitemate. She smokes "socially" when out with friends but denies alcohol use due to her father's history of alcohol abuse. She also denies any illicit drug use. She is currently a junior kinesiology major and hopes to attend physical therapy school on completion of her degree. She is also on the University Dance line. Allie states that she is sexually active with her boyfriend of 8 months. They use condoms as a method of birth control, although inconsistently.

### Meds

Acetaminophen 650 mg po PRN headache or menstrual cramps
Benzoyl peroxide 2.5% cream topically daily PRN acne

### All

Penicillin—"all-over body rash"

### ROS

No fever, chills, myalgia, chest pain, or shortness of breath; no nausea, vomiting, or diarrhea

### Physical Examination

*Gen*

Well-developed, thin female in NAD

*VS*

BP 104/68 mm Hg, P 64, RR 14, T 37°C; Wt 50 kg, Ht 5′6″

*HEENT*

PERRLA, conjunctivae clear, TMs intact. No epistaxis or nasal discharge. No sinus swelling or tenderness, and mucous membranes are moist. There are no oropharyngeal lesions.

*Neck/Lymph Nodes*

Supple without adenopathy or thyromegaly

*Chest*

(−) Rhonchi, rales, increased fremitus, wheezing, or egophony; negative bronchophony

*CV*

RRR without MRG

*Abd*

Soft, nontender, (+) BS

*Genit/Rect*

Deferred

*MS/Ext*

Pulses 2+ throughout

*Neuro*

A & O × 3; 2+ reflexes throughout, 5/5 strength; CN II–XII intact

### Labs

| | | | |
|---|---|---|---|
| Na 140 mEq/L | Hgb 14 g/dL | WBC 6 × $10^3$/mm$^3$ | Monos 6% |
| K 4.5 mEq/L | Hct 38% | Segs 55% | Eos 2% |
| Cl 102 mEq/L | RBC 5.0 × $10^6$/mm$^3$ | Bands 3% | Basos 1% |
| $HCO_3$ 24 mEq/L | Plt 250 × $10^3$/mm$^3$ | Lymphs 33% | |
| BUN 14 mg/dL | | | |
| SCr 0.7 mg/dL | | | |
| FPG 88 mg/dL | | | |

### Sputum Culture

No pathogens isolated

### Assessment

1. Presumed acute bronchitis.
2. Sexual/reproductive health issues should be further explored and addressed.
3. (+) Smoking history, although patient states, "I only smoke when I'm out, so I can stop at any time."

# QUESTIONS

## Problem Identification

1.a. Create a list of the patient's drug therapy problems.

1.b. What information (signs, symptoms, laboratory values) indicates the presence or severity of acute bronchitis?

1.c. What additional information must be considered before deciding whether antimicrobial therapy is indicated?

## Desired Outcome

2. What are the goals of pharmacotherapy in this case?

## Therapeutic Alternatives

3.a. What nondrug therapies might be useful for this patient?

3.b. What feasible pharmacotherapeutic alternatives are available for treatment of uncomplicated acute bronchitis?

3.c. What are the most likely alternatives for smoking cessation?

3.d. What sexual/reproductive health considerations are applicable to this patient?

3.e. What psychosocial considerations are applicable to this patient?

## Optimal Plan

4.a. What drugs, dosage form, dose, schedule, and duration of therapy are best to alleviate this patient's symptoms of acute bronchitis?

4.b. What medication and dosage should be recommended for this patient's smoking cessation plan?

## Outcome Evaluation

5. What clinical and laboratory parameters are necessary to evaluate the therapy for achievement of the desired outcome and to detect or prevent adverse effects?

## Patient Education

6. What information should be provided to the patient to enhance adherence, ensure successful therapy, and minimize adverse effects?

## FOLLOW-UP QUESTION

1. What vaccinations should this patient receive?

## SELF-STUDY ASSIGNMENTS

1. Outline a treatment plan for a patient with chronic bronchitis presenting with an acute exacerbation, and contrast how this treatment would differ from treatment for a patient with a new diagnosis of acute bronchitis.
2. Prepare a patient education pamphlet on acute bronchitis. Be sure to address why antibiotics are not usually first-line therapy for uncomplicated acute bronchitis.
3. Discuss the differences in presentation and treatment, if any, of uncomplicated acute bronchitis for a child versus an adult versus an elderly patient.

## CLINICAL PEARL

Many patients who present with symptoms of acute bronchitis expect to receive an antibiotic. Therefore, time should be spent with the patient to explain what goes into the decision to not prescribe an antibiotic, and why excessive use of unnecessary antibiotics could harm the community at large.

## REFERENCES


1. Braman SS. Chronic cough due to acute bronchitis: ACCP evidence-based clinical practice guidelines. Chest 2006;129:95S–103S.
2. Wenzel RP, Fowler AA. Acute bronchitis. N Engl J Med 2006;355:2125–2130.
3. Smucny J, Flynn C, Becker L, Glazier R. $\beta_2$-agonists for acute bronchitis. Cochrane Database Syst Rev 2006;(4).
4. Gonzales R, Bartlett JG, Besser RE, et al. Principles of appropriate antibiotic use for treatment of uncomplicated acute bronchitis: background. Ann Intern Med 2001;134:521–529.
5. Phillips TG, Hickner J. Calling acute bronchitis a chest cold may improve patient satisfaction with appropriate antibiotic use. J Am Board Fam Pract 2005;18:459–463.
6. Brunton S, Carmichael BP, Colgan R, et al. Acute exacerbation of chronic bronchitis: a primary care consensus guideline. Am J Manag Care 2004;10:689–696.
7. Irwin RS, Baumann MH, Boulet L, et al. Diagnosis and management of cough executive summary: ACCP evidence-based clinical practice guidelines. Chest 2006;129:1S–23S.
8. Centers for Disease Control and Prevention. Recommended adult immunization schedule—United States, 2010. MMWR 2010;59(1):1–4.


# 119

# COMMUNITY-ACQUIRED PNEUMONIA

Fever with a Cough . . . . . . . . . . . . . . . . . . . . Level II


**Trent G. Towne, PharmD, BCPS (AQ-ID)**

**Sharon M. Erdman, PharmD**


## LEARNING OBJECTIVES

After completing this case study, the reader should be able to:

- Recognize the typical signs, symptoms, physical examination, and laboratory/radiographic findings in a patient with community-acquired pneumonia (CAP).
- Describe the most common causative pathogens of CAP, including their frequency of occurrence and susceptibility to commonly used antimicrobials.
- Discuss the risk stratification strategies that can be employed to determine whether a patient with CAP should be treated as an inpatient or outpatient.
- Provide recommendations for initial empiric antibiotic therapy for an inpatient or outpatient with CAP based on clinical presentation, severity of infection, age, presence of comorbidities, and presence of allergies.
- Define the goals of antimicrobial therapy for a patient with CAP, including monitoring parameters that should be used to assess the response to therapy as well as the occurrence of adverse effects.
- Describe the clinical parameters that should be considered when changing a patient from IV to oral antimicrobial therapy in the treatment of CAP.

## PATIENT PRESENTATION

### Chief Complaint

"I have been short of breath and have been coughing up rust-colored mucus for the past 3 days."

### HPI

James Thompson is a 55-year-old man with a 3-day history of worsening shortness of breath, subjective fevers, chills, right-sided chest pain, and a productive cough. The patient states that his initial symptom of shortness of breath began approximately 1 week ago after delivering mail on an extremely cold winter day. After several days of not feeling well, he went to an immediate care clinic and received a prescription for levofloxacin 750 mg orally once daily for 5 days, which he did not fill due to financial reasons. He has been taking acetaminophen and an over-the-counter cough and cold preparation, but feels that his symptoms are getting "much worse." The patient began experiencing pleuritic chest pain and a productive cough over the past 3 days, and feels that he has been feverish with chills, although he did not take his temperature. On presentation to the ED, he is febrile and appears visibly short of breath.

### PMH

Hypertension × 15 years
Type 2 diabetes mellitus × 10 years

### SH

Lives with wife and four children
Employed as a mail carrier for the US Postal Service
Denies alcohol, tobacco, or intravenous drug use

### Home Medications

*Prescription*

Patient states that he only sporadically takes his medications due to financial reasons.
Lisinopril 10 mg orally once daily.
Hydrochlorothiazide 25 mg orally once daily.
Metformin 1,000 mg orally twice daily.

*Over-the-Counter*

Acetaminophen 650 mg orally every 6 hours as needed for pain
Guaifenesin/dextromethorphan (100 mg/10 mg/5 mL) two teaspoonfuls every 4 hours as needed for cough

### All

Amoxicillin (rash—as a child). Patient has received Keflex as an adult without problem.

### ROS

Patient is a good historian. He has been experiencing shortness of breath, a productive cough with rust-colored sputum, subjective fevers, chills, and pleuritic chest pain that is "right in the middle of my chest." He denies any nausea, vomiting, constipation, or problems urinating.

### Physical Examination

*Gen*

Patient is a well-developed, well-nourished, African-American man in moderate respiratory distress appearing somewhat anxious and uncomfortable.

*VS*

BP 155/85, P 127, RR 30, T 39.5°C; Wt 110 kg, Ht 5′11″

*Skin*

Warm to the touch; poor skin turgor

*HEENT*

PERRLA; EOMI; dry mucous membranes

*Neck/Lymph Nodes*

No JVD; full range of motion; no neck stiffness; no masses or thyromegaly; no cervical lymphadenopathy

*Lungs/Thorax*

Tachypneic, labored breathing; coarse rhonchi throughout right lung fields; decreased breath sounds in right middle and right lower lung fields

*CV*

Audible $S_1$ and $S_2$; tachycardic with regular rate and rhythm; no MRG

*Abd*

NTND; (+) bowel sounds

*Genit/Rect*

Deferred

*Extremities*

No CCE; 5/5 grip strength; 2+ pulses bilaterally

*Neuro*

A & O × 3; CN II–XII intact

### Labs on Admission

| | | |
|---|---|---|
| Na 140 mEq/L | Hgb 12.1 g/dL | WBC 23.1 × $10^3$/mm$^3$ |
| K 4.3 mEq/L | Hct 35% | Neutros 67% |
| Cl 102 mEq/L | RBC 3.8 × $10^6$/mm$^3$ | Bands 15% |
| $CO_2$ 22 mEq/L | Plt 220 × $10^3$/mm$^3$ | Lymphs 12% |
| BUN 42 mg/dL | MCV 91 μm$^3$ | Monos 6% |
| SCr 1.4 mg/dL | MCHC 35 g/dL | |
| Glu 295 mg/dL | | |

### ABG

pH 7.38; $pCO_2$ 29; $pO_2$ 70 with 87% $O_2$ saturation in room air

### Chest X-Ray

Right middle and right lower lobe airspace disease, likely pneumonia. Left lung is clear. Heart size is normal.

### Chest CT Scan Without Contrast

No axillary, mediastinal, or hilar lymphadenopathy. The heart size is normal. There is consolidation of the right lower lobe and lateral segment of the middle lobe, with air bronchograms. No significant pleural effusions. The left lung is clear.

### Sputum Gram Stain

>25 WBC/hpf, <10 epithelial cells/hpf, many Gram (+) cocci in pairs

### Sputum Culture

Pending

### Blood Cultures × Two Sets

Pending

### Assessment

Probable multilobar CAP involving the RML and RLL
Hypoxemia

## QUESTIONS

### Problem Identification

1.a. Create a list of the patient's drug therapy problems.

1.b. What clinical, laboratory, and radiographic findings are consistent with the diagnosis of CAP in this patient?

1.c. What are the common causative bacteria of CAP?

1.d. What clinical, laboratory, and physical examination findings should be considered when deciding on the site of care for a patient with CAP (inpatient or outpatient)?

### Desired Outcome

2. What are the goals of pharmacotherapy in the treatment of CAP?

### Therapeutic Alternatives

3. What feasible pharmacotherapeutic alternatives are available for treatment of CAP?

### Optimal Plan

4.a. What drug, dose, route of therapy, dosing schedule, and duration of treatment should be used in this patient?

## CLINICAL COURSE

While in the ED, the patient was placed on 4 L NC of $O_2$, and his oxygen saturation improved to 98%. The patient was initiated on ceftriaxone 1 g IV daily and azithromycin 500 mg IV daily and admitted to the hospital. Over the next 48 hours, the patient's clinical status improved with decreasing fever, tachypnea, tachycardia, and shortness of breath. On hospital day 2, the sputum culture demonstrated growth of *Streptococcus pneumoniae* that was resistant to erythromycin (MIC ≥1), but susceptible to penicillin (MIC ≤2), ceftriaxone (MIC ≤1), levofloxacin (MIC ≤0.5), and vancomycin (MIC ≤1).

4.b. Given this new information, what changes in the antimicrobial therapy would you recommend?

4.c. What oral antibiotic would be suitable to complete the course of therapy for CAP? When is it appropriate to convert a patient from IV to oral therapy for the treatment of CAP?

## Outcome Evaluation

5. What clinical and laboratory parameters should be monitored to ensure the desired therapeutic outcome and to detect or prevent adverse effects?

## Patient Education

6. By hospital day 4, the patient's clinical symptoms of pneumonia had almost completely resolved, and the patient was discharged home on oral antibiotics to complete a 7-day course of treatment. What information should be provided to the patient about his oral outpatient antibiotic therapy to enhance adherence, ensure successful therapy, and minimize adverse effects?

## SELF-STUDY ASSIGNMENTS

1. Review the most recent practice guidelines for the treatment of CAP published by the Infectious Diseases Society of America (IDSA)/American Thoracic Society, and evaluate changes from the last published guidelines.
2. Review national, regional, and local patterns of *S. pneumoniae* susceptibility and compare the data to what is seen at your institution or clinic setting.
3. Describe the role of short-course antibiotic therapy in the management of CAP.

## CLINICAL PEARL

Influenza and pneumococcal vaccines for appropriate patient types are important components in the prevention of CAP as well as for reducing the morbidity and mortality associated with CAP.

## REFERENCES


1. Mandell LA, Wunderink RG, Anzueto A, et al. Infectious Diseases Society of America/American Thoracic Society consensus guidelines on the management of community-acquired pneumonia in adults. Clin Infect Dis 2007;44(Suppl 2):527–572.
2. Infections of the lower respiratory tract. In: Forbes BA, Sahm DF, Weissfeld AS, eds. Diagnostic Microbiology, 11th ed. St. Louis, MO, Mosby Inc, 2002:884–898.
3. Miyashita N, Shimizu H, Ouchi K, et al. Assessment of the usefulness of sputum gram stain and culture for diagnosis of community-acquired pneumonia requiring hospitalization. Med Sci Monit 2008;14(4):CR171–CR176.
4. Segreti J, House HR, Siegel RE. Principles of antibiotic treatment of community-acquired pneumonia in the outpatient setting. Am J Med 2005;118(7A):21S–28S.
5. Bochud PY, Moser F, Erard P, et al. Community-acquired pneumonia: a prospective outpatient study. Medicine 2001;80(2):75–87.
6. File TM. Community-acquired pneumonia. Lancet 2003;362: 1991–2001.
7. Aujesky D, Auble TE, Yealy DM. Prospective comparison of three validated prediction rules for prognosis in community-acquired pneumonia. Am J Med 2005;118:384–392.
8. Fine MJ, Auble TE, Yealy DM, et al. A prediction rule to identify low-risk patients with community-acquired pneumonia. N Engl J Med 1997;336:243–250.
9. Lim WS, van der Eerden MM, Laing R, et al. Defining community-acquired pneumonia severity on presentation to hospital: an international derivation and validation study. Thorax 2003;58: 377–382.
10. Centers for Disease Control and Prevention. 2009. Active Bacterial Core Surveillance Report, Emerging Infections Program Network, *Streptococcus pneumoniae*, 2008.
11. Clinical and Laboratory Standards Institute. 2009. Performance standards for antimicrobial susceptibility testing. Approved standard M100-120. Wayne, PA, Clinical and Laboratory Standards Institute.
12. Mandell LA, File TM. Short-course treatment of community-acquired pneumonia. Clin Infect Dis 2003;37:761–763.
13. Fine MJ, Stone RA, Singer DE, et al. Process and outcomes of care for patients with community-acquired pneumonia: results from the Pneumonia Patients Outcomes Research Team (PORT) cohort study. Arch Intern Med 1999;159:970–980.


# 120

# HOSPITAL-ACQUIRED PNEUMONIA

The Happening . . . . . . . . . . . . . . . . . . . . . . . Level III

**Kendra M. Atkinson, PharmD**

## LEARNING OBJECTIVES

After completing this case study, the reader should be able to:

- Recognize the signs and symptoms of hospital-acquired pneumonia (HAP).
- Identify the most common causative organisms associated with HAP, and recognize the impact of bacterial resistance on the etiology and treatment of HAP.
- Design an appropriate empiric antimicrobial therapy regimen for a patient with HAP.
- Formulate a list of alternative antimicrobial therapy options for the treatment of HAP based on the most common causative organisms.
- Recommend a directed/targeted antimicrobial therapy regimen for a patient with HAP based on patient-specific data and final microbiology culture and susceptibility results.

## PATIENT PRESENTATION

### Chief Comsplaint

"I can't catch my breath, and this cough is getting worse."

### HPI

Justin Case is a 60-year-old man with a past medical history significant for myocardial infarction who was admitted to the hospital 5 days ago to undergo a scheduled surgical procedure following a recent diagnosis of colorectal adenocarcinoma with metastatic lesions to the liver. The patient was taken to the OR on hospital day 2 and underwent an exploratory laparotomy, diverting ileostomy, and Hickman port placement in preparation for chemotherapy. Postoperatively, the patient was transferred to the PICU for his recovery without complication. The patient had no new complaints until hospital day 5 when he complained of retrosternal crushing chest pain radiating to the left shoulder and left jaw, shortness of breath, and a worsening cough with sputum production. The patient was noted to be in respiratory distress with an RR of 43, HR 153, BP 162/103, and $O_2$ saturation of 87%. The patient was then transferred to the medical ICU and underwent endotracheal intubation. Cardiac markers were obtained, given the patient's symptoms and history of MI. Blood and sputum cultures were obtained after patient transfer.

## PMH

Coronary artery disease, S/P MI 3 years ago for which he did not undergo any surgical intervention

## SH

Lives with his wife
Smokes one ppd × 40 years
Denies alcohol or illicit drug use

## Meds

Patient states that he did not take any medications at home. Hospital medications include:

- Aspirin 325 mg po daily
- Enoxaparin 30 mg subcutaneously every 12 hours
- Esomeprazole 40 mg po daily
- Fentanyl 25 mcg/h IV continuous infusion
- Lorazepam 2 mg/h IV continuous infusion
- Metoprolol 25 mg po every 12 hours
- Morphine 1–2 mg IV every 1–2 hours as needed for chest pain
- Nicotine patch 21 mg per day applied daily

## All

NKDA

## ROS

Patient is experiencing significant chest pain, shortness of breath, and a cough with sputum production. He denies nausea, vomiting, or difficulty urinating. He complains of mild abdominal pain near his ostomy and incision sites.

## Physical Examination

### Gen

WDWN Caucasian man, initially anxious, ill-appearing, and in moderate respiratory distress; now, S/P endotracheal intubation and in NAD

### VS

BP 162/103, P 147, RR 42, T 38.5°C; Wt 70 kg, Ht 5′6″

### Skin

Warm; no rash; no skin breakdown

### HEENT

PERRLA; moist mucous membranes

### Neck/Lymph Nodes

Supple; no lymphadenopathy

### Lungs/Thorax

Scattered rhonchi with expiratory wheezing; diffuse bilateral crackles; decreased breath sounds in bilateral bases; right IJ port-a-cath intact without erythema

### CV

Tachycardic with regular rhythm; no MRG

### Abd

Soft; mildly distended; hypoactive BS; large liver palpated in RUQ; ileostomy in RLQ is pink and functioning; surgical incision is C/D/I.

### Genit/Rect

Deferred

### MS/Ext

1+ pitting edema; 2+ pulses bilaterally; good peripheral perfusion

### Neuro

Prior to intubation, was A & O × 3; CN II–XII intact; patient is now intubated and sedated.

## Labs

| Lab Parameter | Admission | Hospital Day 5 |
|---|---|---|
| Na (mEq/L) | 130 | 141 |
| K (mEq/L) | 4.1 | 5.1 |
| Cl (mEq/L) | 92 | 110 |
| $CO_2$ (mEq/L) | 24 | 19 |
| BUN (mg/dL) | 22 | 34 |
| Cr (mg/dL) | 1 | 1.1 |
| Glu (mg/dL) | 113 | 148 |
| Ca (mg/dL) | 9.4 | 9.2 |
| WBC ($mm^{-3}$) | $9.5 \times 10^3$ | $17 \times 10^3$ |
| Neutros (%) | 89 | 88 |
| Bands (%) | 0 | 5 |
| Lymphs (%) | 5 | 4 |
| Monos (%) | 6 | 3 |
| Eos (%) | 0 | 0 |
| Hgb (g/dL) | 11.9 | 12.4 |
| Hct (%) | 35 | 37 |
| Plts ($mm^{-3}$) | $448 \times 10^3$ | $584 \times 10^3$ |

## Cardiac Markers

CK 871 IU/L, Troponin-I 1.23 ng/mL

## ABG

pH 7.39; $pCO_2$ 30; $pO_2$ 51 with 87% $O_2$ saturation in room air (pre-intubation)

pH 7.44; $pCO_2$ 29; $pO_2$ 89 with 100% $O_2$ saturation in 40% inspired oxygen (postintubation)

## Chest X-Ray

New bilateral opacities are noted in the left upper lobe and right middle lobe; likely infectious process. Some increased alveolar infiltrates in a perihilar location and involving the lower lobes.

## Chest CT Scan with IV Contrast

No evidence of pulmonary embolism. The heart size is normal. There are small mediastinal and axillary lymph nodes; none are pathologically enlarged. There are small bilateral pleural effusions with adjacent atelectasis. There are pleural-based airspace opacities within the left upper lobe and right middle lobe; this is most consistent with an acute infectious process.

## EKG

Sinus tachycardia, low voltage QRS, septal infarct (age undetermined); ST- and T-wave abnormality; consider inferior ischemia. Inverted T waves noted in the inferior leads.

### Sputum Gram Stain

>25 WBC/hpf, <10 epithelial cells/hpf, 1+ (few) gram-positive cocci, 3+ (many) gram-negative rods

### Sputum Culture

Pending

### Blood Cultures × Two Sets

Pending

### Assessment

Presumed bilobar HAP involving the LUL and RML
Postoperative NSTEMI

# QUESTIONS

## Problem Identification

1.a. Create a list of the patient's drug therapy problems.

1.b. What subjective and objective data are consistent with the diagnosis of HAP in this patient?

1.c. What are the most common causative organisms associated with HAP?

## Desired Outcome

2. What are the goals of pharmacotherapy in the treatment of this patient's HAP?

## Therapeutic Alternatives

3. What feasible pharmacotherapeutic alternatives are available for treatment of HAP?

## Optimal Plan

4.a. What drug (s), dosage form, dose, dosing schedule, and duration of therapy represent(s) an appropriate empiric antimicrobial therapy for this patient?

4.b. What alternative antimicrobial therapy options exist in the event the initial therapy fails or is not tolerated by the patient?

## CLINICAL COURSE

Following endotracheal intubation, the patient experienced improved oxygen saturation and a normalization of his respiratory and heart rates. The patient was initiated on therapy for NSTEMI per cardiology. The patient was initiated on appropriate empiric antimicrobial therapy while awaiting the results of sputum and blood cultures. On hospital day 7, the blood and sputum cultures revealed *Escherichia coli*. The organism's susceptibility profile is provided below. Over the next 72 hours, the patient's clinical status improved with decreased sputum production, oxygen requirement, temperature, and WBC count, and improvement in chest x-ray findings were also noted, resulting in extubation on hospital day 8. The patient was transferred to the PICU for his continued recovery.

| Antimicrobial Agent | MIC (mg/L) | Interpretation |
|---|---|---|
| Ampicillin | ≥32 | Resistant |
| Ampicillin/sulbactam | ≥32 | Resistant |
| Piperacillin/tazobactam | ≤4 | Susceptible |
| Cefazolin | 32 | Intermediate |
| Ceftriaxone | ≤1 | Susceptible |
| Cefepime | ≤1 | Susceptible |
| Meropenem | ≤0.25 | Susceptible |
| Gentamicin | ≤1 | Susceptible |
| Tobramycin | ≤1 | Susceptible |
| Ciprofloxacin | ≤0.25 | Susceptible |
| Levofloxacin | ≤0.12 | Susceptible |
| Trimethoprim/sulfamethoxazole | ≥320 | Resistant |

4.c. Based on the new data listed above, provide a recommendation for directed/targeted therapy for this patient's HAP.

## Outcome Evaluation

5. What clinical and laboratory parameters are necessary to monitor for the achievement of the desired therapeutic outcome as well as to detect or prevent adverse effects of the antimicrobial therapy?

## Patient Education

6. What information should be provided to the patient to enhance adherence, ensure successful therapy, and minimize adverse effects?

## SELF-STUDY ASSIGNMENTS

1. Review national, regional, and local patterns of bacterial susceptibility for the most common causative organisms associated with HAP to determine appropriate empiric antimicrobial therapy choices for your geographic location.
2. Evaluate the literature to determine the most appropriate duration of therapy for HAP according to the causative microorganism.
3. Evaluate the literature to determine the most appropriate recommendations for the medical management of CAD, given the patient's recent NSTEMI and PMH of MI 3 years ago.

## CLINICAL PEARL

Delays in initiation of appropriate antimicrobial therapy have been associated with significant increases in hospital lengths of stay, health care costs, and mortality among patients with HAP.

## REFERENCES

1. ATS/IDSA Therapeutics Work Group. Guidelines for the management of adults with hospital-acquired, ventilator-associated, and healthcare-associated pneumonia. Am J Respir Crit Care Med 2005;171:388–416.
2. Lancaster JW, Lawrence KP, Fong JJ, et al. Impact of an institution-specific hospital-acquired pneumonia protocol on the appropriateness of antibiotic therapy and patient outcomes. Pharmacotherapy 2008;28(7):852–862.
3. Peleg AY, Hooper DC. Hospital-acquired infections due to gram-negative bacteria. N Engl J Med 2010;362:1804–1813.
4. Gastermeier P, Sohr D, Geffers C, Ruden H, Vonberg RP, Welte T. Early and late-onset pneumonia: is this still a useful classification? Antimicrob Agents Chemother 2009;53(7):2714–2718.
5. Ferrer M, Liapikou A, Valendia M, et al. Validation of the American Thoracic Society–Infectious Diseases Society of America guidelines for hospital-acquired pneumonia in the intensive care unit. Clin Infect Dis 2010;50:945–952.

6. Niederman MS. Use of broad-spectrum antimicrobials for the treatment of pneumonia in seriously ill patients: maximizing clinical outcomes and minimizing selection of resistant organisms. Clin Infect Dis 2006;42:S72–S81.
7. Chastre J, Wolff M, Fagon J, et al. Comparison of 8 vs 15 days of antibiotic therapy for ventilator-associated pneumonia in adults. JAMA 2003;290(19):2588–2598.

# 121

# OTITIS MEDIA

## Up To My Ears with Ear Infections . . . . . . . . . Level II

**Rochelle Rubin, PharmD, BCPS**

## LEARNING OBJECTIVES

After completing this case study, the reader should be able to:

- Identify the signs and symptoms of acute otitis media (AOM).
- Identify risk factors associated with an increased incidence of AOM.
- Identify the pathogens most commonly causing AOM.
- Recommend an effective and economical treatment regimen including specific agent(s), route of administration, and dose(s) of antibiotics and analgesic medications.
- Recognize the role of delaying antibiotic therapy for AOM.
- Educate parents about recommended drug therapy using appropriate nontechnical terminology.

## PATIENT PRESENTATION

### Chief Complaint

Per patient's mom: "I've had it up to my ears with his ear infections!"

### HPI

Seth Jacobs is a 16-month-old boy who is brought to his pediatrician by his distraught mother on a Monday morning in early March. Mom describes a 1-day history of tugging at his right ear and crying, and a 2-day history of decreased appetite, decreased playfulness, and difficulty sleeping. Mom states that his temperature last night was elevated by electronic axial thermometer (39.5°C), so she gave him 5 mL ibuprofen every 12 hours × 2 doses. When Seth is asked if anything hurts, he does not respond. Mom requests all recommendations be written as prescriptions (even ibuprofen) for daycare administration. She also notes that it is tax season and she needs Seth to be able to return to daycare immediately so she can return to work as an accountant.

### PMH

Former full-term, NSVD, 3.0-kg healthy infant at birth, breastfed for 6 months.

Immunizations are up-to-date, including four doses of seven-valent pneumococcal conjugate vaccination (Prevnar).

First episode of AOM at age 4 months treated with amoxicillin without adverse effects. Recurrent AOM × 3 over the past year; most recent episode 2 weeks ago treated with high-dose amoxicillin for 10 days without adverse effects.

Seth was seen approximately 1 month ago for persistent nonproductive cough of 5-day duration. A diagnosis of acute bronchitis was made and symptoms improved with ibuprofen treatment, fluids, and rest.

### FH

Both parents in good health. Two siblings, 3 and 6 years old, in good health.

### SH

Seth lives at home with his parents and two sisters. Both parents are employed and work out of the house. Seth and his 3-year-old sister attend daycare. His elder sister attends elementary school. There is a pet dog in the home. Seth uses a pacifier regularly throughout the day.

### Meds

Ibuprofen suspension 100 mg/5 mL, 5 mL Q 12 h × 2 doses in the last 24 hours.

### All

NKDA

### ROS

Head: no drainage from ears; ears nontender to the touch; however, per mom, patient has been tugging them.

Respiratory: (per mom) denies wheezing; lingering, mild cough still present, no sputum production.

### Physical Examination

*Gen*

WDWN Caucasian male, now crying

*VS*

BP 104/60, HR 130, RR 26, T 38.8°C; Wt 9.0 kg, Ht 30″

*HEENT*

Both TMs erythematous (with R > L); right TM is bulging with limited mobility, copious cerumen and purulent fluid behind TM; left TM landmarks appear normal including the pars flaccida, the malleus, and the light reflex below the umbo. However, the right TM landmarks are difficult to visualize and the fluid is obstructing visualization of the umbo. Throat is erythematous; nares patent.

*Neck*

Supple

*Chest*

Mild crackles at bases bilaterally, improved since bronchitis visit 1 month ago

*CV*

RRR

*Abd*

Soft, nontender

*Genit*

Tanner stage I

*Ext*

No CCE; moves all extremities well; warm, pink, no rashes

*Neuro*

Responsive to stimulation, DTR 2+ no clonus, CN intact

#### Assessment

Right ear AOM

## QUESTIONS

### Problem Identification

1.a. Create a drug therapy problem list for this patient.

1.b. What subjective and objective data support the diagnosis of AOM, and is the diagnosis certain or uncertain in this case?

1.c. How would you distinguish AOM from OME?

1.d. How is the severity of otitis media determined?

1.e. What risk factors for AOM are present in this child?

### Desired Outcome

2. What are the goals of pharmacotherapy for AOM in this child?

### Therapeutic Alternatives

3.a. What organisms typically cause AOM?

3.b. What pharmacotherapeutic alternatives are available for treatment of AOM in this patient?

3.c. Should this patient receive antibiotic therapy at this time, or should watchful waiting (observation) be the course of action? Defend your answer.

3.d. What measures are available to prevent AOM infections in children?

### Optimal Plan

4.a. If antibiotics are indicated, which of the alternatives would you recommend to treat this child's AOM? Include the dose, duration of therapy, and rationale for your selection.

4.b. What other therapies would you recommend to treat this child's symptoms?

### Outcome Evaluation

5. How should the therapy you recommended be monitored for efficacy and adverse effects?

### Patient Education

6. How would you provide important information about this therapy to the child's mother?

## SELF-STUDY ASSIGNMENTS

1. Describe a scenario in which it would be appropriate to use azithromycin to treat AOM.
2. Review the literature for evidence supporting antibiotic prophylaxis in children with frequent ear infections.

## CLINICAL PEARL

*Streptococcus pneumoniae* has been shown to cause 25–50% of childhood AOM cases. First-line treatment remains amoxicillin despite significant resistance because the high dose used is generally effective against susceptible, intermediate, and often resistant pneumococci and it is a low-cost, safe, acceptable tasting therapeutic option with a narrow microbiologic spectrum.

## REFERENCES


1. American Academy of Pediatrics Subcommittee on Management of Acute Otitis Media. Diagnosis and management of acute otitis media. Pediatrics 2004;113:1451–1465.
2. American Academy of Pediatrics, American Academy of Otolaryngology-Head and Neck Surgery, and American Academy of Pediatrics Subcommittee on Otitis Media with Effusion. Otitis media with effusion. Pediatrics 2004;113:1412–1429.
3. Hendley JO. Otitis media. N Engl J Med 2002;347:1169–1174.
4. Spiro DM, Tay KY, Arnold DH, Dziura JD, Baker MD, Shapiro ED. Wait-and-see prescription for the treatment of acute otitis media. JAMA 2006;196:1235–1241.
5. Bertin L, Pons G, d'Athis P, et al. A randomized, double-blind, multicentre controlled trial of ibuprofen versus acetaminophen and placebo for symptoms of acute otitis media in children. Fundam Clin Pharmacol 1996;10:387–392.
6. Neto JFL, Hemb L, Silva DB. Systematic literature review of modifiable risk factors for recurrent otitis media in childhood. J Pediatr 2006;82:87–96.
7. Klein JO, Pelton S. Acute otitis media in children: prevention of recurrence. In: Rose BD, ed. UpToDate. Waltham, MA, UpToDate, 2010.
8. Prymula R, Peeters P, Chrobok V, et al. Pneumococcal capsular polysaccharides conjugated to protein D for prevention of acute otitis media caused by both *Streptococcus pneumoniae* and non-typable *Haemophilus influenzae*: a randomised double-blind efficacy study. Lancet 2006;367:740–748.


# 122

# RHINOSINUSITIS

Sick Sinus . . . . . . . . . . . . . . . . . . . . . . . . . . . . Level II

**Michael B. Kays, PharmD, FCCP**

## LEARNING OBJECTIVES

After completing this case study, the reader should be able to:

- Compare and contrast the clinical signs and symptoms of acute viral and bacterial rhinosinusitis in a given patient, noting the cardinal symptoms of acute rhinosinusitis.
- Differentiate viral from bacterial etiology in rhinosinusitis based on a patient's symptoms.
- Identify the most common pathogens that cause acute bacterial rhinosinusitis.
- Identify adult patients with a diagnosis of acute bacterial rhinosinusitis who may be candidates for observation without use of antibiotics.

- Formulate a treatment plan for a patient with acute bacterial rhinosinusitis based on duration of symptoms, severity of symptoms, and history of previous antibiotic use.
- Revise the treatment plan for a patient who fails the initially prescribed therapy.

## PATIENT PRESENTATION

### Chief Complaint

"I feel awful and congested, and my head hurts. I think my sinus infection is back."

### HPI

Kyle Rhiner is a 49-year-old man who presents to his primary care physician with fever, purulent nasal discharge from the left naris, facial pain (L>R), nasal congestion, headache, and fatigue. He states that his symptoms began 7 days ago, but the symptoms initially improved over the first 2–3 days. However, the symptoms have become progressively worse over the last few days. He also complains of intense facial pressure when he bends forward to tie his shoes or to pick up something. He has noticed a decreased ability to smell and states that foods do not taste the same as before. He has experienced occasional episodes of dizziness, tremors, and palpitations for the last week. He has been taking ibuprofen as needed and Claritin-D every 12 hours but has received little relief from his symptoms. He denies nausea, vomiting, diarrhea, chills, diaphoresis, dyspnea, productive cough, or allergies. Mr Rhiner states that he was treated for a sinus infection about 3 weeks ago with an antibiotic that he only had to take one time but he does not remember the drug name (later determined to be azithromycin extended-release oral suspension 2 g). When questioned further, he states that he presented to an urgent care clinic complaining of a runny nose, congestion, sneezing, cough, and a sore throat of 3-day duration. He was leaving the following day for a business trip and asked the physician for an antibiotic prescription. His symptoms slowly improved over several days, and he was symptom-free for a few days before his current symptoms began 7 days ago. He states that he rarely gets sick and has not had an infection in at least last 15 years prior to these episodes.

### PMH

Sinus infection 3 weeks ago
Hypertension (well controlled with medication)
Hypercholesterolemia

### FH

Father died of MI at 64 years of age.
Mother with hypertension and diabetes mellitus.

### SH

Smokes cigars on occasion (one to two per week). Denies cigarette smoking and illicit drug use. Drinks socially (three to four beers and one bottle of red wine per week). He is divorced with two children (23-year-old son, 21-year-old daughter).

### Meds

Lisinopril 20 mg po daily
Hydrochlorothiazide 25 mg po daily
Simvastatin 40 mg po daily
Ibuprofen 200–400 mg po as needed
Claritin-D 12 hours (desloratadine 2.5 mg/pseudoephedrine 120 mg) po Q 12 h

### All

None

### ROS

Patient with a 7-day history of fever, purulent nasal drainage, congestion, facial pain, headache, fatigue, hyposmia, and occasional dizziness and palpitations. The symptoms improved initially but have progressively worsened over the last few days. In addition, the patient complains of insomnia, which may be contributing to the fatigue. He has hypertension and hypercholesterolemia, and he was treated for sinusitis 3 weeks ago.

### Physical Examination

*Gen*

Tired-looking, overweight white man in mild distress; appears uncomfortable

*VS*

BP 158/102, P 90, RR 16, T 39.0°C; Wt 113 kg, Ht 6′1″

*Skin*

Warm to touch; good skin turgor; no other abnormalities

*HEENT*

NC/AT; PERRLA; EOMI; funduscopic exam normal; injected conjunctivae; anicteric sclerae. Thick, purulent, yellow-green nasal discharge; mucosal hypertrophy (L > R) without evidence of nasal polyps. Facial pain over left maxillary and frontal sinuses. No oral lesions; no periorbital swelling. Tympanic membranes intact, nonerythematous, nonbulging. Throat erythematous.

*Neck/Lymph Nodes*

Supple, no JVD, mild lymphadenopathy

*Lungs/Thorax*

CTA; no crackles or wheezing

*CV*

Slightly tachycardic; normal $S_1$ and $S_2$, no MRG

*Abd*

Soft, nontender; bowel sounds present; no masses

*Genit/Rect*

Deferred

*MS/Ext*

No CCE

*Neuro*

A & O × 3; CN II–XII intact

### Labs

None drawn

### Assessment

Recurrent rhinosinusitis
Hypertension
Dizziness, tremors, palpitations

## QUESTIONS

### Problem Identification

1.a. Create a drug therapy problem list for this patient.

1.b. What subjective and objective data support the diagnosis of acute bacterial rhinosinusitis versus viral rhinosinusitis?

1.c. What are the three cardinal symptoms of acute rhinosinusitis?

1.d. What other diagnostic studies (cultures, radiographs, sinus CT, etc.), if any, would you suggest before recommending therapy?

1.e. Should the patient have been treated with an antibiotic for his initial presentation 3 weeks ago? Why or why not? If yes, what antibiotic should the patient have received?

### Desired Outcome

2. What are the goals of pharmacotherapy for this patient?

### Therapeutic Alternatives

3.a. What are the most likely causative bacterial pathogens in this patient?

3.b. Based on the patient's current symptoms, is he a candidate for watchful waiting (i.e., observation without antibiotic therapy) as a therapeutic option in his treatment plan?

3.c. What antibiotics and dosage regimens are appropriate treatment options for the patient at this time?

3.d. What are the most likely reasons why this patient has an infection despite receiving previous antibiotic therapy?

### Optimal Plan

4.a. Based on the patient's clinical presentation, what antibiotic would you recommend for therapy? Include drug name, dosage form, schedule, and duration of therapy.

4.b. What adjunctive measures can be employed to optimize the patient's medical therapy?

4.c. What alternatives, if any, would be appropriate if the patient fails to respond to the initial regimen?

### Outcome Evaluation

5. How should the therapy you recommend be monitored for efficacy and adverse effects?

### Patient Education

6. What information should be provided to the patient to ensure successful therapy, enhance adherence, and minimize adverse effects?

## ■ SELF-STUDY ASSIGNMENTS

1. Determine if a change in mucus color from clear to yellow or green is an indication of a bacterial infection or if it is the natural course of a viral infection.
2. If the patient had a penicillin allergy, review the likelihood of an allergic reaction if he had received a cephalosporin.
3. Review the pharmacokinetic and pharmacodynamic properties of antibacterial agents commonly used in the treatment of acute bacterial rhinosinusitis.
4. Review the most common mechanisms of bacterial resistance in pathogens frequently encountered in acute bacterial rhinosinusitis.

## CLINICAL PEARL

The etiology of most cases of acute rhinosinusitis is viral; however, an antibiotic is prescribed in 85–98% of cases. In patients with a clinical diagnosis of acute bacterial rhinosinusitis, the spontaneous resolution rate is 50–60%. This information is important to consider when evaluating antimicrobial efficacy from comparative clinical studies.

## REFERENCES


1. Rosenfeld RM, Andes D, Bhattacharyya N, et al. Clinical practice guidelines: adult sinusitis. Otolaryngol Head Neck Surg 2007;137:S1–S31.
2. Rosenfeld RM. Clinical practice guideline on adult sinusitis. Otolaryngol Head Neck Surg 2007;137:365–377.
3. Pearlman AN, Conley DB. Review of current guidelines related to the diagnosis and treatment of rhinosinusitis. Curr Opin Otolaryngol Head Neck Surg 2008;16:226–230.
4. Anon JB. Upper respiratory tract infections. Am J Med 2010;123:S16–S25.
5. Garau J, Dagan R. Accurate diagnosis and appropriate treatment of acute bacterial rhinosinusitis: minimizing bacterial resistance. Clin Ther 2003;25:1936–1951.
6. Benninger MS, Payne SC, Ferguson BJ, Hadley JA, Ahmad N. Endoscopically directed middle meatal cultures versus maxillary sinus taps in acute bacterial maxillary rhinosinusitis: a meta-analysis. Otolaryngol Head Neck Surg 2006;134:3–9.
7. Martin CL, Njike VY, Katz DL. Back-up antibiotic prescriptions could reduce unnecessary antibiotic use in rhinosinusitis. J Clin Epidemiol 2004;57:429–434.
8. Benninger M, Brook I, Farrell DJ. Disease severity in acute bacterial rhinosinusitis is greater in patients infected with *Streptococcus pneumoniae* than in those infected with *Haemophilus influenzae*. Otolaryngol Head Neck Surg 2006;135:523–528.
9. Karageorgopoulos DE, Giannopoulou KP, Grammatikos AP, Dimopoulos G, Falagas ME. Fluoroquinolones compared with β-lactam antibiotics for the treatment of acute bacterial sinusitis: a meta-analysis of randomized controlled trials. CMAJ 2008;178:845–854.
10. Van Bambeke F, Tulkens PM. Safety profile of the respiratory fluoroquinolone moxifloxacin. Drug Saf 2009;32:359–378.


# 123

# ACUTE PHARYNGITIS

A Serious Pain in the Neck . . . . . . . . . . . . . . . . Level I

**John L. Lock, PharmD**

## LEARNING OBJECTIVES

After completing this case study, the reader should be able to:

- Evaluate the need for antibiotic therapy in a patient with pharyngitis based on signs and symptoms as well as microbiological and immunological diagnostic studies.
- Identify the most common organisms responsible for causing pharyngitis.

- Select an appropriate pharmacologic regimen for a patient with acute pharyngitis, including route, frequency, and duration.
- List the suppurative and nonsuppurative complications of acute pharyngitis, as well as the prevalence of these complications, and the measures to prevent occurrence.

## PATIENT PRESENTATION

### Chief Complaint

"It hurts to swallow."

### HPI

David Jacobs is a 5-year-old boy who presents to his pediatrician complaining of sore throat. His mother states he has had fever and has been sleeping more than usual over the past 2 days. He has refused to eat anything solid since this time. Mother states he does not have a cough, shortness of breath, or difficulty breathing. The patient states that both his stomach and head ache, but his mother states that he has not vomited. Mother notes no illness in the family, but she heard parents in daycare talking about "strep."

### PMH

The patient has had prior cases of otitis media, his last over a year ago. Otherwise he is healthy. His mother states that he is up-to-date on all vaccinations.

### FH

Noncontributory

### SH

David lives with his parents and infant sister. He attends a local daycare and preschool.

### Meds

None

### All

NKDA

### ROS

Negative except for complaints noted in the HPI

### Physical Examination

*Gen*

WDWN 5-year-old male, clearly fatigued

*VS*

BP 104/70, P 92, RR 22, T 38.8°C, Wt 21 kg, Ht 45″

*Skin*

Pale, warm, no sign of rash

*HEENT*

PERRLA; tonsils erythematous with associated white exudates; uvula edematous; soft palate with notable petechiae, TM normal

*Neck/Lymph Nodes*

Enlarged anterior cervical lymph nodes

*Lungs/Thorax*

CTA bilaterally, (−) shortness of breath, (−) cough

*CV*

RRR, normal $S_1$ and $S_2$

*Abd*

Soft, nontender, nondistended, (+) BS

*Genit/Rect*

Deferred

*Neuro*

CN I–XII intact

### Labs

RADT: positive

### Assessment

A 5-year-old male presents to the pediatrician with GABHS pharyngitis.

## QUESTIONS

### Problem Identification

1.a. List the patient's drug therapy problem(s).

1.b. What are the signs and symptoms in this patient that are indicative of GABHS infection?

1.c. What diagnostic tool(s) may be used to facilitate a diagnosis?

### Desired Outcome

2. List the goals of therapy.

### Therapeutic Alternatives

3.a. What nonpharmacologic therapies are available for treatment of GABHS acute pharyngitis?

3.b. What are the pharmacologic options for GABHS acute pharyngitis?

### Optimal Plan

4.a. What is the preferred treatment for DJ's acute pharyngitis? Include dose, route, frequency, and duration.

4.b. Which option would be most appropriate if DJ reported a penicillin allergy?

### Outcome Evaluation

5.a. What should be monitored to evaluate successful therapy and/or development of adverse effects?

5.b. What would be the appropriate treatment if DJ's infection did not resolve?

### Patient Education

6. What information should be shared with DJ and his parents regarding his drug therapy?

## SELF-STUDY ASSIGNMENTS

1. Create a table that lists the preferred and alternative therapeutic options for GABHS pharyngitis and includes the following comparative data:
   - Drug
   - Dose
   - Frequency
   - Duration
   - Available dosage forms
   - Adverse effects
   - Cost
2. Prepare a one-page paper that describes the signs, symptoms, and onset of scarlet fever, rheumatic fever, and poststreptococcal glomerulonephritis.

## CLINICAL PEARL

Immediate administration of antibiotics is not necessary to treat pharyngitis because even untreated, most signs and symptoms of pharyngitis are absent within 3–4 days, treatment with antibiotics decreases length of illness only by approximately 24 hours, and antibiotic therapy can be withheld for over 1 week without significantly increasing risk of rheumatic fever.

## REFERENCES


1. Gerber MA, Baltimore RS, Eaton CB, et al. Prevention of rheumatic fever and diagnosis and treatment of acute streptococcal pharyngitis. *Circulation* 2009;119:1541–1551.
2. Bisno AL, Gerber MA, Gwaltney JM Jr, Kaplan EL, Schwartz RH. Practice guidelines for the diagnosis and management of group A streptococcal pharyngitis. Clin Infect Dis 2002;35:113–125.
3. Bisno AL. Acute pharyngitis. N Engl J Med 2001;344(3):205–211.
4. Vincent MT, Celestin N, Hussain AN. Pharyngitis. Am Fam Physician 2004;69:1465–1470.
5. Snow V, Mottur-Pilson C, Cooper RJ, Hoffman JR. Principles of appropriate antibiotic use of acute pharyngitis in adults. Ann Intern Med 2001;134:506–508.
6. McIsaac WJ, Goel V, To T, Low DE.The validity of a sore throat score in family practice. CMAJ 2000;163(7):811–815.
7. Tanz RR, Shulman ST, Shortridge VD, et al. Community-based surveillance in the United States of macrolide-resistant pediatric pharyngeal group A streptococci during 3 respiratory disease seasons. Clin Infect Dis 2004;39:1794–1801.


# 124

# INFLUENZA

Run Over by the Flu .................... Level II

**Margarita V. DiVall, PharmD, BCPS**

## LEARNING OBJECTIVES

After completing this case study, the reader should be able to:

- Recognize the clinical presentation of influenza.
- Discuss influenza-related complications.
- Develop a patient-specific treatment plan for influenza.
- Identify appropriate target populations for vaccination against influenza.
- Compare and contrast available options for preventing influenza.
- Discuss strategies to control influenza outbreaks.

## PATIENT PRESENTATION

### Chief Complaint

"I feel like a truck ran over me. Every muscle and bone hurts, and I am burning up."

### HPI

Vladimir Kharitonov is a 57-year-old Russian man who presents in mid-December to an urgent care clinic with complaints of 1-day history of fever, up to 39°C (102.2°F), muscle and bone aches, feeling tired, and headache. He has not had anything to eat in the past 12 hours due to loss of appetite and has not taken his glyburide this morning. He has been in his usual state of health previously and reports that some of his coworkers have been sick with the "flu." He decided to come to the clinic in hopes that an antibiotic can allow him to recover sooner since his son is getting married next weekend. He missed his regular physical appointment 1 month ago because he was "too busy."

### PMH

Type 2 DM for 14 years
Hyperlipidemia
HTN

### SH

Lives at home with his wife; works full time; quit smoking 10 years ago, but smokes occasionally when really stressed or in a social setting; drinks alcohol in a social setting—mostly vodka

### Meds

Aspirin 81 mg po daily
Hydrochlorothiazide 25 mg po daily
Glyburide 5 mg po every morning
Metformin 1 g po twice daily
Lantus 35 units SC at bedtime
Lipitor 10 mg po daily
Centrum Silver one tablet po daily

### All

NKDA

### ROS

Patient complains of severe fatigue, body aches, alternating between being too cold and sweating, sore throat, nonproductive cough, and a headache. He denies nasal congestion, nausea, vomiting, or diarrhea.

### Physical Examination

*Gen*

WDWN overweight man in NAD

*VS*

BP 145/85, P 95, RR 18, T 38.5°C; Wt 95.5 kg, Ht 5′10″

*Skin*

Warm and moist secondary to diaphoresis, no lesions

*HEENT*

PERRLA; EOMI; TMs intact; wears dentures; mild pharyngeal erythema with no exudates

*Neck/Lymph Nodes*

Neck is supple and without adenopathy; no JVD

*Lungs/Thorax*

CTA; no crackles or wheezing

*CV*

RRR; normal $S_1$, $S_2$; no murmurs

*Abd*

Soft, slightly obese; NT/ND; normal BS

*Genit/Rect*

Not performed

*MS/Ext*

Muscle strength and tone 4–5/5; no CCE

*Neuro*

A & O × 3; CN II–XII intact; decreased sensation to light touch of the lower extremities (both feet)

### Labs

| | | | |
|---|---|---|---|
| Na 138 mEq/L | Hgb 13.2 g/dL | WBC 10 × $10^3$/mm$^3$ | *Fasting lipid profile* |
| K 3.8 mEq/L | Hct 41% | Neutros 50% | T. chol 177 mg/dL |
| Cl 98 mEq/L | Plt 275 × $10^3$/mm$^3$ | Bands 4% | LDL 110 mg/dL |
| $CO_2$ 24 mEq/L | | Eos 0% | HDL 35 mg/dL |
| BUN 26 mg/dL | | Lymphs 39% | Trig 160 mg/dL |
| SCr 1.3 mg/dL | | Monos 7% | |
| Glu 185 mg/dL | | | |
| A1C 8.5% | | | |

### Diagnostic Tests

QuickVue Influenza test—positive

### Assessment

A 57-year-old man with diabetes, hypertension, and hyperlipidemia presents with influenza.

# QUESTIONS

## Problem Identification

1.a. Create a list of patient's drug therapy problems.

1.b. What information (signs, symptoms, laboratory values) indicates the presence of influenza?

1.c. What diagnostic tests are available to confirm and differentiate seasonal influenza from H1N1 influenza? What is the clinical utility of differentiating the two types of influenza?

1.d. What influenza-related complications is this patient at risk for developing?

## Desired Outcome

2. What are the goals of pharmacotherapy in this case?

## Therapeutic Alternatives

3.a. List available options for treating influenza in this patient. Include the drug name, dose, dosage form, route, frequency, and treatment duration. Are these options affected by the type of influenza that this patient experiences (i.e., seasonal vs. H1N1)?

3.b. What other therapies are available to help this patient with his symptoms?

3.c. Should all patients with confirmed influenza receive treatment with antiviral medications?

## Optimal Plan

4.a. Provide your individualized treatment recommendations for treating this patient's influenza, including symptom management.

4.b. Outline your plans for managing each of the patient's other drug therapy problems.

## Outcome Evaluation

5. What clinical and laboratory parameters are necessary to evaluate the therapy for achievement of the desired therapeutic outcome and detect or prevent adverse effects?

## Patient Education

6. What information should be provided to the patient to enhance adherence, ensure successful therapy, and minimize adverse effects?

# CLINICAL COURSE

In October of the following year, Mr Kharitonov presents for his routine physical exam. He has been doing very well. His diabetes, hypertension, and hyperlipidemia are well controlled.

## Follow-Up Questions

1. What indications does this patient have for administration of the seasonal influenza and H1N1 vaccines?
2. If the vaccine(s) is (are) desirable, what is the optimal time frame for this patient to receive vaccination(s)?
3. List available options for vaccination against seasonal and H1N1 influenza. If not available as coformulation, could both vaccines be administered simultaneously?
4. Provide your individualized recommendations for protecting this patient against seasonal and H1N1 influenza virus infections.

# SELF-STUDY ASSIGNMENTS

1. Prepare an educational pamphlet on influenza prevention and treatment directed at both patients and general practice physicians. Be sure to include recommendations for controlling influenza outbreaks.
2. Investigate the expanded role of pharmacists as immunization providers.
3. Investigate the threat of human infection with avian influenza viruses. Are currently available influenza prevention strategies effective against avian flu?

# CLINICAL PEARL

Development of antibodies takes approximately 2 weeks after influenza vaccination in adults, during which time they remain at high risk for influenza infection. If the immunization occurs during an influenza outbreak, chemoprophylaxis with antiviral agents can be administered for 2 weeks immediately after vaccination to minimize the risk of infection.

## REFERENCES


1. Centers for Disease Control and Prevention. Prevention and control of seasonal influenza with vaccines: recommendations of the Advisory Committee on Immunization Practices (ACIP). MMWR Recomm Rep 2010;59:1–62.
2. Dawood FS, Jain S, Finelli L, et al. Emergence of a novel swine-origin influenza A (H1N1) virus in humans. N Engl J Med 2009;360(25): 2605–2615 [Epub May 7, 2009].
3. Harper SA, Bradley JS, Englund JA, et al. Seasonal influenza in adults and children—diagnosis, treatment, chemoprophylaxis and institutional outbreak management: clinical practice guidelines of the Infectious Diseases Society of America for seasonal influenza in adults and children. Clin Infect Dis 2009;48:1003–1032.
4. United States Centers for Disease Control and Prevention. H1N1 clinical and public health guidance. Available at: *http://www.cdc.gov/h1n1flu/guidance/*. Accessed May 12, 2010.
5. Cooper NJ, Sutton AJ, Abrams KR, et al. Effectiveness of neuraminidase inhibitors in treatment and prevention of influenza A and B: systematic review and meta-analyses of randomised controlled trials. BMJ 2003;326:1235.
6. Jefferson T, Demicheli V, Deeks J, et al. Neuraminidase inhibitors for preventing and treating influenza in healthy adults. Cochrane Database Syst Rev 2000;3:CD001265.
7. American Diabetes Association. Standards for medical care in diabetes—2010. Diabetes Care 2010;33(Suppl 1):S11–S61.
8. Chobanian AV, Bakris GL, Black HR, et al. The seventh report of the Joint National Committee on Prevention, Detection, and Treatment of High Blood Pressure. JAMA 2003;289:2560–2572.
9. Jones P, Kafonek S, Laurora I, et al. Comparative dose efficacy study of atorvastatin versus simvastatin, pravastatin, lovastatin, and fluvastatin in patients with hypercholesterolemia (the CURVES study). Am J Cardiol 1998;81:582–587.
10. Relenza. Patient information leaflet. Research Triangle Park, NC, GlaxoSmithKline, 2010.
11. FluMist. Package insert. Gaithersburg, MD, Medimmune Vaccines Inc, 2009.


# 125

# CELLULITIS

A Pain in the Butt. . . . . . . . . . . . . . . . . . . . . . . Level II

**Jarrett R. Amsden, PharmD, BCPS**

## LEARNING OBJECTIVES

After completing this case study, the reader should be able to:

- Evaluate the signs and symptoms of cellulitis.
- Recommend appropriate empiric pharmacologic and nonpharmacologic treatment options for patients presenting with cellulitis.
- Differentiate between the definition and clinical manifestations of uncomplicated versus complicated cellulitis.
- Compare and contrast the clinical characteristics and presentation of cellulitis due to MRSA versus other causative organisms.
- Design an antimicrobial treatment regimen for an MRSA cellulitis.
- Develop a list of alternative therapeutic options for the treatment of uncomplicated cellulitis and refractory (complicated) cellulitis.
- Identify treatment modalities for decolonization of a patient with recurrent MRSA infections.

## PATIENT PRESENTATION

### Chief Complaint

"I have a boil on my butt, and I cannot sit down for class."

### HPI

Jimmie Chipwood is a 19-year-old college student who presents to the ED with a new-onset "boil" on his right buttock. He noticed some pain and irritation in the right buttock area over the past week, but thought it was due to having slid into second base during a baseball game. The pain gradually increased over the next few days, and he went to the student health center, where they cleaned the wound and gave him a prescription for clindamycin 300 mg QID for 7 days. They recommended that he try to keep the area covered until the antibiotic began to work. Today, Jimmie returned to the student health center for further evaluation and was referred to the ED for further care for his continued cellulitis. At the ED, Jimmie says the area on his buttock is worse, and he cannot sit down for class. He reports only partial adherence to the clindamycin regimen, because he often forgets to take it and says it makes him nauseous.

### PMH

Right gluteal cellulitis, diagnosed approximately 1 week ago (Rx for clindamycin was given but the patient reports nonadherence).

### Surgical History

2002—appendectomy
2005—repair of left ACL

### SH

Denies any alcohol or illicit drug use

### Meds

Clindamycin 300 mg po QID × 7 days (prescribed at student health center visit 1 week ago; patient did not complete full course).

### All

Penicillin (hives as a child)

### Immunizations

Up to date per student health center records

### ROS

Negative except for complaints noted in HPI

### Physical Examination

*Gen*

WDWN Caucasian male in no acute distress, but with noticeable pain when he walks and tries to sit

*VS*

BP 129/74, P 96, RR 16, T 37.7°C; Wt 77.5 kg, Ht 6′0″

*Skin*

Right gluteal area: red, erythematous, warm, and tender to touch; localized fluid collection that appears fluctuant, consistent with a carbuncle and surrounding cellulitis

*HEENT*

PEERLA; EOMI, oropharynx clear

*Neck/Lymph Nodes*

Supple, no lymphadenopathy

*Lungs/Thorax*

CTA, no rales or wheezing

*CV*

RRR, no MRG

*Abd*

Soft, NT/ND; (+) BS

*Genit/Rect*

Large 2 cm × 4 cm red swollen area over the right buttock, with surrounding erythema

*MS/Ext*

Upper extremities: WNL
Lower extremities: could not be adequately assessed due to patient's inability to sit; 2+ pulses bilaterally

*Neuro*

A & O × 3

### ■ Labs

| | | |
|---|---|---|
| Na 138 mEq/L | Hgb 15.5 g/dL | WBC 14.3 × $10^3$/mm$^3$ |
| K 3.2 mEq/L | Hct 44% | Neutros 81% |
| Cl 98 mEq/L | Plt 279 × $10^3$/mm$^3$ | Lymphs 18% |
| $CO_2$ 23 mEq/L | | Monos 1% |
| BUN 33 mg/dL | | |
| SCr 0.9 mg/dL | | |
| Glu 95 mg/dL | | |
| Ca 9.4 mg/dL | | |

### ■ Urine Drug Screen

(−) Alcohol, (−) marijuana, (−) cocaine and other substances

### ■ Assessment

Progressive right gluteal cellulitis with focal area of fluctuance/fluid

## QUESTIONS

### Problem Identification

1.a. Classify this patient's cellulitis as either "complicated" or "uncomplicated" and as either "mild–moderate" or "moderate–severe."

1.b. What subjective and objective clinical data are consistent with the diagnosis of cellulitis?

1.c. What are the most common causative organisms of cellulitis?

### Desired Outcome

2.a. What are the goals of nonpharmacologic management of this patient's cellulitis?

2.b. What are the goals of pharmacotherapy for the treatment of this patient's cellulitis?

### Therapeutic Alternatives

3.a. Create a list of nonpharmacologic treatment or supportive options for this patient in the treatment of cellulitis.

3.b. What feasible antimicrobial options are available for the treatment of cellulitis?

### Optimal Plan

4.a. What is the best treatment course for this patient (pharmacologic vs. nonpharmacologic)?

4.b. What antimicrobial agent, dosage form, dose, schedule, and duration of therapy are best for this patient?

## ■ CLINICAL COURSE

The patient was treated in the ED with I&D alone and was given wound care instructions. The fluid was not sent for culture and sensitivity. He returns 8 days later with a recurrent boil in the same right buttock area. On physical exam, the patient is found to have a new area of fluid collection (1 cm × 3 cm) and surrounding erythema. An MRI of the gluteal area was negative for deep tissue involvement and extension to other adjacent areas. Two sets of blood cultures were drawn and are pending, and a second I&D of the area was performed. The patient did have his nares and inguinal area cultured for MRSA, but the results are pending. The patient has reported mild fevers without chills, but he has not taken his temperature at home. His current temperature is 37.8°C, and all other vital signs are stable. Given the current information, the ED physician does not think Jimmie needs to be admitted.

### Microbiology

Blood cultures × 2 sets: pending
Culture of abscess fluid from right buttock: pending
Nares swab: pending
Inguinal swab: pending

### Imaging Studies

Negative for deep tissue involvement; localized area of inflammation and fluid consistent with an abscess

4.c. Was surgical debridement (I&D) alone an appropriate management strategy for the initial presentation of this patient case?

4.d. Based on the above information, the patient has failed oral clindamycin (arguably) and an initial I&D. What antimicrobial regimen would you now recommend for this patient, s/p the second I&D? (Please specify dose, schedule, and duration of therapy.)

4.e. What are some nonpharmacologic measures (outside of proper local/wound care) you could recommend for Jimmie to use at home/school/in the locker room? (Focus on hygiene.)

4.f. What decolonization measures could be considered for Jimmie, if his nares and/or inguinal culture(s) is/are positive for MRSA? (Please discuss the relative options for both, if you would treat them differently.)

## Outcome Evaluation

5. What clinical and laboratory parameters are necessary to evaluate the therapy for its effectiveness in treating this patient's cellulitis?

## Patient Education

6. What information should be provided to the patient to ensure successful therapy?

## ■ SELF-STUDY ASSIGNMENTS

1. Compare and contrast the therapeutic alternatives for the treatment of inpatient and outpatient MRSA skin and skin structure infections and complicated and uncomplicated skin and skin structure infections.
2. Prepare a table that differentiates the presentation, signs, and symptoms of the patient in this case with that of a patient presenting with erysipelas, diabetic foot infection, as well as necrotizing fasciitis and also the organisms involved in each infection, respectively.

## CLINICAL PEARL

In cases of cellulitis where there is frank fluid collection(s) (i.e., pus), surgical debridement is essential. The use of antibiotics in addition to surgical debridement is controversial for initial treatment, but would be indicated for recurrent infections as in the case above. The antibiotic agent(s) should be directed primarily toward *Staphylococcus aureus* (including MRSA), but also *Streptococcus* species.

## REFERENCES


1. Stevens DL, Bisno AL, Chambers HF, et al. Practice guidelines for the diagnosis and management of skin and soft-tissue infections. Clin Infect Dis 2005;41:1373–1406.
2. Pendland SL, Fish DN, Danziger LH. Skin and soft tissue infections. In: DiPiro JT, Talbert RL, Yee GC, et al, eds. Pharmacotherapy: A Pathophysiologic Approach, 7th ed. New York, McGraw-Hill, 2008:1801–1819.
3. Ubbink DT, Vermeulen H, Goossens A, Kelner RB, Schreuder SM, Lubbers MJ. Occlusive vs gauze dressings for local wound care in surgical patients: a randomized clinical trial. Arch Surg 2008;143: 950–955.
4. Healy B, Freedman A. ABC of wound healing: infections. BMJ 2006;332:838–841.
5. Stryjewski ME, Chambers HF. Skin and soft-tissue infections caused by community-acquired methicillin-resistant *Staphylococcus aureus*. Clin Infect Dis 2008;46:S368–S377.
6. Moran GJ, Krishnadasan A, Gorwitz RJ, et al. Methicillin-resistant *S. aureus* infections among patients in the emergency department. N Engl J Med 2006;55:666–674.
7. Rybak MJ, LaPlante KL. Community-associated methicillin-resistant *Staphylococcus aureus*: a review. Pharmacotherapy 2005:25:74–85.
8. Stryjewski ME, Graham DR, Wilson SE, et al. Telavancin versus vancomycin for the treatment of complicated skin and skin-structure infections caused by gram-positive organisms. Clin Infect Dis 2008;46:1683–1693.
9. Ruhe JJ, Smith N, Bradsher RW, et al. Community-onset methicillin-resistant *Staphylococcus aureus* skin and soft-tissue infections: impact of antimicrobial therapy on outcome. Clin Infect Dis 2007;44: 777–784.
10. Rajendran PM, Young D, Maurer T, et al. Randomized, double-blind, placebo-controlled trial of cephalexin for treatment of uncomplicated skin abscesses in a population at risk for community-acquired methicillin-resistant *Staphylococcus aureus* infection. Antimicrob Agent Chemother 2007;51:4044–4048.
11. Miller LG, Diep BA. Colonization, fomites, and virulence: rethinking the pathogenesis of community-associated methicillin-resistant *Staphylococcus aureus* infection. Clin Infect Dis 2008;46:752–760.
12. Barrett TW, Moran GJ. Update on emerging infections: news from the Centers for Disease Control and Prevention. Methicillin-resistant *Staphylococcus aureus* infections among competitive sports participants—Colorado, Indiana, Pennsylvania, and Los Angeles County, 2000–2003. Ann Emerg Med 2004;43:41–45.
13. McConeghy KW, Mikolich DJ, LaPlante KL. Agents for the decolonization of methicillin-resistant *Staphylococcus aureus*. Pharmacotherapy 2009;29:263–280.


# 126

# DIABETIC FOOT INFECTION

Let's Nail That Infection . . . . . . . . . . . . . . . . . . Level II

**Renee-Claude Mercier, PharmD, BCPS, PhC**

**Paulina Deming, PharmD, PhC**

## LEARNING OBJECTIVES

After completing this case study, the reader should be able to:

- Recognize the signs and symptoms of diabetic foot infections and identify the risk factors and the most likely pathogens associated with these infections.
- Recommend appropriate antimicrobial regimens for diabetic foot infections, including for patients with drug allergies or renal insufficiency.
- Recommend appropriate home IV therapy and proper counseling to patients.
- Outline monitoring parameters for achievement of the desired pharmacotherapeutic outcomes and prevention of adverse effects.
- Counsel diabetic patients about adequate blood glucose control as part of an overall plan for good foot health.

## PATIENT PRESENTATION

### ■ Chief Complaint

As per the Spanish interpreter: "He had an ingrown toe nail that became infected several weeks ago, and now the whole foot is swollen."

### ■ HPI

Jesus Chavez is a 67-year-old Hispanic man, Spanish-speaking only, who presents to the ED complaining of a sore and swollen foot. Three weeks ago he noticed that his right great toe became swollen and red due to an ingrown toenail. The patient tried to fix the nail with scissors and tweezers, but the swelling got worse, and thick, foul-smelling drainage became noticeable approximately 2 weeks ago. The patient was visiting family in Mexico at the time and now has just returned home to New Mexico. History is per translation by a hospital interpreter. The patient is accompanied by his wife who also only speaks Spanish.

Primary care physician is Dr Martinez at First Choice Clinic in Albuquerque.

## PMH

Type 2 DM × 18 years
Hospitalized 2 months ago for HHS
Hospitalized 7 months ago with MI, received PCI with bare metal stents placed in the RCA and LAD
Left second toe amputation 1 year ago secondary to diabetic foot infection
Hyperlipidemia
Hypertension
Chronic renal insufficiency

## FH

Father is deceased (56 yo) secondary to MI, type 2 DM, HTN
Mother is deceased secondary to breast cancer (41 yo)
One daughter, alive and well, 42 yo

## SH

The patient lives with his wife in Albuquerque, New Mexico. He denies tobacco and illicit drug use; however, he admits to a long history of drinking four to five beers per day and states he quit after his MI several months ago. He admits to nonadherence with his medications and glucometer.

## Meds

Novolin 70/30 60 units Q AM and Q PM
Metformin 1,000 mg po twice daily
Aspirin 81 mg po once daily
Lisinopril 20 mg po once daily
Simvastatin 40 mg po once daily
Clopidogrel 75 mg po once daily

## All

Sulfa—severe rash

## ROS

Negative except as noted in the HPI

## Physical Examination

### *Gen*

Patient is a thin Hispanic man who appears very concerned about losing his foot.

### *VS*

BP 126/79, P 92, RR 20, T 38.4°C; Wt 60 kg, Ht 5′10″

### *Skin*

Warm, coarse, and very dry

### *HEENT*

PERRLA; EOMI; funduscopic exam is normal with absence of hemorrhages or exudates. TMs are clouded bilaterally but with no erythema or bulging. Oropharynx shows poor dentition but is otherwise unremarkable.

### *Neck/Lymph Nodes*

Neck is supple; normal thyroid; no JVD; no lymphadenopathy

### *Chest*

CTA

### *Heart*

RRR, normal $S_1$ and $S_2$

### *Abd*

Distended, (+) BS, no guarding, no hepatosplenomegaly or masses felt

### *Ext*

2+ edema with markedly diminished sensation of the right foot. Significant swelling and induration extend from first metatarsal to midfoot. Purulent drainage expressed from great toe wound. Wound probe 2 cm deep. Pedal pulses present but diminished. Normal range of motion. Poor nail care with some fungus and overgrown toenails.

### *Neuro*

A & O × 3; CN II–XII intact. Motor system intact (overall muscle strength 4–5/5). Sensory system exam showed a decreased sensation to light touch of the lower extremities (both feet); intact upper body sensation.

## Labs

| | |
|---|---|
| Na 136 mEq/L | Hgb 14.1 g/dL |
| K 3.6 mEq/L | Hct 42.3% |
| Cl 98 mEq/L | Plt 390 × $10^3$/mm$^3$ |
| $CO_2$ 24 mEq/L | WBC 17.3 × $10^3$/mm$^3$ |
| BUN 30 mg/dL | PMNs 78% |
| SCr 2.1 mg/dL | Lymphs 17% |
| Glu 181 mg/dL | Monos 5% |
| A1C 11.8% | |
| ESR 73 mm/h | |

## X-Ray

Right foot: There is soft tissue swelling from first metatarsal to midfoot consistent with cellulitis. No fluid collection noted. No evidence of adjacent periosteal reactions or erosions to suggest radiographic evidence of osteomyelitis. No definite subcutaneous air is evident. Presence of vascular calcifications.

## Assessment

Diabetic foot infection in a patient with poorly controlled diabetes mellitus

## Clinical Course

On the day of admission, the patient went to surgery for I&D. Blood and tissue specimens were sent for culture and sensitivity testing.

# QUESTIONS

## Problem Identification

1.a. Create a list of the patient's drug therapy problems.

1.b. What signs, symptoms, or laboratory values indicate the presence of an infection?

1.c. What risk factors for infection does the patient have?

1.d. What organisms are most likely involved in this infection?

## Desired Outcome

2. What are the therapeutic goals for this patient?

## Therapeutic Alternatives

3.a. What nondrug therapies might be useful for this patient?

3.b. What feasible pharmacotherapeutic alternatives are available for the empiric treatment of diabetic foot infection?

3.c. What economic and social considerations are applicable to this patient?

## Optimal Plan

4. Outline a drug regimen that would provide optimal initial empiric therapy for the infection.

## Outcome Evaluation

5.a. What clinical and laboratory parameters are necessary to evaluate your therapy for achievement of the desired therapeutic outcomes and monitoring for adverse effects?

## ■ CLINICAL COURSE

Mr Chavez received the empiric therapy you recommended until the tissue cultures were reported positive for *Bacteroides fragilis* and *Staphylococcus aureus*, and reported sensitive to vancomycin, linezolid, quinupristin/dalfopristin, and daptomycin and resistant to oxacillin (and other β-lactams), tetracycline, erythromycin, clindamycin, and sulfamethoxazole/trimethoprim. Susceptibilities are not available for *B. fragilis*. The blood cultures were all found to have no growth. The patient remained hospitalized for an additional 10 days and received a more directed antimicrobial regimen and multiple surgical debridements of the wound. The cellulitis slowly improved over this time, and multiple x-rays did not suggest osteomyelitis. He was then discharged to complete his antimicrobial regimen on an outpatient basis. Over the next 2 weeks, he received wound care at home and showed significant but slow progress in healing of the wound.

5.b. What therapeutic alternatives are available for treating this patient after results of cultures are known to contain MRSA and *B. fragilis*?

5.c. Design an optimal drug treatment plan for treating the mixed infection while he remains hospitalized.

5.d. Design an optimal pharmacotherapeutic plan for completion of his treatment after he is discharged from the hospital.

## Patient Education

6. What information should be provided to the patient to enhance adherence, ensure successful therapy, and minimize adverse effects with IV vancomycin and oral metronidazole?

## ■ SELF-STUDY ASSIGNMENTS

1. Review in more detail different therapeutic options available for home IV therapy, including the antimicrobial agents suitable for use, types of IV lines available, and contraindications to home IV therapy.
2. Outline the patient counseling you would provide for successful home IV therapy.
3. Describe how you would educate this diabetic patient about proper foot care to prevent further skin or tissue breakdown.

## CLINICAL PEARL

Treatment of diabetic foot infections with antimicrobial agents alone is often inadequate; local wound care (incision, drainage, debridement, and amputation), good glycemic control, and immobilization of the limb are often required.

## REFERENCES


1. Lipsky BA, Berendt AR, Deery G, et al. Diagnosis and treatment of diabetic foot infections. Clin Infect Dis 2004;39:885–910.
2. Levin ME. Management of the diabetic foot: preventing amputation. South Med J 2002;95:10–20.
3. Rybak JM, LaPlante KL. Community-associated methicillin-resistant *Staphylococcus aureus*: a review. Pharmacotherapy 2005;25:74–85.
4. Lipsky BA, Tabak YP, Johannes RS, Vo L, Hyde L, Weigelt JA. Skin and soft tissue infections in hospitalised patients with diabetes: culture isolates and risk factors associated with mortality, length of stay and cost. Diabetologia 2010;53:914–923.
5. Herwaldt LA. Control of methicillin-resistant *Staphylococcus aureus* in the hospital setting. Am J Med 1999;106:11S–18S [discussion 48S–52S].
6. Asensio A, Guerrero A, Quereda C, Lizán M, Martinez-Ferrer M. Colonization and infection with methicillin-resistant *Staphylococcus aureus*: associated factors and eradication. Infect Control Hosp Epidemiol 1996;17:20–28.
7. Wieman TJ, Smiell JM, Su Y. Efficacy and safety of a topical gel formulation of recombinant human platelet-derived growth factor-B (becaplermin) in patients with chronic neuropathic diabetic ulcers. A phase III randomized, placebo-controlled, double-blind study. Diabetes Care 1998;21:822–827.
8. Weigelt J, Itani K, Stevens D, Lau W, Dryden M, Knirsch C. Linezolid versus vancomycin in the treatment of complicated skin and soft tissue infections. Antimicrob Agents Chemother 2005;46:2260–2266.
9. Nicolau DP, Stein GE. Therapeutic options for diabetic foot infections: a review with an emphasis on tissue penetration characteristics. J Am Podiatr Med Assoc 2010;100:52–63.
10. Cruciani M, Lipsky BA, Mengoli C, de Lalla F. Granulocyte-colony stimulating factors as adjunctive therapy for diabetic foot infections. Cochrane Database Syst Rev 2009;3:CD006810.


# 127

# INFECTIVE ENDOCARDITIS

Toxic Choices . . . . . . . . . . . . . . . . . . . . . . . . . . Level II


**Tonya L. Crawford, PharmD, BCPS**

**Manjunath P. Pai, PharmD**

**Keith A. Rodvold, PharmD, FCCP**


## LEARNING OBJECTIVES

After completing this case study, the reader should be able to:

- Differentiate the signs and symptoms of infective endocarditis compared to bacteremia.
- Analyze the risks/benefits of the addition of aminoglycosides for treatment of MRSA endocarditis.

- Select appropriate antimicrobial therapy based on a particular organism, the patient's drug allergies, and the patient's social limitations.
- Recognize severe adverse reactions experienced by a patient receiving therapy for infective endocarditis and revise the therapeutic plan.
- Establish monitoring parameters for a selected drug therapy in the treatment of a patient with infective endocarditis.

## PATIENT PRESENTATION

### Chief Complaint

"My heart feels like it is skipping a beat."

### HPI

Zoë French is a 37-year-old woman well known to the ED staff who was found unconscious, cyanotic, and in respiratory distress by EMS personnel. She was revived with a dose of naloxone and transported to the ED. Ms French relays a history of fever, chills, shortness of breath, and chest pain that developed 1 week ago but worsened after injecting heroin a few hours ago. She has been seen in the ED twice this month for chest pain after "snorting" cocaine. She was also admitted 2 months ago for treatment of upper extremity cellulitis.

### PMH

Intermittent asthma (diagnosed 2 years ago)
Hypertension (diagnosed 3 years ago)

### FH

Noncontributory

### SH

Unemployed and homeless; resides in shelters during the winter
Active cocaine and heroin abuse; denies ETOH use, smokes one to two cigarettes per day for past year

### Meds

Propranolol 40 mg po BID
Albuterol inhaler two puffs Q 4 h PRN shortness of breath

### All

Penicillin

### ROS

Noncontributory except for complaints noted in HPI

### Physical Examination

*Gen*

Patient is a caucasian woman in moderate distress. She is alert and oriented to person but not place or date.

*VS*

BP 152/92, P 119, RR 22, T 38.9°C; Wt 62 kg, Ht 5′7″

*Skin/Nails*

Painful, tender, erythematous nodules on pads of fingers, 6–8 mm in size. Painless, erythematous lesions (1–2 mm in size) on lower, right abdomen.

*HEENT*

Nonicteric sclerae, myosis in both eyes, pink conjunctivae, dry oral mucosa, no Roth spots; poor dentition

*Neck/Lymph Nodes*

No lymphadenopathy, JVD, or thyromegaly

*Lungs*

Clear to auscultation; no wheezing

*CV*

RRR, normal $S_1$ and $S_2$, $S_3$ present, III/VI holosystolic murmur

*Abd*

Nontender, nondistended with painless, erythematous lesions (1–2 mm in size) on lower, right abdomen

*Genit/Rect*

Normal; guaiac-negative stool

*Ext*

Reflexes bilaterally 4/5 UE, 3/5 LE; no edema

*Neuro*

Nonfocal; alert and oriented × 1; negative asterixis

### Labs

| | | |
|---|---|---|
| Na 136 mEq/L | Hgb 7.2 g/dL | WBC 13.3 × $10^3$/mm$^3$ |
| K 4.1 mEq/L | Hct 21.6% | Neutros 78% |
| Cl 102 mEq/L | Plt 220 × $10^3$/mm$^3$ | Bands 8% |
| $CO_2$ 25 mEq/L | RDW 14.2% | Lymphs 12% |
| BUN 15 mg/dL | MCV 81.1 μm$^3$ | Monos 2% |
| SCr 0.8 mg/dL | MCH 26.3 pg/cell | Alb 2.1 g/dL |
| Glu 98 mg/dL | MCHC 34 g/dL | INR 1.0 |
| ESR 140 mm/h | | |

### Rapid HIV Test

Pending

### ECG

Nonspecific T-wave changes; prolonged QTc interval

### Chest X-Ray

Normal heart size. Lungs well expanded without opacities or infiltrates.

### Two-Dimensional Echocardiogram (Transthoracic)

Vegetations not visualized on heart valves

### Transesophageal Echocardiogram

Six-millimeter vegetation on the tricuspid valve with severe tricuspid regurgitation. No perivalvular abscess noted. (See Fig. 127-1 for location of heart valves and other cardiac structures.)

### Blood Cultures

Three of three sets (+) for *Staphylococcus aureus* (collection times: 03:40, 03:41, 04:30).

### Assessment

A 37-year-old woman with a history of actively abusing heroin and cocaine, hypertension, asthma, and recent hospitalization for cellulitis presents with *S. aureus* endocarditis (vegetation on tricuspid valve).

Additional problems include uncontrolled hypertension and anemia.

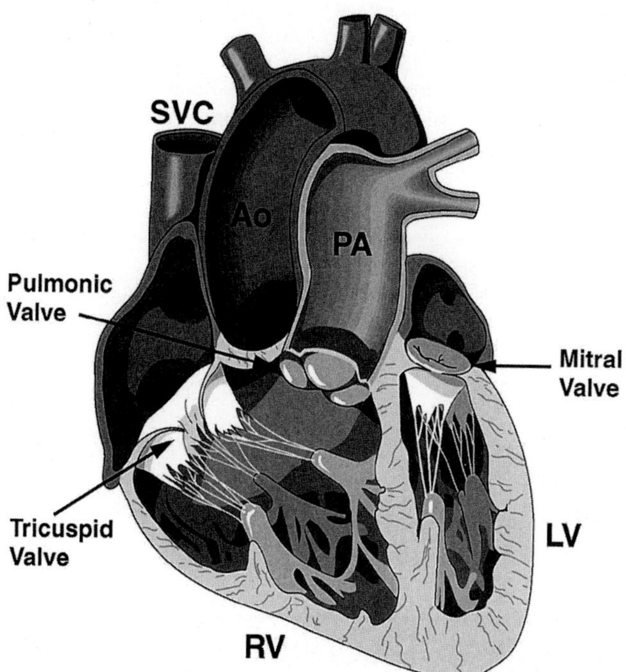


**FIGURE 127-1.** Diagram illustrating the location of the tricuspid, pulmonic, and mitral valves. Ao, aorta; LV, left ventricle; PA, pulmonary artery; RV, right ventricle; SVC, superior vena cava.

## QUESTIONS

### Problem Identification

1.a. Create a list of the patient's drug therapy problems.

1.b. What signs, symptoms, and other information indicate the presence of endocarditis in this patient?

1.c. What risk factors does this patient have for developing endocarditis?

1.d. Based on this patient's risk factors and location of the vegetation, does this patient have right- or left-sided endocarditis, and what is the prognostic relevance of left-sided versus right-sided endocarditis?

1.e. What additional information (laboratory tests or patient information) is needed to satisfactorily assess this patient?

### Desired Outcome

2. What are the goals of pharmacotherapy for infective endocarditis?

### ■ CLINICAL COURSE

The patient was started on empiric vancomycin and gentamicin until susceptibilities for the *S. aureus* isolate became available. Susceptibility testing subsequently showed the organism to be resistant to oxacillin, but sensitive to vancomycin, trimethoprim–sulfamethoxazole, telavancin, quinupristin/dalfopristin, linezolid, tigecycline, and daptomycin. Her HIV antibody EIA test is negative and the Western blot is pending.

### Therapeutic Alternatives

3.a. What nondrug therapies might be useful to treat a patient diagnosed with endocarditis?

3.b. What economic and social considerations are applicable to this patient?

3.c. Identify the therapeutic alternatives for the treatment of *S. aureus* endocarditis based on the organism's susceptibilities. Include the drug names, doses, dosage forms, schedules, and durations of therapy in your answer.

### ■ CLINICAL COURSE

Due to a vancomycin MIC of 2.0 μg/mL, vancomycin is switched to daptomycin 6 mg/kg per day within 48 hours of hospitalization. On Day 5, the patient developed acute kidney injury and gentamicin was discontinued. Her serum creatinine increased from 0.8 to 2.0 mg/dL.

3.d. What information supported the possibility of therapeutic failure in this clinical scenario?

3.e. What clinical literature supports the discontinuation of vancomycin and gentamicin?

3.f. What clinical and laboratory parameters are necessary to evaluate the therapy for achievement of the desired therapeutic outcome and to detect or prevent adverse effects?

### ■ CLINICAL COURSE

MRSA bacteremia clears on Day 5 of therapy and the patient remains on daptomycin 6 mg/kg per day. Her serum creatinine decreased over 7 days and stabilized to 1.4 mg/dL. The patient is transferred to a skilled nursing facility on Day 16. The therapeutic plan is for the patient to complete an additional 2 weeks of therapy. On Day 18, the patient develops symptoms of myopathy. CPK is measured and was recorded to be over 1,000 IU/L.

3.g. Based on your assessment of this patient's response and her past history, what alternatives are available for completing her course of therapy?

### Optimal Plan

4. What drug, dosage form, dose, schedule, and duration of therapy are best for this patient?

### Outcome Evaluation

5.a. What clinical and laboratory parameters are necessary to detect or prevent adverse effects?

### ■ CLINICAL COURSE

While receiving her therapy, the patient's serum creatinine increases from 1.4 to 2.8 mg/dL.

5.a. Based on your assessment of this patient's response, would you recommend changing the patient's current therapeutic plan?

### ■ CLINICAL COURSE

The patient concluded her 4 weeks of therapy (as recommended in response to question 8). Blood cultures continue to report no growth to date. She remains afebrile (24-hour maximum temperature: 36.5°C), her white cell count is normalizing (WBC $8.1 \times 10^3/mm^3$ with no bands), and her ESR has decreased to 18 mm/h. She has been normotensive (BP: 130/80 mm Hg) throughout her hospital and skilled nursing facility stay. She states that she would like to leave the nursing facility. The patient will be discharged later on in the afternoon and has appointments for a follow-up visit with the outpatient clinic.

## Patient Education

6. Prior to the patient being discharged from the nursing facility, what information should be provided to her regarding her outpatient care?

## SELF-STUDY ASSIGNMENTS

1. Evaluate the clinical literature that assesses the risk of nephrotoxicity associated with higher doses of vancomycin (≥4 g per day) and targeted vancomycin concentrations.
2. Compare and contrast the potential safety concerns with the use of linezolid, daptomycin, or telavancin to treat MRSA-related infections for a greater than 14-day duration of therapy.
3. Analyze the clinical literature reporting the clinical outcomes of patients who receive high-dose (≥8 mg/kg) daptomycin for treatment of *S. aureus* infections.

## CLINICAL PEARL

Initiation of gentamicin for treatment of native valve infective *S. aureus* is optional.[2] Recent clinical literature reports an increased risk of nephrotoxicity with the combination therapy of gentamicin and vancomycin or antistaphylococcal agents in comparison to daptomycin monotherapy.[7] Routine use of gentamicin for treatment of native valve endocarditis should be avoided.

## REFERENCES


1. Yung D, Kottachci D, Neupane B, Haider S, Loeb M. Antimicrobials for right-sided endocarditis in intravenous drug users: a systemic review. J Antimicrob Chemother 2007;60(5):921–928.
2. Bonow RO, Carabello BA, Chatterjee K, et al. 2008 focused update incorporated into the ACC/AHA 2006 guidelines for the management of patients with valvular heart disease: a report of the American College of Cardiology/American Heart Association Task Force on Practice Guidelines. Circulation 2008;118(15):e523–e661.
3. Rybak M, Lomaestro B, Rotschafer JC, et al. Therapeutic monitoring of vancomycin in adult patients: a consensus review of the American Society of Health-System Pharmacists, the Infectious Diseases Society of America, and the Society of Infectious Diseases Pharmacists. Am J Health Syst Pharm 2009;66(1):82–98.
4. Fowler VG, Boucher HW, Corey GR, et al. Daptomycin versus standard therapy for bacteremia and endocarditis caused by *Staphylococcus aureus*. N Engl J Med 2006;355(7):653–665.
5. Markowitz N, Quinn EL, Saravolatz LD. Trimethoprim–sulfamethoxazole compared with vancomycin for the treatment of *Staphylococcus aureus* infection. Ann Intern Med 1992;117(5):390–398.
6. Sakoulas G, Moise-Broder PA, Schentag J, Forrest A, Moellering R, Eliopoulos GM. Relationship of MIC and bactericidal activity to efficacy of vancomycin for treatment of methicillin-resistant *Staphylococcus aureus* bacteremia. J Clin Microbiol 2004;42(6):2398–2402.
7. Cosgrove SE, Vigliani GA, Fowler VG Jr, et al. Initial low-dose gentamicin for *Staphylococcus aureus* bacteremia and endocarditis is nephrotoxic. Clin Infect Dis 2009;48(6):713–721.
8. Madrigal AG, Basuino L, Chambers HF. Efficacy of telavancin in a rabbit model of aortic valve endocarditis due to methicillin-resistant *Staphlyococcus aureus* or vancomycin-intermediate *Staphylococcus aureus*. Antimicrob Agents Chemother 2005;49(8):3163–3165.
9. Hidayat LK, Hsu DI, Quist R, Shriner KA, Wong-Beringer A. High-dose vancomycin therapy for methicillin-resistant *Staphylococcus aureus* infections: efficacy and toxicity. Arch Intern Med 2006;166(19):2138–2144.
10. Stryjewski ME, Graham DR, Wilson SE, et al. Telavancin versus vancomycin for the treatment of complicated skin and skin-structure infections caused by gram-positive organisms. Clin Infect Dis 2008;46(11):1683–1693.


# 128

# TUBERCULOSIS

Close Encounters . . . . . . . . . . . . . . . . . . . . . . . Level II

**Sharon M. Erdman, PharmD**

**Kendra M. Atkinson, PharmD**

## LEARNING OBJECTIVES

After completing this case study, the reader should be able to:

- Recognize the typical signs and symptoms of pulmonary tuberculosis.
- Design a therapeutic regimen for the treatment of a patient with newly diagnosed pulmonary tuberculosis based on the presenting signs and symptoms of infection, history of present illness, subjective and objective clinical findings, and desired clinical response.
- Develop a monitoring plan that should be employed during the treatment of pulmonary tuberculosis to ensure efficacy and prevent toxicity.
- Provide patient education on the proper administration of drug therapy for pulmonary tuberculosis including directions for use, the administration of therapy in relation to meals, the importance of adherence, and potential side effects of the medications.
- Recognize potential drug interactions that may occur with agents used in the treatment of pulmonary tuberculosis.

## PATIENT PRESENTATION

### Chief Complaint

"I have been coughing up blood for the past 3 days."

### HPI

Jose Rodriguez is a 35-year-old Hispanic man who presents to the emergency department at the county hospital in Indianapolis, Indiana, with a 3- to 4-week history of a productive cough, which was originally productive of yellow sputum but is now accompanied by the presence of blood in the sputum for the past 3 days. Along with the cough, the patient also complains of subjective fevers, chills, night sweats, dyspnea, pleuritic chest pain, fatigue, and an unintentional 20-lb weight loss over the past several weeks. The patient moved to the United States from Mexico 4 years ago and has not recently traveled.

### PMH

None

## FH

Mother has DM and HTN.
Father died of MI 6 months ago.

## SH

Patient has a 10 pack-year history of smoking but quit several weeks ago when the current illness started. The patient denies illicit drug use, but does report drinking alcohol on weekends.

Patient is a laborer and is currently working for cash on a new home construction project in close contact with other workers. Several of his coworkers have recently moved to the United States from Mexico and have similar respiratory symptoms. The patient does not have any medical insurance.

Patient is homeless and stays at homeless shelters or friends' houses as needed.

## Meds

OTC antitussives, which have not provided any relief

## All

No known drug allergies

## ROS

Patient complains of a productive cough with hemoptysis for the past few days. He also complains of shortness of breath that worsens with exertion, pleuritic chest pain, subjective fevers, chills, night sweats, fatigue, and a 20-lb weight loss over the past several weeks.

## Physical Examination

### *Gen*

Somewhat thin-appearing Hispanic male in mild respiratory distress

### *VS*

BP 131/70, P 94, RR 24, T 38.8°C, 93% $O_2$ saturation in room air; Wt 68 kg, Ht 5′9″

### *Skin*

No lesions

### *HEENT*

PERRLA, EOMI, no scleral icterus

### *Neck*

Supple

### *Chest*

Bronchial breath sounds in RUL

### *CV*

Slightly tachycardic, no MRG

### *Abd*

Soft NTND; (+) bowel sounds; no hepatosplenomegaly

### *Ext*

No CCE, pulses 2+ throughout; full ROM

### *Neuro*

A & O × 3; CN II–XII intact; reflexes 2+, sensory and motor levels intact

## Labs

| | | | |
|---|---|---|---|
| Na 143 mEq/L | Hgb 11.6 g/dL | WBC 12.3 × $10^3$/mm$^3$ | Bili 0.6 mg/dL |
| K 3.7 mEq/L | Hct 34.8% | Neutros 74% | Alk phos 120 U/L |
| Cl 106 mEq/L | RBC 3.8 × $10^6$/mm$^3$ | Bands 8% | ALT 45 IU/L |
| $CO_2$ 22 mEq/L | Plt 269 × $10^3$/mm$^3$ | Lymphs 10% | AST 34 IU/L |
| BUN 21 mg/dL | MCV 92 μm$^3$ | Monos 8% | |
| SCr 0.9 mg/dL | MCHC 33 g/dL | | |
| Glu 101 mg/dL | | | |

PPD skin test result: Pending
Sputum AFB stain: Numerous AFB (Fig. 128-1)

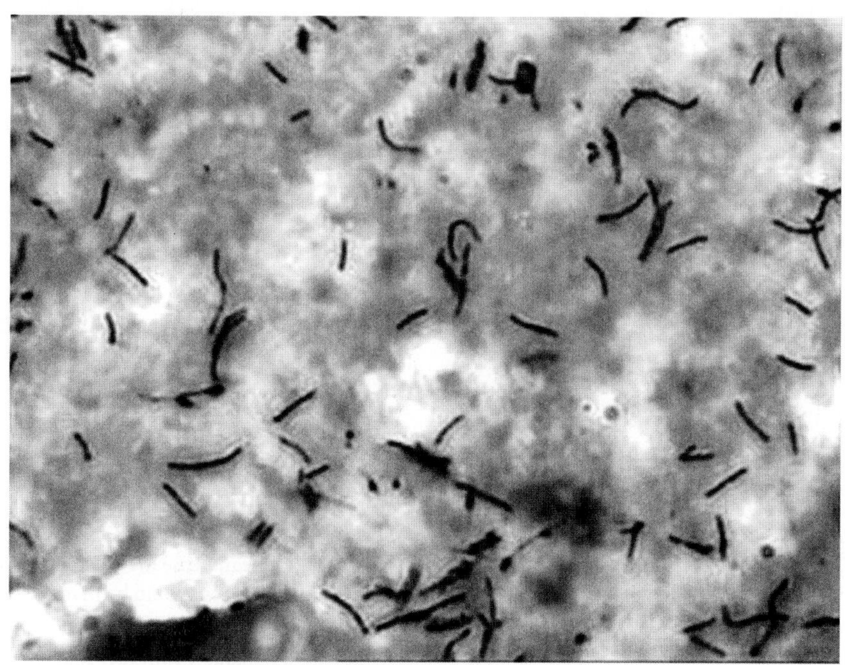

**FIGURE 128-1.** Acid-fast bacilli (AFB) smear. AFB (*shown as thin rods*) are tubercle bacilli.

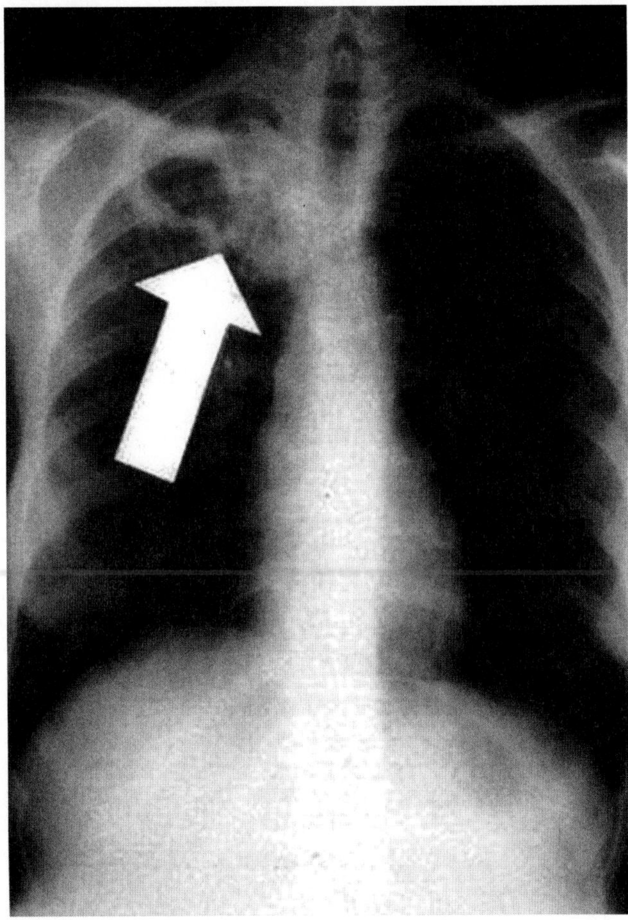

**FIGURE 128-2.** Chest radiograph. *Arrow* points to cavitation in patient's upper right lobe.

Sputum AFB culture: Pending
HIV antibody test (ELISA and Western blot): Pending

### Radiology

CXR: RUL consolidation and cavitary lesion (Fig. 128-2)

Chest CT: Focal airspace disease in the RUL, including a cavitary lesion measuring 3.5 cm × 3.5 cm. Right hilar lymphadenopathy with scattered mediastinal lymphadenopathy. There is no pleural effusion or pneumothorax. Findings are consistent with active tuberculosis infection.

### Assessment

Active pulmonary tuberculosis

## QUESTIONS

### Problem Identification

1.a. What clinical, laboratory, and radiographic findings are consistent with the diagnosis of active pulmonary tuberculosis in this patient?

1.b. What factors place this patient at increased risk for acquiring TB?

### Desired Outcome

2. What are the therapeutic goals in the treatment of active pulmonary tuberculosis?

### Therapeutic Alternatives

3.a. What nonpharmacologic therapies should be considered in the management of a patient with active pulmonary tuberculosis?

3.b. What are the general principles of therapy in the management of active pulmonary tuberculosis?

3.c. What pharmacologic therapies and dosing strategies are available for the treatment of active pulmonary tuberculosis?

### Optimal Plan

4.a. What specific drug regimen should be used for the treatment of this patient's active pulmonary tuberculosis, including the drugs, dosage forms, doses, schedules, and duration of therapy? Include regimens that employ twice- or thrice-weekly administration of antituberculosis medications.

4.b. What economic and social considerations are applicable to this patient?

4.c. How should other close contacts of the patient be evaluated and treated?

### Outcome Evaluation

5. What clinical and laboratory parameters should be monitored to evaluate the efficacy of therapy and to detect or prevent adverse effects?

### Patient Education

6. What information should be provided to the patient to ensure successful therapy, enhance adherence, minimize adverse effects, and avoid drug interactions?

## CLINICAL COURSE

The patient was admitted to the hospital for appropriate management, including placement in a negative-pressure hospital room to provide respiratory isolation. Because the initial sputum sample demonstrated the presence of numerous AFB, the patient was started on the antituberculosis therapy you recommended while waiting for the results of culture and susceptibility tests. On hospital day 2, his PPD skin test was positive measuring 20 mm, and his HIV test was negative. The patient tolerated the antituberculosis regimen during the initial weeks of therapy, and subsequent sputum AFB smears became negative 2 weeks after the initiation of therapy. The sputum AFB culture eventually grew *Mycobacterium tuberculosis*, which was susceptible to isoniazid, rifampin, pyrazinamide, ethambutol, and streptomycin. During the third week of antituberculosis therapy, an increase in the patient's AST and ALT was noted, although the patient appeared asymptomatic. The AST increased to 140 IU/L, and the ALT increased to 120 IU/L. The total bilirubin and alkaline phosphatase remained within normal limits. Follow-up mycobacterial sputum cultures obtained after 2 months of antituberculosis therapy were negative.

## FOLLOW-UP QUESTIONS

1. How should the results of the susceptibility report of this patient's *M. tuberculosis* isolate influence his drug therapy?
2. How should the increase in AST and ALT in this patient be managed? What changes should be made to the current antituberculosis regimen and/or monitoring plan?
3. How should a patient with AST and ALT elevations greater than five times the upper limit of normal be managed?

## SELF-STUDY ASSIGNMENTS

1. Review the safety and efficacy of rifapentine in the management of active pulmonary tuberculosis.
2. Perform a literature search to determine the national and regional rates of isoniazid resistance in clinical isolates of *M. tuberculosis*. How do these rates compare to those reported in other areas of the world where tuberculosis is endemic?
3. Review the management strategies of active pulmonary tuberculosis in an HIV-infected patient on antiretroviral therapy, with special attention to potential drug interactions between first-line antituberculosis agents and the non-nucleoside reverse transcriptase inhibitors or protease inhibitors.

## CLINICAL PEARL

The treatment of tuberculosis in patients with HIV infection is often modified based on the many drug interactions that can occur among the rifamycins and antiretroviral agents.

## REFERENCES

1. Quast TM, Browning RF. Pathogenesis and clinical manifestations of pulmonary tuberculosis. Dis Mon 2006;52:413–419.
2. American Thoracic Society, Centers for Disease Control and Prevention, Infectious Diseases Society of America. Controlling tuberculosis in the United States. Am J Respir Crit Care Med 2005;172:1169–1227.
3. American Thoracic Society. Targeted tuberculin testing and treatment of latent tuberculosis infection. Am J Respir Crit Care Med 2000; 161:S221–S247.
4. American Thoracic Society, Centers for Disease Control and Prevention, Infectious Diseases Society of America. Treatment of tuberculosis. Am J Respir Crit Care Med 2003;167:603–662.
5. Gleeson TD, Decker CF. Treatment of tuberculosis. Dis Mon 2006; 52:428–434.
6. Palomino JC. Newer diagnostics for tuberculosis and multi-drug resistant tuberculosis. Curr Opin Pulm Med 2006;12:172–178.
7. Munsiff SS, Kambili C, Ahuja SD. Rifapentine for the treatment of pulmonary tuberculosis. Clin Infect Dis 2006;43:1468–1475.
8. Chang KC, Leung CC, Yew WW, Chan SL, Tam CM. Dosing schedules of 6-month regimens and relapse for pulmonary tuberculosis. Am J Respir Crit Care Med 2006;174:1153–1158.
9. Saukkonen JJ, Cohn DL, Jasmer RM, et al. An official ATS statement: hepatotoxicity of antituberculosis therapy. Am J Respir Crit Care Med 2006;174:935–952.

# 129

# *CLOSTRIDIUM DIFFICILE* INFECTION

*C. diff*-icult to Treat. . . . . . . . . . . . . . . . . . . . . . Level II

**Michael J. Gonyeau, BS, PharmD, BCPS**

## LEARNING OBJECTIVES

After completing this case study, the reader should be able to:

- Identify signs and symptoms of clostridium difficile infection (CDI).
- Discuss CDI complications.
- Evaluate treatment options and develop an optimal patient-specific treatment plan for initial and recurrent CDI including drug, dose, frequency, route of administration, and duration of therapy.
- Develop a pertinent monitoring plan for a CDI regimen from a therapeutic and toxic standpoint.
- Discuss novel agents being developed for CDI treatment.

## PATIENT PRESENTATION

### Chief Complaint

"I have been having to go to the bathroom a lot more frequently, and my stomach hurts a lot."

### HPI

John Quinn, a 73 yo man, is transferred to your medical team from the MICU after being admitted for urosepsis and hypotension requiring pressor support. Over the past 2 days, he has been complaining of frequent foul-smelling stools. One week prior to being transferred to your team, he was admitted to the hospital complaining of urinary frequency and urgency for 3 days, nausea, vomiting, and left-sided flank pain, as well as lightheadedness and dizziness. In the ED, the patient was noted to be hypotensive (BP 92/63 mm Hg) and tachycardic (HR 112–124), with an elevated lactate level and leukocytosis. He was transferred to the MICU for pressor support and started on an empiric regimen of ceftriaxone 2 g IV daily, levofloxacin 750 mg IV daily, and vancomycin 1 g IV Q 12 h for diagnosed urosepsis. Urine (×2) and blood (×3) cultures were subsequently found to be growing *E. coli* and enteric gram-negative rods, respectively, and antibiotic coverage was narrowed to ceftriaxone 2 g IV daily on day 5. The patient's blood pressure was stabilized, and he was transferred to the internal medicine service on day 7 of hospitalization. He is now complaining of new-onset diarrhea and abdominal pain, as described above.

### PMH

Type 2 DM
Hyperlipidemia
HTN
s/p MI 2003

### SH

Lives at home alone, lifetime smoker (half pack per day for 54 years), drinks alcohol socially

### Medications

Metoprolol XL 100 mg po once daily
Amlodipine 5 mg po once daily
Pravastatin 20 mg po once daily
Omeprazole 20 mg po once daily
Metformin 500 mg po twice daily

### All

NKDA

### Physical Examination

*Gen*

Patient is overweight and complains of abdominal discomfort.

*VS*

BP 139/85; P 98; RR 20; T 38.8°C; Ht 5′8″; Wt 87.2 kg

*Skin*

Warm and moist secondary to diaphoresis, no lesions

*HEENT*

PERRLA; EOMI; TMs intact; clear oropharynx, moist oral mucosa

*Neck/Lymph Nodes*

Neck is supple and without adenopathy; no JVD

*Lungs/Thorax*

CTA

*CV*

RRR; normal $S_1$, $S_2$; no murmurs

*Abd*

Abdomen is soft and nondistended, diffusely tender to palpation. Slight rebound and guarding. Positive bowel sounds.

*Genit/Rect*

Not performed

*MS/Ext*

Muscle strength and tone 5/5 in upper and lower; no C/C/E

*Neuro*

A & O × 3; CN II–XII intact

### Labs

| | | | |
|---|---|---|---|
| Na 138 mEq/L | Hgb 16.1 g/dL | WBC 16.9 × $10^3$/mm$^3$ | T. chol 205 mg/dL |
| K 3.5 mEq/L | Hct 49.8% | Neutros 50% | LDL 137 mg/dL |
| Cl 102 mEq/L | Plt 375 × $10^3$/mm$^3$ | Bands 9% | HDL 29 mg/dL |
| $CO_2$ 22 mEq/L | A1C 7.9% | Eos 0% | Trig 197 mg/dL |
| BUN 36 mg/dL | | Lymphs 34% | |
| SCr 1.8 mg/dL (baseline 0.9 mg/dL) | | Monos 7% | |
| Glu 181 mg/dL | | | |
| Alb 1.9 mg/dL | | | |

**CXR:** Clear
**EKG:** NSR, unchanged from previous
***Clostridium difficile* toxin EIA test:** A/B toxin assay positive
**Fecal leukocytes:** Not performed

### Assessment

A 73 yo man presents with frequent, foul-smelling stools for 2 days with recent history of having received broad-spectrum antibiotics and currently receiving ceftriaxone for urosepsis (day 9); *C. difficile* toxin positive.

# QUESTIONS

## Problem Identification

1.a. Create a list of the patient's drug therapy problems.

1.b. How common is CDI in hospitalized patients?

1.c. What risk factors for CDI are present in this patient?

1.d. What information (signs, symptoms, laboratory values) indicates the presence of CDI?

1.e. Which antibiotics are most likely to cause CDI?

## Desired Outcome

2. What are the goals of pharmacotherapy in this case?

## Therapeutic Alternatives

3.a. What nonpharmacologic strategies would be prudent to implement in this patient?

3.b. List available options for treating CDI in this patient. Include the drug name, dose, dosage form, route, frequency, and treatment duration.

# CLINICAL COURSE

Metronidazole 500 mg po every 8 hours was initiated. Two days after starting metronidazole, the patient continued to have frequent foul-smelling stools, diffuse cramping and abdominal pain, and mild fever. A subsequent *C. difficile* toxin EIA test remained positive. At that time, metronidazole was changed to 500 mg po every 6 hours and cholestyramine 2 g po every 8 hours was initiated.

## Optimal Plan

4.a. Your medical team wants to start the patient on loperamide 2 mg po after each bowel movement. Do you agree with this course of action? Why or why not?

4.b. Was the initial therapy appropriate in this case? Why or why not?

4.c. Outline your plans for managing each of the patient's other drug therapy problems.

## Outcome Evaluation

5. What clinical and laboratory parameters are necessary to evaluate the therapy for achievement of the desired therapeutic outcome and detect or prevent adverse effects?

## Patient Education

6. What information should be provided to the patient to enhance adherence, ensure successful therapy, and minimize adverse effects?

# FOLLOW-UP QUESTIONS

1. What if our patient does not respond to initial therapy?
2. What if our patient develops similar signs and symptoms 3 weeks after successful CDI treatment?

# SELF-STUDY ASSIGNMENTS

1. Develop a plan for assessing need for rehydration therapy in patients presenting with CDI, and discuss the pros and cons of available drug and nondrug options.
2. Conduct a literature search and develop a policy regarding infection control procedures to reduce the risk of CDI.
3. Conduct a literature search and outline treatment options for a patient who develops fulminant *C. difficile* colitis.
4. Conduct a literature search to assess the potential role of tolevamer in the treatment of CDI.

## CLINICAL PEARL

CDIs are an increasing concern in hospitalized patients due to increased incidence of highly toxigenic and treatment-resistant strains. There are a number of additional antibiotics or antiprotozoal agents under investigation for treatment of CDI including nitazoxanide, tinidazole, fidaxomicin, and ramoplanin. Their clinical effectiveness looks promising, but their place in therapy is still to be determined.[17,18]

## REFERENCES

1. Loo VG, Poirier L, Miller MA. A predominantly clonal multi-institutional outbreak of *Clostridium difficile*-associated diarrhea with high morbidity and mortality. N Engl J Med 2005;353:2442–2449 [erratum, N Engl J Med 2006;354:2200].
2. Voelker R. Increased *Clostridium difficile* virulence demands new treatment approach. JAMA 2010;303(20):2017–2019.
3. Warny M, Pepin J, Fang A. Toxin production by an emerging strain of *Clostridium difficile* associated with outbreaks of severe disease in North America and Europe. Lancet 2005:366(9491):1079–1084.
4. McDonald LD, Owings M, Jernigan DB. *Clostridium difficile* infection in patients discharged from US short-stay hospitals, 1996–2003. Emerg Infect Dis 2006;12:409–415.
5. McDonald LC, Killgore GE, Thompson A, et al. An epidemic, toxin gene–variant strain of *Clostridium difficile*. N Engl J Med 2005;353:2433–2441.
6. Cohen SH, Gerding DN, Johnson S et al. Clinical practice guidelines for *Clostridium difficile* infection in adults: 2010 update by the Society for Healthcare Epidemiology of America (SHEA) and the Infectious Diseases Society of America (IDSA). Infect Control Hosp Epidemiol 2010;31:431–455.
7. Musher DM, Aslam S, Logan N, et al. Relatively poor outcome after treatment of *Clostridium difficile* colitis with metronidazole. Clin Infect Dis 2005;40:1586–1590.
8. Zar FA, Bakkanagari SR, Moorthi KM, Davis MB. A comparison of vancomycin and metronidazole for the treatment of *Clostridium difficile*–associated diarrhea, stratified by disease severity. Clin Infect Dis 2007;45(3):302–307.
9. Aas J, Gessert CE, Bakken JS. Recurrent *Clostridium difficile* colitis: case series involving 18 patients treated with donor stool administered via a nasogastric tube. Clin Infect Dis 2003;36(5):580–585.
10. Louie T, Gerson M, Grimard D, et al. Results of a phase III trial comparing tolevamer, vancomycin and metronidazole in patients with *Clostridium difficile*–associated diarrhea (CDI). In: 47th Annual Interscience Conference on Antimicrobial Agents and Chemotherapy Meeting, Chicago, IL, September 17–20, 2007 [abstract].
11. Cone LA, Lopez C, Tarleton HL, et al. A durable response to relapsing *Clostridium difficile* colitis may requires combined therapy with high dose oral vancomycin and intravenous immune globulin. Infect Dis Clin Pract 2006;14:217–220.
12. Johnson S, Schriever C, Galang M, Kelly CP, Gerding DN. Interruption of recurrent *Clostridium difficile*–associated diarrhea episodes by serial therapy with vancomycin and rifaximin. Clin Infect Dis 2007;44(6):846–848.
13. American Diabetes Association. Executive summary: standards of medical care in diabetes—2010. Diabetes Care 2010;33(Suppl 1):S4–S10.
14. Joint National Committee on Prevention, Detection, Evaluation, Treatment of High Blood Pressure. The seventh report of the Joint National Committee on Prevention, Detection, Evaluation, Treatment of High Blood Pressure. Arch Intern Med 2003;42:1206–1252.
15. Expert Panel on Detection, Evaluation, and Treatment of High Blood Cholesterol in Adults. Executive summary of the third report of the National Cholesterol Education Program (NCEP) Expert Panel on Detection, Evaluation, and Treatment of High Blood Cholesterol in Adults (Adult Treatment Panel III). JAMA 2001;285:2486–2497.
16. Kelly C. A 76-year-old man with recurrent *Clostridium difficile*–associated diarrhea. JAMA 2009;301(9):954–962.
17. Bartlett JG. New drugs for *Clostridium difficile* infection. Clin Infect Dis 2006;43:428–431.
18. Hecht DW, Galang MA, Sambol SP, et al. In vitro activities of 15 antimicrobial agents against 110 toxigenic *Clostridium difficile* clinical isolates collected from 1983 to 2004. Antimicrob Agents Chemother 2007;51:2716–2719.

# 130

# INTRA-ABDOMINAL INFECTION

Like Mother, Like Son . . . . . . . . . . . . . . . . . . . Level II

**Renee-Claude Mercier, PharmD, BCPS, PhC**

**Paulina Deming, PharmD, PhC**

## LEARNING OBJECTIVES

After completing this case study, the reader should be able to:

- Recognize the clinical manifestations of bacterial peritonitis.
- Identify the normal microflora found in the various segments of the GI tract.
- List the goals of antimicrobial therapy for bacterial peritonitis.
- Recommend appropriate empiric and definitive antibiotic therapy for primary bacterial peritonitis (also known as spontaneous bacterial peritonitis).
- Monitor antibiotic therapy for safety and efficacy.
- Recommend secondary prophylaxis for primary bacterial peritonitis.
- Establish a long-term plan for the patient regarding alcohol abuse and hepatitis C, including monitoring parameters and counseling.

## PATIENT PRESENTATION

### Chief Complaint

"My belly hurts so bad I can barely move."

### HPI

John Chavez is a 47-year-old Hispanic man who was brought to the ED by his wife. She stated that he has been suffering from nausea, vomiting, and severe abdominal pain, and has been acting "goofy" for the last 2–3 days. His intake of food and fluids has been minimal over the past several days. He is a well-known patient of the ED who often presents with alcohol intoxication and severe hepatic encephalopathy.

### PMH

Cirrhosis with ascites for the last 2 years
Hepatic encephalopathy
GERD
HTN
Cholecystectomy 15 years ago

Hepatitis C+ × 4 years
Spontaneous bacterial peritonitis—one episode 9 months ago

### FH

Mother was alcoholic; died 10 years ago in car accident. Father's history unknown.

### SH

Retired construction worker; ETOH abuse with 10–12 cans of beer per day × 25 years; denies use of tobacco or illicit drugs; has several nonprofessional tattoos; poor adherence to medications and dietary restrictions

### Meds

Lactulose 30 mL po QID PRN
Amlodipine 10 mg po once daily
Inderal LA 80 mg po once daily
Spironolactone 100 mg po once daily
Omeprazole 20 mg po once daily
Maalox 30 mL po QID PRN

### All

NKDA

### ROS

As noted in the HPI

### Physical Examination

*Gen*

Elderly man who appears older than his stated age and is in severe pain

*VS*

BP 154/82, P 102, RR 32, T 38.2°C; current Wt 92 kg, IBW 68 kg

*Skin*

Jaundiced, warm, coarse, and very dry. Spider angiomata present.

*HEENT*

Yellow sclerae; PERRLA; EOMI; funduscopic exam is normal. Tympanic membranes are clouded bilaterally, but with no erythema or bulging. Oropharynges show poor dentition but are otherwise unremarkable.

*Neck/Lymph Nodes*

Supple; normal size thyroid; no JVD or palpable lymph nodes

*Chest*

Lungs are CTA; shallow and frequent breathing

*Heart*

Tachycardia, normal $S_1$ and $S_2$ with no $S_3$ or $S_4$

*Abd*

Distended; pain on pressure or movements; pain is sharp and diffuse throughout abdomen; (+) guarding. (+) HSM. Decreased bowel sounds.

*Genit/Rect*

Prostate normal size; guaiac (−) stool

*Ext*

Unremarkable

*Neuro*

Oriented × 2 (time and person); lethargic and apathetic, slumped posture, slowed movements. CN II–XII intact. Motor system intact; overall muscle strength equal to 4–5/5; poor coordination and gait. Sensory system intact. Reflexes 3+.

### Labs

| | | |
|---|---|---|
| Na 142 mEq/L | Hgb 13.1 g/dL | AST 290 IU/L |
| K 3.9 mEq/L | Hct 40.6% | ALT 320 IU/L |
| Cl 96 mEq/L | Plt 101 × $10^3$/mm$^3$ | Alk phos 350 IU/L |
| $CO_2$ 20 mEq/L | WBC 12.25 × $10^3$/mm$^3$ | T. bili 3.2 mg/dL |
| BUN 44 mg/dL | Neutros 73% | D. bili 1.4 mg/dL |
| SCr 1.1 mg/dL | Bands 9% | Albumin 2.8 g/dL |
| Glu 101 mg/dL | Lymphs 13% | INR 1.34 |
| | Monos 5% | |

### Abdominal X-Ray

No evidence of free air

### Chest X-Ray

No infiltrates; heart normal size and shape

### Blood Cultures

Pending × 2

### Paracentesis

Ascitic fluid: leukocytes 720/mm$^3$, protein 2.8 g/dL, albumin 1.6 g/dL, pH 7.28, lactate 30 mg/dL. Gram stain: numerous PMNs, no organisms.

### Assessment

Primary bacterial peritonitis

## CLINICAL COURSE

Because of the recent low intake of food and fluids and the high BUN-to-creatinine ratio, the patient was thought to be dehydrated and was given 1 L/h of 0.9% NaCl IV in the ED. His breathing became progressively worse, and he had to be intubated and transferred to the intensive care unit.

## QUESTIONS

### Problem Identification

1.a. Create a list of the patient's drug therapy problems.

1.b. What signs, symptoms, and laboratory values indicate the presence of primary bacterial peritonitis?

1.c. What risk factors for infection are present in this patient?

1.d. Which organisms are the most likely cause of this infection?

### Desired Outcome

2. What are the therapeutic goals for this patient?

### Therapeutic Alternatives

3.a. What nondrug therapies might be useful for this patient?

3.b. What feasible pharmacotherapeutic alternatives are available for the treatment of primary bacterial peritonitis?

## Optimal Plan

4.a. Given this patient's condition, which drug regimens would provide optimal therapy for the infection?

4.b. In addition to antimicrobial therapy, what other drug-related interventions are required for this patient?

## Outcome Evaluation

5. What clinical and laboratory parameters are necessary to evaluate the therapy for achievement of the desired therapeutic outcome and to detect or prevent adverse effects?

## Patient Education

6. What information should be provided to the patient to enhance adherence, ensure successful therapy, and minimize adverse effects?

## CLINICAL COURSE

After 48 hours of IV antibiotics, Mr Chavez was extubated. The blood cultures were reported positive for *Klebsiella pneumoniae*, resistant to ampicillin and ampicillin/sulbactam, and sensitive to aztreonam, ceftriaxone, levofloxacin, and piperacillin/tazobactam. The ascitic fluid culture grew *K. pneumoniae* as well. He received cefotaxime 2 g IV Q 8 h for a total of 10 days. After 3 days of antimicrobial treatment, repeat blood cultures were negative. He rapidly improved, and on discharge his mental status had returned to baseline.

## SELF-STUDY ASSIGNMENTS

1. Develop a table that illustrates the primary differences (clinical manifestations, pathogens involved, diagnosis methods, and treatment) between primary and secondary bacterial peritonitis.
2. Describe risk factors, clinical signs and symptoms, modes of transmission, diagnostic methods, prognosis, and therapeutic options associated with hepatitis C.

## CLINICAL PEARL

Bacteremia is present in up to 75% of patients with primary peritonitis caused by aerobic bacteria but is rarely found in those with peritonitis caused by anaerobes. Ascitic fluid cultures are often negative and a diagnosis of SBP is frequently made based on ascitic fluid PMN counts and the patient's clinical presentation.

## REFERENCES

1. Runyon BA, McHutchison JG, Antillon MR, Akriviadis EA, Montano AA. Short-course versus long-course antibiotic treatment of spontaneous bacterial peritonitis: a randomized controlled study of 100 patients. Gastroenterology 1991;100:1737–1742.
2. Runyon BA. American Association for the Study of Liver Diseases (AASLD) practice guidelines: management of adult patients with ascites due to cirrhosis: an update. Hepatology 2009;49:2087–2107.
3. Parsi MA, Atreja A, Zein NN. Spontaneous bacterial peritonitis: recent data on incidence and treatment. Cleve Clin J Med 2004;71:569–576.
4. Felisart J, Rimola A, Arroyo V, et al. Cefotaxime is more effective than is ampicillin–tobramycin in cirrhotics with severe infections. Hepatology 1985;5:457–462.
5. Garcia-Tsao G, Lim J, Veterans Affairs Hepatitis C Resource Center Program. Management and treatment of patients with cirrhosis and portal hypertension: recommendations from the department of Veterans Affairs Hepatitis C Resource Center Program and the National Hepatitis C Program. Am J Gastroenterol 2009;104:1802–1829.
6. Such J, Runyon BA. Spontaneous bacterial peritonitis. Clin Infect Dis 1998;27:669–676.
7. Sort P, Navasa M, Arroyo V, et al. Effect of intravenous albumin on renal impairment and mortality in patients with cirrhosis and spontaneous bacterial peritonitis. N Engl J Med 1999;341:403–409.
8. Sigal SH, Stanca CM, Fernandez J, Arroyo V, Navasa M. Restricted use of albumin for spontaneous bacterial peritonitis. Gut 2007;56:597–599.

# 131

# LOWER URINARY TRACT INFECTION

Where Is the Bathroom? . . . . . . . . . . . . . . . . . . Level I

Sharon M. Erdman, PharmD

Keith A. Rodvold, PharmD, FCCP

## LEARNING OBJECTIVES

After completing this case study, the reader should be able to:

- Recognize the typical signs and symptoms of an uncomplicated UTI in females.
- Design a therapeutic regimen for the treatment of a patient with acute uncomplicated cystitis after consideration of symptoms, medical history, allergies, objective findings, and desired clinical response.
- Describe parameters that should be monitored during the treatment of acute uncomplicated cystitis to ensure efficacy and prevent toxicity.
- Provide patient education on the proper administration of drug therapy for acute uncomplicated cystitis, including directions for use, the administration of therapy in relation to meals, the importance of medication adherence (including the need to complete the entire prescribed course), proper storage, and potential side effects of the medication.

## PATIENT PRESENTATION.

### Chief Complaint

"It burns when I urinate, and I am urinating all the time."

### HPI

Sarah Ramsey is a 26-year-old woman who presents to a family practice clinic in Seattle with complaints of dysuria, urinary frequency and urgency, and suprapubic tenderness for the past 2 days.

### PMH

Patient has been diagnosed with three UTIs over the past 8 months based on symptoms, each treated with TMP–SMX.

### FH

Mother has DM; remainder of FH is noncontributory.

### SH

Denies smoking but admits to occasional marijuana use and social ETOH use. Patient has been sexually active with one partner for the past 9 months and typically uses spermicide-coated condoms for contraception.

### Meds

None

### All

No known allergies

### ROS

Patient reports urethral pain and burning with urination, as well as mild suprapubic tenderness. Patient denies systemic symptoms such as fever, chills, vomiting, or back pain, and does not report any urethral or vaginal discharge. Patient notes that the UTIs seemed to have started soon after she met her boyfriend, and she does not always completely empty her bladder after sexual intercourse.

### Physical Examination

*Gen*

Cooperative woman in no acute distress

*VS*

BP 110/60, P 68, R 16, T 36.8°C; Wt 57 kg, Ht 5′5″

*Skin*

No skin lesions

*HEENT*

PERRLA; EOMI; TMs intact

*Neck/Lymph Nodes*

Supple without lymphadenopathy

*Chest*

CTA

*CV*

RRR, no MRG

*Back*

No CVA tenderness

*Abd*

Soft; (+) bowel sounds; no organomegaly or tenderness

*Pelvic*

No vaginal discharge or lesions; LMP 2 weeks ago; mild suprapubic tenderness

*Ext*

Pulses 2+ throughout; full ROM

*Neuro*

A & O × 3; CN II–XII intact; reflexes 2+; sensory and motor levels intact

### Labs

*Urinalysis from Urine Sample Taken in Clinic*

Yellow, cloudy; pH 5.0; WBC 10–15 cells/hpf; RBC 1–5 cells/hpf; protein neg; trace blood; glucose (−); leukocyte esterase (+); nitrite positive; many bacteria (Fig. 131-1)

*Urine Culture*

Not performed

### Assessment

Acute uncomplicated cystitis (Fig. 131-2)

## QUESTIONS

### Problem Identification

1.a. What clinical and laboratory findings are consistent with the diagnosis of acute uncomplicated cystitis in this patient?

1.b. How is the clinical presentation and diagnostic approach to acute uncomplicated cystitis different from that of urethritis (caused by *Chlamydia trachomatis*, *Neisseria gonorrhoeae*, or herpes simplex virus) or vaginitis (caused by *Candida* or *Trichomonas* species)?

1.c. Should urine cultures be obtained in patients with in acute uncomplicated cystitis?

1.d. What are the most common causative pathogens of acute uncomplicated cystitis in females including their frequency of causing infection?

1.e. What are the risk factors for the development of acute uncomplicated cystitis?

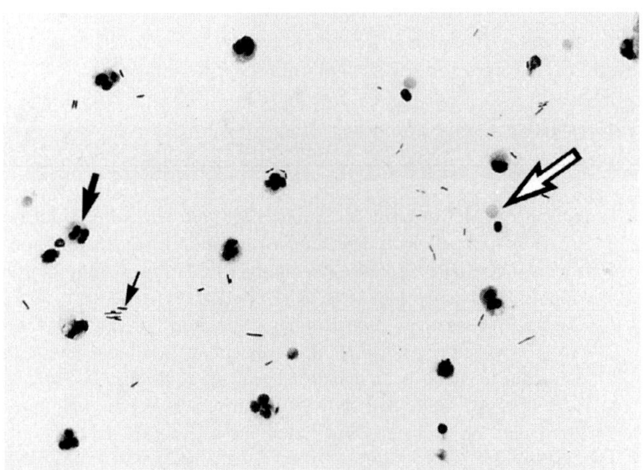

**FIGURE 131-1.** Urine sediment with neutrophils (*solid arrow*), bacteria (*small arrow*), and occasional red blood cells (*open arrow*) (Wright–Giemsa × 1,650). (*Photo courtesy of Lydia C. Contis, MD.*)

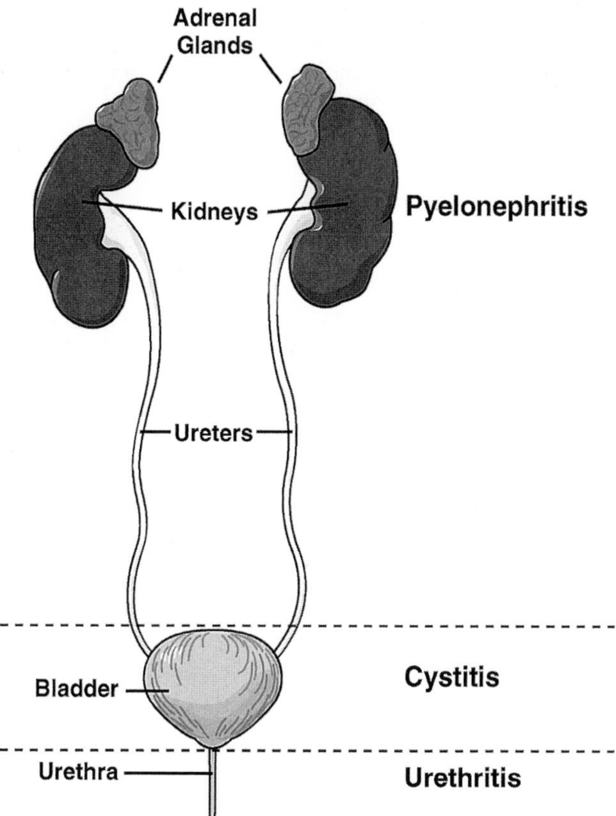


**FIGURE 131-2.** Anatomy and associated infections of the urinary tract.

## Desired Outcome

2. What are the therapeutic goals in the treatment of acute uncomplicated cystitis?

## Therapeutic Alternatives

3.a. What are the important characteristics of an antibiotic that should be considered in the treatment of acute uncomplicated cystitis?

3.b. What nonpharmacologic therapies may be useful in treating or preventing acute uncomplicated cystitis?

3.c. What pharmacotherapeutic alternatives are available for empiric first- and second-line treatment of acute uncomplicated cystitis?

## Optimal Plan

4.a. What drug, dosage form, dose, schedule, and duration of therapy are best for the treatment of this patient's acute uncomplicated cystitis?

4.b. What long-term treatment strategies could be employed for this patient with recurrent acute uncomplicated cystitis?

4.c. How should this patient be managed if she presents with continuing symptoms of a UTI 3 days after she finished the antibiotic treatment originally prescribed?

## Outcome Evaluation

5. What clinical and laboratory parameters should be monitored to evaluate the efficacy of therapy and to detect or prevent adverse effects?

## Patient Education

6. What information should be provided to the patient to enhance adherence, ensure successful therapy, and minimize adverse effects?

# ■ SELF-STUDY ASSIGNMENTS

1. Review the safety and efficacy of single-dose and 3- and 7-day antimicrobial therapy for the treatment of acute uncomplicated cystitis.
2. Perform a literature search to obtain current data on the national and regional rates of resistance of outpatient urinary tract isolates of *Escherichia coli* to TMP–SMX and fluoroquinolone antibiotics. How do these rates compare to those reported at your institution, your clinic, or your geographic area?
3. Provide an assessment and recommendation on the role of phenazopyridine in treatment of UTIs.

## CLINICAL PEARL

UTIs occur rarely in young males, unless there is an underlying structural abnormality or instrumentation of the urinary tract.

## REFERENCES

1. Hooton TM. The current management strategies for community-acquired urinary tract infection. Infect Dis Clin North Am 2003;17:303–332.
2. Fihn SD. Acute uncomplicated urinary tract infection in women. N Engl J Med 2003;349:259–266.
3. Wagenlehner FM, Weidner W, Naber KG. An update on uncomplicated urinary tract infections in women. Curr Opin Urol 2009;19:368–374.
4. Karlowsky JA, Kelly LJ, Thornsberry C, Jones ME, Sahm DF. Trends in antimicrobial resistance among urinary tract infection isolates of *Escherichia coli* from female outpatients in the United States. Antimicrob Agents Chemother 2002;46:2540–2545.
5. Stapleton A. Novel approaches to prevention of urinary infections. Infect Dis Clin North Am 2003;17:457–471.
6. Guay DR. Cranberry and urinary tract infections. Drugs 2009;69(7):775–807.
7. Warren JW, Abrutyn E, Hebel JR, Johnson JR, Schaeffer AJ, Stamm WE. Guidelines for antimicrobial treatment of uncomplicated acute bacterial cystitis and acute pyelonephritis in women. Infectious Diseases Society of America (IDSA). Clin Infect Dis 1999;29:745–758.
8. Gupta K, Hooton TM, Roberts PL, Stamm WE. Short-course nitrofurantoin for the treatment of acute uncomplicated cystitis in women. Arch Intern Med 2007;167:2207–2212.
9. Hooton TM. Recurrent urinary tract infection in women. Int J Antimicrob Agents 2001;17:259–268.
10. Gupta K, Sahm DF, Mayfield D, Stamm WE. Antimicrobial resistance among uropathogens that cause community-acquired urinary tract infections in women: a nationwide analysis. Clin Infect Dis 2001;33:89–94.
11. Zhanel GG, Hisanaga TL, Laing NM, et al. Antibiotic resistance in *Escherichia coli* outpatient urinary tract isolates: final results from the North American Urinary Tract Infection Collaborative Alliance (NAUTICA). Int J Antimicrob Agents 2006;27:468–475.
12. Wright SW, Wrenn KD, Haynes ML. Trimethoprim–sulfamethoxazole resistance among urinary coliform isolates. J Gen Intern Med 1999;14:606–609.
13. Gupta K. Emerging antibiotic resistance in urinary tract pathogens. Infect Dis Clin North Am 2003;17:243–259.

# 132

# PYELONEPHRITIS

Resistant Rod . . . . . . . . . . . . . . . . . . . . . . . . . . Level II

**Elizabeth A. Coyle, PharmD, FCCM, BCPS**

## LEARNING OBJECTIVES

After completing this case study, the reader should be able to:

- Differentiate the signs, symptoms, and laboratory findings associated with pyelonephritis from those seen in lower urinary tract infections.
- Recognize patient risk factors that predispose to development of pyelonephritis.
- Recognize the prevalence of resistant *Escherichia coli* infections, and be able to recommend appropriate antibiotic therapy for resistant infections.
- Recommend appropriate empiric antimicrobial and symptomatic pharmacotherapy for a patient with suspected pyelonephritis.
- Make appropriate adjustments in pharmacotherapy based on patient response and culture results.
- Design a monitoring plan for a patient with pyelonephritis that allows objective assessment of the response to therapy.

## PATIENT PRESENTATION

### Chief Complaint

"I am freezing and my back is killing me."

### HPI

Isabella Toms is a 22-year-old college student with type 1 diabetes, who presents to the ER complaining that she has had pain in her right flank region over the last 24 hours, as well as pain in her abdomen. She complains of some nausea and reports that she woke up this morning with severe stomach and back pain, but has not vomited. The patient states she has not eaten for 24 hours, but has been able to drink water and non–diet soda, and has continued to keep her insulin pump on, but has not given any additional regular insulin. The patient reports she recently started treatment for a urinary tract infection about 2 days ago with trimethoprim/sulfamethoxazole. She states that she has been feeling feverish and has the chills. She reports no substernal chest pain, shortness of breath, cough, or sputum production. She denies any diarrhea or rash.

### PMH

Type 1 diabetes, diagnosed at age 11; has an insulin pump

### FH

Mother and father are in their 40s and healthy; one sister with asthma, and an older brother with Crohn's disease

### SH

Nonsmoker, no IVDA, drinks alcohol socially. Single, but has a steady boyfriend and is sexually active. Currently is a first-year law student at the local university.

### Meds

Ortho-Novum 7/7/7 one tablet daily
Insulin pump; regular insulin basal rate of 28 units per day
Regular insulin 2 units with breakfast, lunch, and supper
Trimethoprim/sulfamethoxazole one double strength tablet twice daily for 3 days (she has completed 2 days of therapy)

### All

Penicillin (develops an itchy rash)

### ROS

She has a history of UTIs and has had two UTIs in the past year, the most recent 2 days ago.

### Physical Examination

*Gen*

Conscious, alert, and oriented young Caucasian woman in mild distress

*VS*

BP 112/68, P 65, RR 16, T 39.0°C, $O_2$ sat 98% room air; Wt 63 kg (IBW 61.1 kg), Ht 5′7″

*Skin*

No tenting; dry skin; no signs of redness or rash

*HEENT*

EOMI; funduscopic examination WNL; pharynx clear and dry

*Neck*

Supple, no JVD

*Chest*

CTA

*CV*

RRR

*Abd*

Soft with suprapubic tenderness to deep palpation; no rebound or guarding; active bowel sounds. There is no hepatosplenomegaly or masses.

*Back*

No paraspinal or spinal tenderness

*Genit/Rect*

Normal female genitalia; no abnormal vaginal discharge; normal sphincter tone; last menstrual period 1 week ago

*Ext*

No CCE; pulses 2+ bilaterally

*Neuro*

A & O × 3; CN II–XII intact; sensory and perception intact

**TABLE 132-1 Laboratory Tests and Urinalyses on Days 1–3 of Hospitalization**

| Parameter (Units) | Day 1 | Day 2 | Day 3 |
|---|---|---|---|
| Serum chemistry | | | |
| Na (mEq/L) | 141 | 139 | 141 |
| K (mEq/L) | 3.9 | 4.0 | 4.1 |
| Cl (mEq/L) | 99 | 101 | 102 |
| $CO_2$ (mEq/L) | 27 | 28 | 28 |
| BUN (mg/dL) | 19 | 14 | 12 |
| SCr (mg/dL) | 1.1 | 1.0 | 1.0 |
| Glucose (mg/dL) | 65 | 92 | 89 |
| Hematology | | | |
| Hgb (g/dL) | 13.9 | 13.8 | 13.6 |
| Hct (%) | 40.6 | 40.3 | 40.5 |
| Plt ($\times 10^3/mm^3$) | 275 | 276 | 276 |
| WBC ($\times 10^3/mm^3$) | 26.3 | 20.4 | 12.5 |
| PMN/B/L/M (%) | 80/13/7/0 | 85/10/5/0 | 86/6/7/1 |
| Urinalysis | | | |
| Appearance | Hazy | | |
| Color | Amber | | |
| pH | 5.0 | | |
| Specific gravity | 1.017 | | |
| Blood | 2+ | | |
| Ketones | Negative | | |
| Leukocyte esterase | 3+ | | |
| Nitrites | 2+ | | |
| Urine protein, qualitative | Trace | | |
| Urine glucose, qualitative | Trace | | |
| WBC/hpf | 487 | | |
| RBC/hpf | 102 | | |
| Bacteria | Many | | |
| WBC casts | 2+ | | |

B, bands; L, lymphocytes; M, monocytes; PMN, polymorphonuclear leukocytes.

### Labs and UA on Admission

See Table 132-1.

### Chest X-Ray

No infiltrates, no consolidation seen

### CT Abdomen with Contrast

*Findings:* Liver, gallbladder, pancreas, spleen, and adrenals are unremarkable. No evidence of ascites or focal areas of fluid collection. The left kidney is unremarkable. A hypoattenuating lesion is seen involving the right kidney from mid- to lower pole.

*Impression:* Hypoattenuating lesion in right kidney consistent with pyelonephritis; correlate with clinical picture.

### Abdominal Ultrasound

*Findings:* There is a hypoechoic region within the lateral cortex of the right kidney, which does not display through transmission.

*Impression:* Focal cortical thickening with decreased echogenicity involving the mid right renal cortex, similar to the recent CT scan, most likely representing focal pyelonephritis. No renal abscess identified. No hydronephrosis.

### Urine Gram Stain

Many gram-negative rods

### Blood Culture

Many gram-negative rods

### Vaginal Swab

Negative

### Assessment

Pyelonephritis
Bacteremia
Type 1 diabetes

# QUESTIONS

## Problem Identification

1.a. Create a list of the patient's drug therapy problems.

1.b. What information (signs, symptoms, laboratory tests) indicates the presence and severity of pyelonephritis in this patient?

1.c. List any potential contributing factors that may have predisposed this patient to developing pyelonephritis.

1.d. What additional information is needed to fully assess the patient?

## Desired Outcome

2. What are the goals of pharmacotherapy in this patient?

## Therapeutic Alternatives

3.a. What nondrug therapies might be useful for this patient?

3.b. What organisms are commonly associated with pyelonephritis?

3.c. How often is antimicrobial resistance to *E. coli* seen in the community?

3.d. What feasible pharmacotherapeutic alternatives are available for the empiric treatment of pyelonephritis?

## Optimal Plan

4. Outline an antimicrobial regimen that will provide appropriate empiric therapy for pyelonephritis in this patient.

## Outcome Evaluation

5.a. What clinical and laboratory parameters are necessary to evaluate the antibiotic therapy for achievement of the desired therapeutic outcomes and to detect or prevent adverse effects?

# CLINICAL COURSE

The patient was started on the empiric antimicrobial regimen you recommended. She required acetaminophen Q 6 h for pain. Her fevers subsided with the initiation of acetaminophen and antibiotics. On day 3 of hospitalization, she was much improved and was ready for discharge. Laboratory tests for days 2 and 3 are included in Table 132-1. Culture results from admission were finalized on day 3 (late in the day) and are shown in Table 132-2.

5.b. What recommendations, if any, do you have for changes in the initial drug regimen?

## Patient Education

6. What information should be provided to the patient on discharge to enhance adherence, ensure successful therapy, and minimize adverse effects?

**TABLE 132-2 Culture Results of Urine and Blood Samples Taken on Day 1 and Reported on Day 3**

| Urine culture | |
|---|---|
| **Result: >100,000 cfu/mL *Escherichia coli*** | |
| **Antibiotic** | **Kirby–Bauer Interpretation** |
| Ampicillin/sulbactam | Intermediate |
| Ampicillin | Resistant |
| Cefazolin | Intermediate |
| Cefuroxime | Sensitive |
| Ceftriaxone | Sensitive |
| Levofloxacin | Sensitive |
| Piperacillin/tazobactam | Sensitive |
| Tobramycin | Sensitive |
| TMP/SMX | Resistant |
| **Day 1 blood cultures × 2 sets** | |
| **Result: Many *E. coli*** | |
| **Antibiotic** | **Kirby–Bauer Interpretation** |
| Ampicillin/sulbactam | Intermediate |
| Ampicillin | Resistant |
| Cefazolin | Intermediate |
| Cefuroxime | Sensitive |
| Ceftriaxone | Sensitive |
| Levofloxacin | Sensitive |
| Piperacillin/tazobactam | Sensitive |
| Tobramycin | Sensitive |
| TMP/SMX | Resistant |
| **Vaginal swab** | |
| No growth × 3 days | |
| **Day 2 blood cultures** | |
| **Results:** No growth to date | |
| **Day 3 blood cultures** | |
| **Results:** No growth to date | |

## SELF-STUDY ASSIGNMENTS

1. Develop a protocol for switching patients from IV to oral therapy when treating pyelonephritis.
2. Perform a literature search to find clinical trials comparing drug therapy in pyelonephritis, and compare inclusion criteria, drug regimens, outcomes, and costs of therapy.
3. Develop a clinical pathway that could be used for the management of suspected pyelonephritis.

## CLINICAL PEARL

Pyelonephritis can be managed with many different drugs; choose drugs that are bactericidal and cleared in the active form by the kidney. Drugs suitable for once-daily therapy help to reduce treatment costs.

## REFERENCES

1. Talan DA, Krishnadasan A, Abrahamian FM, Stamm WE, Moran GJ. Prevalence and risk factor analysis of trimethoprim–sulfamethoxazole and fluoroquinolone-resistant *Escherichia coli* infection among emergency department patients with pyelonephritis. Clin Infect Dis 2008;47:1150–1158.
2. Warren JW, Abrutyn E, Hebel JR, Johnson JR, Schaeffer AJ, Stamm WE. Guidelines for antimicrobial treatment of uncomplicated acute bacterial cystitis and acute pyelonephritis in women. Infectious Diseases Society of America (IDSA). Clin Infect Dis 1999;29: 745–758.
3. Neal DE. Complicated urinary tract infections. Urol Clin North Am 2008;35:13–22.
4. Talan DA, Stamm WE, Hooton TM, et al. Comparison of ciprofloxacin (7 days) and trimethoprim–sulfamethoxazole (14 days) for acute uncomplicated pyelonephritis in women. A randomized trial. JAMA 2000;283:1583–1590.
5. Peterson J, Kaul S, Khashab M, Fisher AC, Kahn JB. A double-blind, randomized comparison of levofloxacin 750 mg once-daily for five days with ciprofloxacin 400/500 mg twice-daily for 10 days for the treatment of complicated urinary tract infections and acute pyelonephritis. Urology 2008;71(1):17–22.
6. Pinson AG, Philbrick JT, Lindbeck GH, Schorling JB. ED management of acute pyelonephritis in women: a cohort study. Am J Emerg Med 1994;12:271–278.
7. Brown P, Moran K, Foxman B. Acute pyelonephritis among adults, cost of illness and considerations for the economic evaluation of therapy. Pharmacoeconomics 2005; 23(11):1123–1142.
8. Wagenlehner FME, Wagenlehner C, Redman R, Weidner W, Naber KG. Urinary bactericidal activity of doripenem versus that of levofloxacin in patients with complicated urinary tract infections or pyelonephritis. Antimicrob Agents Chemother 2009;53(4): 1567–1573.

# 133

# PELVIC INFLAMMATORY DISEASE AND OTHER SEXUALLY TRANSMITTED INFECTIONS

Frankie and Jenny Were Lovers . . . . . . . . . . . Level II

**Denise L. Howrie, PharmD**

**Pamela J. Murray, MD, MHP**

## LEARNING OBJECTIVES

After completing this case study, the reader should be able to:

- Identify relevant information from patient history, physical examination, and laboratory data suggestive of the diagnosis of a sexually transmitted infection (STI).
- List major complications of STIs and appropriate strategies for prevention and/or treatment.
- Discuss other health issues that may be present in patients referred for treatment of STIs, including immunization needs.
- Provide appropriate treatment plans for patients with STIs, including drug(s), doses, and monitoring.
- Develop patient counseling strategies regarding drug treatment and possible adverse effects.
- Recognize opportunities and provide appropriate recommendations for immunizations, including human papillomavirus (HPV) vaccine.

## PATIENT PRESENTATION 1

### Chief Complaint

"My lady and I don't feel good."

### HPI

Frankie Mason is a 24-year-old man who presents to a health clinic with complaints of 5 days of painful urination and increasing amounts of discolored urethral discharge. Today, he noted four painful blisters on the penis. He is single, is sexually active with two to three concurrent partners, and admits to unprotected sex "at least once" in the past 2 weeks. He does not know the sexual histories of his current or past sexual partners or their sexual partners, and he admits to over 15 lifetime sexual partners. He denies IV drug use, is heterosexual, and has no active medical problems. He denies oral or rectal intercourse.

### PMH

History of genital herpes 2 years ago. He has not undergone testing for HIV. He has been immunized against hepatitis B but has not been immunized against HPV as "it's only for women." He is unaware of hepatitis A or C as infectious diseases, asking "Do you get that from sex or restaurant food?"

### FH

Noncontributory

### SH

Denies cigarette use; has two to four beers "on weekends"; may be unreliable in keeping follow-up appointments because he states, "I don't like doctors."

### Meds

None

### All

Ciprofloxacin ("makes me dizzy")

### ROS

Occasional headaches; denies stomach pain, constipation, vision problems, night sweats, weight loss, or fatigue

### Physical Examination

*Gen*

Patient is a well-developed male in NAD, very talkative.

*VS*

BP 104/80, HR 72, RR 12, T 37.6°C; Wt 78 kg

*Skin*

No rashes or other lesions seen

*HEENT*

No erythema of pharynx or oral ulcers

*Neck/Lymph Nodes*

No lymphadenopathy; neck supple

*Chest*

Normal breath sounds; good air entry

*CV*

RRR; no murmurs

*Abd*

No tenderness or rebound; no HSM

*Genit/Rect*

Tanner stage V; testes descended, nontender, without erythema. Thick gray-white urethral discharge; four small erupting vesicles on penile tip and glans; negative rectal examination; no scrotal tenderness or swelling. No genital growths visualized.

*MS/Ext*

No inguinal or other lymphadenopathy; no lesions or rashes; muscle strength and tone normal

*Neuro*

CN II–XII intact; DTRs 2+ bilaterally and symmetric

### Urethral Smear

15 WBC/hpf; Gram stain (+) for intracellular gram-negative diplococci; rare flagellated organisms by saline prep microscopy—sample sent for gonorrhea culture and sensitivity

### Other Tests

A urine specimen was sent for NAAT for gonococcus and chlamydia.

### Assessment

1. Urethritis caused by gonococcal and *Trichomonas* infections
2. Recurrent genital herpes

## PATIENT PRESENTATION 2

### Chief Complaint

"I feel sick to my stomach."

### HPI

Jenny Klein is a 20-year-old female sexual partner of Frankie who reports a 1-day history of increasingly severe dysuria, lower abdominal pain, fever, nausea, emesis × 2, and vaginal discharge. She is sexually active with "only Frankie," has no previous history of urinary or genital infection, and denies IV drug use. She is unaware of Frankie's multiple sexual partners. Her last menses ended 10 days ago and last intercourse was 7 days ago without use of a condom. She noted the vaginal discharge yesterday, which she describes as thick and yellow. She denies oral or rectal intercourse. She admits to three lifetime sexual partners.

### PMH

Negative with no pregnancies. She has received a complete hepatitis B series. She has not been immunized against hepatitis A and has not received the HPV vaccine series, because her mother did not consent to the vaccine. She believes she is "low risk" for HPV.

### FH

HTN in maternal grandmother

■ SH

Denies nicotine or recreational drug use; occasional one to two glasses of wine; does not use hormonal or other contraception, reports occasional use of condoms; no routine medical care

■ Meds

None

■ All

NKDA

■ ROS

Occasional painful menses self-treated with acetaminophen

■ Physical Examination

*Gen*

Well-developed woman in moderate-to-severe abdominal discomfort

*VS*

BP 110/76, HR 100, RR 16, T 39.2°C; Wt 62 kg

*Skin*

No rashes seen

*HEENT*

No erythema of pharynx or oral ulcers

*Neck/Lymph Nodes*

No lymphadenopathy; neck supple

*Chest*

Normal breath sounds; good air entry; breasts Tanner stage V

*CV*

Tachycardia; regular rhythm; no murmurs

*Abd*

Guarding of right and mid–lower quadrants with palpation

*Genit/Rect*

Pubic hair Tanner stage V; vulva with no ulcers visible; moderate erythema with mild excoriations. Vagina with large amount of thick yellow-white discharge and mild erythema. Cervix shows erythema and extensive yellow-white discharge from the os; no masses on bimanual examination; cervical motion tenderness; adnexal tenderness and fullness. No genital growths visualized.

*MS/Ext*

No adenopathy, lesions, or rashes; no arthritis or tenosynovitis

*Neuro*

CN II–XII intact, DTRs 2+ and symmetric bilaterally

■ Labs

| | | |
|---|---|---|
| Na 138 mEq/L | Hgb 12.2 g/dL | WBC 12.75 × $10^3$/mm$^3$ |
| K 4.2 mEq/L | Hct 37% | Neutros 66% |
| Cl 102 mEq/L | Plt 250 × $10^3$/mm$^3$ | Bands 12% |
| BUN 22 mg/dL | | Lymphs 10% |
| SCr 0.9 mg/dL | | Monos 12% |
| Glu 106 mg/dL | | |

■ Other

Examination of vaginal discharge: pH 6.0, no yeast or hyphae seen; KOH prep negative, "whiff" test negative; motile flagellated organisms and increased WBC seen by saline prepared microscopy; negative for clue cells

■ UA

Rare WBC/hpf; protein 100 mg/dL; Gram stain (−)

■ Assessment

PID and *Trichomonas*

Infection of the genital tract: upper tract, cervicitis, vaginitis, and urethritis

## QUESTIONS

### Problem Identification

1.a. For each patient, create a list of drug therapy problems.

1.b. What information indicates the presence or severity of each STI in each patient?

1.c. Should any additional tests be performed in these patients?

1.d. What complications of infection can be reduced or avoided with appropriate therapy for each patient?

### Desired Outcome

2. State the goals of treatment for each patient.

### Therapeutic Alternatives

3. What therapeutic options are available for treatment of each patient?

### Optimal Plan

4.a. What treatment regimen (drug, dosage form, dose, schedule, and duration) is appropriate for these patients?

4.b. What alternatives would be appropriate if the initial therapy cannot be used?

### Outcome Evaluation

5.a. What clinical and laboratory parameters are necessary to evaluate the therapy for achievement of the desired outcome and to detect or prevent adverse effects?

## ■ CLINICAL COURSE

One day later, *Chlamydia* and gonorrhea NAAT-positive test results received on samples from both patients.

Two days later, bacterial cultures of urethral discharge (Frankie) are reported positive for *Neisseria gonorrhoeae*; β-lactamase negative.

5.b. What changes, if any, in antibacterial therapy are required?

### Patient Education

6. What information should be provided to Frankie to enhance adherence, ensure success of therapy, and minimize adverse effects?

## SELF-STUDY ASSIGNMENTS

1. Review insurance coverage available through health insurance providers in your locale for immunizations for HPV, hepatitis A, and hepatitis B for adults 21–35 years of age. Are there restrictions to access? What are anticipated costs of copayment or other out-of-pocket expenses?
2. Public and private health insurers may frequently restrict formulary access to anti-infectives for STIs, leading to refusal of prescribed medications or requirements for authorizations that may lead to delayed treatments. Select two to three insurers in your community and determine impact of formulary restrictions on anti-infective prescribing for Frankie.
3. Review the legal status of expedited partner therapy (EPT) in your area of practice. Discuss the ethical implications of this practice (see *www.cdc.gov/std/ept*).

## CLINICAL PEARLS

1. Partner notification and treatment may be enhanced through "EPT" strategies in which the sexual partner receives medication(s) or prescription(s) from the patient with a documented STI, in addition to information and referral for evaluation.
2. Health care providers should view a diagnosis of STI as an immunization opportunity to enhance care of the individual while furthering public health initiatives for disease prevention.

## REFERENCES


1. Centers for Disease Control and Prevention. Sexually transmitted diseases treatment guidelines, 2006. MMWR Morb Mortal Wkly Rep 2006;55(RR-11):1–94.
2. Centers for Disease Control and Prevention. Update to CDC's sexually transmitted diseases treatment guidelines 2006: fluoroquinolones no longer recommended for treatment of gonococcal infections. MMWR Morb Mortal Wkly Rep 2007;56:332–336.
3. Greer L, Wendel GD. Rapid diagnostic methods in sexually transmitted infections. Infect Dis Clin North Am 2008;22:601–617.
4. Lareau SM, Beigi RH. Pelvic inflammatory disease and tubo-ovarian abscess. Infect Dis Clin North Am 2008;22:693–708.
5. Trigg BG, Kerndt PR, Aynalem G. Sexually transmitted infections and pelvic inflammatory disease in women. Med Clin North Am 2008;92:1083–1113.
6. Akhter S, Beckmann K, Gorelick M. Update on sexually transmitted infections, 2008. Pediatr Emerg Care 2009;25:608–615.
7. Hollier LM, Workowski K. Treatment of sexually transmitted infections in women. Infect Dis Clin North Am 2008;22:665–691.
8. Hogben M, Burstein GR, Golden MR. Partner notification in the clinician's office: patient health, public health and interventions. Curr Opin Obstet Gynecol 2009;21:365–370.
9. Centers for Disease Control and Prevention. Expedited Partner Therapy in the Management of Sexually Transmitted Diseases. Atlanta, GA, US Department of Health and Human Services, 2006.
10. Centers for Disease Control and Prevention. Quadrivalent human papillomavirus vaccine: recommendations of the Advisory Committee on Immunization Practices. MMWR Morb Mortal Wkly Rep 2007;56 (RR-02):1–24.
11. Centers for Disease Control and Prevention. FDA licensure of bivalent human papillomavirus vaccine (HPV2, Cervarix) for use in females and updated HPV vaccination recommendations from the Advisory Committee on Immunization Practices (ACIP). MMWR Morb Mortal Wkly Rep 2010;59:626–629.
12. Centers for Disease Control and Prevention. FDA licensure of quadrivalent human papillomavirus vaccine (HPV4, Gardasil) for use in males and guidance from the Advisory Committee on Immunization Practices. MMWR Morb Mortal Wkly Rep 2010;9:630–632.


# 134

# SYPHILIS

Here Today … Gone Tomorrow? . . . . . . . . . . . Level I

**John S. Esterly, PharmD, BCPS**

**Marc H. Scheetz, PharmD, MSc, BCPS**

## LEARNING OBJECTIVES

After completing this case study, the reader should be able to:

- Discuss the diagnosis of syphilis and differentiate among the temporal stages of the disease.
- Develop a pharmacotherapeutic treatment plan individualized for the patient's stage of syphilis.
- Recommend alternate treatment regimens when the primary therapeutic option is contraindicated.
- Describe appropriate monitoring, follow-up, and counseling of patients with a syphilitic infection to ensure success of treatment.

## PATIENT PRESENTATION

### Chief Complaint

"This rash started 3–4 days ago on my back and stomach. My whole left side has been hurting, and I've also been feeling weaker than usual lately."

### HPI

John Rutherford, a 27-year-old man with a past medical history of HIV on HAART, presents with left upper quadrant/left back/left side pain and a diffuse rash. He states the rash started 3–4 days ago, and is mostly on his chest, abdomen, and arms. He also has seven macules on his scalp. The rash is nonpainful and nonpruritic, except on his scalp where he has developed a few scabs from itching; no drainage from any lesions is noted. He also has been having some chest pain that is worse with breathing. He notes nausea, though no vomiting, and reports ongoing nonbloody diarrhea for months. He presents to the ED primarily because of pain in his upper left back that radiates around his left side. His urine is very dark, brownish-red; however, he has no dysuria. The patient also states that he has felt weaker than usual for the past few days.

### PMH

Hepatitis B, now immune

HIV diagnosed 6 months ago, on HAART

### FH

Both parents with hypertension, still living

### SH

Unemployed

Tobacco 1.5 ppd since early teens

Social alcohol usage (average four drinks per week)

Occasional methamphetamine use—both smoked and injected (with clean needles)
Previous MSM Hx (four partners in last 6 months) with inconsistent use of condoms

## Meds

Tenofovir/emtricitabine 300/200 mg po once daily
Raltegravir 400 mg po BID
Acetaminophen–hydrocodone 325/5 mg po Q 6 hours PRN

## All

Codeine

## ROS

Constitutional: reports weakness and malaise; denies fever.
Eyes: denies vision changes.
ENT: denies sore throat, rhinorrhea, or sinus pressure.
Lymphatic: denies lymph node swelling.
Respiratory: denies shortness of breath, dyspnea on exertion, or cough.
Cardiovascular: reports some chest pain on inspiration.
GI: reports intermittent nausea, no vomiting, and consistent diarrhea.
Neurologic: denies neuropathy symptoms.
MS: reports arthralgias and myalgias.
Skin: rash on scalp, abdomen, arms, and legs present.
Pain: reports persistent abdominal and left side pain.

## Physical Examination

### *Gen*

Awake and alert, NAD. Appropriate. Oriented to person, place, and year.

### *VS*

T 98.4°F, BP 114/70, HR 92, RR 16, $O_2$ sat 98; Ht 68 in, Wt 59 kg

### *Skin*

Numerous palpable, blanchable macules mostly ~5 mm with one area of confluence on the left lower abdomen. Macules present on both arms, chest, and back. Four to five scabs with surrounding erythema on scalp.

### *HEENT*

Moist mucous membranes, neck supple. No cervical, postauricular, or supraclavicular lymphadenopathy. No obvious oral lesions. Mild icterus.

### *Neck/Lymph Nodes*

Supple; no lymphadenopathy, bruits, JVD, or thyromegaly

### *Chest*

CTA bilaterally. No crackles or wheezes.

### *CV*

RRR; $S_1$, $S_2$; no m/r/g

### *Abd*

Soft, nondistended. Diffuse tenderness with minimal localization to the RUQ and more prominent on the epigastrium, LUQ, and back. (+) BS. No rebound or guarding.

### *Extremities*

Warm, well perfused, no edema. 2+ DP and PT pulses.

### *GU*

Rash extending to penis; no other lesions present. Moderate inguinal lymphadenopathy.

### *Rectal*

Scar from recently healed ulcer noted

### *Musculoskeletal*

No joint swelling, or effusions

### *Neuro*

CN II–XII grossly intact. No dysmetria. Strength 5/5 on all four extremities.

## Labs

| | |
|---|---|
| Na 138mEq/L | WBC 9.3 × $10^3$/mm$^3$ |
| K 3.9 mEq/L | Plt 391 × $10^3$/mm$^3$ |
| Cl 96 mEq/L | ALT 66 IU/L |
| $CO_2$ 28 mEq/L | AST 95 IU/L |
| BUN 7 mg/dL | Alk phos 1271 IU/L |
| SCr 0.7 mg/dL | T-bili 5.0 mg/dL |
| Glu 100 mg/dL | CD4 460 cells/mm$^3$ |
| Hgb 12.3 g/dL | HIV VL <48 copies/mL |
| Hct 36.9% | |

## Other

RPR: Titers positive at 1:256.
FTA-ABS: Positive.
Hepatitis B: HBsAB positive, HBsAG negative.
Hepatitis C: RNA negative.
CT abdomen and pelvis: Mild hepatosplenomegaly with minimal intrahepatic biliary ductal dilatation and prominence of the common duct. There are multiple tortuous perirectal vessels that may represent varices secondary to portal hypertension. Proctitis is present with innumerable reactive perirectal and pelvic lymph nodes.

## Assessment

1. The patient is a 27-year-old man with a history of HIV and newly diagnosed syphilis that appears to be in a secondary stage based on signs, symptoms, and report of sexual history.
2. This patient may be at higher risk for disease progression, specifically neurosyphilis, due to HIV coinfection.

# QUESTIONS

## Problem Identification

1.a. Which populations are most at risk for syphilis?

1.b. What information (signs, symptoms, laboratory values) indicates the presence or stage of syphilis?

1.c. What laboratory tests are used in the diagnosis of syphilis, and how should they be interpreted?

## Desired Outcome

2. What are the goals of pharmacotherapy in this case?

## Therapeutic Alternatives

3.a. What pharmacotherapeutic alternatives are available for this patient?

3.b. What nondrug measures should be implemented in this case?

## Optimal Plan

4. What is the recommended treatment (drug, dose, and duration) for this patient?

## Outcome Evaluation

5. What clinical and laboratory parameters are necessary to evaluate the therapy for achievement of the desired therapeutic outcome and to detect or prevent adverse effects?

## Patient Education

6.a. What information should be provided to the patient to enhance adherence, ensure successful therapy, and minimize adverse effects?

6.b. What information should be provided to the patient to prevent a future sexually transmitted disease?

## SELF-STUDY ASSIGNMENTS

1. Describe the differences in syphilis presentation in relation to disease progression.
2. Discuss the tests or procedures that should be used to diagnose and monitor the progression/regression of syphilis over time.
3. Identify potential confounding factors that may impact test results in HIV-infected patients.

## CLINICAL PEARL

Patients undergoing penicillin therapy for syphilis will frequently experience the Jarisch–Herxheimer reaction within the first 24 hours of treatment. This is an inflammatory response to the breakdown of spirochetes and subsequent release of endotoxins. Usually manifesting as fever, chills, myalgias, arthralgias, and headache, it is generally self-limiting and may be treated with analgesics and antipyretics as needed.

## REFERENCES


1. Centers for Disease Control and Prevention. Sexually Transmitted Disease Surveillance, 2008. Atlanta, U.S. Department of Health and Human Services, November 2009. Available at: *www.cdc.gov*. Accessed May 23, 2010.
2. Centers for Disease Control and Prevention. Sexually transmitted diseases treatment guidelines. MMWR Morb Mortal Wkly Rep 2006;55(RR-11):22–35. Available at: *www.cdc.gov*. Accessed May 23, 2010.
3. Tramont EC. *Treponema pallidum* (syphilis). In: Mandell GL, Bennett JE, Dolin R, eds. Principles and Practice of Infectious Diseases, 7th ed. Philadelphia, Churchill Livingstone, 2009:3035–3054.
4. Mofenson LM, Brady MT, Danner SP, et al. Guidelines for the prevention and treatment of opportunistic infections in HIV-infected adults and adolescents: recommendations from CDC, the National Institutes of Health, and the HIV Medicine Association of the Infectious Diseases Society of America. MMWR Recomm Rep 2009;58(RR-4):1–207.
5. Hook EW 3rd, Behets F, Van Damme K, et al. A phase III equivalence trial of azithromycin versus benzathine penicillin for the treatment of early syphilis. J Infect Dis 2010;201(11):1729–1735.
6. Warwick Z, Dean G, Fisher M. Should syphilis be treated differently in HIV-positive and HIV-negative individuals? Treatment outcomes at a university hospital, Brighton, UK. Int J STD AIDS 2009;20(4): 229–230.
7. See S, Scott EK, Levin MW. Penicillin-induced Jarisch–Herxheimer reaction. Ann Pharmacother 2005;39(12):2128–2130.


# 135

# GENITAL HERPES, GONOCOCCAL, AND CHLAMYDIAL INFECTIONS

Triple Threat . . . . . . . . . . . . . . . . . . . . . . . . . . . Level II

**Suellyn J. Sorensen, PharmD, BCPS**

## LEARNING OBJECTIVES

After completing this case study, the reader should be able to:

- Identify subjective and objective data consistent with genital herpes, gonorrhea, and chlamydia.
- Recommend appropriate therapies for the treatment of genital herpes, gonorrhea, and chlamydia.
- Provide effective and comprehensive counseling for patients with genital herpes, gonorrhea, and chlamydia.
- Identify drug interactions of clinical significance and provide recommendations for managing them.

## PATIENT PRESENTATION

### Chief Complaint

"I have painful sores in my genital area, and I have terrible headaches and muscle aches."

### HPI

Megan Thompson is a 19-year-old nulligravida woman who presents to the county health STD clinic for evaluation of genital lesions that have been present for 3 days. She has also noticed a white nonodorous vaginal discharge that has lasted 14 days. She admits to anal and vaginal intercourse with two regular partners in the last 60 days. It has been 5 days since her last sexual encounter.

### PMH

Recurrent UTIs; most recent 3 months ago
Vaginal candidiasis; most recent 6 months ago
Gonorrhea 5 years ago
*Trichomonas vaginalis* 2 years ago

### FH

Mother with type 2 DM; father died at age 50 of an acute MI

## SH

Lives with her boyfriend and works at a local grocery store. She admits to occasional use of alcohol and marijuana.

## Meds

Junel 21 1/20 one tablet po daily
Multivitamin with iron one tablet po daily
Ibuprofen 200 mg po PRN
Ciprofloxacin 250 mg po once daily

## All

Penicillin (hives and tongue swelling)

## ROS

(−) Cough, night sweats, weight loss, dysuria, or urinary frequency; (+) diarrhea and anorectal pain; LMP 6 weeks ago

## Physical Examination

*Gen*

Thin, young woman in NAD

*VS*

BP 136/71, P 78, RR 17, T 37.8°C; Wt 51 kg, Ht 5′5″

*Skin*

Dry, no lesions, normal color and temperature

*HEENT*

PERRLA, EOMI without nystagmus

*Neck*

Supple; no adenopathy, JVD, or thyromegaly

*Chest*

Air entry equal; no crepitations or wheezing

*CV*

RRR, normal $S_1$ and $S_2$; no $S_3$ or $S_4$; no murmurs or rubs

*Abd*

Soft, mild tenderness to palpation in RLQ, (+) bowel sounds, no HSM

*Genit/Rect*

Tender inguinal adenopathy. External exam clear for nits and lice, several extensive shallow small painful vesicular lesions over vulva and labia, swollen and red. Vagina red, rugated, moderate amounts of creamy white discharge. Cervix pink, covered with above discharge, nontender, ~3 cm. Corpus nontender, no palpable masses. Adnexa with no palpable masses or tenderness. Rectum with no external lesions; (+) diffuse inflammation and friability internally, no masses.

*Ext*

Peripheral pulses 2+ bilaterally, DTRs 2+, no joint swelling or tenderness

*Neuro*

Alert and oriented, CN II–XII intact

## Labs

| | | | |
|---|---|---|---|
| Na 135 mEq/L | Hgb 12.9 g/dL | WBC 6.3 × $10^3$/mm$^3$ | RPR nonreactive |
| K 4.0 mEq/L | Hct 37.3% | PMNs 64% | Preg test: hCG pending |
| Cl 102 mEq/L | Plt 255 × $10^3$/mm$^3$ | Bands 2% | |
| $CO_2$ 27 mEq/L | | Eos 1% | HIV serology: ELISA pending |
| BUN 11 mg/dL | | Lymphs 24% | |
| SCr 0.9 mg/dL | | Monos 9% | |
| Glu 72 mg/dL | | | |

## Other

Vaginal discharge—"whiff" test (−); pH <4.5; wet mount *Trichomonas* (−), clue cells (−), yeast (+)

## Clinical Course

The following results were reported 2 days later:
- Vulval swab DFA monoclonal stain: HSV-2 isolated
- Vaginal and rectal swab gonorrhea NAAT (PCR): *Neisseria gonorrhoeae* (+)
- Vaginal and rectal swab chlamydia NAAT (PCR): *Chlamydia trachomatis* (+)

## Assessment

A 19-year-old woman who may be pregnant and has primary genital HSV-2 infection, vaginal candidiasis, and gonococcal and chlamydial infections of the vagina, cervix, and rectum

# QUESTIONS

## Problem Identification

1.a. Create a list of the patient's drug therapy problems.

1.b. What subjective and objective clinical data are consistent with a primary genital herpes infection?

1.c. Could any of the patient's problems have been caused by drug therapy?

## Desired Outcome

2. What are the goals of pharmacotherapy in this case?

## Therapeutic Alternatives

3.a. What nondrug therapies might be useful for this patient?

3.b. What feasible pharmacotherapeutic alternatives are available for treatment of genital herpes, chlamydia, and gonorrhea?

## Optimal Plan

4.a. What drug, dosage form, dose, schedule, and duration of therapy are best for treating this patient's genital herpes, chlamydial, and gonococcal infections?

4.b. If a NAAT (also called PCR) test was negative for chlamydia but positive for gonorrhea, would treatment for chlamydia still be warranted?

## Outcome Evaluation

5. What clinical and laboratory parameters are necessary to evaluate the therapy for achievement of the desired therapeutic outcome and to detect or prevent adverse effects?

## Patient Education

6. What information should be provided to the patient to enhance adherence, ensure successful therapy, and minimize adverse effects?

## FOLLOW-UP QUESTIONS

1. Six months later, Megan calls the STD clinic complaining of genital lesions that look and feel the same as the lesions she had 6 months earlier when seen and treated in the clinic. Should this episode of recurrent genital herpes be treated? If so, what therapies would be appropriate?
2. Is daily suppressive therapy indicated because she had a recurrent episode?
3. When is herpes treatment indicated for sexual partners?
4. When is chlamydia and gonorrhea treatment indicated for sexual partners?
5. What additional pharmacotherapeutic interventions should be made to address the drug therapy problems that were identified in question 1.a.?

## SELF-STUDY ASSIGNMENTS

1. Determine whether there is a role for vaccines in the future management of herpes simplex disease.
2. Recommend alternative agents for the treatment of acyclovir-resistant herpes.
3. Explain the relationship between herpes simplex and HIV infections. Is there a role for herpes simplex virus–suppressive therapy in preventing HIV transmission?
4. Describe herpes simplex complications that may require hospitalization, and recommend an appropriate treatment regimen.

## CLINICAL PEARL

Most genital herpes infections are transmitted by persons who have asymptomatic viral shedding and are unaware that they have the infection. Systemic antiviral drugs control the signs and symptoms of genital herpes infection, but they do not eradicate latent virus.

## REFERENCES

1. Centers for Disease Control and Prevention. 2010 S.T.D treatment guidelines. MMWR Morb Mortal Wkly Rep 2010:59(RR-12):1–110. Available at: *www.cdc.gov/std/treatment*. Accessed Feb 19, 2011.
2. Valtrex Caplets Package Insert. Research Triangle Park, NC, GlaxoSmithKline, March 2010.
3. Comparative Drug Prices. Available at: *www.drugstore.com*. Accessed July 1, 2010.
4. Famvir Tablets Package Insert. East Hanover, NJ, Novartis Pharmaceuticals Corporation, December 2009.
5. Workowski KA, Berman SM. Centers for Disease Control and Prevention sexually transmitted diseases treatment guidelines. Clin Infect Dis 2007;44(Suppl 3):S73–S174.
6. Centers for Disease Control and Prevention. Update to CDC's sexually transmitted diseases treatment guidelines, 2006: fluoroquinolones no longer recommended for treatment of gonococcal infections. MMWR Morb Mortal Wkly Rep 2007;56:332–336. Available at: *http://www.cdc.gov/mmWR/preview/mmwrhtml/mm5614a3.htm*. Accessed Feb 19, 2011.
7. CDC. Updated recommended treatment regimens for gonococcal infections and associated conditions—United States, April 2007. Available at: *www.cdc.gov/std/treatment*. Accessed Feb 19, 2011.
8. Corey L, Wald A, Patel R, et al. Once daily valacyclovir to reduce the risk of transmission of genital herpes. N Engl J Med 2004;350:11–20.

# 136

# OSTEOMYELITIS AND SEPTIC ARTHRITIS

## The Soccer Kick that Packed a Powerful Punch . . . . . . . . . . . . . . . . . Level I

**Edward P. Armstrong, PharmD, FASHP**

**Allan D. Friedman, MD, MPH**

## LEARNING OBJECTIVES

After completing this case study, the reader should be able to:

- Compare the most common presenting signs and symptoms of acute osteomyelitis and septic arthritis.
- Recommend a treatment plan for empiric therapy of acute osteomyelitis and septic arthritis in a pediatric patient.
- Develop alternative treatment approaches for acute osteomyelitis and septic arthritis in a pediatric patient if the initial treatment regimen fails.
- Create monitoring parameters for antibacterial treatment of osteomyelitis and septic arthritis, including efficacy and toxicity of therapy.

## PATIENT PRESENTATION

### Chief Complaint

"My knee is killing me."

### HPI

Miles Diaz is a 4-year-old boy who complains of persistent right knee pain after being kicked in the leg and knee during a soccer game. The day after the incident, the patient was seen in the emergency department at his local hospital because of right leg pain and was discharged to his parents with a recommendation to use ibuprofen and warm compresses.

His parents brought him back to the emergency department 2 weeks later, because he continued to complain of leg pain just above the knee when trying to walk. His parents reported that if he took Advil, he was able to walk a little. During this visit, laboratory tests and x-rays were obtained.

At that time he had a WBC count of $6.0 \times 10^3/mm^3$, an ESR of 40 mm/h, a CRP of 41 mg/L, and on physical exam, he had tenderness over the right lateral femoral condyle. His x-rays confirmed the diagnosis of osteomyelitis of the distal right femur (Fig. 136-1). He was referred to the Pediatric Infectious Disease Clinic where he underwent aspiration of both the knee joint and the bone where

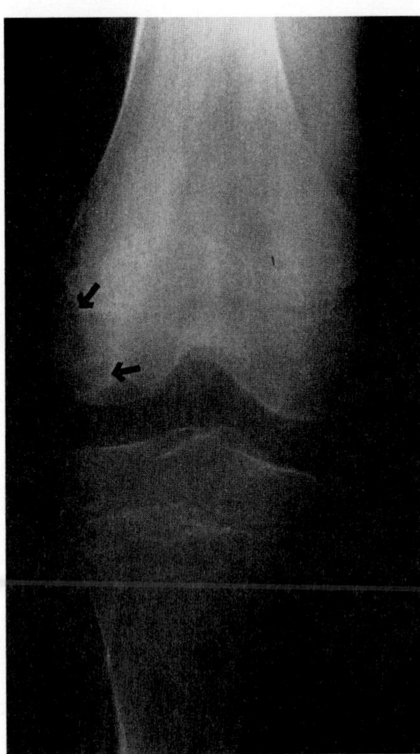

**FIGURE 136-1.** Lytic lesion of the distal right femur indicating osteomyelitis (*arrows*).

it was most tender. There was purulent fluid in the bone. He was started on home IV therapy with cefuroxime 1,000 mg every 8 hours. His pain began to improve after 3 days.

### PMH

No prior history of serious diseases; however, the parents do not know if any of his immunizations are up-to-date.

### FH

No family history of early childhood deaths secondary to severe infection

### SH

Mother and father live in the household and are healthy.

### Meds

Cefuroxime 1,000 mg IV Q 8 h

### All

NKA

### ROS

No positive findings with regard to head, eyes, ears, nose, throat, cardiorespiratory systems, skin lesions, or recent illness. No other significant trauma besides the recent kick to the right leg he received during a soccer game.

### Physical Examination

*Gen*

His general appearance is that of a thin, apprehensive boy in no distress apart from the tenderness in his right leg just above the knee.

*VS*

BP 100/70, P 102, RR 18, T 36.0°C; Wt 22 kg, Ht 4′6″

*Skin*

No lesions, but redness on right leg near the knee

*HEENT*

Within normal limits

*Neck/Lymph Nodes*

No lymphadenopathy or thyromegaly

*Lungs/Thorax*

Chest is clear to percussion and auscultation

*CV*

Normal $S_1$ and $S_2$; no murmurs present

*Abd*

Soft without hepatosplenomegaly

*Genit/Rect*

Genitalia are normal; circumcised male

*MS/Ext*

Swollen, slightly tender right leg just above the knee. He has difficulty walking on the leg.

*Neuro*

Reflexes 2+; plantar reflexes downgoing; no cerebellar or sensorial abnormalities; normal strength and tone except where not measurable at the right knee

### Assessment

Osteomyelitis in the distal femur probably due to a staphylococcal infection.

## QUESTIONS

### Problem Identification

1.a. Create a list of the patient's drug therapy problems.

1.b. What information (signs, symptoms, laboratory values) indicates the presence or severity of acute osteomyelitis?

1.c. What information (signs, symptoms, laboratory values) would indicate if septic arthritis might also be present?

### Desired Outcome

2. What are the goals of pharmacotherapy in this case?

### Therapeutic Alternatives

3.a. What nondrug therapies might be useful for this patient?

3.b. What feasible pharmacotherapeutic alternatives are available for the empiric treatment of acute osteomyelitis?

### Optimal Plan

4. What drug, dosage form, dose, schedule, and duration of therapy are best for this patient?

## Outcome Evaluation

5. What clinical and laboratory parameters are necessary to evaluate the therapy for achievement of the desired therapeutic outcome and to detect or prevent adverse effects?

## Patient Education

6. What information should be provided to the patient's caregiver to enhance adherence, ensure successful therapy, and minimize adverse effects?

## CLINICAL COURSE

A subsequent x-ray showed the presence of a bone lesion (Fig. 136-2), but the clinical signs and symptoms were markedly improved. With the clinical improvement, the patient was successfully converted to an oral regimen of cefuroxime after 1 week of IV therapy.

Two weeks later, the patient was again seen in the Pediatric Infectious Disease Clinic where clinical evaluation revealed no additional new findings. The patient continued to be afebrile, his CRP was down to 6 mg/L, and his ESR was down to 12 mm/h. He still had difficulty walking without ibuprofen. He had been tolerating the oral antibiotic regimen without apparent abdominal discomfort, diarrhea, or rash. Oral cefuroxime was to be continued for a total of 6 weeks.

## SELF-STUDY ASSIGNMENTS

1. Plan alternative IV and oral treatment regimens in the event that the patient could not tolerate the antibiotic initially used.
2. Compare optimal oral treatment strategies for osteomyelitis in adults with those in children.

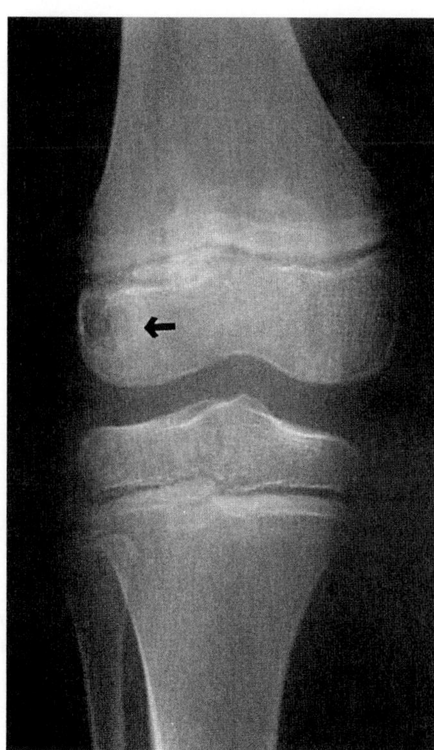

**FIGURE 136-2.** Persistent lesion of the distal right femur (*arrow*) after low-dose antibiotic treatment.

## CLINICAL PEARL

The ultimate prognosis of acute osteomyelitis and septic arthritis is based on the speed of diagnosis, prompt initiation of appropriate antimicrobial therapy, and surgical drainage, if needed.

## REFERENCES


1. Gutierrez K. Bone and joint infections in children. Pediatr Clin North Am 2005;52:779–794.
2. Goergens ED, McEvoy A, Watson M, Barrett IR. Acute osteomyelitis and septic arthritis in children. J Paediatr Child Health 2005;41:59–62.
3. Unkila-Kallio L, Kallio MJ, Eskola J, Peltola H. Serum C-reactive protein, erythrocyte sedimentation rate, and white blood cell count in acute hematogenous osteomyelitis of children. Pediatrics 1994;93:59–62.
4. Lazzarini L, Lipsky BA, Mader JT. Antibiotic treatment of osteomyelitis: what have we learned from 30 years of clinical trials? Int J Infect Dis 2005;9:127–138.
5. Weichert S, Sharland M, Clarke NMP, Faust SN. Acute haematogenous osteomyelitis in children: is there any evidence for how long we should treat? Curr Opin Infect Dis 2008;21:258–262.
6. Zaoutis T, Localio AR, Leckerman K, Saddlemire S, Bertoch D, Keren R. Prolonged intravenous therapy versus early transition to oral antimicrobial therapy for acute osteomyelitis in children. Pediatrics 2009;123:636–642.
7. Daver NG, Shelburne SA, Atmar RL, et al. Oral step-down therapy is comparable to intravenous therapy for *Staphylococcus aureus* osteomyelitis. J Infect 2007;54:539–544.


# 137

# SEPSIS

Question the Source . . . . . . . . . . . . . . . . . . . . Level III


**Christopher M. Scott, PharmD, BCPS, FCCM**

**Tate N. Trujillo, PharmD, BCPS, FCCM**


## LEARNING OBJECTIVES

After completing the case study, the reader should be able to:

- Differentiate between systemic inflammatory response syndrome (SIRS), sepsis, septic shock, and severe sepsis with an understanding of the continuum that exists between them.
- List the variables (general, inflammatory, hemodynamic, organ dysfunction, and tissue) used by health care professionals to diagnose sepsis.
- List the hemodynamic parameters that should be met during the first 6 hours of the diagnosis or identification of sepsis.
- Discuss the different components of the Surviving Sepsis Campaign as they relate to pharmacotherapy.

## PATIENT PRESENTATION

### Chief Complaint

The patient's primary caregiver reports that the patient has been vomiting a lot in the last few days.

### HPI

Jessica Lauver is a 74-year-old woman with a PMH significant for asthma and HTN who was sent from subacute care facility with hypokalemia reports of nonbloody, nonbilious emesis (three to four episodes per day for 2–3 weeks), loose stools, decreased appetite, and chills. Patient denies dysuria/hematuria, chest pain, or dyspnea.

### PMH

Asthma
DM
HTN
Morbid obesity
Depression

### PSH

Partial SBO/ventral hernia repair 3 months ago
Cholecystectomy (date unknown)

### FH

No HTN, DM, CA, or vascular disease

### SH

One to two cigarettes every other day; stopped in the 1980s. Also stopped drinking alcohol in the 1980s.

### Meds PTA

Albuterol MDI two puffs Q 6 h PRN
Metformin 850 mg po BID
Fluticasone inhaler two puffs BID
Lisinopril 10 mg po daily
Mirtazapine 15 mg po at bedtime
Promethazine 25 mg po Q 6 h PRN nausea/vomiting

### All

NKDA

### Physical Examination

*Gen*

Morbidly obese, white female in moderate distress

*VS*

BP 87/43, P 120–153, RR 14–33, T 37.8°C, $SpO_2$: 94% on 4 L NC, ins/outs (24 hours): 8,489 mL/25 mL; Wt 145.5 kg, Ht 5′2″

*HEENT*

NCAT, PERRLA, no JVD, cap refill >3 seconds

*Chest*

Positive for expiratory wheezes throughout; tachypnea

*CV*

Tachycardia, regular rhythm; NL $S_1/S_2$, no MRG

*Abd*

(+) Pannus, unable to palpate organs, tenderness to deep palpation

*Ext*

No cyanosis/edema, 2+ pedal pulses

*Neuro*

A & O × 2 (not oriented to place)

### Labs

| | | | |
|---|---|---|---|
| Na 133 mEq/L | Mg 2.5 mg/dL | Hgb 13.6 g/dL | pH 7.14 |
| K 2.9 mEq/L | Phos 2.5 mg/dL | Hct 42% | $pCO_2$ 26 mm Hg |
| Cl 98 mEq/L | Alb 2.1 g/dL | Plt 261 × $10^3/mm^3$ | $pO_2$ 189 mm Hg |
| $CO_2$ 12 mEq/L | Alk phos 127 IU/L | WBC 25.5 × $10^3/mm^3$ | $HCO_3$ 8.9 mmol/L |
| BUN 13 mg/dL | T. bili 0.2 mg/dL | PMNs 58% | Base deficit –9.3 mmol/L |
| SCr 1.1 mg/dL | AST 11 IU/L | Bands 15% | Lactate 9.8 mmol/L |
| Glu 230 mg/dL | ALT 7 IU/L | Lymphs 22% | |
| Ca 6.9 mg/dL | | Monos 5% | |

EKG: sinus tach (113), but with artifacts, QRS 98/QT–$QT_c$ 358/425

### Clinical Course

After spending several hours waiting in the ED for a ward bed, Ms Lauver developed hypotension (systolic blood pressures in the low 60–70s) refractory to fluids, altered mental status, and decreased urine output. Ms Lauver also required intubation and was placed on the mechanical ventilator at that time secondary to respiratory failure and the inability to protect her airway. The primary team is concerned about septic shock. Over the next 30 minutes to 1 hour, she was started on the following medications:

Norepinephrine 20 mcg/min
Vasopressin 0.03 units/min
Propofol 25 mcg/kg/min
Fentanyl 50 mcg/h
Levofloxacin 500 mg IV daily

### Assessment

A 74-year-old female in septic shock with acute respiratory and renal failure; probable intra-abdominal infection

## QUESTIONS

### Problem Identification

1.a. Create a list of this patient's drug therapy and disease state problems.

1.b. What information (signs, symptoms, laboratory values) indicates the presence or severity of the problem or disease?

### Desired Outcome

2. What are the goals of patient care in this case?

### Therapeutic Alternatives

3.a. What interventions and/or therapies should be accomplished within the first 6 hours of all septic shock or severe sepsis patients?

3.b. What type of fluid should be recommended to appropriately resuscitate patients with septic shock and/or severe sepsis?

3.c. When should vasopressor agents be considered in the treatment of hypotension related to sepsis, and which agents are appropriate?

3.d. When should you consider inotropic agents in this patient's therapy, and which agents are appropriate?

3.e. When are corticosteroids used to treat septic shock?

3.f. When would you recommend recombinant human activated protein C (rhAPC) or drotrecogin alfa (activated) (Xigris) for this patient?

3.g. What other supportive care issues should be implemented for all severe sepsis patients?

3.h. What economic and ethical considerations are applicable to this patient?

## Optimal Plan

4. The surgical critical care team has determined that Ms Lauver has severe sepsis with a possible intra-abdominal source. Design an optimal sepsis treatment regimen for Ms Lauver.

## Outcome Evaluation

5. What clinical and laboratory parameters are necessary to evaluate the therapy for achievement of the desired therapeutic outcome and to detect or prevent an adverse effect?

## SELF-STUDY ASSIGNMENTS

1. Design evidence-based usage criteria for drotrecogin alfa (activated) taking into account the contraindications, precautions, and the patient population in whom this agent may be most beneficial.
2. Compare and contrast the available literature supporting the use of corticosteroids in severe sepsis focusing on the dosing and diagnosis of relative adrenal insufficiency.

## CLINICAL PEARL

Propofol often precipitates hypotension in patients who do not have adequate intravascular volumes. Alternative sedative agents should be sought when hypotension is encountered with propofol. Propofol may cause other problems in severe sepsis patients because it is formulated in a lipid emulsion that may contribute to the inflammatory process as well as provide unnecessary calories from fat (1.1 kcal/mL).

## REFERENCES


1. Levy MM, Fink MP, Marshall JC, et al. 2001 SCCM/ESICM/ACCP/ATS/SIS International Sepsis Definitions Conference. Crit Care Med 2003;31:1250–1256.
2. Rivers E, Nguyen B, Havstad S, et al. Early goal-directed therapy in the treatment of severe sepsis and septic shock. N Engl J Med 2001;345:1368–1377.
3. Dellinger RP, Levy MM, Carlet JM, et al. Surviving Sepsis Campaign: international guidelines for management of severe sepsis and septic shock: 2008. Crit Care Med 2008;36(1):296–327.
4. Sprung CL, Annane D, Keh D, et al. Hydrocortisone therapy for patients with septic shock. N Engl J Med 2008;358:111–124.
5. Eli Lilly and Company. Xigris package insert. Indianapolis, IN, October 2008. Available at: *www.xigris.com*. Accessed July 28, 2010.
6. Bernard GR, Vincent JL, Laterre PF, et al. Efficacy and safety of recombinant human activated protein C for severe sepsis. N Engl J Med 2001;344:699–709.
7. Finfer S, Chittock DR, Su SY, et al, NICE-SUGAR Study Investigators. Intensive versus conventional glucose control in critically ill patients. N Engl J Med 2009;360:1346–1349.
8. ASHP therapeutic guidelines on stress ulcer prophylaxis. ASHP Commission on Therapeutics and approved by the ASHP board of directors on November 14, 1998. Am J Health Syst Pharm 1999;56:347–379.
9. Solomkin JS, Mazuski JE, Bradley JS, et al. Diagnosis and management of complicated intra-abdominal infection in adults and children: guidelines by the Surgical Infection Society and the Infectious Diseases Society of America. Clin Infect Dis 2010;50:133–164.


# 138

# DERMATOPHYTOSIS

Toeing the Line. . . . . . . . . . . . . . . . . . . . . . . . . Level I

**Scott J. Bergman, PharmD, BCPS**

## LEARNING OBJECTIVES

After completing this case study, the reader should be able to:

- Recognize the signs and symptoms of a dermatophyte infection.
- Evaluate the risk factors for developing a dermatophyte infection.
- Recommend an appropriate treatment plan for a dermatophyte infection.
- Explain the best way for the patient to use a selected antifungal product.

## PATIENT PRESENTATION

### Chief Complaint

"My feet itch."

### HPI

Dave Harvester is a 41-year-old man who presents to the local pharmacy because of recent itching in the area of his feet. He is an assistant manager at a local retail store who plays basketball at the YMCA for exercise three times a week. He sweats profusely during games and always showers before going home. He has not changed laundry detergent recently, but he admits that he does not always wash his athletic clothes between workouts. He says his feet have always smelled bad, but he first started to notice the burning and itching about 6 weeks ago. He started applying some deodorizing spray to his feet a week ago, but thus far it has only made a slight improvement in itching. Now his groin is starting to itch as well.

### PMH

Appendectomy 20 years ago
GERD diagnosed 5 years ago
Type 2 diabetes mellitus diagnosed 1 year ago
High cholesterol diagnosed 1 year ago

### SH

Recent sexual activity (within past month)
Denies tobacco use
Drinks beer on weekends and after games or practice

■ Meds

Pantoprazole 40 mg daily
Simvastatin 20 mg daily
Metformin 500 mg twice daily
Men's multivitamin daily

■ All

Penicillin (rash as a baby)

■ ROS

Denies fever and chills. Fatigued only after basketball practice. Reports frequent trauma to feet while playing in games. Complains of itching between his toes and groin area.

■ Physical Examination (Limited)

*Gen*

An obese, but healthy-looking man wearing sandals, shorts, and a T-shirt

*VS*

BP 118/78, P 60, RR 18; Wt 105 kg, Ht 5′11″

*Skin*

Visible regions are soft and moist.

*Abd*

Fat rolls can be seen around his belly.

*Genit/Rect*

Not directly examined, but patient reports pruritus and burning of skin around groin, not on penis or scrotum. Redness can be seen on the medial aspects of the upper thighs.

*MS/Ext*

Foul-smelling, dry, scaling feet with white flaking between toes. Toenails on both feet appear to have yellow-brown discoloration. The nails of some of the toes appear to be thicker than the rest, particularly on the right foot.

■ Labs

None available, but patient states his cholesterol and blood sugars are "good."

■ Assessment of Current Problems

1. Athlete's foot (tinea pedis)
2. Jock itch (tinea cruris)
3. Possible onychomycosis
4. Unsanitary foot and body hygiene

## QUESTIONS

### Problem Identification

1.a. What are this patient's drug therapy problems?

1.b. What information leads you to this conclusion?

1.c. What risk factors does the patient have for these conditions?

1.d. What pathogen is most likely to cause these infections?

1.e. What tests could be done at a physician's office to confirm diagnosis of these conditions?

### Desired Outcome

2. What are the goals of treatment in this case?

### Therapeutic Alternatives

3.a. What nonpharmacologic measures should be recommended to this patient?

3.b. What pharmacologic treatments can be sold to this patient without a prescription for these conditions? Include drug, formulation, route of administration, and duration.

3.c. What additional pharmacologic treatments for these conditions could be used if a prescription is obtained from the patient's physician? Include drug, formulation, and route of administration.

## ■ CLINICAL COURSE

You recommend an OTC product and see the patient in your pharmacy 2 months later. He tells you that his itching has stopped, but his toenails have grown thick and crusty. They are also darker yellow than before. He has an appointment with his physician next week.

### Optimal Plan

4.a. What treatment option would you recommend for this patient's onychomycosis and why? Include drug, dosage form, strength, frequency, and duration of therapy.

4.b. If this treatment fails to work or is not tolerated, what alternatives exist?

### Outcome Evaluation

5.a. How would you determine whether your treatment succeeded?

5.b. What side effects can occur with oral and topical antifungal treatments, and how should you monitor for the occurrence of such side effects?

### Patient Education

6. What would you say to the patient (in layman's terms) when counseling on how to treat his condition with the selected antifungal product? Include how to take the medication and what to expect from it in terms of efficacy and possible side effects.

## ■ FOLLOW-UP QUESTIONS

1. What is "pulse" therapy for superficial fungal infections, and what are its advantages and disadvantages?
2. What are the differences between appropriate treatment of onychomycosis and tinea pedis?
3. If itraconazole had been prescribed for this patient, what could be some possible reasons for lack of efficacy?

## ■ SELF-STUDY ASSIGNMENTS

1. Explain the situations where it is necessary to refer a patient to a physician for the treatment of tinea infections and when oral therapy is preferred over topical agents.
2. Compare and contrast the mechanisms of action for the azole and allylamine antifungals.
3. Review the rates and precipitating factors of oral terbinafine– and oral itraconazole–associated hepatotoxicity.

## CLINICAL PEARL

Over 70% of the population will experience a mycotic infection of the skin, hair, or nail at some point in their lifetime.

## REFERENCES


1. Nadalo D, Montoya C, Hunter-Smith D. What is the best way to treat tinea cruris? J Fam Pract 2006;55:256–258.
2. Gupta AK, Ryder, Chow M, Cooper EA. Dermatophytosis: the management of fungal infections. Skinmed 2005;4:305–310.
3. Singal A, Pandhi D, Agrawal S, Das S. Comparative efficacy of topical 1% butenafine and 1% clotrimazole in tinea cruris and tinea corporis: a randomized, double-blind trial. J Dermatolog Treat 2005;16:331–335.
4. Patel A, Brookman SD, Bullen MU, et al. Topical treatment of interdigital tinea pedis: terbinafine compared with clotrimazole. Australas J Dermatol 1999;40:197–200.
5. Crawford F, Young P, Godfrey C, et al. Oral treatments for toenail onychomycosis: a systematic review. Arch Dermatol 2002;138:811–816.
6. Cost of topical products for tinea pedis. Med Lett Drugs Ther 2010;52:35–36.
7. Topical treatment of superficial fungal infections. Pharm Lett Prescriber Lett 2009;(8):250806.
8. Crawford F, Hollis S. Topical treatments for fungal infections of the skin and nails of the foot. Cochrane Database Syst Rev 2007;(3):CD001434.
9. Gupta AK, Tu LQ. Therapies for onychomycosis. Dermatol Clin 2006;24:375–379.
10. Penzak SR, Gubbins PO, Gurley BJ, Wang PL, Saccente M. Grapefruit decreases the systemic availability of itraconazole capsules in healthy volunteers. Ther Drug Monit 1999;21:304–309.


# 139

# BACTERIAL VAGINOSIS

Competition among Bacteria. . . . . . . . . . . . . . . Level I

**Charles D. Ponte, BS, PharmD, BC-ADM, BCPS, CDE, CPE, FAPhA, FASHP, FCCP**

## LEARNING OBJECTIVES

After completing this case study, the reader should be able to:

- Identify predisposing factors associated with bacterial vaginosis.
- List the common clinical and diagnostic findings associated with bacterial vaginosis.
- Develop a therapeutic plan for the management of bacterial vaginosis.
- Describe the role of the pharmacist in the overall management of infectious vaginitis.

## PATIENT PRESENTATION

### Chief Complaint

"I think I might have a yeast infection."

### HPI

Judy Heyman is a 30-year-old female graduate student who comes to the Family Practice Center for an acute visit. She states that 1 month ago she was seen at an urgent care center for severe facial pain and headache. She was diagnosed with an acute sinus infection and given a prescription for a 2-week course of doxycycline (100 mg po BID). During treatment, she developed a vaginal yeast infection. She self-treated it with a nonprescription antifungal cream that alleviated her symptoms. She states that she completed her course of doxycycline despite some mild diarrhea attributed to the drug. Presently, she complains of some mild vaginal discomfort (worse with intercourse) and a "fishy" vaginal odor. Her last period was approximately 5 weeks ago. She admits to inconsistent use of a diaphragm and foam for contraception.

### PMH

Venereal warts—1999
GERD

### FH

Noncontributory

### SH

Is a graduate student in the College of Business and Economics. Has multiple sexual partners (including women); male partners rarely use condoms. Has smoked one pack of cigarettes per day since age 16. Alcohol use consists of a glass of wine nightly and occasional beer. Smokes an occasional marijuana joint.

### Meds

Prilosec 20 mg po QHS
Multivitamin one po daily
Calcium supplement with vitamin D one po daily

### All

Cats → itchy eyes and sneezing; house dust → watery eyes, sneezing; penicillin → hiveslike pruritic rash, some tightness in her chest; topical clindamycin → facial rash when used to treat acne 15 years ago

### ROS

Noncontributory except that she has noticed a small amount of thin, white mucus on her underclothing and her period is approximately 7 days late

### Physical Examination

Limited because of acute visit for specific gynecologic complaint

*Gen*

Patient is a healthy-appearing 30-year-old woman in NAD.

*VS*

BP 130/75, P 90, RR 16, T 37.4°C; Wt 51.5 kg, Ht 5′3″

*Genit/Rect*

External genitalia WNL; no discharge expressed from the urethra, vagina with a small amount of thin white mucus; positive "whiff" test; pH 5.0. Cervix—not completely visualized; appears clear with a small amount of mucoid discharge from the os. Uterus is slightly enlarged, nontender, retroflexed, no cervical motion tenderness. Adnexa without tenderness or masses.

**TABLE 139-1** Characteristics of Different Types of Vaginitis

| Characteristic | *Candida* | Bacterial | *Trichomonas* | Chemical |
|---|---|---|---|---|
| Pruritus | ++ | +/− | +/− | ++ |
| Erythema | + | +/− | +/− | + |
| Abnormal discharge | + | + | +/− | − |
| Viscosity | Thick | Thin | Thick/thin | − |
| Color | White | Gray | White, yellow, green-gray | − |
| Odor | None | Foul, "fishy" | Malodorous | − |
| Description | Curdlike | Homogeneous | Frothy | − |
| pH | 3.8–5.0 | >4.5 | 5.0–7.5 | − |
| Diagnostic tests | Potassium hydroxide preparation shows long, threadlike fibers of mycelia microscopically | (+) "Whiff test," "clue cells" | Pear-shaped protozoa, cervical "strawberry" spots | − |

### Labs

Microscopic examination of vaginal secretions: 20–25 WBC/hpf; 10–15 clue cells/hpf; 0 lactobacilli/hpf; 15–20 squamous epithelial cells/hpf
Serum pregnancy test—negative

### Assessment

Vaginal candidiasis—resolved
Bacterial vaginosis

## QUESTIONS

### Problem Identification

1.a. Create a list of the patient's drug therapy problems.

1.b. What clinical or laboratory information indicates the presence of bacterial vaginosis (Table 139-1)?

1.c. What is the pathophysiologic basis for the development of bacterial vaginosis?

1.d. Could the patient's problem have been caused by drug therapy?

### Desired Outcome

2. What are the goals of pharmacotherapy in this case?

### Therapeutic Alternatives

3.a. What feasible pharmacotherapeutic alternatives are available for the treatment of bacterial vaginosis?

3.b. What economic, psychosocial, and ethical considerations are applicable to this patient?

### Optimal Plan

4.a. What drug, dosage form, dose, schedule, and duration of therapy are best for this patient?

4.b. What alternatives would be appropriate if the initial therapy fails or cannot be used?

### Outcome Evaluation

5. What clinical and laboratory parameters are necessary to evaluate the therapy for achievement of the desired therapeutic outcome and to detect or prevent adverse effects?

### Patient Education

6. What information should be provided to the patient to enhance adherence, ensure successful therapy, and minimize adverse effects?

## CLINICAL COURSE

After completion of the treatment you recommended, the patient returns to the clinic in 10 days for follow-up. She voices no complaints except that she has been experiencing some vaginal itching, dysuria, and continued painful intercourse. Physical examination reveals a thick, whitish material adherent to the vaginal mucosa. The vulva appears erythematous with excoriations on the labia majora. Microscopic analysis of vaginal secretions revealed hyphae and budding yeast. No white cells are noted. Vaginal pH is normal. The patient is diagnosed with vaginal candidiasis.

### Follow-Up Questions

1. What is the most likely cause of this patient's vaginal candidiasis?
2. What other issues should be addressed with the patient during this follow-up visit?
3. What is the role of the pharmacist in the management of patients with infectious vaginitis?

## SELF-STUDY ASSIGNMENTS

1. Discuss the management of a patient who fails a specific course of treatment for bacterial vaginosis.
2. Discuss the pros and cons of screening asymptomatic pregnant women for the presence of bacterial vaginosis.
3. Describe the best therapeutic approach for a woman diagnosed with bacterial vaginosis who is breastfeeding her infant.
4. Discuss the role of sexual transmission in the pathogenesis of bacterial vaginosis.

## CLINICAL PEARL

Patients should be counseled that oral metronidazole may cause a mild disulfiram (Antabuse)–like reaction if alcohol is consumed during therapy. Symptoms may include flushing, GI distress, sweating, thirst, and blurred vision. Advise patients to abstain from alcoholic beverages during therapy and for 72 hours following its completion.

## REFERENCES

1. Biggs WS, Williams RM. Common gynecologic infections. Prim Care 2009;36:33–51.
2. Tam MT, Yungbluth M, Myles T. Gram stain method shows better sensitivity than clinical criteria for detection of bacterial vaginosis

in surveillance of pregnant, low-income women in a clinical setting. Infect Dis Obstet Gynecol 1998;6:204–208.

3. Nyirjesy P. Vulvovaginal candidiasis and bacterial vaginosis. Infect Dis Clin North Am 2008;22:637–652.
4. McCormack WM. Bacterial vaginosis. In: Mandell GL, Bennett JE, Dolin R, eds. Mandell, Douglas, and Bennett's: Principles and Practice of Infectious Diseases, Vol 1, 7th ed. Philadelphia, PA, Elsevier, 2009:1502–1504.
5. Centers for Disease Control and Prevention. Diseases characterized by vaginal discharge. Sexually transmitted diseases treatment guidelines, 2010. MMWR Morb Mortal Wkly Rep 2010;59(RR-12):1–109. Available at: *www.cdc.gov*. Accessed Feb 19, 2011.
6. Sobel JD. What's new in bacterial vaginosis and trichomoniasis? Infect Dis Clin North Am 2005;19:387–406.
7. Swidsinski A, Mendling W, Loening-Baucke V, et al. An adherent *Gardnerella vaginalis* biofilm persists on the vaginal epithelium after standard therapy with oral metronidazole. Am J Obstet Gynecol 2008;198:e1–e6.
8. Okun N, Gronau KA, Hannah ME. Antibiotics for bacterial vaginosis or *Trichomonas vaginalis* in pregnancy: a systematic review. Obstet Gynecol 2005;105:857–862.
9. Nygren P. Evidence on the benefits and harms of screening and treating pregnant women who are asymptomatic for bacterial vaginosis: an update review for the U.S. Preventive Services Task Force. Ann Intern Med 2008;148:220–233.

# 140

# *CANDIDA* VAGINITIS

It's Back. . . . . . . . . . . . . . . . . . . . . . . . . . . . . . . Level I

**Rebecca M.T. Law, BS Pharm, PharmD**

## LEARNING OBJECTIVES

After completing this case study, the reader should be able to:

- Distinguish *Candida vaginitis* (vulvovaginal candidiasis [VVC]) from other types of vaginitis.
- Know when to refer a patient with symptoms of vaginitis to a physician for further evaluation and treatment.
- Choose an appropriate treatment regimen for the patient with VVC.
- Choose appropriate alternatives for the patient with recurrent VVC, while considering issues relating to non-*albicans* VVC.
- Educate patients with vaginitis about proper use of pharmacotherapeutic treatments and nonpharmacologic management strategies.

## PATIENT PRESENTATION

### Chief Complaint

"I'm having the same problem I had 2 weeks ago, and my doctor is away until next Monday. Can you give me some more of these suppositories?"

### HPI

Sophie Kim is a 32-year-old woman who presents to your pharmacy with the above complaint. On further questioning, you find that she was diagnosed 3 weeks ago by her physician as having another vaginal *Candida* infection. She was prescribed nystatin suppositories 100,000 units intravaginally for 14 nights, which was the same as what she had been prescribed for her previous episode of vaginal candidiasis 2 months earlier. She stated that she had finished the prescription 1 week ago and had felt better then. However, 3 days ago she began to notice mild vaginal itching again. She thought it was her new control-top pantyhose and stopped wearing them, but the itching got worse and became fairly severe with a burning sensation. There was also a white, dry, curdlike vaginal discharge that was nonodorous. This seemed to be identical to what she had experienced 3 weeks ago. Her physician is away until next week, and she wondered if the pharmacy can give her some more suppositories.

### PMH

Diabetes type 1 since age 11. Her blood glucose is well controlled, and her physician is keeping a close eye due to her pregnancy.

Recurrent leg ulcers and foot infections for which she has been prescribed antibiotics on a frequent basis. Currently, there are no ulcers or infections, and she is not on antibiotics.

Last month, she began using tights (with an adjustable waist) to help prevent varicose veins.

### SH

Nonsmoker; drinks alcohol in moderate amounts (one to two drinks maximum) at social functions. She is married and is 7.5 months pregnant.

### Meds

Insulin glargine 15 units SC Q AM for past year

Insulin lispro 6 units SC 15 minutes prior to breakfast, 8 units 15 minutes prior to lunch, and 10 units 15 minutes prior to dinner, for past 4 months

Materna one po Q AM

### All

NKDA

### ROS

Not performed

### Physical Examination

*VS*

BP 120/78; Wt 70 kg, Ht 5′5″

*Note:* No further assessments performed.

### Labs

Not available

## QUESTIONS

### Problem Identification

1.a. What signs and symptoms indicate the presence and severity of VVC (*Candida* vaginitis) (Table 140-1)?

**TABLE 140-1** Characteristics of Different Types of Vaginitis

| Characteristic | *Candida* | Bacterial | *Trichomonas* | Chemical |
|---|---|---|---|---|
| Pruritus | ++ | +/− | +/− | ++ |
| Erythema | + | +/− | +/− | + |
| Abnormal discharge | + | + | +/− | − |
| Viscosity | Thick | Thin | Thick/thin | − |
| Color | White | Gray | White, yellow, green-gray | − |
| Odor | None | Foul, "fishy" | Malodorous | − |
| Description | Curdlike | Homogeneous | Frothy | − |
| pH | 3.8–5.0 | >4.5 | 5.0–7.5 | − |
| Diagnostic tests | Potassium hydroxide preparation shows long, threadlike fibers of mycelia microscopically | (+) "Whiff" test, "clue cells" | Pear-shaped protozoa, cervical "strawberry" spots | − |

For some discussion of above conditions and diagnostic considerations, see: *Centers for Disease Control and Prevention, Workowski KA, Berman SM. Diseases characterized by vaginal discharge. Sexually transmitted diseases treatment guidelines, 2010. MMWR 2010;59(RR-12),1–109. Available at: http://www.cdc.gov/std/treatment/2010/vaginal-discharge.htm. Accessed Feb 19, 2011.*

1.b. What predisposing factors for VVC might exist in this patient?

1.c. How common is VVC?

## Desired Outcome

2. What are the goals of therapy for this patient?

## Therapeutic Alternatives

3. What pharmacotherapeutic alternatives are available for the treatment of VVC?

## Optimal Plan

4. Design a pharmacotherapeutic plan for this patient.

## Outcome Evaluation

5. What parameters should be monitored to assess the efficacy of the treatment and to detect adverse effects?

## Patient Education

6. What information should the patient receive about her treatment?

## CLINICAL COURSE

The recommended treatment was successful. Two months later, Sophie had another episode of VVC, which was again successfully treated. She delivered a healthy 7-lb baby boy born at term. A month after that, she had another episode of VVC, and she is now nursing.

## Follow-Up Question

1. What is the most appropriate course of action for management of this patient's recurrent VVC?

## SELF-STUDY ASSIGNMENTS

1. Obtain information on tests used to diagnose different types of vaginitis.
2. Compare the retail cost of nonprescription vaginitis treatments in your area.
3. Outline your plans for communicating your treatment recommendations to the patient's physician.

## CLINICAL PEARL

Patients with symptoms suggestive of bacterial vaginosis or sexually transmitted disease (fever, abdominal or back pain, foul-smelling discharge) should be referred to a physician for further evaluation and treatment.

## REFERENCES


1. Centers for Disease Control and Prevention, Workowski KA, Berman SM. Diseases characterized by vaginal discharge. Sexually transmitted diseases treatment guidelines, 2010. MMWR 2010;59(RR-12): 1–109.
2. Section 4: Management and treatment of specific syndromes: vaginal discharge (bacterial vaginosis, vulvovaginal candidiasis, trichomoniasis). In: Canadian Guidelines on Sexually Transmitted Infections, 2008 ed. Ottawa, Ontario, Public Health Agency of Canada. Available at: *http://www.phac-aspc.gc.ca/std-mts/sti-its/guide-lignesdir-eng.php*. Accessed May 30, 2010.
3. Young GL, Jewell D. Topical treatment for vaginal candidiasis (thrush) in pregnancy [review]. In: The Cochrane Library, Issue 5 [search updated October 1, 2009]. Chichester, UK, John Wiley & Sons Ltd, 2010. Abstract available at: *http://www2.cochrane.org/reviews/en/ab000225.html*. Accessed on May 30, 2010.
4. Pappas PG, Rex JH, Sobel JD, et al. Guidelines for treatment of candidiasis. Clin Infect Dis 2004;38:161–189.
5. Sobel JD, Chaim W, Nagappan V, Leaman D. Treatment of vaginitis caused by *Candida glabrata*: use of topical boric acid and flucytosine. Am J Obstet Gynecol 2003;189:1297–1300.
6. Briggs, GG, Freeman RK, Yaffe SJ. Drugs in Pregnancy and Lactation, 7th ed. Baltimore, MD, Williams and Wilkins, 2005.
7. Sanchez JM, Moya G. Fluconazole teratogenicity. Prenat Diagn 1998;18:862–863.
8. Jick SS. Pregnancy outcomes after maternal exposure to fluconazole. Pharmacotherapy 1999;19:221–222.
9. Falagas ME, Betsi GI, Athanasiou S. Probiotics for prevention of recurrent vulvovaginal candidiasis: a review. J Antimicrob Chemother 2006;58:266–272.
10. Hilton E, Isenberg HD, Alperstein P, France K, Borenstein MT. Ingestion of yogurt containing *Lactobacillus acidophilus* as prophylaxis for candidal vaginitis. Ann Intern Med 1992;116:353–357.
11. Ray D, Goswami R, Banerjee U, et al. Prevalence of *Candida glabrata* and its response to boric acid vaginal suppositories in comparison with oral fluconazole in patients with diabetes and vulvovaginal candidiasis. Diabetes Care 2007;30:312–317.
12. Wooltorton E. Drug advisory: the interaction between warfarin and vaginal miconazole. CMAJ 2001;165(7):938. Available at: *http://www.cmaj.ca/cgi/content/full/165/7/938-b*. Accessed May 30, 2010.

13. Devaraj A, O'Beirne JP, Veasey R, Dunk AA. Drug points: interaction between warfarin and topical miconazole cream. BMJ 2002;325:77. Available at: *http://www.bmj.com/cgi/content/full/325/7355/77*. Accessed May 30, 2010.

# 141

# INVASIVE FUNGAL INFECTIONS

The Brewer's Yeast . . . . . . . . . . . . . . . . . . . . . Level II

**Douglas Slain, PharmD, BCPS, FCCP**

## LEARNING OBJECTIVES

After completing this case study, the reader should be able to:

- Construct a prudent, empiric, antifungal regimen for a patient with candidemia.
- Determine situations to use echinocandins for invasive Candida infections.
- Discuss how the identification of non-albicans Candida species can influence antifungal selection.

## PATIENT PRESENTATION

### Chief Complaint

"I am burning up and feel like I have the flu."

### HPI

August Hops is a 50-year-old man who has been experiencing fever and chills and has not been feeling well over the past 4 days. He was admitted to our hospital yesterday. He was at home receiving home intravenous therapy with daptomycin 700 mg IV once daily (day 12 of 14 of daptomycin therapy) via PICC line for MRSA bacteremia, which he developed after having an appendectomy at an outside community hospital about a month ago. During that hospitalization, he also received a course of piperacillin–tazobactam for his appendicitis. His postoperative stay was complicated by a surgical site infection and MRSA bacteremia. He had his catheter removed at that time and was started on vancomycin, until he developed a rash and possible neutropenia. He was then switched to (and eventually sent home on) daptomycin. Prior to being discharged from the outside hospital, Mr Hops also received 7 days of fluconazole 200 mg po daily for a urine sample from a Foley catheter that grew 100,000 colonies/mL of *C. glabrata*. He never grew *Candida* from any other site.

A set of blood cultures was drawn on admission to our hospital and is showing no growth at 24 hours. His surgical site does not look infected. His PICC line was removed, and blood and urine cultures were drawn. Piperacillin–tazobactam was added to the daptomycin empirically on admission.

### PMH

GERD
Hyperlipidemia
HTN
Chronic knee pain (bilateral)

### PSH

S/P hernia repair
S/P appendectomy 1 month ago

### FH

Father died of CHF, mother still alive with no major medical problems

### SH

He is the brewmaster at the local brewery. Married, has four adult children. Denies smoking or excessive ethanol use.

### Home Meds

Omeprazole 40 mg po once daily
Simvastatin 40 mg po once daily
Metoprolol XL 50 mg po once daily
Ibuprofen 600 mg po TID PRN

### All

Vancomycin—reaction: neutropenia and rash

### Physical Examination

*Gen*

Patient is an obese 50-year-old Caucasian man who is resting somewhat comfortably in bed. Weight: 125 kg; height: 5′11″.

*VS*

BP 130/85, P 70, RR 20, T 38.5°C, $O_2$ sat 97%

*Skin*

Mildly clammy, no Janeway lesions or Osler's nodes

*HEENT*

PERRLA, EOMI, nares patent

*Neck/Lymph Nodes*

Neck supple; no lymphadenopathy

*Lungs/Thorax*

CTA

*Heart*

EKG: Regular rate and rhythm. No murmurs.

*Abd*

Bowel sounds faint, mildly distended. Has not had BM for 2 days.

*GU*

Grossly normal, UA pending

*MS/Ext*

No abnormalities

*Neuro*

Intact

**Labs**

| | | | |
|---|---|---|---|
| Na 137 mEq/L | Hgb 12.9 g/dL | WBC 13.4 × $10^3$/mm$^3$ | AST 35 IU/L |
| K 4.3 mEq/L | Hct 40% | PMNs 70% | ALT 30 IU/L |
| Cl 99 mEq/L | Plt 332 × $10^3$/mm$^3$ | Bands 10% | Alk phos 140 IU/L |
| $CO_2$ 27 mEq/L | CK 56 IU/L | Lymphs 14% | T. bili 1.1 mg/dL |
| BUN 7 mg/dL | | Monos 5% | |
| SCr 0.8 mg/dL | | Eos 1% | |
| Glu 98 mg/dL | | Lipase 92 units/L | |
| Mg 2.2 mg/dL | | Amylase 112 units/L | |

**Chest X-Ray**

No infiltrates

**Assessment**

1. Infection? (New source vs. nonresponding MRSA bacteremia.)
2. Constipation.

**Plan**

1. Infection:
   - ✓ Continue daptomycin 700 mg IV daily and piperacillin–tazobactam 3.375 mg IV Q 8 hours.
   - ✓ Order an abdominal CT.
   - ✓ Order a TEE.
2. Constipation:
   - ✓ Senna/docusate tablet po now and daily PRN
   - ✓ Docusate sodium capsule 100 mg po daily

## CLINICAL COURSE

TEE shows no signs of vegetation. CT of abdomen showed no signs of intra-abdominal infection. Despite 2 more days of continued daptomycin therapy, the patient continues to be febrile with leukocytosis, but WBC is slightly improved.

Culture and sensitivity data are now available:

- *Blood cultures* positive at 72 hours (drawn on admission):
  - ✓ PICC line catheter: Rare budding yeast and rare coagulase-negative staphylococci
  - ✓ Left peripheral: Rare budding yeast

The lab states that it appears to be germ tube negative. The team added fluconazole 400 mg IV daily and discontinued piperacillin–tazobactam. They also ordered a funduscopic eye exam to check the patient for *Candida* endophthalmitis.

## QUESTIONS

### Problem Identification

1.a. Create a list of the patient's drug therapy problems.

1.b. What information (signs, symptoms, laboratory values) indicates the presence or severity of each of the drug therapy problems?

### Desired Outcome

2. What are the goals of pharmacotherapy for this patient's drug therapy problems?

### Therapeutic Alternatives

3.a. What nondrug therapies might be useful for this patient?

3.b. What feasible pharmacotherapeutic alternatives are available for treating this infection?

### Optimal Plan

4. What drug, dosage form, dose, schedule, and duration are best for this patient?

### Outcome Evaluation

5. What clinical and laboratory parameters are necessary to evaluate the therapy for achievement of the desired therapeutic outcome and to detect or prevent adverse effects?

### Patient Education

6. What information should be provided to the patient and/or the patient's caregiver to enhance adherence, ensure successful therapy, and minimize adverse effects?

## FOLLOW-UP QUESTIONS

1. What risk factors does Mr Hops have for developing candidemia?
2. What duration of antifungal therapy should be prescribed for Mr Hops?

## SELF-STUDY ASSIGNMENTS

1. Explain how use of PNA FISH technology in the microbiology laboratory can reduce antifungal drug expenditures.
2. Explain how this patient's therapy would be different if he developed signs of endophthalmitis.
3. Research available literature to determine whether any antifungal agents have displayed useful activity against *Candida* in biofilm.

## CLINICAL PEARL

Despite the general enhanced in vitro *Candida* activity of voriconazole over fluconazole, therapy with voriconazole may be affected by azole-class resistance mechanisms.

## REFERENCES


1. Parkins MD, Sabuda DM, Elsayed S, Laupland KB. Adequacy of empirical antifungal therapy and effect on outcome among patients with invasive *Candida* species infections. J Antimicrob Chemother 2007;60:613–618.
2. Pappas PG, Kauffman CA, Andes D, et al. Clinical practice guidelines for the management of candidiasis: 2009 update by the Infectious Diseases Society of America. Clin Infect Dis 2009;48:503–535.
3. Gubbins PO, Heldenbrand S. Clinically relevant drug interactions of current antifungal agents. Mycoses 2010;53:95–113.
4. Heelan JS, Siliezar D, Coon K. Comparison of rapid testing methods for enzyme production with the germ tube method for presumptive identification of *Candida albicans*. J Clin Microbiol 1996;34:2847–2849.
5. Cauda R. Candidemia in patients with an inserted medical device. Drugs 2009;69(Suppl):33–38.

6. Chen SC, Sorrell TC. Antifungal agents. Med J Aust 2007;187: 404–409.
7. Cleary JD, Schwartz M, Rogers PD, de Mestral J, Chapman SW. Effects of amphotericin B and caspofungin on histamine expression. Pharmacotherapy 2003;23:966–973.

# 142

# INFECTIONS IN IMMUNOCOMPROMISED PATIENTS

Making a Rash Decision . . . . . . . . . . . . . . . . . Level II

**Aaron Cumpston, PharmD**
**Douglas Slain, PharmD, BCPS, FCCP**

## LEARNING OBJECTIVES

After completing this case study, the reader should be able to:

- Construct a prudent empiric antibiotic regimen for a febrile neutropenic patient.
- Determine appropriate situations to use vancomycin in empiric antimicrobial regimens for the treatment of febrile neutropenic episodes.
- Describe situations in which antibiotic monotherapy versus combination therapy would be warranted in the empiric treatment of febrile neutropenia.

## PATIENT PRESENTATION

### Chief Complaint

"I have a fever and chills."

### HPI

Scarlet Hives is a 60-year-old woman with a history of IgG kappa multiple myeloma who is undergoing an autologous hematopoietic cell transplant. Her stem cells were collected by peripheral blood collection, which were mobilized with cyclophosphamide and filgrastim. During collection she developed a vesicular rash involving her left lower abdominal quadrant, which was documented by PCR analysis to be herpes zoster. This was treated with valacyclovir. Her preparative regimen for transplant was high-dose melphalan, followed by stem cell rescue with her peripheral blood stem cells. Eight days after stem cell infusion, she spiked a fever of 38.6°C (101.5°F). She now also complains of chills and nausea.

### PMH

IgG kappa multiple myeloma
GERD
HTN
Hyperlipidemia
CAD
Peripheral neuropathy
Type 2 DM
Chronic back pain

### Surgical History

Hysterectomy—17 years ago

### FH

Mother died of CAD at early age; father died at age 67 from lung cancer; has one sister and one brother, both living and well.

### SH

High school cafeteria manager of 22 years, now retired. She is married and lives with her husband. She has three children. Denies smoking or ethanol use.

### Home Meds

Esomeprazole 40 mg po once daily
Atorvastatin 80 mg po once daily
Fentanyl patch 75 mcg every 48 hours
Neurontin 800 mg po TID
Lisinopril 5 mg po once daily
Metoprolol 75 mg po BID
Multivitamin po once daily
Oxycodone IR 15 mg every 6 hours PRN pain
Pioglitazone 15 mg po once daily
Promethazine 25 mg po every 6 hours PRN nausea
Valacyclovir 500 mg po once daily, after receiving 1,000 mg TID × 7 days for treatment course
Fluconazole 400 mg po once daily
Levofloxacin 500 mg po once daily
Filgrastim 480 mcg subcutaneously daily

### All

Ceftazidime—bad rash

### ROS

(+) Fever/chills, (+) nausea; denies vomiting, cough, diarrhea

### Physical Examination

*Gen*

Patient is a 60-year-old Caucasian woman who appears alert and oriented.

*VS*

BP 115/83, P 115, RR 16, T 38.6°C, $O_2$ sat 98%; Wt 191 lb, Ht 5′1″

*Skin*

Warm and dry. No erythema or induration around port on left chest. Resolving herpes zoster rash on abdomen; lesions are crusted and healing.

*HEENT*

PERRLA, EOMI, (−) tonsillar erythema, (−) rhinorrhea, (−) mucositis

*Neck/Lymph Nodes*

Neck supple; no lymphadenopathy

*Lungs/Thorax*

Normal; no wheezes, crackles, or rhonchi

*Heart*

Tachycardic but regular rhythm; no murmurs, rubs, or gallops

*Abd*

Soft, NT, (+) bowel sounds

*Genit/Rect*

Deferred

*MS/Ext*

No deformity, mild weakness, no peripheral edema

*Neuro*

A & O × 3; CN II–XII grossly intact

### Labs

| | | |
|---|---|---|
| Na 135 mEq/L | WBC 0.2 × $10^3$/mm$^3$ | AST 16 IU/L |
| K 3.6 mEq/L | PMNs 14% | ALT 15 IU/L |
| Cl 95 mEq/L | Bands 5% | Alk phos 38 IU/L |
| $CO_2$ 21 mEq/L | Lymphs 81% | LDH 187 IU/L |
| BUN 16 mg/dL | Hgb 8.9 g/dL | T. bili 0.6 mg/dL |
| SCr 1.0 mg/dL | Hct 25.3% | |
| Glu 149 mg/dL | RBC 2.6 × $10^6$/mm$^3$ | |
| Ca 8.0 mg/dL | Plt 21 × $10^3$/mm$^3$ | |

### UA

Pending

### Blood Cultures

PICC line: Pending
Peripheral: Pending

### Chest X-Ray

Interval presence of a 2.2-cm oval-shaped density projecting at the level of the retrocardiac aspect of the medial left lung base

### CT Scan with IV Contrast

Normal, no evidence of pulmonary nodule that was a concern on chest x-ray

### Assessment

1. Multiple myeloma s/p autologous stem cell transplant
2. Neutropenic fever
3. Concern for possible pneumonia, ruled out by CT scan

### Plan

1. Begin empiric antimicrobials:
   Piperacillin–tazobactam 4.5 g IV Q 8 h (infused over 30 minutes)
2. Discontinue prophylactic levofloxacin.
3. Monitor for rash due to history of ceftazidime allergy.
4. Monitor renal function and hydrate with IV fluids due to IV contrast with CT scan.
5. Continue home medications.

## QUESTIONS

### Problem Identification

1.a. Create a list of the patient's drug therapy problems.

1.b. What information (signs, symptoms, laboratory values) indicates the presence or severity of each of the drug therapy problems?

### Desired Outcome

2. What are the goals of pharmacotherapy in this patient's case?

### Therapeutic Alternatives

3.a. What nondrug therapies might be useful for this patient?

3.b. What feasible pharmacotherapeutic alternatives are available for treating this febrile episode?

### Optimal Plan

4. What drug(s), dosage form(s), dose(s), schedule, and duration of therapy are best for the empiric treatment of this febrile episode in this patient?

### Outcome Evaluation

5. What clinical and laboratory parameters are necessary to evaluate the therapy for achievement of the desired therapeutic outcome and to detect or prevent adverse effects?

### Patient Education

6. What information should be provided to the patient to enhance adherence, ensure successful therapy, and minimize adverse effects?

## CLINICAL COURSE

On day 2 of admission, the patient is still febrile and the following laboratory results are reported: SCr 2.1 mg/dL, Hgb 8.4 g/dL, Hct 22.8%, and platelets 9 × $10^3$/mm$^3$. The WBC is 0.2 × $10^3$/mm$^3$.

BP 120/75, P 100, RR 18, T 38.3°C, $O_2$ sat 98% RA

Urine and blood cultures (PICC line and peripheral): No growth at 24 hours

The team continued to monitor the patient as planned. She started developing a systemic erythematous rash. On day 3, her piperacillin–tazobactam was changed to imipenem–cilastatin due to the presumed drug rash. Her rash continued to worsen while taking imipenem. On day 5 (WBC = 0.3 × $10^3$/mm$^3$) of the admission, caspofungin was added for empiric coverage of persistent fevers. On day 6, her WBC was 0.6 × $10^3$/mm$^3$ with an ANC of 0.520 × $10^3$/mm$^3$. At this time, her blood cultures (from the PICC line) became positive for gram-positive cocci in pairs and chains. The team added vancomycin 1,500 mg Q 24 h and stopped the imipenem–cilastatin since the rash was still worsening and the patient was no longer neutropenic. The PICC line was removed, and caspofungin was also discontinued the next day. The final identification of the organism in the blood was reported on day 8 as *Enterococcus faecalis*, sensitive to ampicillin and vancomycin. The patient became afebrile after initiation of vancomycin. Her creatinine had normalized by this time, she was no longer neutropenic, and her rash was starting to resolve. She was discharged to complete a 2-week course of vancomycin. All subsequent blood and urine cultures were negative for microbial growth.

### Follow-Up Questions

1. What other antibiotic therapies could have been used for the treatment of Mrs Hives's bacteremia?
2. What is the possibility of cross-reactivity between ceftazidime and aztreonam?
3. When should vancomycin be considered as an initial empiric agent in febrile neutropenic patients?

## SELF-STUDY ASSIGNMENTS

1. Review the criteria for classification of febrile neutropenic patients as either "low" or "high" risk. What types of neutropenic

patients would be considered "low risk" and might benefit from oral antibiotic regimens?

2. Construct a treatment algorithm for treating neutropenic patients with bloodstream infections caused by vancomycin-resistant *Enterococcus faecium* (VRE). The algorithm should include decisions based on renal function and drug contraindications.

## CLINICAL PEARL

Bacterial infections in neutropenic patients have evolved from the historical isolation of gram-negative pathogens to the most common bacteria isolated currently being gram-positive organisms. This is especially true when fluoroquinolone prophylaxis is used.

## REFERENCES


1. Klastersky J. Science and pragmatism in the treatment and prevention of neutropenic infection. J Antimicrob Chemother 1998;41(Suppl D):13–24.
2. Hughes WT, Armstrong D, Bodey GP, et al. 2002 guidelines for the use of antimicrobial agents in neutropenic patients with cancer. Clin Infect Dis 2002;34:730–751.
3. Mermel LA, Farr BM, Sherertz RJ, et al. Guidelines for the management of intravascular catheter-related infections. Clin Infect Dis 2009;49:1–45.
4. Paul M, Soares-Weiser K, Leibovici L. Beta lactam monotherapy versus beta lactam-aminoglycoside combination therapy for fever with neutropenia: systematic review and meta-analysis. BMJ 2003;326:1111–1119.
5. Del Favero A, Menichetti F, Martino P, et al. A multicenter, double-blind, placebo-controlled trial comparing piperacillin–tazobactam with and without amikacin as empiric therapy for febrile neutropenia. Clin Infect Dis 2001;33:1295–1301.
6. Donowitz GR, Maki DG, Crnich CJ, Pappas PG, Rolston KV. Infections in the neutropenic patient: new views of an old problem. Hematology 2001;(Suppl):113–139.
7. National Comprehensive Cancer Network (NCCN) Clinical Practice Guidelines in Oncology (v2.2009). Available at: *http://www.nccn.org/professionals/physician_gls/PDF/infections.pdf*. Accessed July 4, 2010.
8. Gilbert DN, Moellering RC, Eliopoulos GM, Chambers HF, Saag MS, eds. The Sanford Guide to Antimicrobial Therapy 2010. Sperryville, VA, Antimicrobial Therapy Inc, 2010.
9. Frumin J, Gallagher JC. Allergic cross-sensitivity between penicillin, carbapenem, and monobactam antibiotics: what are the chances? Ann Pharmacother 2009;43:304–315.


# 143

# ANTIMICROBIAL PROPHYLAXIS FOR SURGERY

In Life, Preparation is Everything .......... Level II

**Curtis L. Smith, PharmD, BCPS**

## LEARNING OBJECTIVES

After completing this case study, the reader should be able to:

- Recommend appropriate antimicrobial prophylaxis for a given surgical procedure.
- Discuss the timing of antimicrobial prophylaxis for surgery, including doses prior to surgery and dosing after surgery.
- Describe the controversy regarding mechanical bowel preparation prior to colorectal surgery.
- Identify the pros and cons to using oral antimicrobial decontamination prior to colorectal surgery.
- Evaluate the need for perioperative β-blocker therapy in a specific surgical patient.

## PATIENT PRESENTATION

### Chief Complaint

"I have colon cancer and i'm here for surgery."

### HPI

Edward Adler is a 72-year-old man who was recently diagnosed with anemia and generalized weakness. The workup for anemia included a colonoscopy, which showed a malignant neoplasm of the proximal ascending colon. The neoplasm was identified, and the biopsy revealed moderately differentiated adenocarcinoma. The patient denies any current abdominal pain or change in bowel habits, but reports a 20-lb weight loss over the past several months. He is eating but has less of an appetite than normal.

### PMH

Positive for HTN, CAD, TIA, and chronic rhinitis; also mild osteoarthritis, for which he has required no regularly scheduled medications in the past. History of gastritis and anemia.

### PSH

Tonsillectomy, left inguinal hernia repair, colonoscopy with biopsy

### SH

Positive for smoking history of one half of a pack daily; quit 20 years ago

### Meds

Atenolol 100 mg po daily
Hydrochlorothiazide 12.5 mg po daily
Sertraline 100 mg po daily
Omeprazole 20 mg po daily
Aspirin 81 mg po daily
Nasacort nasal spray, two sprays in the morning
Ferrous sulfate 325 mg po TID
Multivitamin one po once daily

### All

None

### ROS

Cardiopulmonary: Denies chest pain, shortness of breath, or wheezing.
Gastrointestinal: Denies history of hepatitis, ulcers, or jaundice.
Genitourinary: He has no history of hematuria or renal calculi.
Musculoskeletal: Positive for arthritis of both wrists and hands.
Psychiatric: Positive for some depression.

### Physical Examination

*Gen*

He has the appearance of a normally developed white man who appears his stated age. He is alert, awake, and in no obvious distress.

*VS*

BP 132/86, P 68, RR 11, T 37.1°C; Wt 69 kg, Ht 5′8″

*Skin*

Warm and dry. Multiple seborrheic dermatomes over the abdomen and chest.

*HEENT*

Face reveals no asymmetry. Pupils are equal. Eyes have no icterus or exophthalmus, extraocular muscles intact. He is wearing corrective lenses.

*Neck/Lymph Nodes*

No adenopathy or thyromegaly. There is no jugular venous distention.

*Lungs/Thorax*

Clear to auscultation

*CV*

Regular rate and rhythm without murmurs

*Abd*

The patient has a faint, left inguinal scar from prior left inguinal hernia repair. The abdomen is without palpable masses, splenomegaly, or hepatomegaly. No tenderness noted.

*Genit/Rect*

Not examined

*MS/Ext*

No scoliosis. He has normal lordotic and kyphotic components to the vertebral curvature. No paravertebral tenderness or spasm. Leg lengths and shoulder heights are grossly equal. He was examined in the sitting and supine positions. Extremities: no gross deformities, rashes, or ecchymoses. 2+ pulses in all four extremities.

*Neuro*

No gross motor or sensory deficits or hyperreflexia. Good grip strength bilaterally.

### Labs

| | | |
|---|---|---|
| Na 132 mEq/L | Hgb 9.9 g/dL | WBC 6.0 × $10^3$/mm$^3$ |
| K 4.1 mEq/L | Hct 30.2% | PMNs 70% |
| Cl 97 mEq/L | RBC 4.06 × $10^6$/mm$^3$ | Bands 0% |
| $CO_2$ 26 mEq/L | Plt 324 × $10^3$/mm$^3$ | Eos 5% |
| BUN 14 mg/dL | MCV 74 μm3 | Lymphs 13% |
| SCr 0.9 mg/dL | MCHC 32.8 g/dL | Monos 12% |
| Glu 93 mg/dL | | |
| Alb 3.9 g/dL | | |

### Assessment

1. Adenocarcinoma of the proximal ascending colon
2. Right hemicolectomy planned

## QUESTIONS

### Problem Identification

1.a. Based on the planned surgical procedure, what is the risk for a surgical wound infection in this patient postoperatively?

1.b. List all of the patient's drug-related problems, including potential postoperative problems.

### Desired Outcome

2. What are the goals of antimicrobial pharmacotherapy for prevention of a surgical wound infection?

### Therapeutic Alternatives

3.a. Discuss the pharmacologic options available for this patient to prevent a surgical wound infection. When would you dose antimicrobials related to the surgical procedure, and how long would you continue antibiotics after the procedure?

3.b. Will a mechanical bowel preparation prior to surgery benefit this patient?

3.c. What are the potential advantages and disadvantages associated with giving oral antibiotics prior to a colorectal surgical procedure?

### Optimal Plan

4.a. What would you recommend for antimicrobial prophylaxis prior to this surgical procedure?

4.b. Will this patient require additional antimicrobial dosing during the procedure? How long would you continue antibiotics following the procedure?

4.c. Should this patient receive perioperative β-blocker therapy?

### Outcome Evaluation

5. What clinical parameters should be monitored to assess the development of a surgical wound infection?

### Patient Education

6. What information should be provided to this patient regarding the risk of surgical wound infections and the use of antibiotics to prevent this risk?

## SELF-STUDY ASSIGNMENTS

1. Construct a chart listing surgical procedures requiring preoperative antimicrobial prophylaxis and the recommended agent(s) to use.
2. Perform a literature search and assess the current information regarding the use of oral antibiotics prior to colorectal surgery.
3. Perform a literature search and assess the current information regarding using perioperative β-blockers (based on both patient characteristics and surgical procedure).

## CLINICAL PEARL

Patients who receive antibiotics for surgical prophylaxis within 3 hours after the surgical incision have a three times higher risk of surgical wound infection compared to patients who receive antibiotics within 2 hours before the incision.

## REFERENCES

1. Edwards JR, Peterson KD, Mu Y, et al. National Healthcare Safety Network (NHSN) report: data summary for 2006 through 2008, issued December 2009. Am J Infect Control 2009;37(10):783–805.
2. Fleisher LA, Beckman JA, Brown KA, et al. 2009 ACCF/AHA focused update on perioperative beta blockade incorporated into the ACC/AHA 2007 guidelines on perioperative cardiovascular evaluation and care for noncardiac surgery: a report of the American College of Cardiology Foundation/American Heart Association Task Force

on Practice Guidelines. Circulation 2009;120(21):e169–e276 [Epub November 2, 2009].
3. Burger W, Chemnitius JM, Kneissl GD, Rücker G. Low-dose aspirin for secondary cardiovascular prevention—cardiovascular risks after its perioperative withdrawal versus bleeding risks with its continuation—review and meta-analysis. J Intern Med 2005;257:399–414.
4. Oscarsson A, Gupta A, Fredrikson M, et al. To continue or discontinue aspirin in the perioperative period: a randomized, controlled clinical trial. Br J Anaesth 2010;104(3):305–312.
5. Geerts WH, Bergqvist D, Pineo GF, et al. Prevention of venous thromboembolism. Chest 2008;133:381S–453S.
6. Bratzler DW, Houck PM. Surgical Infection Prevention Guidelines Writers Workgroup. Antimicrobial prophylaxis for surgery: an advisory statement from the National Surgical Infection Prevention Project. Clin Infect Dis 2004;38:1706–1715.
7. Scher KS. Studies on the duration of antibiotic administration for surgical prophylaxis. Am Surg 1997:63:59–62.
8. Nelson RL, Glenny AM, Song F. Antimicrobial prophylaxis for colorectal surgery. Cochrane Database Syst Rev 2009;(1):CD001181.
9. Antimicrobial prophylaxis for surgery. Treat Guidel Med Lett 2009;7(82):47–52.
10. Classen DC, Evans RS, Pestotnik SL, Horn SD, Menlove RL, Burke JP. The timing of prophylactic administration of antibiotics and the risk of surgical-wound infection. N Engl J Med 1992;326:281–286.
11. Guenaga KK, Matos D, Wille-Jørgensen P. Mechanical bowel preparation for elective colorectal surgery. Cochrane Database Syst Rev 2009;(1):CD001544.

# 144

# PEDIATRIC IMMUNIZATION

Back to School . . . . . . . . . . . . . . . . . . . . . . . . . Level II

**Jean-Venable "Kelly" R. Goode, PharmD, BCPS, FAPhA, FCCP**

## LEARNING OBJECTIVES

After completing this case study, the reader should be able to:

- Develop a plan for administering any needed vaccines, when given a patient's age, immunization history, and medical history.
- Describe appropriate use of pediatric vaccines.
- Educate a child's parents on the risks associated with pediatric vaccines and ways to minimize adverse effects.
- Recognize *inappropriate* reasons for deferring immunization.

## PATIENT PRESENTATION

### Chief Complaint

"My daughter is here for the 'Back to School' program."

### HPI

Allison Showalter is a 4-year-old girl who is generally healthy. She presents today (August 30, 2010) to the pharmacy with her mother for evaluation and to receive any needed immunizations. Allison will be entering junior kindergarten in the fall, and she needs to have an updated immunization record.

### PMH

Some prenatal care, delivered at 42 weeks' gestation via uncomplicated vaginal delivery; birth weight 7 lb, 4 oz. Mother states that her child has had several ear infections and three or four "colds," no other illnesses.

### FH

Mother is 4 months pregnant.

### SH

Lives with mother, age 30, and father, age 32. No siblings. Mother works part-time. Father works as an electrician.

### Meds

Amoxicillin suspension 540 mg po Q 8 h
No recent OTC medication use

### All

NKDA

### ROS

Negative

### Physical Examination

*Gen*

Alert, happy, appropriately developed 4-year-old child in NAD. Wt 18 kg (75th percentile), height 40 in (50th percentile).

*VS*

BP 105/65, P 110, RR 28, T 36.7°C (axillary)

*HEENT*

AF open, flat; PERRL; funduscopic exam not performed; ears slightly red; normal looking TMs, landmarks visualized, no effusion present; nose clear; throat normal

*Lungs*

Clear bilaterally

*Cor*

RRR, no murmurs

*Abd*

Soft, nontender, no masses or organomegaly; normal bowel sounds

*Genit/Rect*

Normal external genitalia; rectal exam deferred, no fissures noted

*Ext*

Normal

*Neuro*

Alert; normal DTRs bilaterally

### Labs

No other labs obtained

### Assessment

Normal-appearing child, in need of immunizations

**IMMUNIZATION RECORD CARD**
**NAME: ALLISON SHOWALTER**

| Vaccine | Dose/Route/ Site | Date | Health Professional | VIS |
|---|---|---|---|---|
| Hepatitis B | 0.5 mL IM thigh | 3/15/2006 | Colter, RN | Hep B |
| Pediarix (DTaP, Hep B, IPV) | 0.5 mL IM thigh | 5/20/2006 | Edwards, RN | Hep B, IPV, DTaP |
| PCV | 0.5 mL IM thigh | 5/20/2006 | Edwards, RN | PCV |
| Hib (HibTITER) | 0.5 mL IM thigh | 5/20/2006 | Edwards, RN | Hib |
| Pediarix | 0.5 mL IM thigh | 7/29/2006 | Edwards, RN | DTaP, Hep B, IPV |
| PCV | 0.5 mL IM thigh | 7/29/2006 | Edwards, RN | PCV |
| Hib (HibTITER) | 0.5 mL IM thigh | 7/29/2006 | Edwards, RN | Hib |
| Pediarix | 0.5 mL IM thigh | 9/30/2006 | Jones, RN | DTaP, Hep B, IPV |
| PCV | 0.5 mL IM thigh | 9/30/2006 | Jones, RN | PCV |
| Hib (HibTITER) | 0.5 mL IM thigh | 9/30/2006 | Jones, RN | Hib |
| DTaP | 0.5 mL IM thigh | 7/1/2007 | Edwards, RN | DTaP |
| Hib (HibTITER) | 0.5 mL IM thigh | 7/1/2007 | Edwards, RN | Hib |
| PCV | 0.5 mL IM thigh | 7/1/2007 | Edwards, RN | PCV |
| MMR | 0.5 mL SC | 7/1/2007 | Edwards, RN | MMR |
| Varicella | 0.5 mL SC | 7/1/2007 | Edwards, RN | Varicella |

# QUESTIONS

## Problem Identification

1. Create a list of the patient's immunization-related problems including any contraindications or precautions for vaccination.

## Desired Outcome

2.a. What immediate goals are reasonable in this case?

2.b. What long-term goals are appropriate for comprehensive management of this patient?

## Therapeutic Alternatives

3.a. How do health care providers determine which vaccines an infant or child needs?

3.b. What is the proper immunization administration technique for children, including location and needle size?

3.c. What vaccines should be administered to this child today, including dose, route, and any alternatives?

## Optimal Plan

4.a. What immunization schedule should be followed for this patient today?

4.b. In addition to immunizations received today, what should be the plan for providing additional immunizations and when should they be administered?

## Outcome Evaluation

5. How should the response to the immunization plan be assessed?

## Patient Education

6. What important information about vaccination needs to be explained to this child's mother?

# FOLLOW-UP QUESTIONS

1. The next year, the mother brings the child to a pediatric influenza immunization clinic. The mother mentions that the child was diagnosed with diabetes about 3 months ago. The child's immunization record reveals influenza vaccine 0.25 mL × 1 dose last fall. What is your recommendation for influenza vaccine for this child?
2. What other immunizations are indicated for this child who now has a chronic condition, diabetes mellitus?

# SELF-STUDY ASSIGNMENTS

1. Search the Internet for the immunization laws and allowed exemptions in your state. What vaccines are required for child-care and school entry?
2. Review the most current immunization recommendations for persons aged 0–6 years, and provide a summary of how your recommendations for this case would be different if a 6-month-old patient in need of immunizations came into your clinic today.
3. Search the Internet for immunization-related Web sites about vaccine-associated adverse effects; compare and contrast these sites, and evaluate them against reliable Web sites for vaccine information.

# CLINICAL PEARL

Currently, all states have immunization laws, although there are differences in the requirements and types of exemptions allowed by the state. Vaccine requirements for school entry help ensure that most people are protected through immunization. Pharmacists should advocate for parents and caregivers to have their children immunized on time to protect them against vaccine-preventable diseases.

# REFERENCES

1. CDC. Advisory Committee on Immunization Practices. Recommended immunization schedules for persons aged 0–18 years—United States, 2010. MMWR 2010;58(51 & 52):1–4 (updated annually at *http://www.cdc.gov/vaccines/recs/schedules/child-schedule.htm#printable*).
2. American Academy of Pediatrics. Active and passive immunization. In: Red Book—Report of the Committee on Infectious Diseases. Elk Grove Village, IL, American Academy of Pediatrics, 2009:1–104.
3. Chen RT, Clark TA, Halperin SA. The yin and yang of paracetamol and paediatric immunizations. Lancet 2009;374:1305–1306.
4. CDC. General recommendations on immunization. Recommendations of the Advisory Committee on Immunization Practices (ACIP). MMWR 2006;55(RR-15):1–37.
5. CDC. Licensure of a 13-valent pneumococcal conjugate vaccine (PCV13) and recommendations for use among children. Advisory Committee on Immunization Practices (ACIP). MMWR 2010;59(09):258–261.
6. Marin M, Broder KR, Temte JL et al. Use of combination measles, mumps, rubella, and varicella vaccine. Recommendations of the Advisory Committee on Immunization Practices (ACIP). MMWR 2010;59(RR-3):1–12.
7. ACIP Provisional Recommendations for the Use of Influenza Vaccines, February 24, 2010. Available at: *http://www.cdc.gov/vaccines/recs/provisional/downloads/flu-vac-mar-2010-508.pdf*. Last accessed June 1, 2010.

# 145

# ADULT IMMUNIZATION

Immunizations: Not Just Kid Stuff . . . . . . . . . Level II

Jean-Venable "Kelly" R. Goode, PharmD, BCPS, FAPhA, FCCP

## LEARNING OBJECTIVES

After completing this case study, the reader should be able to:

- Develop a plan for administering any needed vaccines when given a patient's age, immunization history, and medical history.
- Recognize appropriate precautions and contraindications for vaccination, including inappropriate reasons for deferring vaccination.
- Explain appropriate administration of vaccines, including timing and spacing of both inactive and live attenuated vaccines.
- Recognize the differences in vaccines for young adults currently in use in the United States.

## PATIENT PRESENTATION

### Chief Complaint

"I'm here to get my new prescription filled."

### HPI

Sandra Williams is a 23-year-old woman who presents to your pharmacy with a new prescription for prednisone 40 mg BID for 10 days in January. She has had a moderate asthma exacerbation. She just started her new job as an elementary school teacher. She is a new patient to your pharmacy. She inquires about your "One less" signs about a new vaccine available.

### PMH

Moderate persistent asthma
Chickenpox at age 5 per patient
Splenectomy secondary to car accident 3 months ago

### FH

One sister—healthy
Mother—healthy
Father with type 2 diabetes

### SH

Does not smoke
Drinks alcohol socially

### Meds

Albuterol MDI two inhalations PRN
Pulmicort DPI two inhalations once daily

### All

NKDA

### Immunization Record

No vaccines since kindergarten except:
- Meningococcal vaccine before she started her freshman year in college
- One dose of hepatitis B vaccine before she started her freshman year in college
- MMR vaccine before she started her freshman year in college Td 10 years ago at her adolescent well check-up

### ROS

WDWN African-American woman in NAD

### VS

BP 120/72 (left arm, large cuff, seated), P 76; Wt 54 kg, Ht 5′5″

### Physical Examination

Deferred

### Assessment

A 23-year-old woman recently treated for a moderate asthma exacerbation. She is in need of immunizations today.

## QUESTIONS

### Problem Identification

1.a. Create a list of the patient's immunization-related problems, including any contraindications or precautions for vaccination.

1.b. Create a list of this patient's drug-related problems.

### Desired Outcome

2.a. What immediate immunization goals are reasonable in this case?

2.b. Provide the rationale for administering each of the recommended vaccines to this patient.

2.c. What long-term goals are appropriate for comprehensive management of this patient?

### Therapeutic Alternatives

3. Identify the therapeutic alternatives for addressing this patient's immunization needs.

### Optimal Plan

4. What immunization schedule should be followed for this patient today, including dose and route of administration and the plan for providing additional immunizations?

### Outcome Evaluation

5. How should the response to the immunization plan be assessed?

### Patient Education

6. What important information about vaccination needs to be explained to this patient?

## FOLLOW-UP QUESTIONS

1. What screening questions should a patient be asked prior to administering any vaccinations?

2. What must be documented after a health care practitioner administers a vaccination?

## SELF-STUDY ASSIGNMENTS

1. Review the most current immunization recommendations for adults, and provide a summary of how your recommendations for this case would be different if this person were 65 years of age.
2. Develop a list of diseases and medications indicating that a patient may be a candidate for immunization.
3. Research the laws in your state to verify which vaccines pharmacists may administer. Also, explore how to implement an immunization service in your practice.
4. Review the guidelines for vaccination of pregnant women.
5. Surf the Internet for immunization-related Web sites about vaccine-associated adverse effects; compare and contrast these sites, and evaluate them against reliable Web sites for vaccine information.

## CLINICAL PEARL

Delays in vaccination put patients at risk of vaccine-preventable diseases. However, there is no need to restart an immunization series if the interval between doses is longer than that recommended in the routine schedule. Instead of starting over, merely count the doses administered (provided that they were given at an acceptable minimum interval) and complete the series.

## REFERENCES

1. Centers for Disease Control and Prevention. General recommendations on immunization. Recommendations of the Advisory Committee on Immunization Practices (ACIP). MMWR 2006;55(RR-15):1–37.
2. Centers for Disease Control and Prevention. Prevention of varicella. Recommendations of the Advisory Committee on Immunization Practices (ACIP). MMWR 2007;56(RR04):1–40.
3. Centers for Disease Control and Prevention. ACIP Provisional Recommendations for Use of Pneumococcal Vaccines, October 28, 2008. Available at: *http://www.cdc.gov/vaccines/recs/provisional/downloads/pneumo-Oct-2008-508.pdf*. Last accessed June 7, 2010.
4. Centers for Disease Control and Prevention. Prevention and control of influenza. Recommendations of the Advisory Committee on Immunization Practices (ACIP). MMWR 2007;56(RR06):1–54.
5. Centers for Disease Control and Prevention. ACIP Provisional Recommendations for the Use of Influenza Vaccines, February 24, 2010. Available at: *http://www.cdc.gov/vaccines/recs/provisional/downloads/flu-vac-mar-2010-508.pdf*. Last accessed June 1, 2010.
6. Centers for Disease Control and Prevention. Quadrivalent human papillomavirus vaccine. Recommendations of the Advisory Committee on Immunization Practices (ACIP). MMWR 2007;56(RR-2):1–23.
7. Centers for Disease Control and Prevention. FDA licensure of bivalent human papillomavirus vaccine (HPV2, Cervarix) for use in females and updated HPV vaccination recommendations from the Advisory Committee on Immunization Practices. MMWR 2010;(20):626–629.
8. Centers for Disease Control and Prevention. Preventing tetanus, diphtheria, and pertussis among adolescents: use of tetanus toxoid, reduced diphtheria toxoid and acellular pertussis vaccine. Recommendations of the Advisory Committee on Immunization Practices (ACIP). MMWR 2006;55(RR-3):1–34.
9. Centers for Disease Control and Prevention. A comprehensive immunization strategy to eliminate transmission of hepatitis B virus infection in the United States. Recommendations of the Advisory Committee on Immunization Practices (ACIP). MMWR 2006;55(RR-16):1–33.
10. Centers for Disease Control and Prevention. Prevention of pneumococcal disease. Recommendations of the Advisory Committee on Immunization Practices (ACIP). MMWR 1997;46(RR-8):1–25.
11. Centers for Disease Control and Prevention. Prevention and control of meningococcal disease: recommendations of the Advisory Committee on Immunization Practices (ACIP). MMWR 2005;54(RR-7):1–21.
12. Centers for Disease Control and Prevention. Updated recommendations from the Advisory Committee on Immunization Practices (ACIP) for revaccination of persons at prolonged increased risk for meningococcal disease. MMWR 2009;58(37):1042–1043.
13. Centers for Disease Control and Prevention. Prevention of hepatitis A through active or passive immunization. Recommendations of the Advisory Committee on Immunization Practices (ACIP). MMWR 2006;55(RR-07):1–23.
14. Centers for Disease Control and Prevention. Haemophilus b conjugate vaccines for prevention of *Haemophilus influenzae* type B disease among infants and children two months of age and older. Recommendations of the ACIP. MMWR 1991;40(RR01):1–7.
15. Centers for Disease Control and Prevention. Recommended adult immunization schedule—United States, 2010. MMWR 2010;59:1.
16. CDC. Advisory Committee on Immunization Practices. Recommended immunization schedules for persons aged 0–18 years—United States, 2010. MMWR 2010;58(51 & 52):1–4 (updated annually at *http://www.cdc.gov/vaccines/recs/schedules/child-schedule.htm#printable*).

# 146

# HIV INFECTION

## The Antiretroviral-Naive Patient . . . . . . . . . . . . Level II

**Rodrigo M. Burgos, PharmD**

**Keith A. Rodvold, PharmD, FCCP**

## LEARNING OBJECTIVES

After completing this case study, the reader should be able to:

- Describe situations in which antiretroviral therapy should be initiated in patients with HIV infection, and determine the desired outcome of such therapy.
- Recommend appropriate first-line antiretroviral therapies for the antiretroviral-naive person.
- Provide patient education on the proper dose, administration, and adverse effects of antiretroviral agents.

## PATIENT PRESENTATION

### Chief Complaint

"I am here for regular care. It hurts to swallow."

### HPI

Jenny Baird is a 42-year-old woman diagnosed with HIV infection 2 years ago during a routine exam. At the time of diagnosis, the patient was asymptomatic. Since her diagnosis, she has been following up regularly every 4 months. She also reports painful and difficult swallowing over the past 2–3 weeks.

Today she returns for a follow-up visit.

## PMH

HIV infection diagnosed 2 years ago; risk factor heterosexual contact
Bronchitis
Asthma
GERD

## FH

Noncontributory

## SH

History of crack cocaine use, last use 1 month ago.
Smokes marijuana once per month mainly as an appetite enhancer.
Tobacco 0.5 ppd, ETOH one to two drinks on weekends.
Unemployed, lives with partner.
Sexually active with stable partner; 100% condom use as sole method of contraception. Partner is HIV (−) and is aware of her HIV status.

## Medications

Multivitamin po once daily
Tums PRN heartburn
Albuterol HFA MDI, two puffs Q 6 h PRN SOB

## All

Bactrim (rash)

## ROS

Difficulty and pain on swallowing

## Physical Examination

*Gen*

Thin, well-developed black female in NAD, alert and oriented × 3

*VS*

BP 110/64, P 80, RR 18, T 35.9°C; Wt 58 kg, Ht 5′5″

*Skin*

Anicteric, has large tattoo on back. No other skin lesions noted.

*HEENT*

(+) Oral lesions and white plaques, sinuses nontender, PERRLA, ears and nose clear

*Neck*

Supple, no thyromegaly, R neck lymph node 0.7 cm in diameter

*Chest*

Lungs clear

*CV*

$S_1$, $S_2$ without $S_3$, $S_4$, or murmur

*Abd*

(+) BS, soft, nontender, without HSM
(+) Bilateral inguinal lymph nodes 0.5 cm in diameter

*GU*

The pelvic exam reveals normal external genitalia. The vaginal vault is within normal limits. Perineum and perianal regions are free of grossly visible lesions. Guaiac (−) stools.

*Ext*

No wasting, no CCE

*Neuro*

No focal deficits

## Labs

See Table 146-1.

**TABLE 146-1** Laboratory Values for the Previous Visit and for Subsequent Visits

| Parameter (Units) | 2 Years Ago | This Visit | 6 Weeks Later | 12 Weeks Later |
|---|---|---|---|---|
| General | | | | |
| Weight (kg) | 65 | 58 | 57 | 60 |
| Hematology | | | | |
| Hgb (g/dL) | 10.9 | 11.1 | 12.2 | 12.9 |
| Hct (%) | 32.9 | 33.6 | 36.5 | 37.3 |
| Plt ($\times 10^3$/mm$^3$) | 234 | 287 | 298 | 311 |
| WBC ($\times 10^3$/mm$^3$) | 7.1 | 5.7 | 6.9 | 7.1 |
| Lymphs (%) | 47.3 | 45.5 | 44.9 | 47.3 |
| Monos (%) | 6.4 | 6.6 | 6.1 | 6.4 |
| Eos (%) | 3.5 | 0.9 | 2.0 | 3.5 |
| Basos (%) | 0.3 | 0.2 | 0.4 | 0.3 |
| Neutros (%) | 42.5 | 46.8 | 46.6 | 42.5 |
| ANC ($\times 10^3$/mm$^3$) | 3.0 | 2.7 | 3.2 | 3.0 |
| Chemistry | | | | |
| BUN (mg/dL) | 5 | 10 | 9 | 7 |
| SCr (mg/dL) | 0.8 | 0.9 | 0.9 | 0.8 |
| T. bili (mg/dL) | 0.5 | 1.6 | – | 0.6 |
| Alb (g/dL) | 3.3 | 3.8 | – | 3.4 |
| AST (IU/L) | 17 | 19 | – | 18 |
| ALT (IU/L) | 12 | 13 | – | 14 |
| Fasting glucose | 115 | 93 | 92 | |
| Fasting lipid profile | | | | |
| T. chol | – | 162 | – | 164 |
| Triglycerides | – | 53 | – | 92 |
| LDL | – | 45 | – | 112 |
| Surrogate markers | | | | |
| CD4 (%) | 38 | 25 | – | 17 |
| CD4 (cells/mm$^3$) | 689 | 335 | – | 529 |
| CD8 (%) | 48 | 48 | – | 59 |
| HIV RNA (RT-PCR)[a] (copies/mL) | 55,000 | 155,000 | 154 | <50 |
| Antiviral resistance test (genotypic resistance test) | L63P | – | – | – |
| Hepatitis virus serologies | | | | |
| HBV Ab | Negative | | | |
| HBV core Ab total | Negative | | | |
| HBV Ag | Negative | | | |
| HCV Ab | Negative | | | |
| HAV Ab | Positive | | | |

[a]Reverse transcriptase polymerase chain reaction assay.

■ Assessment

A 42-year-old woman with HIV infection, shows steady decline in CD4 cell count and rising levels of HIV viremia since her initial diagnosis 2 years ago, presenting with painful swallowing and white plaques on posterior pharynx and mouth consistent with esophageal and oropharyngeal candidiasis

# QUESTIONS

## Problem Identification

1.a. What information (signs, symptoms, laboratory values) indicates the severity of HIV disease?

1.b. Is prophylactic therapy for any associated opportunistic pathogen indicated in this patient? Why or why not?

1.c. What is your recommendation regarding antiretroviral therapy for this patient?

## Desired Outcome

2. What are the goals of pharmacotherapy in this case?

## Therapeutic Alternatives

3.a. What therapeutic options are available for treating this antiretroviral-naive patient?

3.b. What economic, psychosocial, racial, and ethical considerations are applicable to this patient?

3.c. How would you evaluate patient readiness for antiretroviral treatment initiation?

## Optimal Plan

4.a. Propose an antiretroviral regimen for this woman. Indicate the drug name, dosage form, dose, schedule, and duration of therapy for the regimen you choose.

4.b. Design an antiretroviral regimen that would be appropriate if the patient informs you that she would like to consider becoming pregnant once her HIV infection is under control.

4.c. Recommend an antiretroviral regimen that would be appropriate if this patient has a history of chronic kidney disease, not requiring hemodialysis.

4.d. Discuss the role of HIV resistance testing in designing a regimen for the antiretroviral treatment-naive patient.

## Outcome Evaluation

5. What clinical and laboratory parameters are necessary to evaluate the clinical efficacy and toxicity of the antiretroviral regimen selected? Specify frequency with which you will monitor these parameters. Indicate therapeutic goal.

## Patient Education

6.a. What important information would you provide to this patient about her therapy?

6.b. Explain in nontechnical terms the surrogate markers and their use in monitoring HIV disease.

6.c. Identify potential barriers to medication adherence, and discuss potential strategies to overcome these barriers and maximize treatment adherence.

# ■ CLINICAL COURSE

The provider and patient accepted your treatment recommendations. The patient returns to the clinic for follow-up 6 and 12 weeks after treatment initiation. Her treatment flow sheet is as follows:

| Parameter | 6 Weeks Later | 12 Weeks Later |
|---|---|---|
| HIV RNA (RT-PCR) (copies/mL) | 154 | <50 |
| CD4-lymphocyte count (cells/mm$^3$) | NA | 529 |
| Symptoms of HIV infection | Asymptomatic | Asymptomatic |
| Adverse events reported | Mild nausea, no vomiting | None |
| Concomitant medications | Oral contraceptive daily<br>MVI daily<br>Dapsone 100 mg daily<br>Albuterol INH PRN<br>Tums PRN | Oral contraceptive daily<br>MVI daily<br>Dapsone 100 mg daily<br>Albuterol INH PRN<br>Tums PRN |

## Follow-Up Questions

1. Provide an assessment of the antiretroviral regimen efficacy at each follow-up visit.
2. Identify potential problems with her concomitant medications and discuss alternatives.

# ■ SELF-STUDY ASSIGNMENTS

1. Review the current literature regarding recommended therapy for the antiretroviral-naive and treatment-experienced individuals. What is the recommended first-line therapy, and what are the indications to change to alternative therapy? What is known about therapy of HIV and survival?
2. Review the current literature regarding the development of HIV resistance to antiretroviral agents and strategies for the prevention and management of resistance.

# CLINICAL PEARL

Despite the increasing body of clinical data to guide initial antiretroviral therapy in treatment-naive patients, the choice of the optimal regimen remains a complex issue. The ideal time to start treatment for asymptomatic patients is constantly revised based on expert opinion and available cohort data. In addition to potency and efficacy factors, clinicians must take into account a wide range of individual factors, including comorbid conditions, transmitted resistant virus, adherence, potential adverse events, drug–drug or drug–food interactions, and consequences of virologic failure for the particular regimen selected. Clinicians should always individualize therapeutic choices based on available data and unique patient factors.

# REFERENCES


1. Centers for Disease Control and Prevention. Revised surveillance case definitions for HIV infection among adults, adolescents, and children aged <18 months and for HIV infection and AIDS among children aged 18 months to <13 years—United States, 2008. MMWR Morb Mortal Wkly Rep 2008;57(RR-10):1–8.
2. Centers for Disease Control and Prevention. Appendix A: AIDS-defining conditions. MMWR Morb Mortal Wkly Rep 2008;57 (RR-10):9.

3. Centers for Disease Control and Prevention. Guidelines for prevention and treatment of opportunistic infections in HIV-infected adults and adolescents: recommendations from CDC, the National Institutes of Health, and the HIV Medicine Association of the Infectious Diseases Society of America. MMWR Morb Mortal Wkly Rep 2009;58(RR-4):1–206. Available at: *www.aidsinfo.nih.gov*. Accessed May 26, 2010.
4. Guidelines for the use of antiretroviral agents in HIV-infected adults and adolescents. Department of Health and Human Services (DHHS) Panel on Antiretroviral Guidelines for Adults and Adolescents, December 1, 2009. Available at: *www.aidsinfo.nih.gov*. Accessed May 26, 2010.
5. Hammer SM, Eron JJ, Reiss P, et al. Antiretroviral treatment for adult HIV infection: 2008 recommendations of the International AIDS Society-USA Panel. JAMA 2008;300:555–570.
6. Hammer SM. Management of newly diagnosed HIV infection. N Engl J Med 2005;353:1702–1710.
7. Aberg JA, Kaplan JE, Libman H, et al. Primary care guidelines for the management of persons infected with human immunodeficiency virus: update by the HIV Medicine Association of the Infectious Diseases Society of America. Clin Infect Dis 2009;49:651–681.
8. Paterson DL, Swindells S, Mohr J, et al. Adherence to protease inhibitor therapy and outcomes in patients with HIV infection. Ann Intern Med 2000;133:21–30.
9. Novak RM, Chen L, MacArthur RD, et al. Prevalence of antiretroviral drug resistance mutations in chronically HIV-infected, treatment-naive patients: implications for routine resistance screening before initiation of antiretroviral therapy. Clin Infect Dis 2005;40:468–474.
10. Little SJ, Holte S, Routy JP, et al. Antiretroviral-drug resistance among patients recently infected with HIV. N Engl J Med 2002;347:385–394.

SECTION 17
# ONCOLOGIC DISORDERS

## 147

## BREAST CANCER

An Opportunity Lost. . . . . . . . . . . . . . . . . . . . Level II

**Bonnie Lin Boster, PharmD, BCOP**

**Chad Barnett, PharmD, BCOP**

### LEARNING OBJECTIVES

After completing this case study, students should be able to:

- Design a pharmacotherapeutic plan for treatment of locally advanced breast cancer.
- Develop an appropriate monitoring plan for patients receiving adjuvant hormonal therapy for treatment of breast cancer.
- Describe appropriate follow-up for patients after definitive treatment of breast cancer.
- Provide patient education on the proper dosing, administration, and adverse effects of capecitabine and ixabepilone.
- Compare and contrast the goals of treatment for locally advanced breast cancer versus metastatic breast cancer.

### PATIENT PRESENTATION

#### Chief Complaint

"I have a lump in my breast."

#### HPI

Rosalita Garza is a 61-year-old woman presenting for evaluation of a new mass in her left breast. She first noticed a palpable breast mass on self-examination approximately 14 months ago but was unable to have this further investigated due to loss of health insurance. The patient describes the mass as intermittently painful. A mammogram was performed prior to her current visit, which was suspicious for malignancy.

#### PMH

Musculoskeletal injury in 2000. Fell from a chair while at work and suffered injuries to her cervical spine. She has required bone grafting from her right hip to her cervical spine. She is taking multiple medications for pain control.

Depression (diagnosed 7 years ago).

#### FH

Sister diagnosed with breast cancer at age 60, now 5 years postsurgery. The patient was unable to recall any further details. No other significant cancer history is noted.

#### SH

Lives with and acts as primary caretaker for her mother, who has dementia. Denies alcohol use and is a nonsmoker. Has a 35-year-old daughter who also lives with her.

#### Endocrine History

Menarche age 13; menopause age 55; first child age 26; $G_1P_1A_0$. Last Pap smear at age 40. Took Premarin as HRT for 5 years after the onset of menopause.

#### Meds

Pepcid 20 mg po BID
Zoloft 50 mg po once daily
Ambien CR 12.5 mg po at bedtime PRN sleep
Neurontin 300 mg po TID
Hydrocodone/acetaminophen 5 mg/500 mg, one to two tablets po Q 6 h PRN pain

#### All

NKDA

#### ROS

Negative except for complaints noted above

#### Physical Examination

*Gen*

WDWN 61-year-old Hispanic female. Awake, alert, in NAD.

*VS*

BP 127/71, P 89, RR 16, T 36.7°C; Wt 137 lb, Ht 5′1″

*HEENT*

NC/AT; PERRLA; EOMI; ear, nose, and throat are clear

*Neck/Lymph Nodes*

Supple. No lymphadenopathy, thyromegaly, or masses. No supraclavicular or infraclavicular adenopathy.

*Breasts*

*Left:* Notable for a 2.5-cm mass at the 6 o'clock position, approximately 3 cm from the nipple margin, not fixated to skin; no nipple retraction or discharge is visualized; the mass is not tender to palpation; 1.5-cm, nontender, palpable mass in the axilla noted.

*Right:* Without mass or lymphadenopathy.

*Lungs*

CTA and percussion

*CV*

RRR; no murmurs, rubs, or gallops

*Abd*

Soft, NT/ND, normoactive bowel sounds. No appreciable hepatosplenomegaly.

*Spine*

Slight tenderness to percussion

*Ext*

No CCE

*Neuro*

No deficits noted

## Labs

| | | | |
|---|---|---|---|
| Na 142 mEq/L | Hgb 12.9 g/dL | WBC 8.7 × $10^3$/mm$^3$ | AST 36 IU/L |
| K 3.7 mEq/L | Hct 37.6% | Neutros 55% | ALT 17 IU/L |
| Cl 102 mEq/L | RBC 4.13 × $10^6$/mm$^3$ | Lymphs 35% | LDH 488 IU/L |
| $CO_2$ 26 mEq/L | Plt 410 × $10^3$/mm$^3$ | Monos 8% | T. bili 0.2 mg/dL |
| BUN 9 mg/dL | PT 11.9 sec | Eos 2% | CA 27.29 36.2 units/mL |
| SCr 0.7 mg/dL | INR 1.09 | | |
| Glu 83 mg/dL | aPTT 30.1 sec | | CEA 1.2 ng/mL |

## Chest X-Ray

Lungs are clear.

## Other

*Diagnostic bilateral mammogram* (Fig. 147-1):

1. American College of Radiology Category V, highly suspicious for malignancy in the left breast. There is a high-density, irregular mass measuring 2.2 cm with indistinct margins seen in the left breast lower hemisphere at 6 o'clock located 3 cm from the nipple.
2. In the right breast, no dominant mass, distortion, or suspicious calcifications are identified.

*Unilateral ultrasound left breast and left axilla with biopsy:*

1. An ill-defined, hypoechoic mass is noted in the 5:00–6:00 region. This measures approximately 2.5 cm × 2.3 cm × 1.5 cm and is located 3 cm from the nipple. A core biopsy of this mass was performed.
2. Suspicious lymph nodes are noted in the axilla. The largest node measures 1.8 cm × 1.8 cm × 1.4 cm. A FNA of this lymph node was performed. In the infraclavicular region, a few hypoechoic lymph nodes were also seen and were located in the lateral aspect. The largest node measured 0.8 cm × 0.8 cm × 0.8 cm. A FNA of this infraclavicular lymph node was performed. No suspicious internal mammary or supraclavicular lymph nodes were seen.

*Core needle biopsy of left breast mass:*

Left breast, 6 o'clock: infiltrating ductal carcinoma, modified Black's nuclear grade II (moderately differentiated), ER 95%, PR 95%, HER2 overexpression 2+, HER2 FISH negative (no amplification), and Ki-67 30% (moderate)

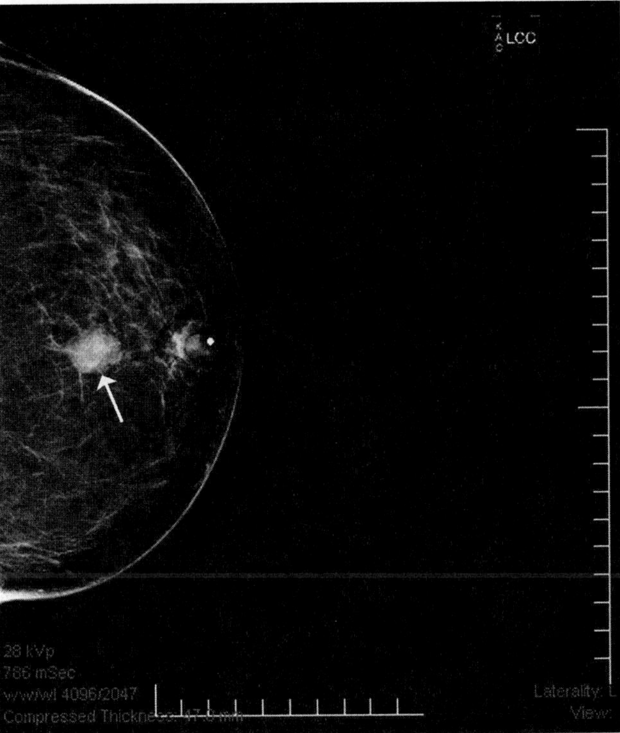


**FIGURE 147-1.** Mammogram of left breast. *Arrow* indicates area of abnormality highly suspicious for malignancy.

*FNA of left axillary and infraclavicular lymph nodes:*

1. Left axillary lymph node: metastatic adenocarcinoma consistent with breast primary
2. Left infraclavicular lymph node: metastatic adenocarcinoma consistent with breast primary

*Bone scan:*

1. No definite evidence of osseous metastases
2. Abnormality in cervical spine consistent with previous history of bone grafting

*Ultrasound liver:*

No lesions suggestive of metastases

*CT chest:*

No evidence of metastases

# QUESTIONS

## Problem Identification

1.a. Create a list of potential drug therapy problems in the patient's medication regimen.

1.b. Given this clinical information, what is this patient's clinical stage of breast cancer?

## Desired Outcome

2.a. What is the primary goal for cancer treatment in this patient?

2.b. What is the prognosis for this patient based on tumor size and nodal status?

2.c. In addition to the stage of disease, what other factors are important for determining the prognosis for breast cancer?

## Therapeutic Alternatives

3. List the treatment modalities available for this patient's breast cancer, and discuss their advantages and disadvantages.

## Optimal Plan

4. Design an appropriate plan for treating this patient's breast cancer, focusing on pharmacologic and nonpharmacologic measures. If the plan includes chemotherapy, identify a specific regimen, and provide your rationale for selecting it.

## Outcome Evaluation

5.a. What parameters should be monitored to evaluate the efficacy and adverse effects of the therapy you recommended?

## ■ CLINICAL COURSE

The patient tolerated your treatment plan well. Twelve months after its completion, the patient returns to clinic complaining of lower back pain for the past 3–4 weeks. She has been taking hydrocodone/acetaminophen more regularly, "about two or three pills per day." This is a significant change since previously she reported not taking any. The patient is restaged with a bone scan, chest x-ray, abdominal CT, chest CT, and laboratory tests. Bone scan reveals metastases to the lumbar spine without spinal cord compression. Chest x-ray is negative. Abdominal CT shows a solitary liver metastasis. Chest CT is negative for metastases. LFTs are within normal limits. Ca 27.29 is 100.7 units/mL. The physician concludes that this patient's breast cancer is now metastatic to the bone and liver. The previous therapy is discontinued, and the patient is started on capecitabine.

5.b. What is this patient's current clinical stage of breast cancer, and what is the primary goal for cancer treatment for this patient now?

5.c. Using this patient's information, calculate her dose and schedule of capecitabine.

5.d. Since the patient has developed bone metastases, what other medication should be added to her treatment plan? At what dose and schedule?

## Patient Education

6. What information should be provided to the patient regarding her new chemotherapy for breast cancer?

## ■ CLINICAL COURSE

Rosalita responded initially to six cycles of capecitabine. She is starting to show signs of palmar plantar erythrodysesthesias, with dry and cracked skin on her hands and feet. She states that her pain has increased and she is now taking four to five pills of hydrocodone/acetaminophen per day. Repeat bone scan and abdominal CT show progression of her bone lesions and stable liver metastasis, respectively. Chest CT is negative for metastases. Due to worsening symptoms and progressive bone metastases, it is decided to discontinue capecitabine and start ixabepilone.

## Additional Case Questions

1. Using this patient's information, calculate her dose and schedule of ixabepilone.
2. What baseline laboratory tests should be considered before starting treatment with ixabepilone?
3. What information should be provided to the patient about her new therapy for breast cancer?

## ■ SELF-STUDY ASSIGNMENTS

1. Perform a literature search to obtain recent information regarding adjuvant clinical trials utilizing trastuzumab in patients with HER2 overexpressing breast cancer.
2. Perform a literature search to obtain recent information regarding adjuvant clinical trials using aromatase inhibitors (anastrozole, letrozole, or exemestane) in patients with hormone receptor–positive breast cancer.
3. Develop a treatment plan for a patient presenting to the emergency center with febrile neutropenia after administration of chemotherapy.
4. Provide educational information regarding genetic testing for a patient with a family history of breast cancer.

## CLINICAL PEARL

Even though metastatic breast cancer is usually considered to be incurable, some patients can live for a relatively long time with hormonal therapy (if hormone receptor–positive) and palliative chemotherapy. These therapies are administered to increase the patient's quality of life and prolong disease progression, and are typically used in a sequential manner until they are no longer effective, or side effects preclude their use. Although the average life span after diagnosis of metastatic disease is a few years, some patients can live a decade or more with the disease.

## REFERENCES


1. Edge SB, Byrd DR, Compton CC, Fritz AG, Greene FL, Trotti A, eds. AJCC Cancer Staging Manual, 7th ed. New York, Springer, 2010.
2. Kaufmann M, Hortobagyi GN, Goldhirsch A, et al. Recommendations from an international expert panel on the use of neoadjuvant (primary) systemic treatment of operable breast cancer: an update. J Clin Oncol 2006;24:1940–1949.
3. Early Breast Cancer Trialists' Collaborative Group (EBCTCG). Effects of chemotherapy and hormonal therapy for early breast cancer on recurrence and 15-year survival: an overview of the randomised trials. Lancet 2005;365:1687–1717.
4. Estevez LG, Munoz M, Alvarez I, et al. Evidence-based use of taxanes in the adjuvant setting of breast cancer. A review of randomized phase III trials. Cancer Treat Rev 2007;33:474–483.
5. Eisen A, Trudeau M, Shelley W, et al. Aromatase inhibitors in adjuvant therapy for hormone receptor positive breast cancer: a systematic review. Cancer Treat Rev 2008;34:157–174.
6. Khatcheressian JL, Wolff AC, Smith TJ, et al. American Society of Clinical Oncology 2006 update of the breast cancer follow-up and management guidelines in the adjuvant setting. J Clin Oncol 2006;24:5091–5097.
7. Winer EP, Hudis C, Burstein HJ, et al. American Society of Clinical Oncology technology assessment on the use of aromatase inhibitors as adjuvant therapy for postmenopausal women with hormone receptor-positive breast cancer: status report 2004. J Clin Oncol 2005;-23:619–629.
8. Hillner BE, Ingle JN, Chlebowski RT, et al. American Society of Clinical Oncology 2003 update on the role of bisphosphonates and bone health issues in women with breast cancer. J Clin Oncol 2003;21:4042–4057.
9. Boehnke Michaud LB. The optimal therapeutic use of ixabepilone in patients with locally advanced or metastatic breast cancer. J Oncol Pharm Pract 2009;15:95–106.

# 148

# NON–SMALL CELL LUNG CANCER

It Takes Your Breath Away . . . . . . . . . . . . . . . . Level II

Julianna V.F. Roddy, PharmD, BCOP

Michelle L. Rockey, PharmD, BCOP

## LEARNING OBJECTIVES

After completing this case study, students should be able to:

- Recognize the most common symptoms of non–small cell lung cancer (NSCLC).
- Identify potential complications associated with NSCLC.
- Design a treatment plan for patients with NSCLC.
- Recommend potential second-line chemotherapy agents for treating refractory NSCLC.
- Design a pharmacotherapeutic plan for the treatment of hypercalcemia.
- Describe appropriate treatment strategies for brain metastases in NSCLC.
- Monitor carboplatin and paclitaxel therapy.
- Educate patients on the anticipated side effects of carboplatin, paclitaxel, and radiation therapy.

## PATIENT PRESENTATION

### Chief Complaint

"I have been coughing up blood."

### HPI

This 64-year-old woman presents to her PCP with complaints of a dry, nonproductive cough for 2 months, dyspnea on exertion, and hemoptysis for 1 week.

### PMH

Dyslipidemia
HTN
Anemia of unknown etiology × 1 year
Type 2 DM
PPD (–)

### FH

Father died of colorectal cancer at age 68.

### SH

Married, lives with son and daughter; 30 pack-year cigarette smoking history (approximately 1 ppd × 30 years); occasional ETOH use; no known recent exposure to TB

### Meds

Folic acid 1 mg po daily
Ferrous sulfate 325 mg po TID
Simvastatin 20 mg po daily
Metformin 500 mg po BID
Pantoprazole 40 mg po daily

### All

Penicillin (rash)

### ROS

(+) For pulmonary symptoms as noted in HPI; no headaches, dizziness, or blurred vision

### Physical Examination

*Gen*

Mildly overweight Caucasian woman in slight distress

*VS*

BP 169/100, P 90, RR 30, T 37.2°C; Wt 75 kg, Ht 5′6″

*Skin*

Patches of dry skin; no lesions

*HEENT*

PERRLA; EOMI; fundi benign; TMs intact

*Neck/Lymph Nodes*

No lymphadenopathy; neck supple

*Lungs*

Wheezing in RUL; remainder of lung fields clear

*Heart*

RRR; slight systolic murmur on left lateral side; normal $S_1$, $S_2$

*Abd*

Soft, nontender; no splenomegaly or hepatomegaly

*Genit/Rect*

Normal female genitalia; guaiac (–) stool

*Neuro*

A & O × 3; sensory and motor intact, 5/5 upper, 4/5 lower; CN II–XII intact; (–) Babinski

### Labs

| | | |
|---|---|---|
| Na 138 mEq/L | Hgb 11.5 g/dL | Ca 9.1 mg/dL |
| K 3.8 mEq/L | Hct 35.6% | Mg 2.0 mg/dL |
| Cl 99 mEq/L | Plt 255 × $10^3$/mm$^3$ | |
| $CO_2$ 23 mEq/L | WBC 9.9 × $10^3$/mm$^3$ | |
| BUN 13 mg/dL | | |
| SCr 1.2 mg/dL | | |
| Glu 125 mg/dL | | |

### Chest X-Ray

PA and lateral views reveal a possible mass in right upper lobe (Fig. 148-1).

### Assessment

A 64-year-old woman with new-onset hemoptysis is admitted for workup of a possible lung mass.

She has anemia and a history of dyslipidemia, DM type 2, and HTN.

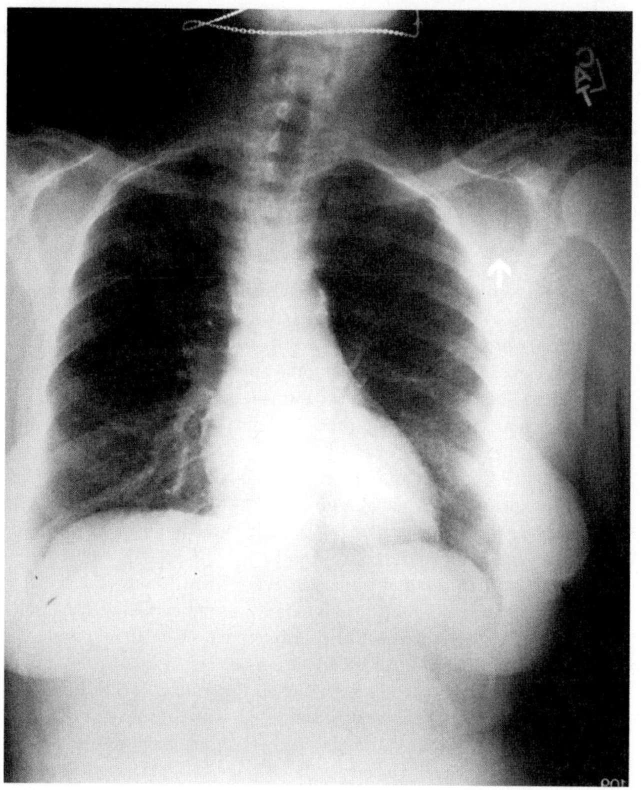

A

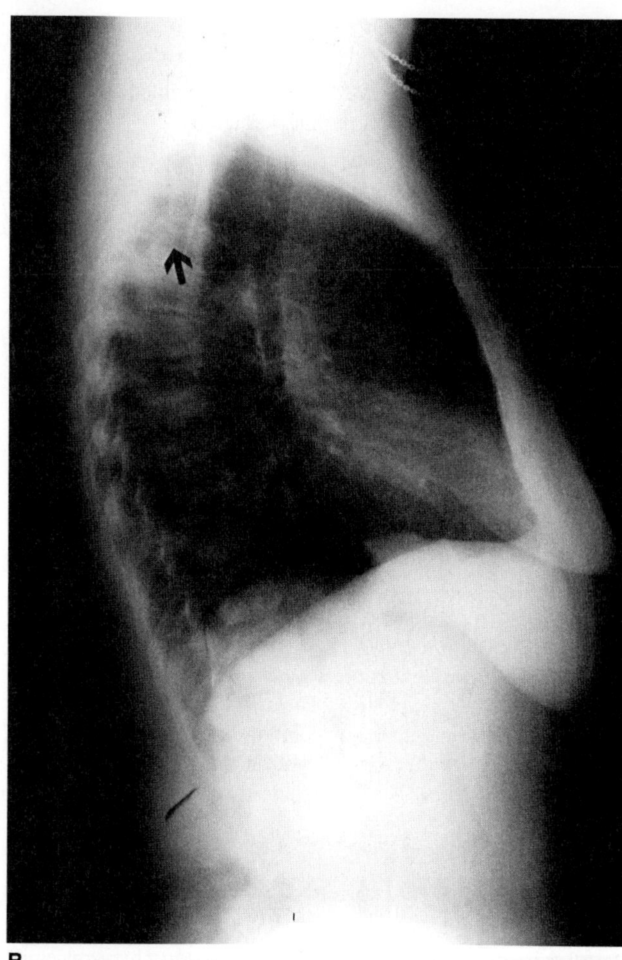

B

**FIGURE 148-1.** Chest x-ray with PA *(A)* and lateral *(B)* views showing a possible mass in the right upper lobe *(arrows)*.

## Clinical Course

The patient was further evaluated for lung cancer on an outpatient basis. A bronchoscopy (with biopsy) was performed that identified squamous cell carcinoma. The chest CT scan revealed a 2.5-cm × 2-cm right lung mass (Fig. 148-2). A mediastinoscopy was performed to determine the resectability of the tumor. The mediastinoscopy and biopsy revealed unresectable stage IIIB NSCLC with metastases to the contralateral mediastinal nodes. EGFR status was positive by IHC. PFTs included $FEV_1$ 1.49 L and FVC 1.9 L. An echocardiogram showed mild LVH with an LVEF of 55%.

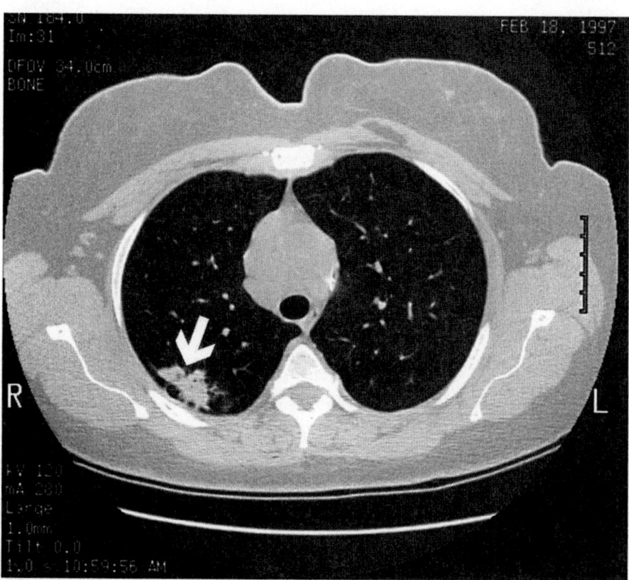


**FIGURE 148-2.** CT scan of the chest revealing a 2.5-cm × 2-cm right lung mass *(arrow)*.

# QUESTIONS

## Problem Identification

1.a. Identify the patient's drug therapy problems.

1.b. What signs, symptoms, and other information indicate the presence of NSCLC in this patient?

## Desired Outcome

2. What is the goal for treatment of NSCLC in this patient? What is the likelihood of achieving this goal?

## Therapeutic Alternatives

3.a. What chemotherapeutic regimens may be considered for NSCLC?

3.b. What nondrug therapies may be used for NSCLC?

## Optimal Plan

4.a. Design a specific chemotherapeutic regimen to treat this patient, and explain why you chose this regimen.

4.b. What additional measures should be taken to ensure the tolerability of the regimen and to prevent adverse effects?

4.c. What additional laboratory and clinical information is needed before administration of the chemotherapy?

4.d. Calculate the patient's BSA, creatinine clearance, and the amount of each drug to be administered based on the regimen chosen.

4.e. Would the treatment plan for this patient change if she had presented initially with stage IV NSCLC? If so, what would the treatment be?

### Outcome Evaluation

5. What clinical and laboratory parameters are necessary to evaluate the therapy for achievement of the desired therapeutic outcome and the occurrence of adverse effects?

### Patient Education

6. What information should be provided to the patient to optimize therapy and minimize adverse effects?

## ■ CLINICAL COURSE

The patient's subsequent courses were further complicated by the occurrence of DVT, weight loss, neutropenic fever, anemia, nausea/vomiting, and infections. At one point, the patient presented with a serum calcium level of 11.5 mg/dL and an albumin of 1.5 g/dL, with symptoms of weakness, confusion, nausea, and vomiting.

### Follow-Up Questions

1. Calculate the patient's corrected calcium level and provide an interpretation of that value.
2. What treatment modalities may be used to correct hypercalcemia?

## ■ CLINICAL COURSE

A repeat chest CT before cycle 3 of carboplatin/paclitaxel shows an increase in the size of the initial mass and several new suspicious lesions.

### Follow-Up Questions

1. What treatment options are available for the patient at this time?
2. Design a specific chemotherapeutic regimen to treat this patient.

## ■ CLINICAL COURSE

Six weeks after beginning the new chemotherapy regimen, the patient presents to the ED with complaints of headache and mental status changes as per the patient's husband and caregiver. An MRI of the head reveals multiple lesions, most likely brain metastases.

### Follow-Up Questions

1. Briefly discuss options (drug and nondrug) to treat brain metastases.
2. What is the role of anticonvulsant agents in the setting of brain metastases?

## ■ SELF-STUDY ASSIGNMENTS

1. Review clinically important drug interactions for cancer patients started on phenytoin. Include appropriate monitoring parameters. Extend your review beyond the medications this patient is currently receiving.
2. The oncologist has decided to place this patient on erlotinib. Design a patient education session for this relatively new drug therapy.

## CLINICAL PEARL

More than 90% of lung cancers are attributable to cigarette smoking. Smoking cessation is the only method proven to decrease the risk of lung cancer.

## REFERENCES


1. National Comprehensive Cancer Network Clinical Practice Guidelines in Oncology. Non-small cell lung cancer, version 2, 2010. Available at: *www.nccn.org/professionals/physician_gls/PDF/nscl.pdf*. Accessed April 10, 2010.
2. Pritchard RS, Anthony SP. Chemotherapy plus radiotherapy compared with radiotherapy alone in the treatment of locally advanced, unresectable, non-small–cell lung cancer. A meta-analysis. Ann Intern Med 1996;125:723–729.
3. Belani CP, Choy H, Bonomi P, et al. Combined chemotherapy regimens of paclitaxel and carboplatin for locally advanced non-small-cell lung cancer: a randomized phase II locally advanced multi-modality protocol. J Clin Oncol 2005;23:5883–5891.
4. Furuse K, Fukuoka M, Kawahara M, et al. Phase III study of concurrent versus sequential thoracic radiotherapy in combination with mitomycin, vindesine, and cisplatin in unresectable stage III non-small-cell lung cancer. J Clin Oncol 1999;17:2692–2699.
5. Fournel P, Robinet G, Thomas P, et al. Randomized phase III trial of sequential chemoradiotherapy compared with concurrent chemoradiotherapy in locally advanced non-small-cell lung cancer: Groupe Lyon-Saint-Etienne d'Oncologie Thoracique-Groupe Francis de Pneumo-Cancerologie NPC 95-01 study. J Clin Oncol 2005;23:5910–5917.
6. Kris MG, Hesketh PJ, Somerfield MR, et al. American Society of Clinical Oncology guideline for antiemetics in oncology: update 2006. J Clin Oncol 2006;24:2932–2947.
7. Rizzo DJ, Somerfield MR, Hagerty KL, et al. Use of epoetin and darbepoetin in patients with cancer: 2007 American Society of Clinical Oncology/American Society of Hematology clinical practice guideline update. J Clin Oncol 2008;26:1–19.
8. Sandler A, Gray R, Perry M, et al. Paclitaxel–carboplatin alone or with bevacizumab for non-small-cell lung cancer. N Engl J Med 2006;355:2542–2550.
9. Weiss GJ, Langer C, Rosell R, et al. Elderly patients benefit from second-line cytotoxic chemotherapy: a subset analysis of a randomized phase III trial of pemetrexed compared with docetaxel in patients with previously treated advanced non-small-cell lung cancer. J Clin Oncol 2006;24:4405–4411.
10. Shepherd FA, Pereira JR, Ciuleanu T, et al. Erlotinib in previously treated non-small-cell lung cancer. N Engl J Med 2005;353:123–132.


# 149

# COLON CANCER

Drug Therapy by Design . . . . . . . . . . . . . . . . . Level II

**Lisa E. Davis, PharmD, FCCP, BCPS, BCOP**

## LEARNING OBJECTIVES

After completing this case study, students should be able to:

- Identify common symptoms associated with colon cancer at presentation and with disease progression.
- Describe the treatment goals associated with early and advanced stages of colon cancer.

- Design an appropriate chemotherapy regimen for colon cancer based on patient-specific data.
- Formulate a monitoring plan for a patient receiving a prescribed chemotherapy regimen for colon cancer based on patient-specific information.
- Recommend alterations in a drug therapy plan for a patient with colon cancer based on patient-specific information.
- Use pharmacogenetic test results to design an appropriate drug therapy plan for a patient with colorectal cancer.
- Educate patients on the anticipated side effects of irinotecan, capecitabine, oxaliplatin, bevacizumab, and epidermal growth factor receptor inhibitors.

## PATIENT PRESENTATION

### Chief Complaint

"The pain below my right ribs is getting worse. Also, I'm having more numbness, cramping, and burning sensations in my hands and feet, especially when I'm working a lot. I don't think I can tolerate it much longer."

### HPI

Peter Robinson is a 56-year-old man who presents with worsening pain in his hands and feet and increasing RUQ pain. He was diagnosed with stage IV colon cancer 11 months ago after presenting with abdominal pain, bloating and distention, a history of intermittent BRBPR, and no BM within the prior 4 days. He presented to the ED where a barium enema revealed an "apple core" lesion in his descending colon that was suggestive of malignancy (Fig. 150-1). An FDG-PET/CT scan showed a complete bowel obstruction and several areas of focal intense uptake in the liver, consistent with metastases. His preoperative CEA was 5.6 ng/mL. He subsequently underwent a laparotomy with a left hemicolectomy and lymphadenectomy. The pathology revealed a moderately differentiated adenocarcinoma with extension through the bowel wall to the serosal surface. The tumor *KRAS* and *BRAF* genes were wild-type. Ten of 13 lymph nodes were positive for tumor. Biopsy of a liver lesion confirmed hepatic metastases. A CT scan of the chest showed no evidence of lung metastases. Seven weeks later, chemotherapy was initiated with capecitabine, oxaliplatin (CapeOx), and bevacizumab. Except for occasional nausea, he generally tolerated the chemotherapy well. However, over the past 2 months he has been experiencing worsening redness and pain on the palms of his hands with numbness and tingling in his fingers and toes. Six days ago he received his 19th cycle of chemotherapy. UGT1A1 testing showed that he was homozygous for the UGT1A1*28 allele.

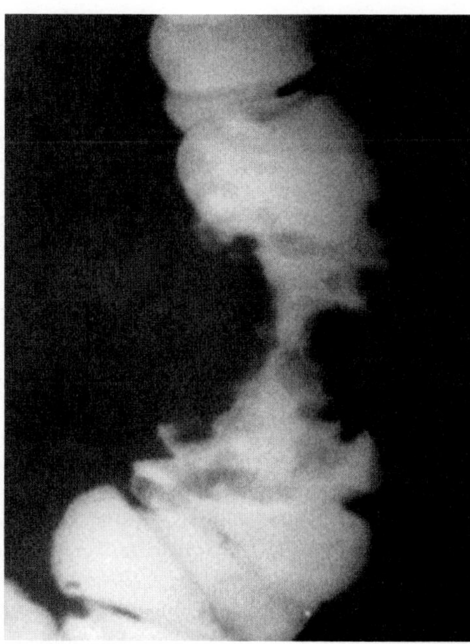

**FIGURE 149-1.** Annular, constricting adenocarcinoma of the descending colon. This radiographic appearance is referred to as an "apple-core" lesion and is always highly suggestive of malignancy. Reprinted with permission from: Mayer RJ. Gastrointestinal Tract Cancer. In: Fauci AS, Kasper DL, Longo DL, et al. Harrison's Principles of Internal Medicine, 17th. Ed. New York: McGraw-Hill; 2008: 577.

### PMH

Type 2 diabetes mellitus × 9 years
Hypertriglyceridemia × 5 years

### FH

The patient is the oldest of three brothers; both siblings are alive and well. He has been married for 26 years and has one daughter who is 20 years old. Both his mother and father are in good health. His paternal grandfather died in his 60s from colon cancer, and his mother died in her 60s from ovarian cancer; he is aware of no other family history of malignancy.

### SH

Self-employed as a graphic designer. He smoked cigarettes, one pack per day, since age 19 but quit 10 years ago. He does not drink alcohol and has never tried illicit drugs.

### Meds

Morphine sustained-release 60 mg po twice daily
Bisacodyl 5 mg po daily as needed
Metformin 750 mg po once daily
Fenofibrate 120 mg po once daily

### All

NKDA

### ROS

The patient reports diffuse abdominal pain that is continuous with a "grabbing, gnawing" sensation and painful redness and swelling on the palms of his hands. He rates the abdominal pain severity as 5–6 out of 10. The numbness, tingling, cramping, and burning sensations in his hands and feet have worsened in frequency and severity over the past 2 months and have not responded well to morphine. He rates the severity of the tingling and burning pain as 6/10. He denies fever, headaches, shortness of breath, cough, nausea, vomiting, or diarrhea. He reports no lesions in his mouth or difficulty swallowing. He has been having fewer bowel movements (about one every 3–4 days), but there is no pain or blood with passage of stool. He denies polyuria, polydipsia, and burning on urination. He has not noticed any bleeding or excessive bruising.

### Physical Examination

*Gen*

Patient is a slightly overweight Caucasian man who appears fatigued.

*VS*

BP 164/93, P 79, RR 22, T 35.6°C; Wt 87 kg, Ht 5′9″

*Skin*

Redness and swelling of the palms of both hands and soles of feet

*HEENT*

PERRLA; EOMI; funduscopic exam without retinopathy; pale conjunctiva; no scleral icterus; moist mucous membranes; no lesions in oral cavity

*Neck/Lymph Nodes*

Supple neck; no lymphadenopathy

*Lungs/Thorax*

Symmetric chest expansion with respiratory effort; clear to A & P; regular breath sounds

*CV*

Normal heart sounds; regular rate and rhythm; no MRG

*Abd*

Well-healed scar on left upper abdomen; diffuse abdominal tenderness to palpation; no rebound tenderness; decreased bowel sounds

*Genit/Rect*

Prostate normal size; no masses palpated; stool heme negative

*MS/Ext*

Full ROM in all four extremities

*Neuro*

A & O × 3; cranial nerves II–XII grossly intact; reduced DTRs bilaterally; reduced feet sensitivity to light touch and pinprick bilaterally in stocking–glove distribution; vibration sensation reduced in distal legs

### Labs

| | | | |
|---|---|---|---|
| Na 137 mEq/L | Hgb 9.6 g/dL | WBC 8.1 × $10^3$/mm$^3$ | AST 52 IU/L |
| K 4.4 mEq/L | Hct 29% | Neutros 40% | ALT 45 IU/L |
| Cl 98 mEq/L | Plt 252 × $10^3$/mm$^3$ | Bands 3% | Alk phos 109 IU/L |
| $CO_2$ 26 mEq/L | MCV 87 μm$^3$ | Eos 4% | LDH 370 IU/L |
| BUN 17 mg/dL | MCHC 33 g/dL | Lymphs 45% | T. bili 1.2 mg/dL |
| SCr 1.0 mg/dL | | Monos 8% | T. chol 199 mg/dL |
| Glu 117 mg/dL | | | CEA 7.9 ng/mL |
| Ca 8.7 mg/dL | | | |
| Phos 3.4 mg/dL | | | |
| Mg 2.3 mg/dL | | | |

### Urinalysis

1+ glucose, (–) ketones, 1+ protein, (–) leukocyte esterase and nitrites; (–) RBC; 2–3 WBC/hpf

### Abdominal CT

Multiple liver metastases, increased approximately 30% in diameter compared to prior scan; multiple new lesions present in both lobes of the liver

### Chest CT

No evidence of pulmonary metastases

### Assessment

Unresectable stage IV colon cancer, with disease progression on CapeOx plus bevacizumab chemotherapy

## QUESTIONS

### Problem Identification

1.a. Identify all of the patient's drug therapy problems.

1.b. What clinical, laboratory, and other information is consistent with colon cancer?

### Desired Outcome

2. What are the goals of pharmacotherapy for this patient?

### Therapeutic Alternatives

3.a. What chemotherapeutic options are appropriate for this patient?

3.b. What treatment modifications are appropriate to address escalating oxaliplatin-induced neuropathy?

### Optimal Plan

4.a. What drugs, dosage forms, treatment schedule, and duration of therapy are best for treating this patient's colon cancer?

4.b. What additional drug treatment interventions should be considered for this patient?

### Outcome Evaluation

5.a. How is the response to the treatment regimen for the colon cancer assessed?

5.b. What acute adverse effects are anticipated with the chemotherapy regimen, and what parameters should be monitored?

5.c. What pharmacologic measures can be instituted to prevent or manage the acute toxicities associated with the chemotherapy regimen?

5.d. What are the potential late-onset toxicities of the chemotherapy regimen, and how can they be detected and prevented?

### Patient Education

6. What information should you provide to the patient to enhance compliance, ensure successful therapy, and minimize adverse effects?

## CLINICAL COURSE

His hypertension resolved after two cycles of the chemotherapy regimen you recommended, and his neuropathic symptoms diminished over time and with drug therapy. He received PRBC transfusions when his hemoglobin dropped below 9 g/dL. His sustained-release morphine dose was increased to 120 mg po every 12 hours, and oral immediate-release morphine sulfate 30 mg, every 4 hours as needed for pain was started. A scheduled regimen of docusate sodium 100 mg orally plus two senna tablets daily maintained a regular pattern of bowel movements. After seven more cycles of chemotherapy, he presented with worsening abdominal pain, fatigue, and new-onset dyspnea. An abdominal CT scan showed the liver lesions increased in size, and a chest CT showed multiple bilateral pulmonary nodules consistent with pulmonary metastases. His ALT and AST increased to five times the upper limit of normal.

### Follow-Up Question

1. What treatment options would be appropriate to consider at this time?

## Additional Case Questions

1. What is the role of UGT1A1 genotyping in the treatment of colon cancer?
2. What is the role of *KRAS* and *BRAF* tumor gene testing in the treatment of colon cancer?
3. How should a patient who develops a thrombotic event during bevacizumab therapy be managed?

## CLINICAL COURSE

The patient expressed interest in receiving further treatment for his colon cancer. After considering limited treatment options with his oncologist, he agreed to participate in a clinical trial. His analgesic therapy was modified, and his pain control was acceptable. His metastatic lesions remained stable (by clinical symptoms and CT scans) for 2 months.

## SELF-STUDY ASSIGNMENTS

1. Develop an algorithm for treatment of colon cancer chemotherapy-induced diarrhea.
2. Develop patient-specific education materials regarding management of cutaneous toxicities of agents used in colon cancer treatment.

## CLINICAL PEARL

There is no available test, including presence of tumor tissue epidermal growth factor receptor expression, that predicts response to cetuximab or panitumumab. However, tumors can be tested for presence of *KRAS* and *BRAF* mutations that are predictive of lack of response to these agents. Patients with tumors that are *KRAS* or *BRAF* mutant are not appropriate candidates for treatment regimens that contain cetuximab or panitumumab.

## REFERENCES


1. Guglielmi AP, Sobrero AF. Second-line therapy for advanced colorectal cancer. Gastrointest Cancer Res 2007;1:57–63.
2. Rougier P, Lepère C. Metastatic colorectal cancer: first and second-line treatment in 2005. Semin Oncol 2005;32(Suppl 8):S15–S20.
3. Tournigand C, André T, Achille E, et al. FOLFIRI followed by FOLFOX6 or the reverse sequence in advanced colorectal cancer: a randomized GERCOR study. J Clin Oncol 2004;22:229–237.
4. Peeters M, Price TJ, Hotko YS, et al. Randomized phase III study of panitumumab with FOLFIRI versus FOLFIRI alone as second-line treatment in patients with metastatic colorectal cancer: PRIME trial. In: 2010 Gastrointestinal Cancer Symposium, January 22–24, 2010, Orlando, FL [abstract 283].
5. Sobrero AF, Maurel J, Fehrenbacher L, et al. EPIC: phase III trial of cetuximab plus irinotecan after fluoropyrimidine and oxaliplatin failure in patients with metastatic colorectal cancer. J Clin Oncol 2008;26:2311–2319.
6. Fuchs CS, Moore MR, Harker G, et al. Phase III comparison of two irinotecan dosing regimens in second-line therapy of metastatic colorectal cancer. J Clin Oncol 2003;21:807–814.
7. Vanhoefer U, Harstrick A, Achterrath W, et al. Irinotecan in the treatment of colorectal cancer: clinical overview. J Clin Oncol 2001; 19:1501–1518.
8. Van Cutsem E, Peeters M, Siena S, et al. Open-label phase III trial of panitumumab plus best supportive care compared with best supportive care alone in patients with chemotherapy-refractory metastatic colorectal cancer. J Clin Oncol 2007;25:1658–1664.
9. Tournigand C, Cervantes A, Figer A, et al. OPTIMOX1: a randomized study of FOLFOX4 or FOLFOX7 with oxaliplatin in a stop-and-go fashion in advanced colorectal cancer—a GERCOR study. J Clin Oncol 2006;24:394–400.
10. Bidard FC, Tournigand C, André T, et al. Efficacy of FOLFIRI-3 (irinotecan D1, D3 combined with LV5-FU) or other irinotecan-based regimens in oxaliplatin-pretreated metastatic colorectal cancer in the GERCOR OPTIMOX1 study. Ann Oncol 2009;20:1042–1047.


# 150

# PROSTATE CANCER

Missed Opportunity . . . . . . . . . . . . . . . . . . . . . Level II

**Diana Hey Cauley, PharmD, BCOP**

## LEARNING OBJECTIVES

After completing this case study, students should be able to:

- Describe typical symptoms associated with prostate cancer at initial diagnosis and at disease progression.
- Describe the standard initial treatment options for androgen-dependent metastatic prostate cancer.
- Recommend a pharmacotherapeutic plan for patients with androgen-independent metastatic prostate cancer.
- Counsel patients regarding the toxicities associated with the pharmacologic agents used in prostate cancer treatment.

## PATIENT PRESENTATION

### Chief Complaint

"I have blood in my urine, I'm using the restroom all the time, and my shoulder is really hurting."

### HPI

Don Walton is a 73-year-old man who usually has yearly physicals and PSA checks by his local physician. The levels have always been in the range of 4–6 ng/mL. He did not go in for his yearly physical last year, and he now presents with painless gross hematuria, shoulder pain, and a PSA level of 35.7 ng/mL. He has had increased urinary symptoms for the last 5 months.

### PMH

Hypercholesterolemia
Congestive heart failure
Diverticulitis
Severe GERD

### SH

Retired highway maintenance employee. Christian by faith, Protestant by denomination. He has an associate degree. He drinks on average one six-pack of beer per day. He smoked 10 cigarettes a day for 21 years; stopped smoking at age 42. He is married with two children. He is an only child. Family history of cancer: father, lung—diagnosed age 71, died age 73; mother, breast—died at age 93. He has a paternal aunt and paternal grandmother who both were diagnosed with unspecified malignancies.

## ROS

He reports significant fatigue and severe pain in right shoulder. No fever, chills, or sweats. No epistaxis or dysphagia. Reports no chest pain, shortness of breath, dyspnea, or cough. No nausea, vomiting, diarrhea, or constipation. He reports dysuria × 5 months with dribbling, nocturia eight times per night, hesitancy, and incomplete voiding. He has recurring hematuria. He denies memory loss, diplopia, or neuropathy; he has had no falls recently. He reports a 15- to 20-year history of tinnitus.

## Meds

Diovan 160 mg po daily
Lasix 40 mg po daily
Klor-Con 10 mEq po daily
Allopurinol 300 mg po daily
Flomax 0.4 mg, two capsules po daily
Prozac 20 mg po daily
Gemfibrozil 600 mg po daily
Tylenol 500 mg po six times daily PRN pain
Motrin 400 mg po four times daily PRN pain
Nexium 40 mg po BID

## All

None

## Physical Examination

### *Gen*

This is a pleasant, elderly gentleman who appears to be in moderate discomfort. Pain is 7 over 10 multifocally. ECOG performance status 1+.

### *VS*

BP 136/61, P 80, RR 20, T 36.9°C; Wt 91.5 kg, Ht 5′6″

### *Skin*

Warm and dry; no lesions or rashes

### *HEENT*

Sclerae are anicteric. PERRLA; EOMI. Tympanic membranes are within normal limits bilaterally.

### *Neck/Lymph Nodes*

No cervical or supraclavicular adenopathy

### *Lungs/Thorax*

Lungs are clear in all fields. Respirations are even and unlabored.

### *CV*

Normal rate and rhythm; $S_1$, $S_2$ normal; no murmurs, gallops, or rubs

### *Abd*

There is a large midline abdominal hernia that does not appear incarcerated. No hepatosplenomegaly.

### *Genit/Rect*

Patient is circumcised with a normal phallus. There are bilaterally descended testicles. No inguinal hernia on examination. Prostate is markedly enlarged and is asymmetric on the right. Texture is firm, but no discrete nodule palpated. Normal rectal tone.

### *MS/Ext*

He has significant pain to touch on the superior aspect of the right shoulder; there is also pain on range of motion. There is tenderness in lumbar area. 1+ ankle and pedal edema is present. Pedal pulses are 2+ bilaterally.

### *Neuro*

CN II–XII grossly normal. Cerebellar function remains intact.

## Labs

| | | | |
|---|---|---|---|
| Na 139 mEq/L | Hgb 9.5 g/dL | WBC 7.2 × $10^3$/mm$^3$ | Total bilirubin 0.2 mg/dL |
| K 4.0 mEq/L | Hct 27.1% | Neutros 70.3% | ALT <12 IU/L |
| Cl 107 mEq/L | RBC 3.6 × $10^6$/mm$^3$ | Baso 0.2% | AST 20 IU/L |
| $CO_2$ 24 mEq/L | Plt 215 × $10^3$/mm$^3$ | Eos 2.3% | LDH 742 IU/L |
| BUN 21 mg/dL | MCV 75 μm$^3$ | Lymphs 16.6% | Alk phos 912 IU/L |
| SCr 0.9 mg/dL | MCHC 35.1 g/dL | Monos 10.6% | Albumin 4 g/dL |
| Glu 114 mg/dL | | PSA 35.7 ng/mL | Calcium 8.7 mg/dL |
| | | Testosterone 276 ng/dL | |

## Bone Scan

Skeletal metastases involving the skull and right shoulder

## Cystoscopy and Bladder Neck Biopsy

High-grade carcinoma consistent with prostatic adenocarcinoma, Gleason score 8 (4 + 4), extensively involving the bladder neck biopsy tissue

## Perineal Prostate Biopsy

Prostatic adenocarcinoma, Gleason score 9 (4 + 5), positive perineural invasion

## CT Abdomen

No significant retroperitoneal adenopathy. Multiple small, external iliac lymph nodes are present, predominantly on the left. Small, deep inguinal lymph nodes are also present.

## Urinalysis

Clear; negative for glucose, ketones, leukocyte esterase, nitrites, and protein; trace hemoglobin; rare bacteria

## Assessment

A 73-year-old man with newly diagnosed T4N1M1b prostate cancer presenting with painless gross hematuria, increased urinary symptoms, and elevated PSA of 35.7 ng/mL. Patient has metastatic androgen-dependent hormone-sensitive disease and is here for consideration of initial treatment options.

# QUESTIONS

## Problem Identification

1. What signs, symptoms, and other information are consistent with metastatic prostate cancer in this case?

## Desired Outcome

2. Considering this patient's disease stage and history, what are reasonable therapeutic goals?

## Therapeutic Alternatives

3. Create a list of the feasible options for initial therapy of this patient's androgen-dependent prostate cancer, including the advantages, potential side effects, and complications associated with each option.

## Optimal Plan

4. Design an optimal pharmacotherapeutic plan for the treatment of this patient's metastatic prostate cancer.

## Outcome Evaluation

5. How should the therapy you recommended be monitored for efficacy and adverse effects?

## Patient Education

6. What information should be provided to the patient about his new therapy?

## ■ CLINICAL COURSE

Mr Walton has been compliant with his treatment plan. The physician also started IV zoledronic acid for the metastatic bone disease and an oral calcium/vitamin D supplement. His testosterone has been castrate since therapy was begun 20 months ago. His PSA 3 months ago was mildly elevated at 0.6 ng/mL, whereas it had been undetectable previously. His PSA has now increased to 38.5 ng/mL, and his testosterone level is 22 ng/mL. He is complaining of increased pain in his pelvis and more bone pain in his ribs and back over the last 2 months, although he is still able to participate in church social activities and play golf on the weekends. A CT of the pelvis shows a soft tissue mass on the posterolateral aspect of the urinary bladder on the right side and multiple blastic lesions in the pelvis and spine. His bone scan shows numerous intense foci in the skull, scapulae, spine, and femurs.

## Follow-Up Questions

1. What pharmacotherapeutic options are available to the patient for his progressive androgen-independent metastatic prostate cancer?
2. What therapeutic options are available for managing this patient's pain?

## ■ SELF-STUDY ASSIGNMENTS

1. Locate information resources that are available to prostate cancer patients and their families.
2. Provide the rationale for intermittent LHRH hormone ablation for locally advanced and metastatic prostate cancer patients.
3. Define the role of secondary hormonal agents (e.g., ketoconazole, estrogens) for metastatic disease relapse.
4. Describe the clinical rationale for starting an antiandrogen 1–4 weeks before giving the first dose of an LHRH agonist.
5. Define the role of bisphosphonates in men with prostate cancer.

## CLINICAL PEARL

Androgen deprivation therapy is not discontinued when a metastatic prostate cancer patient progresses from an androgen-dependent to an androgen-independent state.

## REFERENCES


1. Klotz L, Boccon-Gibod L, Shore N, et al. The efficacy and safety of degarelix: a 12-month, comparative, randomized, open-label, parallel-group phase III study in patients with prostate cancer. BJU Int 2008;102:1531–1538.
2. NCCN Clinical Practice Guidelines in Oncology, V2, 2010. Prostate Cancer. Available at: *http://www.nccn.org/professionals/physician_gls/PDF/prostate.pdf*. Accessed June 1, 2010.
3. Sooriakumaran P, Khaksar SJ, Shah J. Management of prostate cancer. Part 2: localized and locally advanced disease. Expert Rev Anticancer Ther 2006;6:595–603.
4. Shah J, Khaksar SJ, Sooriakumaran P. Management of prostate cancer. Part 3: metastatic disease. Expert Rev Anticancer Ther 2006;6:813–821.
5. Kantoff P, Higano CS, Berger ER, et al. Updated survival results of the IMPACT trial of sipuleucel-T for metastatic castration-resistance prostate cancer (CRPC). In: 2010 Genitourinary Cancers Symposium Fairfax, VA [abstract 8] .
6. Tannock IF, de Wit R, Berry WR, et al. Docetaxel plus prednisone or mitoxantrone plus prednisone for advanced prostate cancer. N Engl J Med 2004;351:1502–1512.
7. Petrylak DP, Tangen CM, Hussain MH, et al. Docetaxel and estramustine compared with mitoxantrone and prednisone for refractory prostate cancer. N Engl J Med 2004;351:1513–1520.
8. Tannock IF, Osoba D, Stockler MR, et al. Chemotherapy with mitoxantrone plus prednisone or prednisone alone for symptomatic hormone-resistant prostate cancer: a Canadian randomized trial with palliative end points. J Clin Oncol 1996;14:1756–1764.
9. NCCN Clinical Practice Guidelines in Oncology, V1, 2009. Adult Cancer Pain. Available at: *http://www.nccn.org/professionals/physician_gls/PDF/pain.pdf*. Accessed February 10, 2010.


# 151

# NON-HODGKIN'S LYMPHOMA

Striking Out Cancer .................... Level II

**Keith A. Hecht, PharmD, BCOP**

## LEARNING OBJECTIVES

After completing this case study, students should be able to:

- Identify and describe the components of the staging workup and the corresponding staging and classification systems for non-Hodgkin's lymphoma (NHL).
- Describe the pharmacotherapeutic treatment of choice and the alternatives available for treating NHL.
- Identify acute and chronic toxicities associated with the drugs used to treat NHL and the measures used to prevent or treat these toxicities.
- Identify monitoring parameters for response and toxicity in patients with NHL.
- Provide detailed patient education for the chemotherapeutic regimen.

## PATIENT PRESENTATION

### ■ Chief Complaint

"What's the next step for my lymphoma?"

### ■ HPI

Homer Bunting is a 58-year-old man who presents to his oncologist's office for recommendations about treatment of a newly diagnosed diffuse, large B-cell lymphoma. He had been in relatively good health other than his long-standing hypertension and chronic heart failure. He initially presented to the ED 2 weeks ago with new onset of shortness of breath and fevers up to 100.8°F (38.2°C). He was then hospitalized for further evaluation and treatment. At that time, he stated that he had lost weight over the past few months. Physical examination findings were significant for decreased breath sounds (worse on the left side than the right) and enlarged, painless supraclavicular lymph nodes on the left side. The largest palpable lymph node measured approximately 2 cm in diameter. Splenomegaly was also noted. Chest x-ray revealed a large heterogeneous mass at the apex of the left lung also involving the mediastinum. Given the patient's lengthy smoking history, he was presumed to have lung cancer. CT-guided biopsy of the mass was performed. Pathology revealed cells consistent with lymphoma, but definitive diagnosis could not be made. An excisional biopsy of the enlarged supraclavicular lymph node was performed. Pathology showed diffuse large non-Hodgkin's B-cell lymphoma. The oncologist on call was consulted, and it was recommended for him to follow up as an outpatient for further evaluation and treatment recommendations.

## PMH

HTN × 10 years
Hypercholesterolemia × 5 years
NYHA Class II CHF × 8 years

## FH

The patient is the oldest of seven children (four brothers and two sisters), all alive and well. He has two children, both in good health. Family history of terminal prostate cancer in his father (died at age 63). No other history of malignancy that he is aware of.

## SH

The patient is employed as an usher at a professional baseball park. He previously smoked one to two ppd for 32 years. He quit when he was diagnosed with CHF, and he complains about the fans who smoke in the section of the ballpark where he works. He drinks one to two beers nightly when working. Diet is mostly ballpark food, heavy on the hot dogs and bratwursts. He states that he does not eat many vegetables, unless popcorn counts. He has been married for 34 years. His wife is with him today in the clinic.

## ROS

The patient reports continuing fever, typically ranging from 100.2 to 101°F (37.9–38.3°C) and cough with occasional hemoptysis. In addition, he describes an unexplained weight loss of approximately 25 lb over the last 3 months. He denies headaches, changes in vision, or fainting episodes. He reports no lesions in his mouth, difficulty swallowing, or nosebleeds. He states that he occasionally has some dyspnea on exertion, but he is able to carry out activities of daily living without limitations. He denies orthopnea, tachycardia, or swelling in the extremities. He also denies burning on urination, frequency, dribbling, or blood in the urine. He has not noticed any additional bleeding or bruising. He has not received any prior transfusions.

## Meds

Lisinopril 20 mg po once daily
Furosemide 20 mg po once daily
Simvastatin 20 mg po at bedtime
Esomeprazole 20 mg po once daily
Temazepam 30mg po at bedtime as needed
Epoetin alfa 40,000 units subQ once weekly

## All

Penicillin—rash

## Physical Examination

*Gen*

Patient is a thin white man in no apparent distress.

*VS*

BP 145/100, P 95, RR 14, T 37.9°C; Wt 72 kg, Ht 5′9″

*Skin*

No rashes or moles noted

*HEENT*

PERRLA; TMs clear; no masses in the tonsils, palate, or floor of the mouth; no stomatitis. Several missing teeth, but no gingival inflammation is noted.

*Neck*

Supple; no masses; no JVD; small scar from excisional biopsy of supraclavicular lymph node noted

*Chest*

Decreased breath sounds bilaterally, more on the left than the right; no wheezes or crackles

*CV*

RRR; no MRG

*Abd*

Soft, NT/ND. Spleen palpable just below the left costal margin. No hepatomegaly. Bowel sounds normoactive.

*Genit/Rect*

Normal male genitalia

*Ext*

Without edema, warm to the touch; pulses 2+ bilaterally

*Neuro*

Symmetric cranial nerve function. Symmetric facial muscle movement, and the tongue is midline. The palate is symmetric. Balance and coordination of the upper extremities are intact, with no evidence of tremor. There is symmetric coordination of rapidly alternating movements. Motor strength in the upper and lower extremities is normal and symmetric.

*Lymph Node Survey*

The lymph node survey is negative for any palpable peripheral nodes in the preauricular, postauricular, cervical, supraclavicular, infraclavicular, or axillary areas. No palpable inguinal nodes present. Small scar noted from excisional biopsy of left supraclavicular node.

## Labs

| | | | |
|---|---|---|---|
| Na 132 mEq/L | Hgb 10.3 g/dL | AST 29 IU/L | Phos 4.0 mg/dL |
| K 4.6 mEq/L | Hct 30% | ALT 27 IU/L | Uric acid 5.6 mg/dL |
| Cl 97 mEq/L | Plt 338 × $10^3$/mm$^3$ | Alk phos 75 IU/L | PT 12.2 sec |
| $CO_2$ 26 mEq/L | WBC 9.9 × $10^3$/mm$^3$ | LDH 623 IU/L | aPTT 21.7 sec |
| BUN 20 mg/dL | Neutros 70% | T. bili 0.6 mg/dL | |
| SCr 0.7 mg/dL | Bands 2% | T. prot 6.3 g/dL | |
| Glu 112 mg/dL | Lymphs 18% | Alb 3.7 g/dL | |
| | Monos 9% | | |
| | Eos 1% | | |

■ CT Chest

Large lobular heterogeneous mass within the left chest and mediastinum that extends from the level of the left lung and apex of the diaphragm

■ Chest X-Ray

Large heterogeneous mass at the apex of the left lung also involving the mediastinum

■ Tumor Pathology

Diffuse large cell lymphoma, B-cell type; CD20+, CD45+, CD3–

■ Tumor Pathology

Diffuse large cell lymphoma. Further staging will include bilateral BM biopsies, PET scan, HIV test, CT of the abdomen, and a baseline cardiac assessment in light of the patient's long-standing history of HTN.

■ Clinical Course

Bone marrow biopsies are negative for lymphoma. PET scanning revealed multiple foci of increased FDG uptake; increased uptake noted in the spleen, mediastinum, and left-side supraclavicular lymph nodes. The HIV test is negative. CT of the abdomen shows large heterogeneous soft tissue mass within the left upper quadrant that may be contiguous with previously noted left chest mass. The mass extends inferiomedially to the tail of the pancreas. There is an additional 4-cm low-density mass near the head of the pancreas. The spleen is enlarged. MUGA scan reveals an LVEF of 45%.

■ Assessment

Diffuse large B-cell lymphoma, stage IIISB; IPI score of 2

# QUESTIONS

## Problem Identification

1.a. Identify all of the drug therapy problems of this patient.

1.b. What clinical and other information is consistent with the diagnosis of NHL?

1.c. Explain what system of staging was used and how his stage of disease was determined.

1.d. What laboratory and clinical features does this patient have that may affect his prognosis? How is the IPI determined?

## Desired Outcome

2. What are the goals of therapy in this case?

## Therapeutic Alternatives

3. What chemotherapy regimens are available for treatment of his NHL?

## Optimal Plan

4.a. What drug, dosage form, schedule, and duration of therapy are best for treating this patient's NHL?

4.b. What other interventions should be made to maintain control of the patient's other concurrent diseases?

4.c. What nondrug therapies might be useful for this patient?

## Outcome Evaluation

5.a. How is the response to the treatment regimen for the NHL assessed?

5.b. What acute adverse effects are associated with the chemotherapy regimen, and what parameters should be monitored?

5.c. What pharmacologic measures should be instituted to treat or prevent the acute toxicities associated with the chemotherapy regimen?

5.d. What are potential late complications of the chemotherapy regimen, and how can they be detected and prevented?

## Patient Education

6. What information would you provide to the patient about the agents used to treat the NHL?

## ■ CLINICAL COURSE

The patient tolerated the first few cycles of chemotherapy well, with only some minimal nausea and vomiting. His antihypertensive medication was modified, increasing the lisinopril to 40 mg daily and maintaining the furosemide 20 mg daily, achieving average systolic BPs in the 120s and average diastolic BPs in the 70s. His fasting lipid panel was checked and was found to be within his goals. One week after completing the fourth cycle of chemotherapy, he presented to the ED with fever (temperature at presentation was 101.3°F [38.5°C]), cough, dyspnea, pain on inspiration, and fatigue. Laboratory evaluation showed an ANC of $0.352 \times 10^3/\text{mm}^3$. He was admitted to the hospital for evaluation and treatment of suspected neutropenic fever with pneumonia. Blood and sputum cultures were negative. The patient was treated with broad-spectrum antibiotics and became afebrile after 3 days. He was discharged from the hospital after the neutropenia resolved, completing a 14-day course of inpatient IV antibiotics. Imaging studies were performed while he was in the hospital to evaluate his lymphoma. PET and CT scans showed that he achieved a complete response.

## Follow-Up Question

1. What measures should be taken to prevent neutropenic fever in subsequent courses of chemotherapy?

## ■ CLINICAL COURSE

The patient completed his planned course of chemotherapy without further event. Eighteen months later, the patient returns to the oncologist office after being diagnosed with relapsed lymphoma during a hospital admission for worsening dyspnea.

## ■ SELF-STUDY ASSIGNMENTS

1. What is the role of radiopharmaceuticals for the treatment of aggressive NHL?
2. What therapeutic options are available for the treatment of relapsed diffuse large B-cell lymphomas?
3. If the patient experienced tumor lysis syndrome, what options are there for treating the hyperuricemia?

## CLINICAL PEARL

The role of CNS prophylaxis in the treatment of aggressive NHL, such as diffuse large B-cell lymphoma, is controversial. Features associated with an increased risk of relapse in the brain include initial presentation in paranasal sinus or testicular involvement and an elevated LDH combined with more than one site of extranodal involvement. Therapeutic options for CNS prophylaxis include intrathecal or high-dose IV methotrexate.

## REFERENCES


1. The International Non-Hodgkin's Lymphoma Prognostic Factors Project. A predictive model for aggressive non-Hodgkin's lymphoma. N Engl J Med 1993;329:987–994.
2. Rodriguez J, Cabanillas F, McLaughlin P, et al. A proposal for a simple staging system for intermediate grade lymphoma and immunoblastic lymphoma based on the "tumor score". Ann Oncol 1992;3:711–717.
3. Fisher RI, Gaynor ER, Dahlberg S, et al. Comparison of a standard regimen (CHOP) with three intensive chemotherapy regimens for advanced non-Hodgkin's lymphoma. N Engl J Med 1993; 328:1002–1006.
4. Vose JM, Link BK, Grossbard ML, et al. Long-term update of a phase II study of rituximab in combination with CHOP chemotherapy in patients with previously untreated, aggressive non-Hodgkin's lymphoma. Leuk Lymphoma 2005;46:1569–1573.
5. Feugier P, Van Hoof A, Sebban C, et al. Long-term results of the R-CHOP study in the treatment of elderly patients with diffuse large B-cell lymphoma: a study by the Groupe d'Etude des Lymphomes de l'Adulte. J Clin Oncol 2005;23:4117–4126.
6. Basser RL, Green MD. Strategies for prevention of anthracycline cardiotoxicity. Cancer Treat Rev 1993;19:57–77.
7. Procrit [Package Insert]. Raritan, NJ, Centocor Ortho Biotech Products, L.P., 2010.
8. Smith TJ, Khatcheressian J, Lyman GH, et al. 2006 update of recommendations for the use of white blood cell growth factors: an evidence-based clinical practice guideline. J Clin Oncol 2006;24:3187–3205.
9. Ganz WI, Sridhar KS, Ganz SS, et al. Review of tests for monitoring doxorubicin-induced cardiomyopathy. Oncology 1996;53:461–470.


# 152

# HODGKIN LYMPHOMA

The Operating Room Nurse . . . . . . . . . . . . . . . Level I

**Cindy L. O'Bryant, PharmD, BCOP**

## LEARNING OBJECTIVES

After completing this case study, students should be able to:

- Recognize the signs and symptoms commonly associated with Hodgkin lymphoma (HL).
- Discuss the pharmacotherapeutic treatment of choice and the alternatives available for treating HL.
- Identify acute and chronic toxicities associated with the medications used to treat HL and the measures used to prevent or treat these toxicities.
- Determine monitoring parameters for response and toxicity in patients with HL.
- Formulate appropriate educational information to provide to a patient receiving chemotherapy treatment for HL.
- Recommend a plan for monitoring the late effects from HL treatment.

## PATIENT PRESENTATION

### Chief Complaint

"I noticed a growth on my chest that has gotten bigger over the last month and won't go away."

### HPI

Tom Montgomery is a 31-year-old man who presents with a 1-month history of a mass on his chest that has gotten progressively bigger. He initially associated the mass with an "elbow in the chest" he received during a basketball game with some of the other operating room staff. He also complains of general fatigue over the last 3 months but has been working extra shifts. He denies any shortness of breath but has experienced fever, night sweats, and weight loss for the past few months. An ultrasound of the mediastinum showed a lymph node that measured approximately 10 cm. On physical exam, enlarged supraclavicular lymph nodes were noted on both the right and left. As a result, a lymph node biopsy was performed that demonstrated classical HL, nodular sclerosing subtype.

### PMH

Appendectomy at age 11 years old

### FH

The patient's parents and one sibling (sister) are all in good health. There is no history of cancer in his family.

### SH

Works as an OR nurse in the local hospital. Drinks socially, about four beers per week. He has never smoked. He does not use street drugs. The patient is married and has one child who is 2 years old.

### Meds

None

### All

NKDA

### ROS

Patient reports fevers, night sweats, and weight loss of approximately 9 kg over the past 3 months. He denies any vision changes, headaches, shortness of breath, or chest pain. He also denies nausea, vomiting, diarrhea, constipation, or urinary symptoms. Generally feels fatigued. All other systems are negative. His performance status is 1 on the Zubrod scale.

### Physical Examination

*Gen*

The patient is a healthy-appearing man in no apparent distress.

*VS*

BP 128/72, P 82, RR 16, T 36.6°C; Wt 81 kg, Ht 5′11″

*Skin*

Soft, diffusely enlarged soft tissue swelling in the middle of the upper chest just below the neck; no erythema or warmth; no rashes

*HEENT*

PERRL; EOMI; TMs intact

*Lymph Nodes*

Supraclavicular lymph nodes are enlarged on both the right and left. The mediastinal mass is palpable. No other lymph nodes are palpable bilaterally.

*Chest*

Respirations with normal rhythm; clear to auscultation

*Breasts*

Normal appearance; no masses on palpation

*CV*

RRR; no JVD, murmurs, or gallops

*Abd*

Soft and nontender with no masses; bowel sounds are normoactive.

*Genit/Rect*

Normal male genitalia; stool is guaiac (–).

*MS/Ext*

Without edema

*Neuro*

A & O × 3; CN II–XII intact; remainder of exam is nonfocal

### Labs

| | | | |
|---|---|---|---|
| Na 135 mEq/L | Hgb 13.1 g/dL | AST 19 IU/L | PT 12.9 s |
| K 4.1 mEq/L | Hct 39.3% | ALT 22 IU/L | aPTT 27.1 s |
| Cl 103 mEq/L | Plt 310 × $10^3$/mm$^3$ | Alk phos 94 IU/L | Phos 3.1 mg/dL |
| $CO_2$ 24 mEq/L | WBC 10.9 × $10^3$/mm$^3$ | LDH 372 IU/L | Magnesium 1.7 mEq/L |
| BUN 14 mg/dL | Neutros 80.5% | T. bili 0.4 mg/dL | Uric acid 4.5 mg/dL |
| SCr 0.6 mg/dL | Lymphs 13.2% | T. prot 7.7 g/dL | ESR 53 mm/h |
| Glu 93 mg/dL | Monos 5.4% | Alb 3.2 g/dL | |
| | Eos 0.9% | | |

### Ultrasound

There are singular, enlarged abnormal lymph nodes in the right and left supraclavicular regions. The largest node on the right measures 2.1 cm × 1.4 cm × 1.8 cm and on the left 1.7 cm × 0.9 cm × 1.1 cm. The large mediastinal node is 10.3 cm × 6.4 cm × 8.7 cm. The nodes contain solid echogenic material and have increased vascular flow.

### Tumor Pathology

Identification of Reed–Sternberg cells classifying this as HL, NS type (see Fig. 152-1). Immunohistochemistry: CD15+, CD30+, CD20–, CD45–.

### PET/Helical CT Scan

Enlarged nodes demonstrating hypermetabolic activity are noted in the bilateral supraclavicular chains. There is involvement of the superior middle mediastinum showing bulky disease and hilar nodal chains within the chest. The bilateral lungs and myocardium are negative for disease. Normal physiologic liver, GI, and urinary activity are noted. Diffuse increased uptake within the bone marrow; it is unclear whether this is lymphoma or hyperplasia.

### Bone Marrow Biopsy

Bilateral biopsies are negative for HL.

### Assessment

Classical HL, nodular sclerosis subtype, stage IIB

## QUESTIONS

### Problem Identification

1.a. What clinical and other information is consistent with the diagnosis of HL?

1.b. Explain what system of staging was used and how his stage of disease was determined.

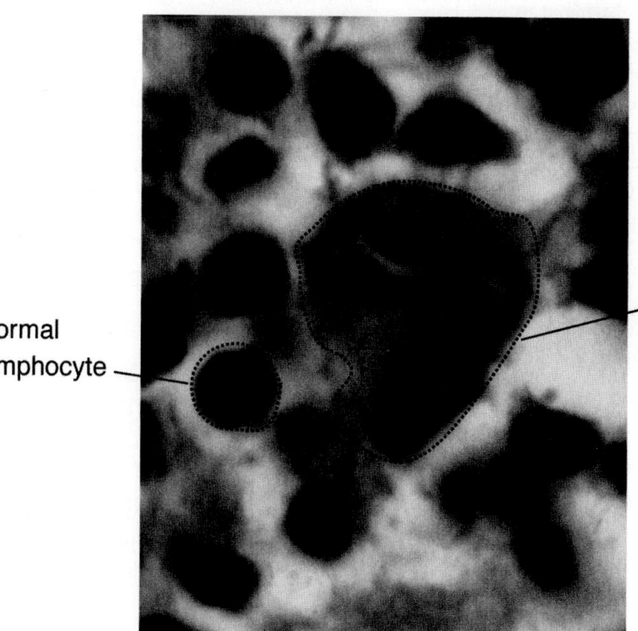


**FIGURE 152-1.** Reed–Sternberg cell (center) surrounded by normal lymphocytes. (*Source: National Cancer Institute.*)

## Desired Outcome

2. What are the goals of therapy in this case?

## Therapeutic Alternatives

3. What treatment options are available for managing this patient's HL?

## Optimal Plan

4.a. What drug, dosage form, schedule, and duration of chemotherapy are best for treating this patient's HL?

4.b. Are additional treatment modalities other than chemotherapy indicated for treating this patient's HL?

## Outcome Evaluation

5.a. What clinical and laboratory parameters are necessary to evaluate the therapy for achievement of the desired therapeutic outcome for treatment of HL?

5.b. What acute adverse effects are associated with the chemotherapy regimen?

5.c. What clinical or laboratory parameters are necessary to detect and prevent acute and long-term adverse events commonly associated with treatment of HL?

## Patient Education

6. What information should be provided to the patient to enhance compliance, ensure successful therapy, and minimize adverse effects for treatment of HL?

## ■ CLINICAL COURSE

The patient's treatment was administered in the outpatient setting. He received day 1 of his first cycle of chemotherapy and experienced acute nausea and vomiting. He also experienced mild mucositis and mild constipation. The patient was instructed to maintain good oral hygiene, use a soft toothbrush, and avoid alcohol and spicy or acidic foods. He was started on a mouthwash (diphenhydramine, lidocaine, and aluminum/magnesium hydroxide) with instructions to swish and spit four times a day. He was instructed to maintain a high-fiber diet and start docusate sodium 50 mg orally once daily for constipation. He returned to the outpatient clinic for the second cycle of chemotherapy, after which he was restaged with a PET/CT scan to assess his response to chemotherapy. Restaging showed the patient had a complete response, and he received two more cycles of chemotherapy and involved-field radiation. On subsequent follow-up, the patient is in remission.

## Follow-Up Question

1. What follow-up and long-term monitoring should this patient receive after completion of his cancer treatment?

## ■ SELF-STUDY ASSIGNMENTS

1. What are unfavorable prognostic factors for early and advanced HL, and how does this influence treatment?
2. What is the antiemetic regimen of choice to prevent acute nausea and vomiting for highly emetogenic chemotherapy?
3. What are the salvage therapy options for patients with relapsing HL?
4. What is the role of bone marrow or stem cell transplantation for HL?

## CLINICAL PEARL

HL can be cured with chemotherapy, even if it is in advanced stages. To achieve a cure, it is essential that a patient receives the appropriate treatment. This is based on several key factors, which include an accurate diagnosis of the type of HL with recommended immunostaining, determination of unfavorable prognostic factors, and use of combined chemotherapy and radiation treatment when appropriate.

## REFERENCES


1. Punnett A, Tsang RW, Hodgson DC. Hodgkin lymphoma across the age spectrum: epidemiology, therapy, and late effects. Semin Radiat Oncol 2010;20:30–44.
2. Engert A, Schiller P, Josting A, et al. Involved-field radiotherapy is equally effective and less toxic compared with extended-field radiotherapy after four cycles of chemotherapy in patients with early stage unfavorable Hodgkin's lymphoma: results of the HD8 trial of the German Hodgkin's Lymphoma Study Group. J Clin Oncol 2003;21:3601–3608.
3. Horning SJ, Hoppe RT, Breslin S, et al. Stanford V and radiotherapy for locally extensive and advanced Hodgkin's disease: mature results of a prospective clinical trial. J Clin Oncol 2002;20:630–637.
4. Henry-Amar M, Friedman S, Hayat M, et al. Erythrocyte sedimentation rate predicts early relapse and survival in early-stage Hodgkin disease: the EORTC Lymphoma Cooperative Group. Ann Intern Med 1991;114:361–365.
5. NCCN Hodgkin Lymphoma Clinical Practice Guidelines in Oncology (Version V.1.2010). Available at: *http://www.nccn.rog*. Accessed March 1, 2010.
6. Hasenclever D, Diehl V. A prognostic score for advanced Hodgkin's disease: International Prognostic Factors Project on Advanced Hodgkin's Disease. N Engl J Med 1998;339:1506–1514.
7. Ganz PA. Survivorship: adult cancer survivors. Prim Care 2009; 36:721–741.


# 153

# OVARIAN CANCER

Family Ties . . . . . . . . . . . . . . . . . . . . . . . . . . . Level II

**Ninh M. La-Beck, PharmD**

**Mark D. Walsh, PharmD**

**William C. Zamboni, PharmD, PhD**

## LEARNING OBJECTIVES

After completing this case study, students should be able to:

- Recognize the signs and symptoms of ovarian cancer.
- Describe the genetic factors associated with ovarian cancer.
- Recommend a pharmacotherapeutic plan for the chemotherapy of newly diagnosed and relapsed ovarian cancer.
- Describe the uses and potential pharmacologic advantages of pegylated liposomal doxorubicin.

- Recognize the dose-limiting and most common toxicities associated with the chemotherapeutic agents used in the treatment of ovarian cancer.

## PATIENT PRESENTATION

### Chief Complaint

"I'm very anxious about getting chemotherapy. My uncles have gone through chemotherapy for colorectal cancer and they became very sick. One of them was even admitted to the hospital due to the side effects. I don't want that to happen to me."

### HPI

Edith Hillebrand is a 56-year-old woman who presents to the Gynecology Oncology clinic 1 week after surgery for stage IIIB (T2c N1 M0) serous epithelial ovarian adenocarcinoma. She originally presented to her PCP's office 1 month ago with complaints of a 3-day progressive worsening of LLE pain, swelling, and redness. The physician ordered a Doppler ultrasound of the LLE. Results indicated that she had a DVT in the popliteal vein extending to the iliac vein. Her last physical exam was performed more than 15 months prior. The physician performed a complete history and physical exam and identified a left adnexal mass, abdominal pain, bloating, and weight gain. CT scans of the abdomen and pelvis showed a large, soft tissue pelvic mass. Laboratory examination revealed CA-125 490 IU/mL.

Mrs Hillebrand underwent an exploratory laparatomy, TAH-BSO, omentectomy, and bilateral pelvic and periaortic lymph node dissection with comprehensive staging by a gynecologic oncologist. On entering the abdomen, there was a relatively small amount of ascitic fluid. A large left adnexal mass measuring 15 cm × 5 cm × 10 cm was discovered and removed. Multiple small tumor nodules (2 cm or less) outside the pelvis were also removed. Numerous adhesions were seen throughout the omentum and surrounding organs. At completion of the surgery, the surgeon noted that the patient was optimally debulked. Ascitic fluid, peritoneal washings, left adnexal mass, left and right ovaries, multiple pelvic and periaortic lymph nodes, and omentum were sent to pathology for further examination.

Gross examination of left and right ovaries revealed multiple adhesions extending from each ovary with interspersed broad regions of necrosis. Each ovary was serially sectioned for microscopic examination, which revealed numerous papillations of tumor cells destructively permeating the stroma (grade 2). Based on this information, Mrs Hillebrand was diagnosed with stage IIIB (T2c N1 M0) serous epithelial ovarian adenocarcinoma.

### PMH

Hypothyroidism × 30 years
HTN × 22 years
Type 2 DM × 17 years
Dyslipidemia × 15 years
GERD × 10 years

### FH

Married × 37 years with two children, a son age 35 and daughter age 32. Her father died of an MI at age 72, and her mother died at age 66 with ovarian cancer. Has two paternal uncles (age 80 and 76 years) but alive with colorectal cancer.

### SH

Consumes one glass of red wine with dinner every evening. Has a 20 pack-year history of cigarette smoking; quit 25 years ago. No recreational drug use.

### Meds

Ibuprofen 200 mg one to two tablets po Q 6 h PRN headaches/muscle aches (OTC)
Levothyroxine 0.1 mg po daily
Pantoprazole 40 mg po daily
Simvastatin/ezetimibe 40 mg/10 mg po daily
Metformin 1,000 mg po twice daily
Glyburide 10 mg po twice daily
Lisinopril 40 mg po daily

### All

Penicillin (hives as a child)
Codeine ("sour stomach")

### ROS

Somewhat fatigued lately, progressively worsening over the last 2 months. Reports to have struggled with weight loss for most of her adult life and reports a 10-kg weight gain over the last 4 months. She also reports requiring more sleep than usual, about 9–10 hours per night, but cannot recall when this change occurred. Her mood is depressed because of concern about her recent cancer diagnosis. She reports occasional headaches (~1 episode per month) relieved by OTC ibuprofen. Denies any changes in sight, smell, hearing, and taste. Also reports constipation and dry skin.

### Physical Examination

*Gen*

The patient appears to be her stated age. Appears anxious in the office on exam.

*VS*

BP 135/85, P 110, RR 18, T 37.0°C; Ht 5′7″, Wt 70 kg

*Skin*

No erythema, rash, ecchymoses, or petechiae

*LN*

No cervical or axillary lymphadenopathy

*HEENT*

PERRLA, EOMI; TMs intact; fundus benign; OP dry

*Breasts*

Without masses, discharge, or adenopathy; no nipple or skin changes

*Cor*

RRR; no M/R/G

*Pulm*

CTA bilaterally

*Abd*

Soft, nontender; no HSM. Surgical wound healing well; no exudate or erythema; covered with 4 × 4 bandage with antibiotic ointment.

*Genit/Rect*

Normal female genitalia; heme (–) dark brown stool; no rectal wall tenderness or masses

*Ext*

No C/C/E. Residual erythema and swelling in LLE from prior DVT; no signs of ulceration.

*Neuro*

CN II–XII intact; sensation decreased to light touch and pinprick below the knees bilaterally; vibration sense diminished at the great toes bilaterally

### Labs

| | | |
|---|---|---|
| Na 140 mEq/L | Hgb 12.8 g/dL | AST 25 IU/L |
| K 3.4 mEq/L | Hct 31% | ALT 40 IU/L |
| Cl 99 mEq/L | Plt 135 × $10^3$/mm$^3$ | T. bili 0.7 mg/dL |
| $CO_2$ 24 mEq/L | WBC 5.2 × $10^3$/mm$^3$ | Alb 4.0 units/L |
| BUN 20 mg/dL | Neutros 60% | CA-125 490 IU/mL |
| SCr 1.1 mg/dL | Bands 3% | |
| Glu 135 mg/dL | Lymphs 30% | |
| Ca 9.8 mg/dL | Monos 5% | |
| Mg 2.0 mg/dL | Eos 1% | |
| Phos 3.5 mg/dL | Basos 1% | |

### UA

WBC 1–5/hpf, RBC 0/hpf, 1+ ketones, 1+ protein, pH 5.0

### Genetic Results

DNA analysis from a blood sample revealed that the patient is a positive for BRCA1 gene mutation.

### Assessment/Plan

Mrs Hillebrand is a 56-year-old woman with advanced stage IIIB (T2c N1 M0) serous epithelial ovarian adenocarcinoma. She underwent optimal surgical debulking by a trained gynecologic oncologist and presents to the clinic for follow-up management. Based on the stage of diagnosis and risk for recurrence, first-line chemotherapy is recommended.

## QUESTIONS

### Problem Identification

1.a. What are the patient's drug therapy problems?

1.b. What information (signs, symptoms, laboratory values) indicates the presence and severity of ovarian cancer?

1.c. What stage of ovarian cancer does this patient have, and how does the stage of disease affect the choice of therapy?

1.d. What is the significance of the size of residual tumor after primary cytoreductive surgery?

### Desired Outcome

2. What are the goals of therapy for this patient?

### Therapeutic Alternatives

3.a. How do her genetic results influence the choice of therapy and prognosis?

3.b. What are the first-line chemotherapy options for this patient?

3.c. What are the specific toxicities and logistical issues related to intraperitoneal (IP) therapy?

### Optimal Plan

4.a. Which first-line chemotherapy regimen and ancillary treatment measures would you recommend for this patient?

4.b. Regardless of whether you recommended intravenous carboplatin, use the Calvert equation to calculate the carboplatin dose required to achieve a target AUC of 5 mg/mL · min.

## CLINICAL COURSE

The patient and oncologist agreed to begin treatment with the combination of IV docetaxel and carboplatin on day 1 every 21 days for six cycles as first-line treatment of her ovarian cancer.

### Outcome Evaluation

5. How would you monitor the therapy for efficacy and adverse effects?

## CLINICAL COURSE

Mrs Hillebrand completed six cycles of docetaxel 75 mg/m$^2$ IV over 1 hour followed by carboplatin AUC 6 IV over 1 hour on day 1 every 21 days. She tolerated therapy very well with no dose reductions or delays. Her serum CA-125 level slowly declined over the course of treatment and was 12 IU/mL 3 weeks after her sixth cycle. Based on her CA-125 level and the negative CT scans following the fourth and sixth cycles, Mrs Hillebrand was defined as a clinical complete response. Her CA-125 levels were followed monthly.

### Patient Education

6. What information would you provide to the patient about this therapy?

## CLINICAL COURSE

Starting 1 month after treatment was discontinued, monthly CA-125 levels were 8, 10, 14, 20, 30, 43, and 88 IU/mL. A CT scan performed at 8 months after treatment discontinuation revealed a pelvic mass (6 cm × 5 cm × 4 cm) arising from the retroperitoneum and a 2-cm mass in the head of the pancreas. Laboratory data were normal except for a CA-125 level of 150 IU/mL. She was diagnosed with recurrent ovarian cancer.

### Follow-Up Questions

1. Is it useful to treat early relapsed disease based only on a rising CA-125 level rather than delaying treatment until there are clinical signs of relapse?
2. What therapeutic options are available for this patient's relapsed disease?

## CLINICAL COURSE

The decision was made to start IV carboplatin AUC 5 and pegylated liposomal doxorubicin 30 mg/m$^2$ on day 1 every 28 days. Mrs Hillebrand received two cycles of carboplatin and pegylated liposomal doxorubicin. Radiologic imaging just prior to the third cycle showed no evidence of disease progression. During her third cycle, she complained of having trouble putting on her shoes and pain in her feet on walking. On physical exam the patient's feet were red, swollen, and cracked. Her CA-125 levels were 155, 158, and 160 IU/mL after each of her first three cycles of carboplatin plus pegylated liposomal doxorubicin.

### Follow-Up Questions

3. Which of the chemotherapeutic regimens would you suggest for the patient's locally relapsed ovarian cancer? Provide the rationale for your answer.

## CLINICAL COURSE

The fourth cycle of therapy was delayed for 2 weeks and restarted when her skin lesions resolved. However, after her fourth cycle radiographic findings revealed evidence of disease progression, and a repeat CA-125 was 288 IU/mL.

## CHAPTER 154

## Follow-Up Questions

4. What are the potential adverse effects of pegylated liposomal doxorubicin therapy that require monitoring and patient education?
5. What options are available for salvage therapy, and which would you choose for this patient? Provide the rationale for your answer.

## SELF-STUDY ASSIGNMENTS

1. What are the pharmacologic advantages of IV therapy versus IP therapy?
2. Why is the size of the residual tumor important with regard to IP therapy?
3. What are the probable causes of paclitaxel and docetaxel hypersensitivity?
4. What are the issues related to maintenance therapy in patients with advanced ovarian cancer after achieving complete response to consolidative chemotherapy?
5. How might cytochrome P450 3A4/5 polymorphism potentially affect docetaxel therapy of ovarian cancer?

## CLINICAL PEARL

Surgical cytoreduction followed by chemotherapy was chosen for Mrs Hillebrand, but what treatments are available for patients whose disease or health status prevents them from undergoing this approach? One option for patients with advanced age or poor performance status is neoadjuvant chemotherapy. Neoadjuvant chemotherapy is given prior to the primary treatment, which is surgery, with the goal of reducing tumor volume in hopes for a greater chance of a cure. It simplifies surgery by decreasing tumor volume, blood loss, and transfusions during surgery and can reduce surgical complications and length of stays.

## REFERENCES


1. The NCCN Clinical Practice Guidelines in Oncology™ Ovarian Cancer (Version 2.2010). © 2009 National Comprehensive Cancer Network Inc. Available at: *NCCN.org*. Accessed June 1, 2010. To view the most recent and complete version of the NCCN guidelines, go online to *NCCN.org*.
2. Boyd J, Sonoda Y, Federici MG, et al. Clinicopathologic features of BRCA-linked and sporadic ovarian cancer. JAMA 2000;283:2260–2265.
3. McGuire WP, Hoskins WJ, Brady MF, et al. Cyclophosphamide and cisplatin compared with paclitaxel and cisplatin in patients with stage III and stage IV ovarian cancer. N Engl J Med 1996;334:1–6.
4. Ozols RF, Bundy BN, Greer BE, et al. Gynecologic Oncology Group. Phase III trial of carboplatin and paclitaxel compared with cisplatin and paclitaxel in patients with optimally resected stage III ovarian cancer: a gynecologic oncology group study. J Clin Oncol 2003; 21:3194–3200.
5. du Bois A, Luck HJ, Meier W, et al, Arbeitsgemeinschaft Gynakologische Onkologie Ovarian Cancer Study Group. A randomized clinical trial of cisplatin/paclitaxel versus carboplatin/paclitaxel as first-line treatment of ovarian cancer. J Natl Cancer Inst 2003;95:1320–1329.
6. Vasey PA, Jayson GC, Gordon A, et al, Scottish Gynaecological Cancer Trials Group. Phase III randomized trial of docetaxel–carboplatin versus paclitaxel–carboplatin as first-line chemotherapy for ovarian carcinoma. J Natl Cancer Inst 2004;96:1682–1691.
7. Armstrong DK, Bundy B, Wenzel L, et al, Gynecologic Oncology Group. Intraperitoneal cisplatin and paclitaxel in ovarian cancer. N Engl J Med 2006;354:34–43.
8. Rustin GJ, van der Burg ME, on behalf of MRC and EORTC Collaborators. A randomized trial in ovarian cancer (OC) of early treatment of relapse based on CA125 level alone versus delayed treatment based on conventional clinical indicators (MRC OV05/EORTC 55955 trials). J Clin Oncol (Meeting Abstracts) 2009;27(18S):1.
9. Parmar MK, Ledermann JA, Colombo N, et al, ICON and AGO Collaborators. Paclitaxel plus platinum-based chemotherapy versus conventional platinum-based chemotherapy in women with relapsed ovarian cancer: the ICON4/AGO-OVAR-2.2 trial. Lancet 2003;361:2099–2106.
10. Pujade-Lauraine E, Mahner S, Kaern J, et al. A randomized, phase III study of carboplatin and pegylated liposomal doxorubicin versus carboplatin and paclitaxel in relapsed platinum-sensitive ovarian cancer (OC): CALYPSO study of the Gynecologic Cancer Intergroup (GCIG). J Clin Oncol (Meeting Abstracts) 2009;27(18S):LBA5509.


# 154

# ACUTE LYMPHOCYTIC LEUKEMIA

Ian's Unexpected Weight Loss. . . . . . . . . . . . . Level II

**Deborah A. Hass, PharmD, BCOP**

## LEARNING OBJECTIVES

After completing this case study, students should be able to:

- Interpret the laboratory values that signify the response of acute lymphocytic leukemia (ALL) to chemotherapy.
- Describe the ancillary medications and supportive care measures that are necessary when administering chemotherapy to patients with ALL.
- Understand the appropriate medications needed to treat neutropenic fever.
- Identify the backbone of therapy for treatment of adult ALL.
- State why CNS prophylaxis is routinely done in adult patients with ALL.

## PATIENT PRESENTATION

### Chief Complaint

Episodic diaphoresis, dizziness, and progressively worsening weakness and dyspnea on exertion × 1 month

### HPI

Ian Hamilton is a 58-year-old man with a past medical history of diabetes, hyperlipidemia, and hypertension who presents with episodic diaphoresis, dizziness, and progressively worsening weakness and dyspnea on exertion for 1 month. He has lost 40 lb in the past 9 months; he recently has been trying to eat more but is still losing 2 lb per week. Flow cytometry done 3 days ago at an outside hospital showed blastic B cells consistent with pre-B-cell lymphoblastic leukemia. The patient was found to have normocytic anemia (Hgb 9.9 g/dL). He also had a CT of the chest/abdomen/pelvis completed at the outside hospital due to weight loss and occasional abdominal pain and sensation that his stomach is "churning," although no report was sent with his records. He denies diarrhea but admits to once having an episode of dry heaving. A CXR was unremarkable. The patient was previously taking Janumet® for type 2 DM, but since this workup began he stopped it and per patient has had blood sugars in the 100s to 130s.

## PMH

DM type 2
HTN
Dyslipidemia

## FH

Father had MI at age 60 and leukemia at age 78, and expired shortly thereafter. Mother is alive with heart disease, skin cancer, an unknown GI malignancy, and a recent diagnosis of lymphoma. He has five brothers and two sisters. One brother died at age 48 from Hodgkin's lymphoma, diagnosed at age 18. Another brother has multiple sclerosis. The other three brothers and both sisters are healthy.

## SH

Denies tobacco, EtOH, and illicit drugs. Drives a waste management truck, has three children and lives with his wife.

## Meds

None

## All

NKDA

## ROS

Constitutional: Positive for sweats, fatigue, anorexia, and weight loss
HEENT: Negative
Respiratory: Positive for dyspnea
CV: Negative
GI: Positive for nausea and abdominal pain
GU: Negative
Heme/lymph: Negative
MS: Negative
Neuro: Positive for dizziness and weakness

## Physical Examination

*Gen*

A & O × 3; NAD

*VS*

BP 124/58, P 106, RR 18, T 37.2°C; Wt 100.8 kg, Ht 5′11″, $SpO_2$: 98% (room air)

*Skin*

Normal, no rashes

*HEENT*

EOMI, no scleral icterus, no conjuctival pallor

*Neck/Lymph Nodes*

No cervical LAD

*Lungs/Thorax*

CTA bilaterally without crackles, wheezes, or rhonchi

*CV*

RRR; normal $S_1$, $S_2$; no murmurs, rubs, or gallops

*Abd*

Soft, obese, NT/ND, normoactive bowel sounds

*Genit/Rect*

Deferred

*MS/Ext*

No CCE

*Neuro*

UE/LE strength 5/5 bilaterally

## Labs

| | | |
|---|---|---|
| Na 137 mEq/L | Hgb 9.9 g/dL | AST 16 IU/L |
| K 4.1 mEq/L | Hct 27.2% | ALT 10 IU/L |
| Cl 100 mEq/L | MCV 93.5 $\mu$mm³ | T. bili 0.5 mg/dL |
| $CO_2$ 28 Eq/L | RDW 17.1% | Alb 3 g/dL |
| BUN 19 mg/dL | Plt 95 × $10^3$/mm³ | Fe 23 mcg/dL |
| SCr 1.2 mg/dL | WBC 7.1 × $10^3$/mm³ | TIBC 252 mcg/dL |
| Glu 93 mg/dL | Segs 35% | T. sat 35% |
| | Bands 0.2% | Ferritin 159 ng/L |
| | Lymphs 5.2% | TSH 3.3 $\mu$IU/mL |
| | Monos 8.6% | PSA 0.52 ng/mL |
| | Myelos 1.6% | $B_{12}$ 311 ng/mL |
| | Blasts 49% | Folate 9.5 ng/mL |

## Peripheral Blood Flow Cytometry

Large population of abnormal blasts, ~49% of leukocyte population expressing CD45. Blasts have precursor B-cell phenotype, express CD19, CD22, CD34, CD38, HLA-DR, and terminal deoxynucleotidyl transferase (TdT). About 59% of blasts express CD20. Blasts are negative for surface IG, T-cell-related antigens, and myeloid antigens. The mature lymphocyte population consists of a mix of unremarkable T and B cells.

## Assessment and Plan

1. Pre-B-cell lymphoblastic leukemia (Philadelphia chromosome negative):
   - Obtain LDH/uric acid.
   - Bone marrow biopsy.
   - MUGA scan.
   - Central catheter placement.
   - Will attempt to obtain CT report from outside hospital.
   - Acute leukemia panel.
2. DM II-pt has controlled BS despite stopping meds recently:
   - Accuchecks QID.
   - Diabetic diet.
   - Obtain UA to check for proteinuria; pt recently on ACE inhibitor but taken off. SCr ranging from 0.9 to 1.2 mg/dL at outside hospital.
3. Nausea:
   - Ondansetron PRN.
4. HTN:
   - Pt recently taken off meds due to weight loss; will monitor pressures and restart meds as needed.

5. Thrombocytopenia:
   - Transfuse to keep platelets greater than $10.0 \times 10^3/mm^3$.
6. Anemia:
   - Transfuse to keep hemoglobin greater than 8 g/dL.
7. FEN:
   - Diabetic diet as above.
   - Maintain K >4 mEq/L and Mg >2 mg/dL.
8. VTE prophylaxis:
   - SCD boots.

## CLINICAL COURSE

Within 2 days of admission, the patient receives a BM biopsy, MUGA (EF = 60%), and PICC line placement. The results of the biopsy were as follows:

> The vast majority of the cells in the aspirate and biopsy are large blasts with fine chromatin and many prominent cytoplasmic vacuoles. Nucleoli are not generally prominent, and flow cytometric studies clearly indicated that this is a neoplasm of immature B cells. In addition, strong TdT expression is seen by immunohistochemistry. CD20 is weakly to strongly expressed in about half of the neoplastic cells.
>
> WHO classification: B lymphoblastic leukemia.

He is started on the following medications:

- Pantoprazole delayed-release tablet 40 mg po daily
- Ondansetron 8 mg po Q 8 h PRN
- 0.9% normal saline by continuous IV infusion
- Allopurinol 300 mg po daily

Following recovery from the PICC line placement, the patient was started on the R-HyperCVAD regimen based on Ht 180 cm, Wt 100.8 kg, and BSA= 2.2 m$^2$.

## CHEMOTHERAPY

*Regimen 1:*

Cyclophosphamide 300 mg/m$^2$ (660 mg) IV over 3 hours every 12 hours for six doses on Days 1–3.

Mesna 600 mg/m$^2$ (1,320 mg) IV over 24 hours on Days 1–3, ending 12 hours after the last dose of cyclophosphamide.

Vincristine 2 mg IV on Days 4 and 11.

Doxorubicin 50 mg/m$^2$ (110 mg) IV on Day 4.

Dexamethasone 40 mg po on Days 1–4 and 11–14.

Rituximab 375 mg/m$^2$ (825 mg) IV on Day 1. (Our patient did not receive it on Day 1 to prevent tumor flare.)

*Regimen 2* (he will alternate cycles every 21 days with the following regimen, for a total of six to eight cycles depending on patient tolerability and disease progression; patient-specific doses will be based on the patient's weight at that time):

Methotrexate 200 mg/m$^2$ IV over 2 hours, followed by 800 mg/m$^2$ IV over 22 hours on Day 1

Leucovorin 25 mg po Q 6 h starting 24 hours after completion of the methotrexate infusion until methotrexate level is <0.05 μmol/mL

Cytarabine 3,000 mg/m$^2$ IV over 2 hours every 12 hours for four doses on Days 2–3

Methylprednisolone 50 mg IV BID on Days 1–3

*CNS prophylaxis:*

Methotrexate 12 mg intrathecally on Day 2

Cytarabine 100 mg intrathecally on Day 8

Repeat with each cycle of chemotherapy, depending on the risk of CNS disease. The CNS prophylaxis is given with both regimens 1 and 2.

**Additional medications with chemotherapy:**

Ondansetron injection 8 mg IV push Q 12 h
Fluconazole 400 mg po daily
Acyclovir 400 mg po Q 12 h
Prochlorperazine 10 mg IV push Q 6 h PRN
Prochlorperazine 10 mg po Q 6 h PRN
Lorazepam 0.5 mg po Q 6 h PRN

## CLINICAL COURSE

*Day 2 of induction chemotherapy:*
Blood glucose remained in the 90s with one reading at 77 early this morning. Patient denies any symptoms of hypoglycemia. Patient was started on a diabetic diet yesterday, which he has been tolerating. Given his recent weight loss, he may no longer have the same degree of insulin resistance as before. Continue to monitor BS levels. Hypoglycemic protocol is in place if patient's BS drops below 70.

*Day 3 of induction chemotherapy:*
Pt c/o mild nausea but still has good appetite and is eating well; encouraged use of PRN antiemetics. Patient tolerated intrathecal chemotherapy. No acute events overnight.

*Day 4 of induction chemotherapy:*
Patient spiked temp to 101°F. Denies any respiratory, urinary, or other symptoms. Started on cefepime 2 g IV Q 8 h and amikacin 15 mg/kg (1,300 mg based on adjusted body weight) IV Q 24 h. Serum amikacin level ordered for 10 hours postdose.

*Day 5 of induction chemotherapy:*
Patient continues to complain of nausea but has not vomited. He is able to tolerate a little solid food but reports that his appetite is not what it was. Reports two episodes of watery, nonbloody diarrhea early this morning with no further episodes since then.

*Day 6 of induction chemotherapy:*
Patient reports that his appetite is improving. He still complains of nausea, which has improved only slightly, but he has had no episodes of vomiting. No further episodes of diarrhea. No acute events overnight. Patient will receive rituximab 375 mg/m$^2$ (825 mg) IV today.

*Day 7 of induction chemotherapy:*
Patient reported chills and shaking during rituximab infusion yesterday. Acetaminophen 650 mg po and diphenhydramine 50 mg IV were given. Patient felt better after that. No further symptoms during the day. Patient's only complaint is lack of bowel movement for 2 days. He is also still nauseated but is able to tolerate a regular meal without any emesis. No acute events overnight.

*Day 8 of induction chemotherapy:*
Patient complains of severe hiccups throughout the day and night yesterday that have prevented him from sleeping. He said that he also has epigastric discomfort associated with the hiccups. He has pain in the epigastric region that he rates as 7/10 in intensity with no radiation. It is neither sharp nor dull and feels like a "knot." He also feels very full and bloated. He says it feels better when he stands up and walks around and also subsides when the hiccups cease. No further episodes of diarrhea and no vomiting. Patient still nauseated but able to tolerate meals. He had one small BM yesterday. No acute events overnight.

*Day 15 of induction chemotherapy:*
The patient was discharged to home. He was instructed to call the hematology fellow on call at any sign of a fever or infection. He was also instructed to stay away from people who have active infections, such as an upper respiratory virus. He was told to avoid large crowds and not to do any gardening. This is all to decrease the risk of infection. He will return to the hospital in 6 days for cycle 2 of chemotherapy. He is sent home with the following prescriptions:

Fluconazole 400 mg po daily
Acyclovir 400 mg po Q 12 h
Prochlorperazine 10 mg po Q 6 h PRN

## QUESTIONS

### Problem Identification

1.a. Create a list of the patient's drug therapy problems. What effect will this chemotherapy regimen have on his diabetes?

1.b. Why was the patient started on allopurinol prior to starting his chemotherapy?

### Desired Outcome

2.a. What are the short-term goals of pharmacotherapy in this patient?

2.b. The patient will receive four cycles of R-HyperCVAD alternating with four cycles of high-dose methotrexate and cytarabine. What are the long-term goals of pharmacotherapy in this patient?

### Therapeutic Alternatives

3.a. What nondrug therapies might be useful for this patient?

3.b. What other pharmacotherapeutic options are available for this patient's ALL?

### Optimal Plan

4.a. Why was the patient started on fluconazole and acyclovir in the doses prescribed?

4.b. Why was the patient started on intrathecal chemotherapy with no current evidence of CNS disease?

4.c. Outline the optimal drug therapy regimen if the initial treatment fails and the alternative therapy you described in question 3.b. is used.

### Outcome Evaluation

5. What laboratory parameters and other diagnostic tests indicate an adequate response to induction therapy?

### Patient Education

6.a. What information should be provided to the patient about the potential beneficial and adverse effects from the chemotherapy agents used during induction therapy?

6.b. Assume that the patient does not understand why he has to have so many courses of chemotherapy. Explain why he cannot be treated with just one cycle of chemotherapy.

## ■ SELF-STUDY ASSIGNMENTS

1. Discuss the value of colony-stimulating factors in the prophylaxis or treatment of therapy-related complications in patients with ALL.
2. Discuss the response criteria used to determine if a patient with ALL has obtained a complete remission or partial remission.
3. Define the terms stable disease and progressive disease as they relate to ALL.

## CLINICAL PEARL

First-line therapy for treatment of ALL must contain the backbone of an anthracycline derivative, vincristine, and a corticosteroid. Asparaginase is also a useful agent in this disease, due to the leukemic cell's unique lack of endogenous asparagine. Patients with Philadelphia chromosome–positive ALL are treated with imatinib or dasatinib *in addition* to the induction chemotherapy regimen, such as R-HyperCVAD which our patient received.

## REFERENCES


1. Kantarjian H, Thomas D, O'Brien S, et al. Long-term follow-up results of hyperfractionated cyclophosphamide, vincristine, doxorubicin, and dexamethasone (Hyper-CVAD), a dose-intensive regimen, in adult acute lymphocytic leukemia. Cancer 2004;101:2788–2801.
2. Thomas DA, Cortes J, O'Brien S, et al. Hyper-CVAD program in Burkitt's-type adult acute lymphoblastic leukemia. J Clin Oncol 1999;17:2461–2470.
3. Hughes WT, Armstrong D, Bodey GP, et al. 2002 guidelines for the use of antimicrobial agents in neutropenic patients with cancer. Clin Infect Dis 2002;34:730–751.
4. Wetzler M, Sanford BL, Kurtzberg J, et al. Effective asparagine depletion with pegylated asparaginase results in improved outcomes in adult acute lymphoblastic leukemia: Cancer and Leukemia Group B Study 9511. Blood 2007;109:4164–4167.


# 155

# CHRONIC MYELOGENOUS LEUKEMIA

Searching for Philadelphia Freedom. . . . . . . . Level II

**Christine M. Walko, PharmD, BCOP**

## LEARNING OBJECTIVES

After completing this case study, students should be able to:

- Identify the presenting signs and symptoms of chronic myelogenous leukemia (CML).
- Identify important prognostic indicators for CML.
- Construct treatment options for newly diagnosed CML and refractory or relapsed CML.
- List appropriate parameters to monitor efficacy and potential adverse effects of treatment for CML.
- Educate patients on treatment complications and the most common side effects of therapy for CML.
- Discuss potential mechanisms of resistance to first-line therapy for CML.

## PATIENT PRESENTATION

### Chief Complaint

"My stomach hurts and I've been having night sweats."

### HPI

Stacey Johnson is a 34 yo woman who complains of left-sided abdominal discomfort and fullness that has resulted in decreased appetite and an unintentional weight loss of about 20 lb over the past 3 months. She also endorses experiencing drenching night sweats for the past 2 months that have progressively gotten worse and more frequent.

### PMH

Seasonal allergies
Wisdom tooth extraction (1999)

### FH

Father is 58 yo with HTN and hypercholesterolemia. Mother is 60 yo with osteoporosis. She has no siblings. No history of cancer.

### SH

Single and works as a nurse in the recovery room at a local community hospital. She has no smoking history but drinks alcohol on social occasions. She denies any illicit drug use.

### Meds

Women's One A Day multivitamin
Loratadine 10 mg po once daily PRN during allergy seasons

### All

Sulfa (mild rash when she was a child)

### ROS

Increased weakness and tiredness. Frequent night sweats, occasional fever and chills; mild shortness of breath on exertion. Denies bleeding, headaches, nausea, vomiting, chest pain, or urinary symptoms.

### Physical Examination

*Gen*

WDWN Caucasian woman in NAD who appears her stated age

*VS*

BP 110/72, P 77, RR 14, T 36.3°C; weight 60.2 kg, Ht 158 cm

*Skin*

No evidence of rash or petechiae

*HEENT*

PERRLA, EOMI, sclerae anicteric, TMs clear. No sinus discharge or tenderness. Oropharynx was clear with trace posterior erythema without exudate. Lips, teeth, and gums were without tenderness.

*Neck*

Supple without masses. No carotid bruits auscultated. No thyromegaly appreciated.

*Lymph Nodes*

No palpable cervical, supraclavicular, axillary, or inguinal adenopathy

*Chest*

CTA bilaterally

*CV*

NSR; normal $S_1$ and $S_2$ without murmurs, rubs, or gallops

*Abd*

Soft, symmetric, and nontender. Spleen palpable 6 cm below costal margin. Normoactive bowel sounds. No hepatomegaly noted.

*Rect*

Deferred

*MS/Ext*

Normal gait, full range of motion in flexion and extension of the upper and lower extremities with 5/5 strength throughout. No joint deformities or peripheral edema. Dorsalis pedis and radial pulses are 2+ and symmetric bilaterally.

*Neuro*

CN II–XII intact; DTRs 1+ throughout; gait steady. A & O × 3.

### Labs

| | | | |
|---|---|---|---|
| Na 139 mEq/L | Hgb 11.2 g/dL | AST 24 IU/L | Ca 8.2 mg/dL |
| K 4.2 mEq/L | Hct 33.8% | ALT 38 IU/L | Mg 2.2 mEq/L |
| Cl 105 mEq/L | Plt 470 × $10^3$/mm$^3$ | Alk phos 72 IU/L | Phos 3.8 mg/dL |
| $CO_2$ 27 mEq/L | WBC 140 × $10^3$/mm$^3$ | LDH 834 IU/L | Uric acid 1.9 mg/dL |
| BUN 28 mg/dL | Segs 26% | T. bili 1.2 mg/dL | LAP absent |
| SCr 0.8 mg/dL | Bands 8% | T. prot 6.9 g/dL | |
| Glu 92 mg/dL | Lymphs 62% | Alb 2.8 g/dL | |
| Retic 2.3% | Myelos 3% | | |
| | Monos 1% | | |

### Bone Marrow Biopsy

Cytogenetic studies revealed a translocation involving the long arms of chromosomes 9 and 22 [t(9q;22q)] (Philadelphia chromosome), with 95% of malignant cells analyzed found to be Ph-positive. The marrow was hypercellular and consisted of 5% myeloblasts, but showed no other blastic abnormalities. This information is consistent with the characteristics of CML-CP.

## QUESTIONS

### Problem Identification

1.a. What information in the patient's history is consistent with a diagnosis of CML-CP? (See Fig. 155-1.)

1.b. Describe the natural progression of CML.

1.c. List factors that signal a poor prognosis for CML patients in chronic phase.

### Desired Outcome

2. What are long-term therapy goals for this patient?

### Therapeutic Alternatives

3. What nonpharmacologic and pharmacologic alternatives should be considered for this newly diagnosed patient?

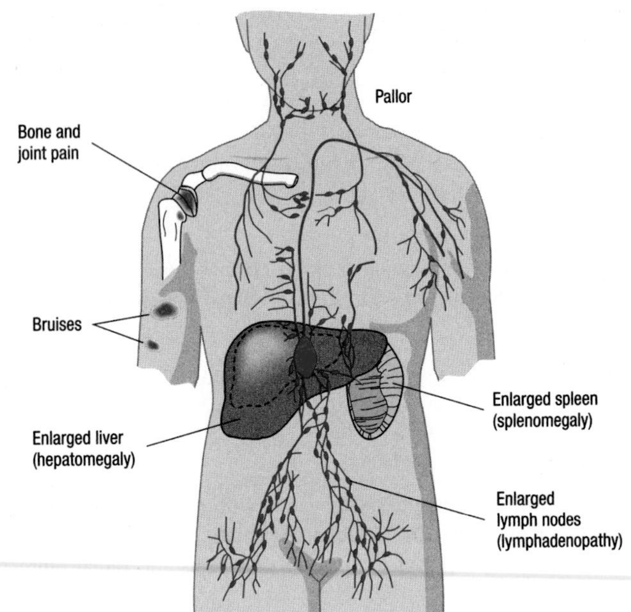


**FIGURE 155-1.** Common signs and symptoms of chronic myelogenous leukemia.

## Optimal Plan

4. Considering all patient factors, describe the optimal initial treatment plan for this patient.

## Outcome Evaluation

5. Describe parameters for monitoring disease response and toxicity for the treatment option you recommended.

## Patient Education

6. What information should be given to the patient prior to treatment?

## CLINICAL COURSE

The regimen you recommended was initiated. At the 2-week follow-up visit, the patient's WBC count was $34 \times 10^3/\text{mm}^3$. At the 4-week follow-up visit, her WBC count had decreased to $9 \times 10^3/\text{mm}^3$. After 3 months of treatment, her WBC count remained stable at $8.2 \times 10^3/\text{mm}^3$ and she had a minimal cytogenetic response as evidenced by a bone marrow biopsy that revealed 70% Philadelphia chromosome–positive metaphases. After 6 months, she remained in complete hematologic response but minor cytogenetic response with 60% positive metaphases. Molecular analysis also showed less than a major response. Because she experienced a suboptimal response, mutation testing was performed and revealed the presence of a Y253F mutation. Also, since beginning treatment with imatinib, the patient has noticed mild periorbital edema, moderate myalgias, and nausea. She presents to clinic today to discuss further treatment options with her physician.

## Follow-Up Questions

1. What are the possible mechanisms of resistance to imatinib?
2. What therapeutic options are available for this patient with a suboptimal response to imatinib 400 mg po daily?
3. Compare and contrast dasatinib and nilotinib in terms of efficacy and toxicity in patients with suboptimal responses to imatinib.
4. What assistance is available for patients receiving imatinib, dasatinib, or nilotinib to help pay for these medications?
5. How would your recommendations differ if the patient had a T315I mutation instead?

## SELF-STUDY ASSIGNMENTS

1. Describe the hematologic and cytogenetic response criteria (complete, partial, minor, and no response) for therapy in patients with CML, including WBC count, splenomegaly, and percent of Ph+ marrow cells.
2. If this patient becomes pregnant, how should her therapy be revised?
3. Discuss the progress being made to develop treatments for patients with the T315I mutation.

## CLINICAL PEARL

Mutation testing in patient with chronic phase CML is generally not performed unless the patient has a suboptimal or lack of response to imatinib because mutations can occasionally be found in patients without resistant disease.

## REFERENCES

1. Baccarani M, Cortes J, Pane F, et al. Chronic myeloid leukemia: an update of concepts and management recommendations of European LeukemiaNet. J Clin Oncol 2009;27:6041–6051.
2. Savage DG, Antman KH. Imatinib—a new oral targeted therapy. N Engl J Med 2002;346:683–693.
3. O'Brien SG, Guilhot F, Larson RA, et al, IRIS Investigators. Imatinib compared with interferon and low-dose cytarabine for newly diagnosed chronic-phase chronic myeloid leukemia. N Engl J Med 2003;348:994–1004.
4. Druker B, Guilhot F, O'Brien SG, et al. Five-year follow-up of patients receiving imatinib for chronic myeloid leukemia. N Engl J Med 2006;355:2408–2417.
5. O'Brien SG, Guilhot F, Goldman J, et al. International randomized study of interferon versus STI571 (IRIS) 7-year follow-up: sustained survival, low rate of transformation and increased rate of major molecular response in patients with newly diagnosed chronic myeloid leukemia in chronic phase treated with imatinib. Blood 2008;112:76 [abstract 186].
6. Devergie A, Apperley JF, Labopin M, et al. European results of matched unrelated donor bone marrow transplantation for chronic myeloid leukemia. Impact of HLA class II matching. Bone Marrow Transplant 1997;20:11–19.
7. Deininger MW, O'Brien SG, Ford JM, et al. Practical management of patients with chronic myeloid leukemia receiving imatinib. J Clin Oncol 2003;21:1637–1647.
8. Druker BJ. Translation of the Philadelphia chromosome into therapy for CML. Blood 2008;112:4808–4817.
9. O'Hare T, Eide CA, Deininger MWN. BCR-ABL kinase domain mutations, drug resistance, and the road to a cure for chronic myeloid leukemia. Blood 2007;110:2242–2249.
10. Talpaz M, Shah NP, Kantarjian H, et al. Dasatinib in imatinib-resistant Philadelphia chromosome-positive leukemias. N Engl J Med 2006;354:2531–2541.
11. Hochhaus A, Baccarini M, Deininger M, et al. Dasatinib induces durable cytogenetic responses in patients with chronic myelogenous leukemia in chronic phase with resistance or intolerance to imatinib. Leukemia 2008;22:1200–1206.
12. Kantarjian H, Giles F, Wunderle L, et al. Nilotinib in imatinib-resistant CML and Philadelphia chromosome-positive ALL. N Engl J Med 2006;354:2542–2551.

# 156

# RENAL CELL CARCINOMA

Molecular Therapies. . . . . . . . . . . . . . . . . . . . Level II

**Michael Newton, PharmD, BCOP**

## LEARNING OBJECTIVES

After completing this case study, students should be able to:

- Describe pharmacotherapeutic options for patients with metastatic renal cell carcinoma (RCC).
- Identify and monitor for toxicities associated with targeted therapies for metastatic RCC.
- Recommend alternative agents for patients who progress on first-line treatment for RCC.
- Provide detailed patient education for targeted treatments used in RCC.

## PATIENT PRESENTATION

### Chief Complaint

"What treatment options do I have?"

### HPI

Tracy DeWitt is a 65-year-old woman who presented 3.5 months ago to her primary care physician with complaints of back pain, cough, and weight loss. She did not respond to an initial course of antibiotics for an assumed pyelonephritis and developed gross hematuria a few days later. She was subsequently referred to a urologist, who detected a mass on renal ultrasound. CT scan of chest, abdomen, and pelvis revealed a 7-cm left upper-pole kidney tumor, and several bilateral lung nodules. She was referred to a nearby cancer center for further evaluation. A core needle biopsy of the kidney mass revealed neoplastic cells, but the sample was too small and heterogeneous to definitively determine a specific histology. In order to relieve worsening symptoms and further elucidate a specific histopathology of the mass, a nephrectomy of the involved left kidney was performed. Pathologic examination revealed clear cell kidney cancer. The patient has recovered from surgery with resolution of back pain and hematuria. Now, 6 weeks after surgery, the patient presents to the medical oncology clinic. A postsurgical CT scan reveals persistent lung metastases, unchanged in number or size. She is interested in pursuing systemic treatment of her metastatic renal carcinoma and would like to know what options she has.

### PMH

Hypertension
Dyslipidemia

### FH

Mother died at age 75 due to complications related to MI. Father died at age 73 due to PE. One brother, age 48, with asthma is alive and otherwise healthy. No family history of cancer.

### SH

Patient is married with one grown son, age 33, who is alive and healthy. Patient reports extensive smoking history (25 pack-years) but quit 5 years ago. She is slightly overweight.

### Meds

Hydrochlorothiazide 25 mg po once daily
Enalapril 5 mg po once daily
Atorvastatin 10 mg po once daily

### All

NKDA

### ROS

No fever or chills; no headaches; no nausea or vomiting; feels very weak since the surgery

### Physical Examination

*Gen*

WDWN Caucasian female in NAD

*VS*

BP 130/84, P 64, RR 18, T 37.0°C; Wt 82.4 kg, Ht 5′6″, BSA 1.96 $m^2$

*Skin*

Olive complexion. Nephrectomy site is fully healed.

*HEENT*

PERRLA, EOMI; oropharynx without lesions

*Neck/Lymph Nodes*

Supple without adenopathy; thyroid without masses

*Lung/Thorax*

Slight wheezing in LUL

*CV*

RRR; normal $S_1$ and $S_2$; no MRG

*Abd*

Soft, NT/ND; (+) BS

*Genit/Rect*

Deferred

*Ext*

No clubbing, cyanosis, or edema

*Neuro*

A & O × 3; CN II–XII intact; DTRs 2+ throughout; motor and sensory levels intact; Babinski (–)

### Labs

| | | | |
|---|---|---|---|
| Na 137 mEq/L | Hgb 12 g/dL | WBC 6.1 × $10^6$/mm$^3$ | T. bili 0.8 mg/dL |
| K 4.0 mEq/L | Hct 36% | Neutros 66% | AST 25 IU/L |
| Cl 99 mEq/L | Plt 325 × $10^3$/mm$^3$ | Bands 4% | ALT 27 IU/L |
| $CO_2$ 25 mEq/L | | Lymphs 26% | Alk phos 125 IU/L |
| BUN 20 mg/dL | | Monos 4% | Alb 3.8 g/dL |
| SCr 2.0 mg/dL | | | LDH 220 IU/L |
| Glu 75 mg/dL | | | Ca 8.5 mg/dL |
| | | | Mg 2.0mg/dL |

### Assessment

A 65-year-old woman with metastatic RCC, S/P resection of primary tumor via nephrectomy. Metastatic lesions in lung persist.

## CLINICAL COURSE

The patient underwent screening for high-dose interleukin-2 (aldesleukin) but was determined to be a poor candidate due to inadequate results of pulmonary function testing (both FVC and $FEV_1$ were <65% of predicted values). She is interested in hearing about other available options.

# QUESTIONS

### Problem Identification

1. What information (signs, symptoms, laboratory values) indicates the presence or severity of RCC?

### Desired Outcome

2. What are the goals of pharmacotherapy in this case?

### Therapeutic Alternatives

3. What feasible antineoplastic options are available for treatment in this case, since aldesleukin is not an option?

### Optimal Plan

4. What drug, dosage form, dose, schedule, and duration of therapy are best for this patient?

### Outcome Evaluation

5. What clinical and laboratory parameters are necessary to evaluate the therapy for achievement of the desired therapeutic outcome and to detect or prevent adverse effects?

### Patient Education

6. What information would you provide to the patient before initiation of treatment?

## ■ CLINICAL COURSE

Mrs DeWitt was started on the treatment you recommended and achieved partial regression of some of her metastatic lesions. She has experienced adverse effects including hypertension (maximum BP was 160/95), hand–foot syndrome, a slight yellowing of her skin, hair depigmentation, and peripheral edema. Hypertension was controlled by increasing her enalapril dosage to 10 mg per day. Unfortunately after 9 months of treatment, today's follow-up CT scan indicates progression of the cancer. The patient expressed a desire to continue treatment with a second-line treatment option.

### Follow-Up Questions

1. Given this situation, what pharmacotherapy regimen would you recommend for the patient? Provide the rationale for your answer.
2. How would you monitor for the potential adverse effects of the treatment you recommended?
3. What education should the patient receive about this new medication?
4. How would you manage this patient's antineoplastic therapy if she were receiving a strong inducer of hepatic CYP3A4 enzymes? What about a strong inhibitor of CYP3A4?

## ■ SELF-STUDY ASSIGNMENTS

1. Discuss the role of high-dose aldesleukin in metastatic RCC.
2. What role, if any, does adjuvant treatment play after surgery for localized RCC?
3. What role does tumor histology play in treatment selection for metastatic RCC?

## CLINICAL PEARL

Until recently, advanced RCC had few effective treatments available. Cytokine therapy with interferon or interleukin is difficult to tolerate and yields mostly disappointing results. Although high-dose interleukin-2 provides a small possibility of prolonged remissions in those who achieve a complete response, many patients are not candidates to receive it. An understanding of the molecular mechanisms in the pathogenesis of RCC has led to a new approach to treatment and a number of available options.

## REFERENCES

1. Hudes G, Carducci M, Tomczak P, et al. Temsirolimus, interferon alfa, or both for advanced renal-cell carcinoma. N Engl J Med 2007;356:2271–2281.
2. Motzer RJ, Hutson TE, Tomczak P, et al. Sunitinib versus interferon alfa in metastatic renal-cell carcinoma. N Engl J Med 2007;356:115–124.
3. Motzer RJ, Hutson TE, Tomczak P, et al. Overall survival and updated results for sunitinib compared with interferon alfa in patients with metastatic renal cell carcinoma. J Clin Oncol 2009;27:3584–3590.
4. Sternberg CN, Davis ID, Mardiak J, et al. Pazopanib in locally advanced or metastatic renal cell carcinoma: results of a randomized phase III trial. J Clin Oncol 2010;28:1061–1068.
5. Rini BI, Halabi S, Rosenberg JE, et al. Bevacizumab plus interferon alfa compared with interferon alfa monotherapy in patients with metastatic renal cell carcinoma: CALGB 90206. J Clin Oncol 2008;26:5422–5428.
6. Escudier B, Szczylik C, Hutson TE, et al. Randomized phase II trial of first-line treatment with sorafenib versus interferon alfa-2a in patients with metastatic renal cell carcinoma. J Clin Oncol 2009;27:1280–1289.
7. NCCN Kidney Cancer Guidelines v.2.2010. Available at: *www.nccn.org*. Accessed April 1, 2010.
8. Motzer RJ, Escudier B, Oudard S, et al. Efficacy of everolimus in advanced renal cell carcinoma: a double-blind, randomized, placebo-controlled phase III trial. Lancet 2008;372:449–456.

# 157

# MELANOMA

You Have Been Exposed . . . . . . . . . . . . . . . . . Level II

**J. Michael Vozniak, PharmD, BCOP**

## LEARNING OBJECTIVES

After completing this case study, the reader should be able to:

- Identify risk factors for developing melanoma.
- Determine chemotherapeutic treatment options for metastatic melanoma.

- Prepare educational information to provide to a patient receiving treatment for metastatic melanoma.
- Discuss ways to prevent melanoma.

## PATIENT PRESENTATION

### Chief Complaint

"I have been getting short of breath walking to work lately."

### HPI

Bobby Chipego is a 52-year-old Caucasian man who presents with increasing shortness of breath and dyspnea on exertion. He denies chest pain and hemoptysis. He reports that he could not walk more than one block without having to stop to catch his breath today. He normally walks 10 blocks to and from work each day and has noted progressive shortness of breath each week for the past 2–4 weeks. He has a history of a left lower leg thrombosis diagnosed 2 months ago after returning home from a trip to Australia. He also has a history of Stage IIA melanoma (T3a, N0, M0) diagnosed 4 years ago.

### PMH

GERD
Type 2 DM
DVT of the LLE, diagnosed 2 months ago
Melanoma (Stage IIA, superficial spreading); diagnosed 4 years ago; left lower back—s/p wide surgical excision—no sentinel lymph node biopsy performed

### FH

Patient is oldest of three children; he has two sisters, both alive; one with type 2 diabetes mellitus. Mother is age 74 with a history of basal cell carcinoma and melanoma skin cancers and heart disease. Father deceased at age 71 secondary to pneumonia.

### SH

The patient is employed as an architect and is married with one daughter (age 17). He has a history of smoking cigarettes, 0.5 pack per day for 4 years in college. He is a social drinker and reports no illicit drug use.

### Meds

Lansoprazole 30 mg po once daily
Glipizide 10 mg po once daily
Metformin 1,000 mg po twice daily
Enoxaparin 150 mg subcutaneously once daily

### All

NKDA

### ROS

Denies fever, chills, rigors, and chest pain; (+) shortness of breath and DOE

### Physical Examination

*Gen*

Slightly overweight Caucasian man in mild respiratory distress

*VS*

BP 129/72, P 92, RR 22, T 37.8°C; Wt 102.2 kg, Ht 5′10″

*Skin*

Fair skin, multiple scattered dysplastic nevi covering trunk and torso; left lower back melanoma excision site noted, which is well healed. Small bruises on abdomen and upper thighs related to enoxaparin injection sites.

*HEENT*

PERRLA, EOMI; normal sclera; clear oropharynx

*Neck/Lymph Nodes*

Supple; no lymphadenopathy or masses

*Lung/Thorax*

Decreased breath sounds in the left lower base

*CV*

RRR; no MRG

*Abd*

NTND; (+) BS

*Genit/Rect*

Deferred

*MS/Ext*

Normal ROM and sensation; LLE slightly larger than RLE

*Neuro*

A & O × 3; normal cranial nerves; normal reflexes and sensation

### Labs

| | | | |
|---|---|---|---|
| Na 135 mEq/L | Hgb 15.8 g/dL | WBC 5.6 × $10^6$/mm$^3$ | T. bili 1.1 mg/dL |
| K 4.1 mEq/L | Hct 46% | Neutros 68% | AST 22 IU/L |
| Cl 100 mEq/L | RBC 5.2 × $10^6$/mm$^3$ | Bands 3% | ALT 28 IU/L |
| $CO_2$ 25 mEq/L | Plt 322 × $10^3$/mm$^3$ | Eos 1% | Alk phos 165 IU/L |
| BUN 9 mg/dL | | Lymphs 26% | Alb 4.2 g/dL |
| SCr 1.0 mg/dL | | Monos 2% | LDH 187 IU/L |
| Glu 75 mg/dL | | | Ca 8.5 mg/dL |
| | | | Mg 2.1 mg/dL |
| | | | $PO_4$ 3.6 mg/dL |

### CT Chest

No pulmonary emboli. Two nodules consistent with metastasis found in the left lower lung; a small- to moderate-sized pleural effusion is also seen in the left lower lung.

### CT Abdomen

Solitary lesion consistent with metastasis seen in the right lobe of the liver

### CT-Guided Lung Biopsy

Tissue taken from left lower lobe is consistent with metastasis from melanoma.

### Assessment

A 52-year old man with recurrent melanoma metastatic to the liver and lungs with shortness of breath and dyspnea on exertion related to his metastatic disease and requires treatment of his disease

# QUESTIONS

## Problem Identification

1.a. Create a list of the patient's drug therapy problems.

1.b. What information (signs, symptoms, laboratory values) indicates the presence or severity of melanoma?

1.c. What risk factor(s) does this patient have for developing melanoma?

## Desired Outcome

2. What are the goals for treatment of melanoma in this patient?

## Therapeutic Alternatives

3.a. What chemotherapeutic regimens are feasible options for this patient?

3.b. What nondrug therapies might be useful for this patient?

## Optimal Plan

4.a. What chemotherapeutic regimen do you suggest for treating this patient's metastatic melanoma?

4.b. Calculate the patient's BSA and the dosage of each drug to be administered.

## Outcome Evaluation

5. What clinical and laboratory parameters are necessary to evaluate the therapy for achievement of the desired therapeutic outcome and to detect or prevent adverse effects?

## Patient Education

6. What information would you provide to the patient about the agent(s) used to treat his metastatic melanoma?

## ADDITIONAL CASE QUESTION

1. Mr Chipego's daughter is concerned that she is at risk for developing melanoma. How can melanoma be prevented?

## SELF-STUDY ASSIGNMENTS

1. Design an antiemetic regimen for the chemotherapeutic regimen you selected.
2. How would you manage this patient's anticoagulation if he were to become thrombocytopenic from his chemotherapy treatment?
3. How long does he need to be anticoagulated for his DVT?
4. What is the ABCD rule in helping to distinguish features of a normal mole from an abnormal mole?

## CLINICAL PEARL

Measurement of serum LDH at the time of Stage IV diagnosis is important in determining prognosis. The 1-year overall survival rate for Stage IV patients with a normal LDH is 65% compared to only 32% in patients with an elevated LDH.

## REFERENCES

1. Balch CM, Gershenwald JE, Soong S, et al. Final version of 2009 AJCC melanoma staging and classification. J Clin Oncol 2009;27:6199–6206.
2. NCCN Melanoma Guidelines v.1.2010. Available at: *www.nccn.org*. Accessed February 21, 2010.
3. Middleton MR, Grob JJ, Aaronson N, et al. Randomized phase III study of temozolomide versus dacarbazine in the treatment of patients with advanced metastatic malignant melanoma. J Clin Oncol 2000;18: 158–166.
4. Serrone L, Zeuli M, Sega FM, Cognetti F. Dacarbazine-based chemotherapy for metastatic melanoma: thirty-year experience overview. J Exp Clin Cancer Res 2000;19:21–34.
5. Atkins MB, Kunkel L, Sznol M, et al. High-dose recombinant interleukin-2 therapy in patients with metastatic melanoma: long-term survival update. Cancer J Sci Am 2000;6(Suppl 1):S11–S14.
6. Atikns MB, Hsu J, Lee S, et al. Phase III trial comparing concurrent biochemotherapy with cisplatin, vinblastine, dacarbazine, interleukin-2, and interferon alfa-2b with cisplatin, vinblastine, and dacarbazine alone in patients with metastatic malignant melanoma (E3695): a trial coordinated by the Eastern Cooperative Oncology Group. J Clin Oncol 2008;26:5748–5754.
7. American Cancer Society. Detailed Guide: Skin Cancer—Melanoma. Available at: *http://www.cancer.org/docroot/CRI/CRI_2_3x.asp?dt=39*. Accessed May 2, 2010.

# 158

# HEMATOPOIETIC STEM CELL TRANSPLANTATION

A T-Cell Firefight. . . . . . . . . . . . . . . . . . . . . . . . Level III

**Patrick J. Kiel, PharmD, BCPS, BCOP**

## LEARNING OBJECTIVES

After completing this case study, students should be able to:

- Understand the regimen-related toxicities of conditioning chemotherapy used for allogeneic stem cell transplantation (SCT).
- Differentiate the presenting features of graft-versus-host disease (GVHD).
- Design appropriate pharmacotherapeutic regimens for patients who are critically ill during the peritransplant period.

## PATIENT PRESENTATION

### Chief Complaint

The patient developed progressive diarrhea complicated by abdominal cramping and persistent nausea on day +22. The patient had grade II mucositis that was managed with parenteral opioids. The patient was also febrile.

### HPI

Jerome O'Byrne is a 33-year-old man who was admitted 27 days ago for an HLA-matched related donor allogeneic marrow transplant for AML. A triple-lumen central venous catheter had been placed prior to this admission. His transplant preparative regimen consisted of total body irradiation 125 cGy per fraction for 11 fractions over 4 days and high-dose cyclophosphamide (60 mg/kg per day) × 2 days. He was supported with aggressive antiemetics, including scheduled doses of a 5-$HT_3$ antagonist with each day of chemotherapy, and dexamethasone for the 2 days of cyclophosphamide. His GVHD prophylaxis consisted of tacrolimus (0.02 mg/kg per day) IV continuous infusion starting on day –3 and a loading dose of sirolimus 12 mg po on day –3 followed by 4 mg po daily. His course has been unremarkable with the exception of grade II mucositis for which he was initiated on a hydromorphone IV infusion and PCA for pain control, elevated liver function tests, and a fever spike on day +5 that prompted the initiation of broad-spectrum antibacterials with cefepime and vancomycin. The patient had already been receiving anti-infective prophylaxis with oral ciprofloxacin (which was discontinued after vancomycin and cefepime were started), fluconazole, and acyclovir.

The patient began to demonstrate signs of engraftment on day +19 when the WBC increased to 0.3 × $10^3$ from <0.2 × $10^3$/$mm^3$ the preceding day. On day +22 the patient's intake and output were negative due to 4 L of diarrhea. The WBC had further increased to 1.1 × $10^3$/$mm^3$ with a differential of 59% polys, 15% bands, and 26% monocytes. As the day progressed, the patient became more nauseated with increased diarrhea. This occurred despite lowering of the hydromorphone PCA from settings the previous day of 0.8 mg/h IV and 0.5 mg IV Q 10 minutes with no lockout to 0.5 mg/h IV and 0.3 mg IV Q 10 minutes with a 4-hour lockout of 5.6 mg. After obtaining stool cultures, a GI Service consult recommended a colonoscopy and an EGD with biopsy.

## PMH

MDS that progressed to AML diagnosed 10 months prior to transplant that was initially treated with induction chemotherapy consisting of cytarabine and daunorubicin (the "7 + 3" regimen). The patient achieved remission, and it was decided that the best course of action was to proceed to an allogeneic SCT on the basis of his poor risk of previous MDS. The patient tolerated the induction chemotherapy with the exception of a *Streptococcus mitis* bacteremia.

## FH

Married with two children. Father is deceased from pulmonary disease.

## Meds (at Day +22)

Fluconazole 400 mg IV daily
Esomeprazole 40 mg IV Q 12 h
Hydromorphone infusion 0.5 mg/h IV with PCA 0.3 mg IV Q 10 minutes; 4-hour lockout of 5.6 mg
Cefepime 2 g IV Q 8 h
Vancomycin 1,000 mg IV Q 12 h
Tacrolimus 0.8 mg per day IV continuous infusion
Chlorhexidine gluconate 0.12% 15 mL swish/spit QID
Acyclovir 375 mg IV Q 12 h
Filgrastim 480 mcg SC daily
Insulin coverage scale
Prochlorperazine 10 mg IV Q 8 h
Sirolimus 2 mg po once daily
D5W + 150 mEq sodium bicarbonate at 125 mL/h
Lorazepam 1 mg IV Q 4 h PRN nausea

## All

Sulfa → rash

## ROS

Progressive abdominal pain, persistent nausea, increasing diarrhea output of 4 L per day

## Physical Examination

*Gen*

Patient is a WDWN Caucasian male.

*VS*

BP 130/82, P 92, T 38.1°C, $O_2$ sat 99% in room air; Wt 75 kg (admission wt 72 kg); Ht 5′10″

*HEENT*

Maculopapular rash on face; grade II oral/esophageal mucositis

*Skin*

Dry; limited rash on face and shoulders

*Neck/Lymph Nodes*

Supple; no thyromegaly

*Lungs*

Clear without wheezes, rhonchi, or crackles

*Heart*

RRR; normal heart sounds; no M/R/G

*Abd*

Slight distention, RUQ tenderness, mild hepatomegaly

*Ext*

Grade I–II edema in LE bilaterally

*Neuro*

A & O × 3

## Labs

| | | |
|---|---|---|
| Na 132 mEq/L | Hgb 8.3 g/dL | AST 55 IU/L |
| K 3.3 mEq/L | Hct 28% | ALT 61 IU/L |
| CL 112 mEq/L | Plt 11 × $10^3$/$mm^3$ | Alk phos 222 IU/L |
| $CO_2$ 18 mEq/L | WBC 1.1 × $10^3$/$mm^3$ | LDH 70 IU/L |
| BUN 22 mg/dL | | T. bili 1.2 mg/dL |
| SCr 0.9 mg/dL | | D. bili 0.4 mg/dL |
| Glu 125 mg/dL | | Alb 2.1 g/dL |

## Blood Cultures

NGTD from day +15 (2/2 containers)

## Other Cultures

All other culture sites (urine, sputum, central venous catheter) are negative.

## Assessment

New-onset abdominal pain, worsening diarrhea, and progressive nausea

# QUESTIONS

## Problem Identification

1.a. What are the likely causes for the patient's worsening diarrhea?

1.b. What are potential causes for development of a skin rash in this patient?

1.c. What are the potential causes of infection in this patient?

**TABLE 158-1 Clinical Grading of Acute Graft-Versus-Host Disease (GVHD)**

| | Skin | Liver | GI Tract |
|---|---|---|---|
| **Symptom stage** | | | |
| Stage 1 | Rash on <25% of skin | Bilirubin 2–3 mg/dL | Diarrhea 500 mL/day or positive biopsy |
| Stage 2 | Rash on 25–50% of skin | Bilirubin >3–6 mg/dL | Diarrhea >1,000 mL/day |
| Stage 3 | Rash on >50% of skin | Bilirubin >6–15 mg/dL | Diarrhea >1,500 mL/day |
| Stage 4 | Generalized erythoderma with bulla formation | Bilirubin >15 mg/dL | Severe abdominal pain with or without ileus |
| **Clinical grade** | | | |
| Grade I | Stage 1–2 | None | None |
| Grade II | Stage 1–3 | Stage 1 | Stage 1 |
| Grade III | Stage 2–3 | Stage 2–3 | Stage 2–3 |
| Grade IV | Stage 2–4 | Stage 2–4 | Stage 2–4 |

## Desired Outcome

2. What are the therapeutic goals in this patient?

## Therapeutic Alternatives

3. What treatment options exist for managing the patient's gastrointestinal disturbance? Outline a treatment plan.

## Optimal Plan

4.a. Outline changes that should be made to the patient's antibiotic regimen.

4.b. What pharmacotherapeutic intervention can be implemented to treat this patient's acute GVHD?

4.c. What drug therapies could be initiated as supportive management for the patient's diarrhea?

## Outcome Evaluation

5. What parameters should you monitor to assess the response to therapy and to detect adverse effects?

## Patient Education

6. What appropriate counseling measures should be used for the patient's family and caregivers?

## ■ CLINICAL COURSE

The antibiotic regimen modifications were implemented as per discussion with pharmacy. The patient underwent a colonoscopy and EGD, and the biopsy revealed: (a) duodenal and sigmoid biopsy with marked apoptotic activity and focal confluent crypt loss, consistent with pathology grade III acute GVHD; (b) stomach biopsy with gastric mucosa with increased apoptotic activity and focal areas of confluent crypt loss; (c) esophagus biopsy with squamous mucosa with scattered basal apoptosis and a mild mixed inflammatory infiltrate, consistent with GVHD. The patient was diagnosed with clinical grade III acute GVHD (Table 158-1). The patient was subsequently started on high-dose corticosteroids with methylprednisolone 75 mg IV BID at 9:00 AM and 2:00 PM and budesonide 9 mg po daily. The dermatology resident was called to obtain a biopsy of the mild red blanching rash on the patient's back. Over the next 48 hours, the patient had an increase in bloody diarrhea to 5.4 L per day. At this time, the patient continued to engraft with the WBC increasing to $3.2 \times 10^3/mm^3$ with an ANC of $1.2 \times 10^3/mm^3$; other labs included Hgb 9.1 g/dL and platelet count $37 \times 10^3/mm^3$, both of which resulted from transfusion. Chemistries were remarkable for BUN 5 mg/dL, SCr 0.6 mg/dL, T. bili 1.5 mg/dL, AST 32 IU/L, ALT 16 IU/L, LDH 138 IU/L, and alk phos 142 IU/L. Bacterial blood cultures have remained negative, and plasma PCR for CMV was <100 copies (negative). The skin biopsy report from dermatopathology came back as grade II GVHD. The patient became afebrile after initiation of methylprednisolone and the patient's abdominal cramping resolved with a decrease to 1 L of nonbloody diarrhea by day +31.

## Follow-Up Questions

1. If the patient fails first-line treatment for GVHD, what further treatment options exist?
2. What are potential antifungal prophylactic options in patients with acute GVHD receiving high-dose corticosteroids?

## ■ SELF-STUDY ASSIGNMENTS

1. What diseases are amenable to treatment with allogeneic SCT?
2. Aside from the complications reviewed in this case, derive a list of potential problems that could occur after allogeneic marrow transplantation.

## CLINICAL PEARL

Allogeneic SCT is often associated with multiple medical conditions and drug interactions requiring careful evaluation to prevent further toxicity.

## REFERENCES


1. Ferrara JL, Levy R, Chao NJ. Pathophysiologic mechanisms of acute graft-vs.-host disease. Biol Blood Marrow Transplant 1999;5:347–356.
2. Przepiorka D, Smith TL, Folloder J, et al. Risk factors for acute graft-versus-host disease after allogeneic blood stem cell transplantation. Blood 1999;94:1465–1470.
3. Tomblyn M, Chiller T, Einsele H, et al. Guidelines for preventing infectious complications among hematopoietic cell transplantation recipients: a global perspective. Biol Blood Marrow Transplant 2009;15:1143–1238.
4. Hughes WT, Armstrong D, Bodey GP, et al. 2002 guidelines for the use of antimicrobial agents in neutropenic patients with cancer. Clin Infect Dis 2002;34:730–751.

5. Ullmann AJ, Lipton JH, Vesole DH, et al. Posaconazole or fluconazole for prophylaxis in severe graft-versus-host disease. N Engl J Med 2007;356:335–347.
6. Marty FM, Lowry CM, Cutler CS, et al. Voriconazole and sirolimus coadministration after allogeneic hematopoietic stem cell transplantation. Biol Blood Marrow Transplant 2006;12:552–559.
7. Lazarus HM, Vogelsang GB, Rowe JM. Prevention and treatment of acute graft-versus-host disease: the old and the new—a report from the Eastern Cooperative Oncology Group (ECOG). Bone Marrow Transplant 1997;19:577–600.
8. Bertz H, Afting M, Kreisel W, Duffner U, Greinwald R, Finke J. Feasibility and response to budesonide as topical corticosteroid therapy for acute intestinal GVHD. Bone Marrow Transplant 1999; 24:1185–1189.
9. Copelan EA. Hematopoietic stem-cell transplantation. N Engl J Med 2006;354:1813–1826.
10. Kim SS. Treatment options in steroid-refractory acute graft-versus-host disease following hematopoietic stem cell transplantation. Ann Pharmacother 2007;41:1436–1444.

SECTION 18
# NUTRITION AND NUTRITIONAL DISORDERS

## 159

## PARENTERAL NUTRITION

Getting Past the Obstruction . . . . . . . . . . . . . . Level III

Michael D. Kraft, PharmD, BCNSP

Melissa Pleva, PharmD, BCPS, BCNSP

## LEARNING OBJECTIVES

After completing this case study, students should be able to:

- Describe how bowel obstruction can lead to nutritional, fluid, and electrolyte abnormalities.
- Characterize the severity of malnutrition based on subjective and objective patient data.
- Identify potential complications related to parenteral nutrition (PN) in patients with malnutrition (e.g., refeeding syndrome) and steps to avoid or manage such complications.
- Design a patient-specific PN prescription that is based on the nutritional diagnosis and other subjective and objective patient data.
- Construct and evaluate appropriate monitoring parameters for a hospitalized patient receiving PN.

## PATIENT PRESENTATION

### Chief Complaint

"My stomach hurts and I can't keep down any food or water."

### HPI

Steven Brown is a 49-year-old man familiar to the GI Surgery Service with a history of a ventral hernia, hypertension, dyslipidemia, and type 2 DM. He presented to the ED earlier today with abdominal pain, nausea, vomiting, and inability to tolerate PO intake. Approximately 2 months ago he underwent an exploratory laparotomy with small bowel resection and primary anastomosis for repair of a ventral hernia with incarcerated small bowel. His postoperative course was complicated by an anastomotic leak, peritonitis, and sepsis, and he was ultimately discharged to home after a 3-week hospital stay. For the past 4 days, he has had worsening abdominal pain and has been unable to tolerate any PO intake. His last bowel movement was 6 days ago. He has lost ~25 lb (~11 kg) from his weight prior to his surgery 2 months ago. This weight loss includes ~14 lb (~6.5 kg) since his prior discharge due to poor appetite and limited PO intake at home.

The surgical team decides to admit Mr Brown to the hospital. On admission, they obtain an abdominal CT scan, which demonstrates dilated loops of small bowel consistent with an SBO and negative for anastomotic leak or abscess. The team believes this SBO is likely due to adhesions from his prior surgery.

### PMH

Ventral hernia
Hypertension
Dyslipidemia
Type 2 DM

### PSH

Exploratory laparotomy, small bowel resection with primary anastomosis for repair of ventral hernia with incarcerated small bowel 2 months ago

### FH

Remarkable for DM in his mother, HTN and CAD in his father

### SH

Married, lives with his wife; construction worker. Drinks two to three alcoholic beverages per week; quit smoking 2 years ago, 25 pack-year history prior to quitting.

### ROS

Reports feeling thirsty, no appetite. Complains of moderate abdominal pain, nausea, and vomiting. Also complains his abdomen feels "crampy" and is very bloated. Complains of not passing flatus or having a bowel movement in 6 days; urinating infrequently over the last 2 days, and urine is dark and concentrated. Feels lightheaded and dizzy if he stands up quickly. Denies chills, fevers, or other pain.

### Meds Prior to Admission

Simvastatin 40 mg po at bedtime
Hydrochlorothiazide 25 mg po daily
Metoprolol 25 mg po twice daily
Glyburide/metformin 10 mg/1,000 mg po twice daily with meals

### All

NKDA

### Physical Examination

*Gen*

African-American man, uncomfortable because of abdominal pain, appears malnourished

*VS*

BP 96/60, P 108, RR 18, T 37.7°C; Wt 71 kg (wt prior to surgery 2 months ago ~83 kg), Ht 71 in (180 cm)

*Skin*

Dry, flaking in some spots, poor turgor

*HEENT*

PERRLA, EOMI, anicteric sclerae, normal conjunctivae, mouth is dry, pharynx is clear, some evidence of wasting noted on temporal lobes, eyes appear sunken in, orbital ridge protruding somewhat.

*Lungs/Thorax*

CTA and percussion bilaterally; bilateral protruding scapulae

*CV*

RRR, no murmurs

*Abd*

Distended; hypoactive (nearly absent) bowel sounds; diffuse tenderness throughout all four quadrants

*Genit/Rect*

No lesions, no internal masses

*MS/Ext*

(–) Cyanosis, (–) edema, 2+ dorsalis pedis and posterior tibial pulses bilaterally, some evidence of wasting in large muscle groups (biceps, triceps, and quadriceps)

*Neuro*

A & O × 3; CN II–XII intact; motor 5/5 upper and lower extremity bilaterally; sensation intact and reflexes symmetric with downgoing toes

### Labs on Admission

| | | | |
|---|---|---|---|
| Na 132 mEq/L | Hgb 12.1 g/dL | AST 24 IU/L | Ca 8.2 mg/dL |
| K 3.3 mEq/L | Hct 35.9% | ALT 21 IU/L | Mg 1.4 mEq/dL |
| Cl 94 mEq/L | Plt 334 × $10^3$/mm$^3$ | Alk phos 41 IU/L | Phos 2.6 mg/dL |
| $CO_2$ 34 mEq/L | WBC 7.5 × $10^3$/mm$^3$ | GGT 45 IU/L | PT 12.3 s |
| BUN 17 mg/dL | | T. bili 0.9 mg/dL | INR 0.8 |
| SCr 0.5 mg/dL | | T. prot 4.9 g/dL | |
| Glu 142 mg/dL | | Alb 2.9 g/dL | |

### Radiology

A CT scan with contrast demonstrates dilated loops of small bowel consistent with SBO; negative for anastomotic leak; negative for abscess.

### Assessment

This is a 49-year-old man with a history of a ventral hernia, hypertension, dyslipidemia and type 2 DM, S/P exploratory laparotomy, small bowel resection with primary anastomosis, and repair of incarcerated ventral hernia 2 months ago, who is admitted with abdominal pain, nausea, vomiting, and inability to tolerate PO intake. His symptoms and CT scan are consistent with SBO. His history and physical exam also demonstrate evidence of malnutrition.

## CLINICAL COURSE

Given that he has had recent abdominal surgery, as well as significant weight loss and evidence of malnutrition, the surgical team elects to manage his SBO conservatively (nonoperatively). Because of recent abdominal surgery, the team would like to avoid reentering the abdomen for surgical intervention at this time (the patient is likely to still have inflammation and adhesions from his prior operation, and additional surgical intervention can further increase inflammation and risk of complications [e.g., adhesions, fistula]). The patient is made NPO, and home PO medications are held for now. An NG tube is placed for gastric decompression, and a PICC is inserted for administration of PN and IV fluids. The team gives the patient a 1,000-mL IV fluid bolus with normal saline followed by normal saline at 100 mL/h. Once PN is initiated and the patient has been resuscitated, IV fluids will be decreased to maintain a total fluid intake of 100 mL/h. The surgical team obtains nutrition and pharmacy consults for PN recommendations.

## QUESTIONS

### Problem Identification

1.a. What clinical and laboratory data indicate the presence of malnutrition in this patient? Characterize the type and severity of malnutrition, and describe why he is at risk for further nutritional abnormalities.

1.b. How can SBO lead to malnutrition? What other disorders related to nutritional status and nutrition support (e.g., fluid, electrolytes, micronutrients) can develop in patients with SBO?

1.c. Create a list of this patient's drug therapy problems, as well as problems related to nutritional status, fluid status, and electrolyte status.

1.d. What are the limitations of serum albumin as an indication of nutritional status in the acute setting?

1.e. What additional nutrition assessment data should you obtain and why?

### Desired Outcome

2. What are the goals of pharmacotherapy and nutrition support therapy in this patient?

### Therapeutic Alternatives

3. What are the therapeutic options for nutrition support intervention in this patient? Is PN indicated? Provide the rationale for your answer.

### Optimal Plan

4.a. What treatment would you recommend for this patient's current drug therapy problems and fluid, electrolyte, and acid–base problems?

4.b. What are the ranges of estimated daily goals for calories (kcal/kg per day), protein (g/kg per day), and hydration (mL per day, mL/kg per day) for this patient?

4.c. Design a goal PN formulation for this patient that includes the total volume (mL per day) and goal rate (mL/h), amino acids (g per day), dextrose (g per day), and lipid emulsion (mL per day). Take into consideration the goals you developed in question 4.b., as well as the underlying nutrition problems identified previously (question 1.c.).

4.d. How would you initiate PN in this patient? How quickly would you advance to the goal infusion rate? Provide the rationale for your answer.

4.e. What other monitoring parameters would you suggest ordering at the initiation of the PN?

### Outcome Evaluation

5.a. What parameters should be monitored to assess the efficacy and safety of PN in this patient? How frequently should each of these be monitored?

5.b. What specific parameter(s) should you monitor to assess this patient's nutritional status?

## Patient Education

6. What information should be provided to the patient and family during his hospitalization regarding the PN?

## ■ CLINICAL COURSE

Mr Brown was managed conservatively with bowel rest, PN, NG tube decompression, and supportive care. His symptoms improved over 4–5 days, and he began having bowel sounds and passing flatus. On hospital day #7, he had a small bowel movement, and the team began to advance his diet and wean the PN.

## Follow-Up Question

1. How should PN be weaned off in this patient? Develop a plan to wean PN based on PO intake in this patient.

## ■ SELF-STUDY ASSIGNMENTS

1. Mr Brown is at risk for a condition called refeeding syndrome. What is the refeeding syndrome? What are its signs, symptoms, and potential complications? How can it be prevented? How should it be treated if signs and symptoms develop?
2. What other specific postoperative complications can develop in surgical patients with moderate to severe malnutrition? How can preoperative nutrition support impact a malnourished surgical patient's risk for postoperative complications?
3. Calculate how many milliliters per day of dextrose 70% and amino acids 10% stock solutions are needed to compound the daily PN prescription you determined for this patient.
4. Using the calculated daily goals for amino acids, dextrose, and IV lipid, determine the minimum PN volume that could be compounded for this patient. Assume it will be compounded using a 10% amino acid solution, 70% dextrose solution, and 20% IV lipid emulsion, and use an estimate of 100 mL for all micronutrients and additives.

## CLINICAL PEARLS

The refeeding syndrome can lead to serious complications, including death. It is one of the few true nutritional emergencies. A good rule of thumb in patients with moderate to severe malnutrition is to "start low and go slow" when initiating nutrition support (PN, enteral nutrition, or even an oral diet) to avoid complications, and aggressively correct electrolyte abnormalities (especially phosphorus, potassium, and magnesium) *before* initiating nutrition support, as well as during therapy.

Achieving appropriate glycemic control and avoiding hyperglycemia can reduce complications and mortality. Van Den Berghe et al first described the potential mortality benefits of tight glycemic control (blood glucose 80–110 mg/dL) with insulin infusions in hospitalized surgical patients (primarily cardiothoracic surgery patients). However, results of subsequent studies have challenged these initial findings, and achieving this goal blood glucose range while avoiding hypoglycemia can be a significant challenge. Although the optimal goal range for serum glucose is debated, an acceptable upper threshold of 145 mg/dL has been suggested (*JAMA* 2003;290:2041–2047).

## REFERENCES


1. A.S.P.E.N. Board of Directors and the Clinical Guidelines Task Force. Guidelines for the use of parenteral and enteral nutrition in adult and pediatric patients. JPEN J Parenter Enteral Nutr 2002;26 (1 Suppl):1SA–138SA.
2. Kudsk KA, Tolley EA, DeWitt RC, et al. Preoperative albumin and surgical site identify surgical risk for major postoperative complications. JPEN J Parenter Enteral Nutr 2003;27:1–9.
3. Kraft MD, Btaiche IF, Sacks GS. Review of the refeeding syndrome. Nutr Clin Pract 2005;20:625–633.
4. Foster NM, McGory ML, Zingmond DS, Ko CY. Small bowel obstruction: a population-based appraisal. J Am Coll Surg 2006;203:170–176.
5. Brown KA, Dickerson RN, Morgan LM, et al. A new graduated dosing regimen for phosphorus replacement in patients receiving nutrition support. JPEN J Parenter Enteral Nutr 2006;30:209–214.
6. The American Society for Parenteral and Enteral Nutrition. Task Force for the Revision of Safe Practices for Parenteral Nutrition. Safe practices of parenteral nutrition. J Parenter Enteral Nutr 2004;28:S39–S70.
7. Sheldon GF, Grzyb S. Phosphate depletion and repletion: relation to parenteral nutrition and oxygen transport. Ann Surg 1975;182:683–689.
8. Van Den Berghe G, Wouters PJ, Weekers F, et al. Intensive insulin therapy in critically ill patients. N Engl J Med 2001;345:1359–1367.
9. Finney SJ, Zekveld C, Elia A, et al. Glucose control and mortality in critically ill patients. JAMA 2003;290:2041–2047.
10. The NICE-SUGAR Study Investigators. Intensive versus conventional glucose control in critically Ill patients. N Engl J Med 2009;360:1283–1297.


# 160

# ADULT ENTERAL NUTRITION

Gut Check. . . . . . . . . . . . . . . . . . . . . . . . . . . . Level III

**Carol J. Rollins, MS, RD, PharmD, BCNSP**

## LEARNING OBJECTIVES

After completing this case study, students should be able to:

- List contraindications to enteral nutrition (EN) therapy.
- Calculate the protein, calorie, and fluid requirements for a patient who is to receive EN therapy.
- Recommend an appropriate enteral formula and feeding route.
- Implement an appropriate monitoring plan to achieve the desired nutritional endpoints and avoid complications.
- Design an appropriate regimen for administering medications via a feeding tube, including recommending alternate dosage forms for medications that cannot be crushed.

## PATIENT PRESENTATION

Craig Baker is a 47-year-old man referred to the nutrition support team for evaluation and possible initiation of parenteral nutrition. The history on the referral states: admission to the hospital 3 days ago with c/o nausea, vomiting, and abdominal pain, primarily in the epigastric and LUQ region. Continued c/o nausea and abdominal pain; no vomiting in the past 24 hours. He is currently NPO except for sips of water for comfort.

## QUESTIONS

### Problem Identification

1.a. What other information is necessary or would be helpful to evaluate the patient and provide recommendations for a nutrition support plan of care?

1.b. What is the appropriate timing for nutrition intervention?

1.c. Based on risk-versus-benefit considerations, is the consult for initiation of parenteral nutrition appropriate for this patient?

## CLINICAL COURSE

After following appropriate procedures, you obtain the following additional information about the patient.

#### HPI

Mr Baker began having symptoms of nausea and epigastric/LUQ pain about a week (per patient) prior to hospital admission. He thought this would "go away on its own; like in the past," and then he began feeling weak and dizzy. He finally asked a friend to take him to the ED after he had several episodes of vomiting the day before admission. His history indicates five episodes with symptoms of nausea and abdominal pain in the past 8 months. With previous episodes, the pain was reported as less severe and lasted only a couple days; nausea occurred, but there was no vomiting; he was not weak or dizzy. He did not go to the hospital with the past episodes since the pain improved on its own.

In the ED, Mr Baker received 6 L of 0.9% NaCl for hydration; D5%/0.45% NaCl + 20 mEq KCl/L has been infusing at 150 mL/h since then. A CT scan in the ED indicated edema of the proximal pancreatic duct with possible stricture and a small pancreatic pseudocyst.

Height: 72 in. Weight: no admission weight available; weight on hospital day 2 was 84 kg. Patient states that he lost a few pounds when he was hospitalized 4 months ago but he "came right back up to 170–175 pounds" where his weight has been for many years.

#### PMH

HTN
GERD
PE 4 months ago for which he receives warfarin 4 mg po daily

#### FH

Mother died from a stroke 8 years ago; she had DM and HTN. Father is healthy and works as an auto mechanic. Per patient, his father's only health complaints are "aching bones" and need for glasses to see his work. All four brothers are "healthy" as far as the patient knows.

#### SH

Divorced; no contact with his ex-wife or two grown children. He works full-time in an auto parts store. He smokes about two packs per week, down from about two packs per day for 15 years prior to the PE; alcohol consumption is typically a beer after work and occasional heavy "party" use (a few times per year). The patient has private health insurance through his employer. Per the case manager, insurance coverage provides a drug benefit for oral medications but follows Medicare Parts A and B for hospitalization and home coverage.

#### ROS

From physician's note today:

Constitutional: Moderate pain and nausea.

ENT: No vision changes or eye pain. No tinnitus or ear pain. No throat pain. No problem with swallowing.

CV: No SOB, DOE, and chest pain.

Resp: No cough or sputum production.

GI: Continued persistent epigastric and LUQ abdominal pain; improved with fentanyl patch and more frequent breakthrough pain coverage. No emesis or diarrhea; complains of intermittent nausea and mild/moderate constipation.

GU: No nocturia or hematuria.

MS: (+) Abdominal pain; no other muscle aches or bone pain.

Skin: No rashes, nodules, or itching. Deep cut on the right heel is red, warm, and swollen; cultures sent today. Mr Baker says he probably stepped on a piece of glass from a cup he dropped the day before coming to the ED.

Neuro: No headaches, dizziness, unsteady gait, or seizures.

Endo: Blood glucose in 100–160 mg/dL range.

Heme/lymph nodes: No recent blood transfusions or swollen glands.

#### Meds

Metoprolol succinate tablet 200 mg po daily
Morphine sulfate, immediate release 4 mg po Q 2 h PRN pain
Fentanyl transdermal patch 50 mcg, change every 72 hours
Lansoprazole 15 mg po every morning
Bisacodyl tablet 5 mg po at bedtime
Moxifloxacin 400 mg po daily × 7 days (start today)
Warfarin 5 mg po daily

#### All

NKDA

#### Physical Examination

*Gen*

Well-developed Caucasian man; alert and conversant

*VS*

BP 144/88, P 88, RR 20, T 37.1°C; Wt 84 kg

*Skin*

No nodules, masses, or rash; no ecchymoses or petechiae. Venous access device in right hand.

*HEENT*

PERRLA; EOMs intact. Eyes anicteric. No mouth lesions; tongue normal size.

*Neck*

Neck supple; no thyromegaly or masses

*Lymph Nodes*

No cervical, supraclavicular, axillary, or inguinal adenopathy

*Heart*

RRR with no gallop, rubs, or murmur

*Lungs*

Clear

*Abd*

Tender to palpation; no masses palpable; no distension

*Genit/Rect*

Deferred

*MS/Ext*

No clubbing or cyanosis; 1+ bilateral ankle edema; 2+ sacral edema; no spine or CVA tenderness

*Neuro*

Cranial nerves intact; DTRs active and equal

### Endoscopy Report

From yesterday: ERCP, unable to enter pancreatic duct due to swelling and edema surrounding the area; suspected stricture although this could not be visualized. Stent placement is not possible at this time. Recommendation for repeat CT in 2–3 weeks to determine if ERCP with stent placement or surgery is more appropriate. Continue patient on NPO except sips of clear liquids.

### Labs

See Table 160-1.

### Other

Peripheral blood smear: anisocytosis 3+, poikilocytosis 2+, macrocytosis 2+, microcytosis 1+, and hypersegmented neutrophils

### Assessment

Acute pancreatitis with pseudocyst, probably secondary to pancreatic duct stricture, possibly related to alcohol. Intolerance to diet; tolerates limited volume (150–200 mL per day) of clear liquids daily. Per GI service note, Mr Baker is to remain NPO except for sips of clear liquids.

## Problem Identification (Continued)

1.d. Create a drug therapy problem list for this patient.

1.e. What information indicates the presence or severity of malnutrition?

1.f. What type and degree of malnutrition does this patient exhibit? What evidence supports your assessment?

## Desired Outcome

2.a. What are the goals of nutrition support in this patient?

2.b. What outcomes should be considered for the patient's other medical problems?

## Therapeutic Alternatives

3.a. What are the potential alternatives for improving nutritional status in this patient other than initiating specialized nutrition support?

3.b. What are the potential routes for specialized nutrition support and the reason(s) why each is or is not appropriate for this patient?

3.c. By postponing invasive therapy (stent or surgery for the stricture) for several weeks, the potential of continuing nutrition support outside the hospital arises. Based on the information now available to you, does this patient meet criteria for home enteral therapy? Recall that his insurance follows Medicare guidelines for home coverage.

## Optimal Plan

4.a. Estimate the protein, calorie, and fluid requirements for this patient.

4.b. What type of formula (e.g., polymeric, monomeric) is most appropriate for this patient?

4.c. What administration regimen should be used for tube feedings?

4.d. Assuming that the patient is to continue his current medications during tube feedings, how should each of these be administered?

## Outcome Evaluation

5. What clinical and laboratory parameters are necessary to evaluate the therapy for detection and/or prevention of adverse effects and to evaluate achievement of the desired response?

## Patient Education

6. What information should be provided to the patient or his caregiver to enhance compliance, ensure successful therapy, and minimize adverse effects of EN therapy?

## CLINICAL COURSE

After presenting literature related to nutrition support during acute pancreatitis to the medical team, EN therapy was discussed with the patient. The patient consented to feeding tube placement. A 1.2-cal/mL, 55.5-g protein/L, 300-mOsm/kg polymeric formula was started using an enteral infusion pump via nasojejunal tube at 35 mL/h for 8 hours, and then advanced to the goal rate of 70 mL/h. Basic metabolic panel results on day 2 of EN revealed electrolyte values WNL. The WBC decreased to $10.6 \times 10^3/mm^3$ with 75% segs, 9% bands, 14% lymphs, and 2% monos. The basic metabolic panel on day 3 of EN showed stable values and a prealbumin of 16 mg/dL. The plan for discharge to home was confirmed and arrangements for home EN were finalized. The plan is for his diet to continue as limited clear liquids (<240 mL per day) and repeat the CT scan in

**TABLE 160-1 Lab Values**

| | | | | |
|---|---|---|---|---|
| Na 140 mEq/L | Hgb 8.5 g/dL | WBC $11.9 \times 10^3/mm^3$ | AST 23 IU/L | T. chol 239 mg/dL |
| K 3.9 mEq/L | Hct 26.7% | Segs 67% | ALT 34 IU/L | Trig 105 mg/dL |
| Cl 109 mEq/L | RBC $2.65 \times 10^6/mm^3$ | Bands 14% | Alk phos 287 IU/L | Ca 7.9 mg/dL |
| $CO_2$ 26 mEq/L | Plt $265 \times 10^3/mm^3$ | Lymphs 17% | LDH 154 IU/L | Mg 1.9 mg/dL |
| BUN 7 mg/dL | MCV 104 $\mu m^3$ | Monos 2% | T. bili 0.9 mg/dL | Phos 3.5 mg/dL |
| SCr 0.9 mg/dL | | | T. prot 7.1 g/dL | Amylase 462 mg/dL |
| Glu 147 mg/dL | | | Alb 2.6 g/dL | Lipase 591 mg/dL |

2–3 weeks to assess the small pancreatic pseudocyst and potentially schedule him for surgery the following week for the pancreatic duct stricture.

## SELF-STUDY ASSIGNMENTS

1. Select a current patient you are following, and design an appropriate regimen for administering medications via a feeding tube, including alternate dosage forms for medications that cannot be crushed and proper dosage adjustments for different forms where necessary.
2. Educate an actual patient or do a mock education with a classmate about medication administration through a feeding tube.
3. Select a current patient you are following, and determine the potential cumulative sorbitol dose if all medications were changed to oral liquid dosage forms.
4. Identify the metabolic changes associated with refeeding syndrome and the characteristics that increase the risk of this complication.

## CLINICAL PEARL

Medications administered through a feeding tube frequently clog the tube; evaluate the medication regimen for alternate dosage forms that do not require crushing or administration through the tube. Adequate flushing of the feeding tube before and after medication administration as well as dilution of thick liquids prior to administration is essential for adequate drug delivery and to reduce the risk of tube occlusion. When a tube clogs, a buffered pancreatic enzyme preparation may be useful for declogging the tube.

## REFERENCES


1. ASPEN Board of Directors and the Clinical Guidelines Task Force. Guidelines for the use of parenteral and enteral nutrition in adult and pediatric patients. J Parenter Enteral Nutr 2002;26(1 Suppl):1SA–138SA.
2. McClave SA, Martindale RG, Vanek VW, et al. Guidelines for the provision and assessment of nutrition support therapy in the adult critically ill patient. Section K. Acute pancreatitis. J Parenter Enteral Nutr 2009;33:277–316.
3. McClave SA, Chang WK, Dhaliwal R, et al. Nutrition support in acute pancreatitis: a systematic review of the literature. J Parenter Enteral Nutr 2006;30:143–156.
4. Tiu A, McClave SA. Pancreatitis. In: Gottschlich MM, ed. The A.S.P.E.N. Nutrition Support Core Curriculum: A Case-Based Approach—The Adult Patient. Silver Spring, MD, American Society for Parenteral and Enteral Nutrition, 2007.
5. Rollins CJ. Home care issues in nutrition support. In: Pharmacotherapy Self-Assessment Program, Module 8: Gastroenterology, Nutrition. Kansas City, MO, American College of Clinical Pharmacy, 2000.
6. Mascarenhas MR, Divito D, McClave S. Pancreatic disease. In: Merritt R, ed. The A.S.P.E.N. Nutrition Support Manual, 2nd ed. Silver Spring, MD, American Society for Enteral and Parenteral Nutrition, 2005:211–230.
7. Bankhead R, Boullata J, Brantley S, et al. Enteral nutrition practice recommendations. J Parenter Enteral Nutr OnlineFirst, published January 27, 2009. Available at: *www.nutritioncare.org*. Accessed January 28, 2010.
8. Makola D, Krenitsky J, Parrish C, et al. Efficacy of enteral nutrition for the treatment of pancreatitis using standard enteral formula. Am J Gastroenterol 2006;101:2347–2355.
9. Burkhardt O, Stass H, Thuss U, et al. Effects of enteral feeding on the oral bioavailability of moxifloxacin in healthy volunteers. Clin Pharmacokinet 2005;44:969–976.
10. Rollins CJ. Drug–nutrient interactions in patients receiving enteral nutrition. In: Boullata JI, Armenti VT, eds. Handbook of Drug–Nutrient Interactions. Totowa, NJ, Humana Press, 2009:515–552.


# 161

# OBESITY

## To Be Single and 23 Again (BMI That Is). . . . Level II

**Dannielle C. O'Donnell, PharmD, BCPS**

## LEARNING OBJECTIVES

After completing this case study, students should be able to:

- Identify common obesity-related comorbidities.
- Calculate body mass index (BMI), and use waist circumference to determine a patient's risk of obesity-related morbidity.
- Develop a pharmacotherapeutic plan and treatment strategy for obese patients.
- Provide patient counseling on the expected benefits, possible adverse effects, and drug interactions with weight loss medications.

## PATIENT PRESENTATION

### Chief Complaint

"I've been through a painful divorce. I think I'm ready to try and get out and meet someone and start over, but I must've eaten my way through all of the stress of the separation and legal proceedings. Who's gonna even look at me when I'm this size? I may have to take up smoking again. It was easy to stay skinny when I smoked."

### HPI

Francine Mallory is a 35-year-old woman who has "yo-yo'd" with her weight over the years. She feels best at 55 kg, which was how much she weighed when she was 23 years old and got married. She states that she was a "chubby" kid who really worked in college to "get healthier" as far as weight was concerned, although that was when she started smoking. She and her ex-husband were smokers and stopped when she was 27 because they wanted a smoke-free home before starting a family. She remembers frustration that while she "did great going cold turkey with the cigs," she put on 12 kg in the first 6 smoke-free months. She "worked out like crazy" and dropped 7 kg before they conceived their first child at the age of 29. She delivered a healthy baby, although her pregnancy was complicated by a diagnosis of gestational diabetes and excessive weight gain (27 kg). Her hyperglycemia resolved postdelivery and she "was happy with how quickly most of the baby weight came off while nursing" but then she plateaued 8 kg above her pre-pregnancy weight and "just couldn't get the rest off. I don't have time to commit to exercising while juggling a job and family." She has now put on more weight during the stress and hectic lifestyle of the divorce, which has left her financially strapped. She now lives in an apartment with her 5-year-old. She says she has tried weight loss shakes as a way to save some money and lose weight, but finds herself just starving and "pigging out" at the end of the day. She says she does not have money for a gym membership or a fancy program where they provide meals for you. She has bought some "herbal stuff" from a coworker that helped with end-of-day hunger, but thinks cigarettes would be even cheaper than that. To economize and work with her hectic single-mom schedule, they eat out quite a bit based on where the "kids eat free" meal nights are (i.e., an all-you-can-eat buffet on Monday nights and a pancake house on Wednesday nights, drive-thru meals at least one other night each week).

### PMH

GDM
Hemorrhoids
Insomnia
Tension headaches

### PSH

None

### FH

Mother had an MI at the age of 62 years; father died in an MVA at the age of 67. Maternal grandmother died at age 62 with diabetes. She states that her mother and grandmother were "big boned," and all women in her family have struggled with their weight. No other family members have a significant medical history, although she states that her 5 year old is "a big boy." She blames his dad, stating that when he has him all they do is eat junk food, and he uses the TV and video games as a babysitter.

### SH

She is a single working mom and a previous smoker (1 ppd × 9 years). Stopped 6 years ago. She denies IVDA. She has previously had success with weight loss by focusing on exercising but is not exercising now.

### Diet

Has never had formal diet instruction. Her diet appears to be low in fiber, high in saturated fat and calories.

### Meds

Tylenol PM PRN sleep (one to two times per week)
Anusol HC PRN
Ibuprofen 600 mg po PRN HA (three to four times per week)
Unknown "herbal" weight loss product—discontinued 3 months ago

### All

Macrolides—rash

### ROS

She complains of general fatigue and periods of weepiness that she attributes to the divorce and a preoccupation with food and her weight and feeling "undesirable." She denies symptoms of cold or heat intolerance; changes in skin, hair, or nails; nervousness; irritability; lethargy; muscle pain or weakness; palpitations; diarrhea or constipation; polyuria; polydipsia; chest pain; or shortness of breath.

### Physical Examination

*Gen*

The patient is in NAD but looks tired and older than her stated age. She is clean in appearance and dressed appropriately for the weather.

*VS*

BP 148/88 (consistent with previous clinic reading), P 80, RR 16, T 36.4°C; Wt 80 kg, waist 100 cm, Ht 5′3″

*Skin*

Warm, with normal distribution of body hair. No significant lesions or discolorations.

*HEENT*

NC/AT; PERRLA; EOMI; TMs intact

*CV*

RRR, $S_1$ and $S_2$ normal; no murmurs, rubs, or gallops

*Pulm*

CTA & P bilaterally

*Abd*

Obese with multiple striae; NT; ND; (+) BS; no palpable masses

*Genit/Rect*

Pelvic and rectal exams deferred

*Ext*

LE varicosities present. Pedal pulses 2+ bilaterally.

*Neuro*

A & O × 3; CN II–XII intact; Romberg test (–); sensory and motor levels intact; 2+ triceps tendons and DTR; Babinski (–)

### Labs (Fasting)

Na 138 mEq/L
K 3.9 mEq/L
Cl 96 mEq/L
$CO_2$ 26 mEq/L
BUN 13 mg/dL
SCr 1.0 mg/dL
Glu 115 mg/dL

AST 24 IU/L
TSH 0.5 mIU/mL
*Fasting lipid profile*
T. chol 208 mg/dL
LDL-C 109 mg/dL
HDL-C 38 mg/dL
Trig 305 mg/dL

# QUESTIONS

## Problem Identification

1.a. Create a drug therapy problem list for this patient.

1.b. Calculate the patient's BMI. By using the BMI and any other markers of adiposity, categorize her obesity and stratify her risk.

1.c. What information (signs, symptoms, laboratory values) indicates the presence or severity of obesity?

1.d. Could any of the patient's problems have been caused by her drug therapy?

1.e. What other medical conditions should be considered to exclude primary causes of her obesity?

## Desired Outcome

2. What are the goals of therapy for the patient's obesity?

## Therapeutic Alternatives

3.a. What nondrug therapies should be recommended for this patient?

3.b. What nonprescription drug product(s) could you recommend for this patient's obesity? Justify your choices.

3.c. What are the primary prescription drug classes to consider when considering prescription drug therapy for obesity?

## Optimal Plan

4.a. What drug(s), dosage form(s), dose(s), schedule(s), and duration would be most appropriate to treat this patient's obesity and why?

4.b. What alternatives would be appropriate if initial therapy fails?

## Outcome Evaluation

5. What clinical and laboratory parameters are necessary to evaluate the therapy for achievement of the desired therapeutic outcome and to detect or prevent adverse effects?

## Patient Education

6. What general and medication-specific information should be provided to the patient to enhance adherence, ensure successful therapy, and minimize adverse effects?

## CLINICAL COURSE

Mrs Mallory returns for her first follow-up visit after 4 months. She never picked up her prescription medication because she states that she could not afford it that first month. She is starting a new job at the school district that will allow her schedule to better mirror her son's schedule as well as a slight pay increase. Additionally, the new job will provide better medical benefits, but she will still be without prescription coverage.

She is now working out at home regularly 30 minutes each evening (typically four nights a week) with a video after her son goes to bed. Although they still eat out a lot, she is making significantly different choices, increasing her lean meats, decreasing carbohydrates and saturated fats, and abstaining from having seconds. She has eliminated sugary beverages (sweet tea, colas) and is having good success sticking to her plan of not eating anything after her son goes to bed. If she is really struggling, she makes herself some hot tea with sugar substitute and eats a rice cake. She found a weight loss group at her church, and they are holding each other accountable for self-reporting weigh-ins since she could not afford the cost of biweekly office visits. She relates progress at each of her weekly weigh-ins, averaging a 1-kg weight loss at each visit through the end of week 8. However, at the 10-week visit she had lost only an additional 0.5 kg.

Since the 3-month point, she has not lost any additional weight. She weighs 73.5 kg, and her waist circumference is 96 cm. Her FBG is now 102 mg/dL, and her fasting lipid profile includes total cholesterol 202 mg/dL, LDL-C 110 mg/dL, HDL-C 45 mg/dL, and triglycerides 235 mg/dL. Her blood pressure has improved to 142/82 mm Hg.

She states that she is as compliant with her lifestyle modifications as in previous weeks and is in much better spirits overall. She has noticed a definite improvement in her clothing fit, but she is starting to become frustrated again and does not like how she looks. She wants to know if there is something she can take that she could afford or if once her new benefits kick in, she could have the Lap-Band procedure. Although she is pleased with the improvement in her blood pressure and glucose, she is frustrated that her cholesterol did not improve more. Before she leaves her current job, she is wondering if it might further help her weight loss efforts if she picked up some of "that herbal dandelion tea from Paraguay" that her coworker sells for weight loss just to help move things along.

## Follow-Up Questions

1. What changes, if any, should be made in her weight loss regimen today?
2. How would you educate her regarding her question about the herbal weight loss tea?
3. What pharmacotherapeutic changes, if any, should be made for her lipids, glucose, and/or blood pressure at this time? Is a medication indicated at this point to prevent or treat diabetes?

## SELF-STUDY ASSIGNMENTS

1. List the limitations of height–weight charts or BMI determinations. What are the most accurate methods for quantifying body fat, and why are they not routinely employed?
2. Assume that you are a member of a pharmacy and therapeutics committee for a managed care corporation. Justify whether anti-obesity drugs should be a covered benefit, and, if so, which specific agent(s) should be added to the formulary.
3. Compile a compendium of common herbal and dietary supplements that claim weight loss benefits, and make a list of the evidence for their safety and efficacy.
4. Identify the control schedule for the various prescription weight loss medications. What are the legal requirements for dispensing the various scheduled weight loss agents in your state?
5. Identify the various surgical interventions currently used for obesity. What are the expected benefits and risks associated with each approach?
6. Make a list of the various prescription weight loss medications that have been introduced and subsequently withdrawn from the US and EU markets and the reasons for the withdrawal.

## CLINICAL PEARL

Taking psyllium with orlistat has been reported to decrease the frequency and severity of orlistat GI side effects such as oily stool and leakage.

## REFERENCES

1. National Institutes of Health. Clinical Guidelines on the Identification, Evaluation and Treatment of Overweight and Obesity in Adults: The Evidence Report. NIH Publication No.: 98-4083, September 1998.
2. Schnee DM, Zaiken K, McCloskey WW. An update on the pharmacological treatment of obesity. Curr Med Res Opin 2006;22:1463–1474.
3. Salem V, Bloom SR. Approaches to the pharmacological treatment of obesity. Expert Rev Clin Pharmacol 2010;3:73–88.
4. Neff LM, Aronne LJ. Pharmacotherapy for obesity. Curr Atheroscler Rep 2007;9:454–462.
5. American Diabetes Association. Standards of medical care in diabetes—2010. Diabetes Care 2010;3(Suppl 1):S11–S61.
6. Samaha FF, Foster GD, Makris AP. Low-carbohydrate diets, obesity, and metabolic risk factors for cardiovascular disease. Curr Atheroscler Rep 2007;9:441–447.
7. Johannsen DL, Redman LM, Ravussin E. The role of physical activity in maintaining a reduced weight. Curr Atheroscler Rep 2007;9:463–471.
8. *http://www.fda.gov/Drugs/DrugSafety/*PostmarketDrugSafetyInformationforPatientsandProviders/DrugSafetyInformationforHeathcareProfessionals/ucm198206.htm. Accessed February 27, 2010.
9. Dunican KC, Adams NM, Desilets AR. The role of pramlintide for weight loss. Ann Pharmacother 2010;44:538–545.

# SECTION 19
# COMPLEMENTARY AND ALTERNATIVE THERAPIES (LEVEL III)

Cydney McQueen, PharmD

## TO THE READER

Although use of many dietary supplements has leveled off or decreased in the last few years (with a few notable and growing exceptions, such as vitamin D and fish oil), many patients are still interested in trying supplements, either in place of (alternative) or along with (complementary) prescription and OTC therapies. As part of providing appropriate care, clinicians have a duty to help individual patients avoid interactions with their drug therapies and prevent use of products unsafe for them because of other disease state contraindications. That is a fairly straightforward task when dealing with prescription and OTC therapies; there is so much information and research available that most problems and risks are well delineated. If a patient is prescribed a contraindicated drug, we can ensure that he or she does not receive it. With dietary supplements, we often do not have enough information to make clear judgments about risks. We also cannot prevent patients from taking supplements we do know are unsafe or risky for them, because we cannot control their access to those therapies. Instead, we are limited to providing as much guidance as possible to help maximize any possible benefit and minimize possible harm.

## CASEBOOK QUESTIONS ABOUT DIETARY SUPPLEMENTS

The following questions regarding supplement therapy aid in the decision-making process and will be addressed in the section "Clinical Course" of the Casebook. It is assumed that necessary information about a patient's medical history and current drug regimen has already been obtained.

**1. What is the known or proposed mechanism of action?**

When there is no or little concrete human evidence for either efficacy or safety, we must often extrapolate based on in vitro or animal data. For example, if a plant extract is shown to improve glucose uptake in tissue studies, then it is reasonable to expect that activity to some extent when taken by human beings. It would also be reasonable to offer cautions about use with sulfonylurea drugs or other hypoglycemic agents, even when no case studies or clinical trials have reported interactions. Depending on the risks if an interaction should happen, appropriate cautions can range from "use with additional monitoring" to "do not use at all in this patient."

**2. How extensive or conclusive are the clinical trial data on effectiveness?**

When clinical trial data conclude that a supplement has beneficial effects, it may be less hazardous for a patient to try a supplement before a prescription drug. When evidence of efficacy is lacking or contradictory, the severity of the patient's condition becomes more important in the risk/benefit equation. For example, a patient wishing to try a supplement for the common cold or athlete's foot is not at great risk of harm if the supplement is not effective—he or she will simply endure some unpleasant symptoms for a time. On the other hand, a patient with severe hypertension who tries a supplement that ends up being ineffective may have increased risk for a cardiovascular event.

**3. What is known about safety?**

This question relates back to what is known about the mechanism of action; because there is a lack of information from long-term clinical trials, decisions about safety must be based on extrapolation from basic science studies and isolated case reports. It must be kept in mind that safety issues can be both overemphasized and underemphasized and that information (and therefore reasonable recommendations) can change fairly rapidly. For example, ginger is often described as being associated with increased risk of bleeding. This is absolutely true when doses exceed 4 g/day but is only a major consideration for patient use at lower doses when there are other medical conditions (e.g., a clotting disorder) or interactions (e.g., warfarin or chronic NSAID use) involved. One safety rule of thumb to keep in mind for counseling patients is that all supplements should be stopped 10–14 days prior to scheduled surgery to minimize risks.

**4. Does the product have any specific quality considerations?**

In general, it is advised that patients purchase products from manufacturers that participate in quality seal programs (such as USP's Dietary Supplement Verification Program) or that have been tested by third-party laboratories (such as ConsumerLab.com). Certain products are more likely to have specific problems with quality or carry additional risk. For example, melatonin is usually produced synthetically, but some products are available that are "natural source" (i.e., extracted from the pituitary glands of cattle). Because of the location of the pituitary gland in the brain, these products do carry a small but real risk of contamination with bovine spongiform encephalopathy. However, the most common consideration for quality is making sure that the product is providing the appropriate standardization or strength and is not subtherapeutic.

**5. Would this be an appropriate treatment choice in this particular patient?**

Each patient may have different motivations to try a treatment. If clinical or basic science supports that a supplement might benefit a given condition, the next thing to consider is the patient's own expectations of therapy and ability to self-monitor for both efficacy and safety. For example, a postmenopausal woman who suffers 10 severe hot flushes a week and wants to end them entirely is likely to be disappointed with black cohosh therapy, whereas another woman who also has severe hot flushes and would like a reduction in their frequency or severity may be very happy with the same therapy. Expectations must be appropriate; rarely will a supplement work as strongly or as quickly as a prescription drug.

**6. If the patient is going to use the product, what counseling information will allow him or her to maximize any possible benefit and minimize any harm?**

Counseling information should cover the same categories of information as prescription drugs: dose, schedule, duration of therapy, side effects, and interactions. Unfortunately, there is usually less information about side effects and interactions, so it is impossible to warn patients about every possibility. It is best to counsel patients to contact their health care providers if anything unexpected or unusual occurs. This provides protection for the patient and allows evaluation of any possible link to the supplement, which aids in expanding the supplement knowledge base.

Specificity is important in counseling. For example, if a patient is going to use *Ginkgo biloba*, he or she needs to be told to watch for easy bruising, not just that the *Ginkgo* may increase bleeding risk. Specificity is even more important in those situations when a patient is choosing to take a supplement that we have counseled against because of known safety issues or interactions with another of his or her medications.

In addition, there are extra categories of information to include in counseling that do not generally have to be addressed with prescription and OTC drugs: using the appropriate product and a high-quality product. For botanical supplements, it is generally necessary to specify information such as the standardization of an extract (e.g., saw palmetto should be 160 mg of extract standardized to 85–95% fatty acids and sterols twice daily). For nonbotanical supplements, the salt form may need to be specified (e.g., glucosamine sulfate has far more evidence of efficacy than glucosamine hydrochloride and so is the preferred form).

## OBTAINING CURRENT AND RELIABLE DIETARY SUPPLEMENT INFORMATION

Decisions made about using supplements are only as good as the information used in making the decisions. Unfortunately, incomplete or wrong information about dietary supplements is abundantly available in both electronic and print media, so using only reliable resources is vital. A brief list of recommended resources is provided at the end of this section, but practitioners need to know what to look for or to avoid as they come across new resources. The following questions and rules of thumb should be kept in mind:

- Avoid resources published or provided by manufacturers; their primary interest is in selling the product.
- Investigate the authors or source of the information; is the resource actually created by trained professionals, or by a ghost-writing group?
- Are recommendations based on careful analysis of the quality of clinical trials? Recommendations based solely on the end results of trial are often wrong; it is not possible to get good decision-making data from a badly designed or conducted trial.
- Are cautions (about interactions, contraindications, or adverse effects) based on all theoretical, animal, or human data available, or only on well-documented human trials or case reports? Although it may seem counterintuitive at first, there is such a lack of high-quality reports and information in humans that use of theoretical (based on in vitro experiments or theorized mechanisms of action) or animal trial data may become more important in generating cautions that help keep patients safe. Often these cautions should not be as strong, of course; if a supplement has been noted to have an effect on glucose utilization in tissue cultures, a diabetic patient starting to take the supplement may be warned appropriately to monitor blood glucose more frequently, whereas a case report of loss of glycemic control in two patients using the supplement would generate a strong warning not to use the supplement.
- Does the resource include up-to-date information? Supplement information changes rapidly, so publication dates can matter tremendously. For example, a well-researched, completely evidenced-based book on herbal toxicology contained an obsolete chapter on St. John's wort (SJW) when it rolled off the printing press in February 2000, due solely to new information about SJW's effects on cytochrome P-450 3A4 published in January 2000.

## RECOMMENDED INFORMATION RESOURCES

One of the most essential resources is a comprehensive literature search, because this can retrieve the most current information. While it is recommended that more than one indexing system be used (such as both Medline and EMBASE), health care students and professionals often do not have access to anything other than Medline. Consequently, it is essential to use very thorough search strategies, discussed as follows:

- Because pertinent articles can be incompletely or wrongly indexed, search using more than just MESH (or EMTREE) terms to ensure proper retrieval. For example, to search for saw palmetto, search the MESH term (*Serenoa*), and then perform keyword searches for the common name (saw palmetto), the botanical name (*Serenoa repens*), and any alternative botanical names (*Sabul serrulata*). Consider searching misspellings; the spelling "saw palmeto" may not be common, but "gingko," instead of "ginkgo," is common. Combining the results of these searches will optimize retrieval.
- Search the relevant disease state and any closely related terms. Continuing the example, search terms such as "BPH," "benign prostatic hyperplasia," "prostatic hyperplasia," and "prostatic hypertrophy." It may also be useful to search symptom or outcome measure terms, such as "urinary retention" or "micturition rate."
- After combining product and disease state searches, if the retrieval set is so large as to be impossible to review, limitations can be used. For clinical decision making, the most useful types of limitations are clinical trials, evidence-based reviews, meta-analyses, and systematic reviews. Because it is not uncommon for articles about dietary supplement trials to report results of both animal and human studies, it is not recommended that a limitation of "human only" be used.

### Electronic Database Resources

Electronic databases available for purchase include:

- Natural Standard (www.naturalstandard.com). It is the most evidence-based clinical recommendations available. It thoroughly discusses the clinical evidence available but includes summaries as well. It is available for purchase by pharmacies and institutions.
- Natural Medicines Comprehensive Database (www. naturaldatabase.com). It is the most comprehensive resource available and includes a very wide range of individual and combination products. It contains evidence-based recommendations and summaries of clinical and basic science information. The site allows for easy checking of supplement–drug interactions. It is available for purchase by individuals as well as institutions. A consumer version is also available.
- ConsumerLab.com (www.consumerlab.com). This is a third-party laboratory that tests dietary supplements for compliance with labeled content and for appropriate dissolution and contaminants. No clinical recommendations are given; the site's utility is limited to aiding in the choice of a high-quality product. It is appropriate for use by consumers.

Free electronic databases include:

- The Health Information site of the National Institutes of Health Office of Dietary Supplements (http://ods.od.nih.gov/Health_Information/Health_Information.aspx). This is a government site with links to several useful informational resources including: (1) fact sheets on a number of dietary supplements; (2) International Bibliographic Information on Dietary Supplements (IBIDS), a database of published medical literature relating to dietary supplements (because the database is focused on medical use of plants, it can be easier to search than other literature databases that contain citations for agricultural-focused studies); (3) Computer Access to Research on Dietary Supplements (CARDS), which is a database of federally funded clinical trials of supplements.
- Memorial Sloan-Kettering Cancer Center Integrative Medicine Service Web site (http://www.mskcc.org/mskcc/html/1979.cfm). It includes a database of individual supplements. Information is specifically focused on use of supplements in cancer patients, a population that has a high rate of use of complementary and alternative medicine therapies. The site includes more discussion of interactions with chemotherapeutic agents than other resources.

### Print Resources

- Because of limitations on the timeliness of information in print resources, it is difficult to make strong recommendations. New print resources should be evaluated according to the criteria listed above to determine their usefulness.

## CASE 25: HYPERLIPIDEMIA

### Garlic and Fish Oil for Hyperlipidemia

*Clinical Course*

Mrs Thorngrass is already taking garlic capsules, but she is not sure about the type or dose. Because you are making changes to her current prescription regimen, you need to investigate the advisability of continuing the garlic. If Mrs Thorngrass does begin a statin drug as indicated, she would not be able to take red yeast rice (duplicative therapy because of mevacolin K content, a lovastatin analog). Would fish oil be a possible option for her?

## FOLLOW-UP QUESTIONS

### Garlic

1. What is the known or proposed mechanism of action?
2. How extensive or conclusive are the clinical trial data on effectiveness?
3. What is known about safety?
4. Does the product have any specific quality concerns?
5. Would this be an appropriate treatment choice in this particular patient?
6. If the patient is going to use the product, what counseling information will allow her to maximize any possible benefit and minimize any harm?

### Fish Oil/Omega-3 Fatty Acids

1. What is the known or proposed mechanism of action?
2. How extensive or conclusive are the clinical trial data on effectiveness?
3. What is known about safety?
4. Does the product have any specific quality concerns?
5. Would this be an appropriate treatment choice in this particular patient?
6. If the patient is going to use the product, what counseling information will allow her to maximize any possible benefit and minimize any harm?

## REFERENCES


1. Khoo YSK, Aziz A. Garlic supplementation and serum cholesterol: a meta-analysis. J Clin Pharm Ther 2009;34:133–145.
2. Brace LD. Cardiovascular benefits of garlic (*Allium sativum* L). J Cardiovasc Nurs 2002;16(4):33–49.
3. Mathew BC, Prasad NV, Prabodh R. Cholesterol-lowering effect of organosulphur compounds from garlic: a possible mechanism of action. Kathmandu Univ Med J 2004;2(2):100–102.
4. Fetrow CW, Avila JR. Professional's Handbook of Complementary & Alternative Medicines. Philadelphia, PA, Lippincott Williams & Wilkins, 2004:342–349.
5. Dhawan V, Jain S. Garlic supplementation prevents oxidative DNA damage in essential hypertension. Mol Cell Biochem 2005;275:85–94.
6. Reinhart KM, Talati R, White CM, Coleman CI. The impact of garlic on lipid parameters: a systematic review and meta-analysis. Nutr Res Rev 2009;22:39–48.
7. Alder R, Lookinland S, Berry JA, Williams M. A systematic review of the effectiveness of garlic as an anti-hyperlipidemic agent. J Am Acad Nurse Pract 2003;15(3):120–129.
8. Reid K, Frank OR, Stocks NP, Fakler P, Sullivan T. Effect of garlic on blood pressure: a systematic review and meta-analysis. BMC Cardiovasc Disord 2008;8:13.
9. Reinhart KM, Coleman CI, Teevan C, Vachhani P, White CM. Effects of garlic on blood pressure in patients with and without systolic hypertension: a meta-analysis. Ann Pharmacother 2008;42:1766–1771.
10. Pittler MH, Ernst E. Clinical effectiveness of garlic (*Allium sativum*). Mol Nutr Food Res 2007;51:1382–1385.
11. Gurley BJ, Gardner SF, Hubbard MA, et al. Cytochrome P450 phenotypic ratios for predicting herb–drug interactions in humans. Clin Pharmacol Ther 2002;72:276–287.
12. Markowitz JS, Devane CL, Chavin KD, et al. Effects of garlic (*Allium sativum* L.) supplementation on cytochrome P450 2D6 and 3A4 activity in healthy volunteers. Clin Pharmacol Ther 2003;74:170–177.
13. Fetterman JW Jr, Zdanowicz MM. Therapeutic potential of *n*-3 polyunsaturated fatty acids in disease. Am J Health Syst Pharm 2009;66:1169–1179.
14. Balk EM, Lichtenstein AH, Chung M, et al. Effects of omega-3 fatty acids on serum markers of cardiovascular disease risk: a systematic review. Atherosclerosis 2006;189(1):19–30.
15. Lewis A, Lookinland S, Beckstrand RL, et al. Treatment of hypertriglyceridemia with omega-3 fatty acids: a systematic review. J Am Acad Nurse Pract 2004;16(9):384–395.
16. Hartweg J, Farmer AJ, Perera R, et al. Meta-analysis of the effects of *n*-3 polyunsaturated fatty acids on lipoproteins and other emerging lipid cardiovascular risk markers in patients with type 2 diabetes. Diabetologia 2007;50(8):1593–1602.
17. Eslick GD, Howe PRC, Smith C, Priest R, Bensoussan A. Benefits of fish oil supplementation in hyperlipidemia: a systematic review and meta-analysis. Int J Cardiol 2009;136:4–16.
18. GISSI-Prevenzione Investigators. Dietary supplementation with *n*-3 polyunsaturated fatty acids and vitamin E after myocardial infarction: results of the GISSI-Prevenzione trial. Lancet 1999;354:447–455.
19. Lavie CJ, Milani RV, Mehra MR, Ventura HO. Omega-3 polyunsaturated fatty acids and cardiovascular diseases. J Am Coll Cardiol 2009;54(7):585–594.
20. Smith SC, Allen J, Blair SN, et al. AHA/ACC guidelines for secondary prevention for patients with coronary and other atherosclerotic vascular disease: 2006 update. Circulation 2006;113:2363–2372.
21. Lovaza [Package Insert]. Liberty Corner, NJ, Reliant Pharmaceuticals Inc, August 2007. Available at: *www.lovaza.com*. Accessed July 2010.

22. Foran SE, Flood JG, Lewandrowski KB. Measurement of mercury levels in concentrated over-the-counter fish oil preparations: is fish oil healthier than fish? Arch Pathol Lab Med 2003;127(12):1603–1605.
23. Smutna M, Kruzikova K, Marsalek P, Kopriva V, Svobodova Z. Fish oil and cod liver as safe and healthy food supplements. Neuroendocrinol Lett 2009;30(Suppl 1):156–162.

## CASE 62: ALZHEIMER'S DISEASE

### Ginkgo biloba for Alzheimer's Disease

*Clinical Course*

Mrs Dale's son, Sam, is concerned about his increasing role in his mother's care, and he has been reading everything he can find about potential treatments for Alzheimer's disease. He has read that *Ginkgo* has improved some symptoms, including apathy and depression, and asks if adding it to her current medicines might help her current issues.

### FOLLOW-UP QUESTIONS

1. What is the known or proposed mechanism of action?
2. How extensive or conclusive are the clinical trial data on effectiveness?
3. What is known about safety?
4. Does the product have any specific quality concerns?
5. Would this be an appropriate treatment choice in this particular patient?
6. If the patient is going to use the product, what counseling information will allow her to maximize any possible benefit and minimize any harm?

## REFERENCES

1. Birks J, Grimley Evans J. *Ginkgo biloba* for cognitive impairment and dementia. Cochrane Database Syst Rev 2007;2:CD003120.
2. White HL, Scates PW, Cooper BR. Extracts of *Ginkgo biloba* leaves inhibit monoamine oxidase. Life Sci 1996;58:1315–1321.
3. Augustin S, Rimbach G, Augustin K, Schliebs R, Wolffram S, Cermak R. Effect of a short- and long-term treatment with *Ginkgo biloba* extract on amyloid precursor protein levels in a transgenic mouse model relevant to Alzheimer's disease. Arch Biochem Biophys 2009;481:177–182.
4. Oken BS, Storzbach DM, Kaye JA. The efficacy of *Ginkgo biloba* on cognitive function in Alzheimer disease. Arch Neurol 1998;55:1409–1415.
5. Kurz A, Van Baelen B. *Ginkgo biloba* compared with cholinesterase inhibitors in the treatment of dementia: a review based on meta-analyses by the *Cochrane* Collaboration. Dement Geriatr Cogn Disord 2004;18:217–226.
6. Dos Santos-Neto LL, de Vilhena Toledo MA, Medeiros-Souza P, de Souza GA. The use of herbal medicine in Alzheimer's disease—a systematic review. eCAM 2006;3:441–445.
7. Napreyenko O, Sonnik G, Tartakovsky I. Efficacy and tolerability of *Ginkgo biloba* extract EGb 761® by type of dementia: analysis of a randomized controlled trial. J Neurol Sci 2009;283:224–229.
8. Scripnikov A, Khomenko A, Napreyenko O. Effects of *Ginkgo biloba* extract EGb 761® on neuropsychiatric symptoms of dementia: findings from a randomized controlled trial. Wein Med Wochenschr 2007;157:295–300.
9. Yancheva S, Ihll R, Nikolova G, Panayotov P, Schlaefke S, Hoerr R. *Ginkgo biloba* extract EGb 761®, donepezil or both combined in the treatment of Alzheimer's disease with neuropsychiatric features: a randomized double-blind, exploratory trial. Aging Ment Health 2009;13:183–190.
10. Markowitz JS, Donovan JL, DeVane CL, et al. Multiple-dose administration of *Ginkgo biloba* did not affect cytochrome P-450 2D6 or 3A4 activity in normal volunteers. J Clin Psychopharmacol 2003;23:576–581.

## CASE 68: PARKINSON'S DISEASE

### Coenzyme Q10 for Parkinson's Disease

*Clinical Course*

Ms Farmer has been taking coenzyme Q10 for about a month before coming in for reevaluation. Unlike the kava and cowage, which could be actively worsening her symptoms or posing other safety problems, coenzyme Q10 might actually have some benefit for Parkinson's disease. The question is whether Ms Farmer should continue taking the supplement.

### FOLLOW-UP QUESTIONS

1. What is the known or proposed mechanism of action?
2. How extensive or conclusive are the clinical trial data on effectiveness?
3. What is known about safety?
4. Does the product have any specific quality concerns?
5. Would this be an appropriate treatment choice in this particular patient?
6. If the patient is going to use the product, what counseling information will allow her to maximize any possible benefit and minimize any harm?

## REFERENCES

1. Shults CW. Therapeutic role of coenzyme $Q_{10}$ in Parkinson's disease. Pharm Ther 2005;107:120–130.
2. Bonakdar RA, Guarneri E. Coenzyme Q10. Am Fam Physician 2005; 72(6):1065–1070.
3. Isobe C, Abe T, Terayama Y. Levels of reduced and oxidized coenzyme Q-10 and 9-hydroxy-2′-deoxyguanosine in the cerebrospinal fluid of patients with living Parkinson's disease demonstrate that mitochondrial oxidative damage and/or oxidative DNA damage contributes to the neurodegenerative process. Neurosci Lett 2010;469:159–163.
4. Shults C, Oakes D, Kieburtz K, et al. Effects of coenzyme $Q_{10}$ in early Parkinson's disease. Arch Neurol 2002;59(10):1541–1550.
5. Muller T, Buttner T, Gholipour A, Kuhn W. Coenzyme $Q_{10}$ supplementation provides mild symptomatic benefit in patients with Parkinson's disease. Neurosci Lett 2003;341(3):201–204.
6. The NINDS NET-PD Investigators. A randomized clinical trial of coenzyme $Q_{10}$ and GPI-1485 in early Parkinson disease. Neurology 2007;68:20–28.
7. Storch A, Jost WH, Vieregge P, et al. Randomized, double-blind, placebo-controlled trial on symptomatic effects of coenzyme $Q_{10}$ in Parkinson disease. Arch Neurol 2007;64:E1–E7.
8. Yang L, Calingasan NY, Wille EJ, et al. Combination therapy with coenzyme Q10 and creatine produces additive neuroprotective effects in models of Parkinson's and Huntington's diseases. J Neurochem 2009;109(5):1427–1439.

## CASE 69: CHRONIC PAIN MANAGEMENT

### α-Lipoic Acid for Chronic Pain

*Clinical Course*

At Ms Adams' next follow-up appointment, she is not completely satisfied with her response to the prescription therapy for her neuropathic pain, although she states that her pain has decreased somewhat. She reports that she read an article on α-lipoic acid in a health magazine last week and wonders if it might be a good product to try. All other disease states are stable on current therapies.

## FOLLOW-UP QUESTIONS

1. What is the known or proposed mechanism of action of α-lipoic acid?
2. How extensive or conclusive are the clinical trial data on effectiveness?
3. What is known about safety?
4. Does the product have any specific quality concerns?
5. Would this be an appropriate treatment choice in this particular patient?
6. If the patient is going to use the product, what counseling information will allow her to maximize any possible benefit and minimize any harm?

## REFERENCES


1. Shay KP, Moreau RF, Smith EJ, Smith AR, Hagen TM. Alpha-lipoic acid as a dietary supplement: molecular mechanisms and therapeutic potential. Biochim Biophys Acta 2009;1790:1149–1160.
2. Packer L, Kraemer K, Rimbach G. Molecular aspects of lipoic acid in the prevention of diabetes complications. Nutrition 2001;17:888–895.
3. Ziegler D, Nowak H, Kempler P, et al. Treatment of symptomatic diabetic polyneuropathy with the antioxidant alpha-lipoic acid: a meta-analysis. Diabet Med 2004;21:114–121.
4. Ziegler D, Hanefeld M, Ruhnau K-J, et al. Treatment of symptomatic diabetic polyneuropathy with the antioxidant α-lipoic acid. Diabetes Care 1999;22:1296–1301.
5. Zeigler D, Ametov A, Barinov A, et al. Oral treatment with alpha-lipoic acid improves symptomatic diabetic polyneuropathy. Diabetes Care 2006;29:2365–2370.
6. Kamenova P. Improvement of insulin sensitivity in patients with type 2 diabetes mellitus after oral administration of alpha-lipoic acid. Int J Endocrinol Metab 2007;5:251–258.
7. Evans JL, Heymann CJ, Goldfine ID, Gavin LA. Pharmacokinetics, tolerability and fructosamine-lowering effect of a novel, controlled-release formulation of alpha-lipoic acid. Endocr Pract 2002;8:29–34.
8. Konrad T, Vicini P, Kusterer K, et al. Alpha-lipoic acid treatment decreases serum lactate and pyruvate concentrations and improves glucose effectiveness in lean and obese patients with type 2 diabetes. Diabetes Care 1999;22:280–287.
9. Packer L, Witt EH, Tritschler HJ. Alpha-lipoic acid as a biological antioxidant. Free Radic Biol Med 1995;19:227–250.
10. Foster TS. Efficacy and safety of α-lipoic acid supplementation in the treatment of symptomatic diabetic neuropathy. Diabetes Educ 2007;33:111–117.


## CASE 71: MIGRAINE HEADACHE

### Butterbur and Feverfew for Prevention of Migraine

*Clinical Course*

While discussing possible changes from her valproic acid therapy, Ms Miller says that a friend who also has migraines had read about some herbal remedies used for migraine prevention. She asks whether any products like that could be used instead of or along with her prescription medications. Ms Miller is very interested in a more "natural" therapy, but only if it could really reduce the number of her migraines.

## FOLLOW-UP QUESTIONS

### Butterbur

1. What is the known or proposed mechanism of action?
2. How extensive or conclusive are the clinical trial data on effectiveness?
3. What is known about safety?
4. Does the product have any specific quality concerns?
5. Would this be an appropriate treatment choice in this particular patient?
6. If the patient is going to use the product, what counseling information will allow her to maximize any possible benefit and minimize any harm?

### Feverfew

1. What is the known or proposed mechanism of action?
2. How extensive or conclusive are the clinical trial data on effectiveness?
3. What is known about safety?
4. Does the product have any specific quality concerns?
5. Would this be an appropriate treatment choice in this particular patient?
6. If the patient is going to use the product, what counseling information will allow her to maximize any possible benefit and minimize any harm?
7. Between the two products, which might be a better choice for Ms Miller?

## REFERENCES


1. Lee DK, Haggart K, Robb FM, Lipworth BJ. Butterbur, a herbal remedy, confers complementary anti-inflammatory activity in asthmatic patients receiving inhaled corticosteroids. Clin Exp Allergy 2004;34:110–114.
2. Agosti R, Duke RK, Chrubasik JE, Chrubasik S. Effectiveness of *Petasites hybridus* preparations in the prophylaxis of migraine: a systematic review. Phytomedicine 2006;13:743–746.
3. Horak S, Koschak A, Stuppner H, Streissnig J. Use-dependent block of voltage-gated Cav2.1 $Ca^{2+}$ channels by petasins and eudesmol isomers. J Pharmacol Exp Ther 2009;330:220–226.
4. Grossmann M, Schmidramsl H. An extract of *Petasites hybridus* is effective in the prophylaxis of migraine. Int J Clin Pharmacol Ther 2000;38:430–435.
5. Lipton RB, Göbel H, Einhäupl KM, et al. *Petasites hybridus* root (butterbur) is an effective preventative treatment for migraine. Neurology 2004;63:2240–2244.
6. Oelkers-Ax R, Leins A, Parzer P, et al. Butterbur root extract and music therapy in the prevention of childhood migraine: an explorative study. Eur J Pain 2008;12:301–313.
7. Pothmann R, Danesch U. Migraine prevention in children and adolescents: results of an open study with a special butterbur root extract. Headache 2005;45:196–203.
8. Diener HC, Rahlfs VW, Danesch U. The first placebo-controlled trial of a special butterbur root extract for the prevention of migraine: reanalysis of efficacy criteria. Eur Neurol 2004;51:89–97.
9. Giles M, Ulbricht C, Khalsa KP, Kirkwood CD, Park C, Basch E. Butterbur: an evidence-based systematic review by the Natural Standard Research Collaboration. J Herb Pharmacother 2005;5:119–143.
10. Anderson N, Meier T, Borlak J. Toxicogenomics applied to cultures of human hepatocytes enabled an identification of novel *Petasites hybridus* extracts for the treatment of migraine with improved hepatobiliary safety. Toxicol Sci 2009;112:507–520.
11. Wang YP, Yan J, Fu PP, Chou MW. Human liver microsomal reduction of pyrrolizidine alkaloid N-oxides to form the corresponding carcinogenic parent alkaloid. Toxicol Lett 2005;155:411–420.
12. Calhoun AH, Hutchinson S. Hormonal therapies for menstrual migraine. Curr Pain Headache Rep 2009;13:381–385.
13. Tassorelli C, Greco R, Morazzoni P, Riva A, Sandrini G, Nappi G. Parthenolide is the component of *Tanacetum parthenium* that inhibits nitroglycerin-induced Fos activation: studies in an animal model of migraine. Cephalalgia 2005;25:612–621.

14. Pittler MH, Ernst E. Feverfew for preventing migraine. Cochrane Database Syst Rev 2000;(3):CD002286.
15. Pfaffenrath V, Diener HC, Fischer M, et al. The efficacy and safety of *Tanacetum parthenium* (feverfew) in migraine prophylaxis—a double-blind, multicentre, randomized placebo-controlled dose-response study. Cephalalgia 2002;22:523–532.
16. Diener HC, Pfeffenrath V, Schnitker J, et al. Efficacy and safety of 6.25 mg t.i.d. feverfew $CO_2$-extract (MIG-99) in migraine prevention—a randomized, double-blind, multicentre, placebo-controlled study. Cephalalgia 2005;25:1031–1041.
17. Unger M, Frank A. Simultaneous determination of the inhibitory potency of herbal extracts on the activity of six major cytochrome P450 enzymes using liquid chromatography/mass spectrometry and automated online extraction. Rapid Commun Mass Spectrom 2004;18:2273–2281.

## CASE 77: MAJOR DEPRESSION

### St. John's Wort for Depression

*Clinical Course*

Mrs Flowers understands that she must stop the SJW she has been taking because of an interaction with her prescribed mirtazapine, but she wonders if it would have been helpful if she had started it when she first began feeling depressed.

### FOLLOW-UP QUESTIONS

1. What is the known or proposed mechanism of action?
2. How extensive or conclusive are the clinical trial data on effectiveness?
3. What is known about safety?
4. Does the product have any specific quality concerns?
5. Would this be an appropriate treatment choice in this particular patient?
6. If the patient is going to use the product, what counseling information will allow her to maximize any possible benefit and minimize any harm?

## REFERENCES

1. Singer A, Wonnemann M, Mueller W. Hyperforin, a major antidepressant constituent of St. John's wort, inhibits serotonin uptake by elevating free intracellular sodium. J Pharmacol Exp Ther 1999;290:1363–1368.
2. Butterweck V. Mechanism of action of St. John's wort in depression: what is known? CNS Drugs 2003;17:539–562.
3. Bennett DA Jr, Phun L, Polk JF, et al. Neuropharmacology of St. John's wort (*Hypericum*). Ann Pharmacother 1998;32:1201–1208.
4. Schrader E. Equivalence of St. John's wort extract (Ze 117) and fluoxetine: a randomized, controlled study in mild–moderate depression. Int Clin Psychopharmacol 2000;15:61–68.
5. Szegedi A, Kohnen R, Dienel A, Kieser M. Acute treatment of moderate to severe depression with *Hypericum* extract WS 5570 (St. John's wort): randomized controlled double blind non-inferiority trial versus paroxetine. BMJ 2005;333:503–506.
6. Bjerkenstedt L, Edman GV, Alken RG, Mannel M. *Hypericum* extract LI 160 and fluoxetine in mild to moderate depression. Eur Arch Psychiatry Clin Neurosci 2005;255:40–47.
7. Randlov C, Mehlsen J, Thomsen CF, et al. The efficacy of St. John's wort in patients with minor depressive symptoms or dysthymia—a double-blind placebo-controlled study. Phytomedicine 2006;13:215–221.
8. Hypericum Depression Trial Study Group. Effect of *Hypericum perofratum* (St. John's wort) in major depressive disorder. JAMA 2002;287:1807–1814.
9. Anghelescu IG, Kohnen R, Szegedi A, Klement S, Kieser M. Comparison of *Hypericum* extract WS 5570 and paroxetine in ongoing treatment after recovery from an episode of moderate to severe depression: results from a randomized multicenter study. Pharmacopsychiatry 2006;39:213–219.
10. Kaspar S, Volz HP, Möller HJ, Dienel A, Kieser M. Continuation and long-term maintenance treatment with *Hypericum* extract WS® 5570 after recovery from an acute episode of moderate depression—a double-blind, randomized, placebo-controlled long-term trial. Eur Neuropsychopharmacol 2008;18:803–813.
11. Shelton RC. St. John's wort (*Hypericum perforatum*) in major depression. J Clin Psychiatry 2009;70(Suppl 5):23–27.
12. Linde K, Berner MM, Kriston L. St. John's wort for major depression. Cochrane Database Syst Rev 2008;(4):CD000448.
13. Rahimi R, Nikfar S, Abdollahi M. Efficacy and tolerability of *Hypericum perforatum* in major depressive disorder in comparison with selective serotonin reuptake inhibitors: a meta-analysis. Prog Neuropsychopharmacol Biol Psychiatry 2009;33:118–127.
14. Fetrow CW, Avila JR. Professional's Handbook of Complementary & Alternative Medicines. Philadelphia, PA, Lippincott Williams & Wilkins, 2004:798–802.
15. Hennessy M, Kelleher D, Spiers JP, et al. St Johns wort increases expression of P-glycoprotein: implications for drug interactions. Br J Clin Pharmacol 2002;53:75–82.
16. Parker V, Wong AH, Boon HS, Seeman MV. Adverse reactions to St John's wort. Can J Psychiatry 2001;46:77–79.
17. Beckman SE, Sommi RW, Switzer J. Consumer use of St. John's wort: a survey on effectiveness, safety, and tolerability. Pharmacotherapy 2000;20(5):568–574.

## CASE 79: GENERALIZED ANXIETY DISORDER

### Kava for Anxiety

*Clinical Course*

Mr Johnson is still worried about both the side effects of prescription drugs to treat his anxiety and whether he will be able to afford them. He states that he has read a lot of information about kava, that "it really works for anxiety." Mr Johnson says, "maybe I was just using a bad product last time I tried it and that's why it didn't help much and hurt my stomach. Should I get a better product and try it again?"

### FOLLOW-UP QUESTIONS

1. What is the known or proposed mechanism of action?
2. How extensive or conclusive are the clinical trial data on effectiveness?
3. What is known about safety?
4. Does the product have any specific quality concerns?
5. Would this be an appropriate treatment choice in this particular patient?
6. If the patient is going to use the product, what counseling information will allow him to maximize any possible benefit and minimize any harm?

## REFERENCES

1. Singh YN, Singh NN. Therapeutic potential of kava in the treatment of anxiety disorders. CNS Drugs 2002;16:731–743.
2. Boonen G, Ferger B, Kuschinsky K, et al. Influence of genuine kavapyrone enantiomers on the GABA-A binding site. Planta Med 1998;64:504–506.
3. Sarris J, Kavanagh DJ. Kava and St. John's wort: current evidence for use in mood and anxiety disorders. J Altern Complement Med 2009;15:827–836.
4. Pittler M, Ernst E. Efficacy of kava extract for treating anxiety: systematic review and meta-analysis. J Clin Psychopharmacol 2000;20:84–89.

5. Pittler M, Ernst E. Kava extract versus placebo for treating anxiety. Cochrane Database Syst Rev 2003;1:CD003383.
6. Witte S, Loew D, Gaus W. Meta-analysis of the efficacy of the acetonic kava-kava WS® 1490 in patients with non-psychotic anxiety disorders. Phytother Res 2005;19:183–188.
7. Woelk H, Kapoula S, Lehrl S, et al. Treatment of patients suffering from anxiety. Double-blind study: kava special extract versus benzodiazepines. Z Allegemeinmed 1993;69:271–277.
8. Boerner RJ, Sommer H, Berger W, et al. Kava-kava extract LI 150 is as effective as opipramol and buspirone in generalised anxiety disorder—an 8-week randomized, double-blind multi-centre clinical trial in 129 out-patients. Phytomedicine 2003;10:38–49.
9. Geier FP, Konstantinowicz T. Kava treatment in patients with anxiety. Phytother Res 2004;18:297–300.
10. Lehrl S. Clinical efficacy of kava extract WS® 1490 in sleep disturbances associated with anxiety disorders. Results of a multicenter, randomized, placebo-controlled, double-blind clinical trial. J Affect Disord 2004;78:101–110.
11. Sarris J, Kavanagh DJ, Byrne G, et al. The kava anxiety depression spectrum study (KADSS): a randomized, placebo-controlled crossover trial using an aqueous extract of *Piper methysticum*. Psychopharmacology 2009;205:399–407.
12. Stevinson C, Huntley A, Ernst E. A systematic review of the safety of kava extract in the treatment of anxiety. Drug Saf 2002;25:251–261.
13. Anonymous. Kava concerns. FDA, Botanical Council raises safety concerns. AWHONN Lifelines 2002;6(1):13–15.
14. Sarris J, Adams J, Wardle JL. Time for a reassessment of the use of kava in anxiety? Complement Ther Med 2009;17:121–122.
15. Zou L, Henderson GL, Harkey MR, Sakai Y, Li A. Effects of kava (kava-kava, 'awa, yaqona, *Piper methysticum*) on c-DNA-expressed cytochrome P450 enzymes and human cryopreserved hepatocytes. Phytomedicine 2004;11:285–294.
16. Mathews JM, Etheridge AS, Valentine JL, et al. Pharmacokinetics and disposition of the kavalactone kawain: interaction with kava extract and kavalactones in vivo and in vitro. Drug Metab Dispos 2005;33:1555–1563.
17. Gurley BJ, Swain A, Hubbard MA, et al. Supplementation with goldenseal (*Hydrastis canadensis*), but not kava kava (*Piper methysticum*), inhibits human CYP3A activity in vivo. Clin Pharmacol Ther 2008;83:61–69.

## CASE 95: MANAGING MENOPAUSAL SYMPTOMS

### Black Cohosh and Soy for Menopausal Symptoms

*Clinical Course*

Because Mrs Peterson is considering stopping her HT due to her family history of breast cancer but still desires some relief from hot flushes, she asks for additional information on other alternatives. She has heard that black cohosh should not be used in women with breast cancer, but she has a friend who also has a family history of breast cancer who has been on black cohosh for about 9 months on the recommendation of her physician, although the friend must have a checkup with lab tests every 6 months. Mrs Peterson asks if black cohosh or soy would be an appropriate option to help keep her hot flushes under control.

## FOLLOW-UP QUESTIONS

### Black Cohosh

1. What is the known or proposed mechanism of action?
2. How extensive or conclusive are the clinical trial data on effectiveness?
3. What is known about safety?
4. Does the product have any specific quality concerns?
5. Would this be an appropriate treatment choice in this particular patient?
6. If the patient is going to use the product, what counseling information will allow her to maximize any possible benefit and minimize any harm?

### Soy

1. What is the known or proposed mechanism of action?
2. How extensive or conclusive are the clinical trial data on effectiveness?
3. What is known about safety?
4. Does the product have any specific quality concerns?
5. Would this be an appropriate treatment choice in this particular patient?
6. If the patient is going to use the product, what counseling information will allow her to maximize any possible benefit and minimize any harm?

## REFERENCES

1. Fetrow CW, Avila JR. Professional's Handbook of Complementary & Alternative Medicines. Philadelphia, PA, Lippincott Williams & Wilkins, 2004:103–107.
2. Borrelli F, Izzo AA, Ernst E. Pharmacological effects of *Cimicifuga racemosa*. Life Sci 2003;73:1215–1229.
3. Kretzchmar G, Nisslein T, Zierau O, Vollmer G. No estrogen-like effects of an isopropanolic extract of Rhizoma Cimicifugae racemosae on uterus and vena cava of rata after 17 day treatment. J Sci Biochem Mol Biol 2005;97:271–277.
4. Ruhlen RL, Haubner J, Tracy JK, et al. Black cohosh does not exert an estrogenic effect on the breast. Nutr Cancer 2007;59:269–277.
5. Osmers R, Friede M, Liske E, et al. Efficacy and safety of isopropanolic black cohosh extract for climacteric symptoms. Obstet Gynecol 2005;105(5 Pt 1):1074–1083.
6. Bai W, Henneicke-van Zepelin H-H, Wang S, et al. Efficacy and tolerability of a medicinal product containing an isopropanolic black cohosh extract in Chinese women with menopausal symptoms: a randomized, double blind, parallel-controlled study versus tibolone. Maturitas 2007;58:31–41.
7. Frei-Kleiner S, Schaffner W, Rahlfs VW, et al. *Cimicifuga racemosa* dried ethanolic extract in menopausal disorders: a double-blind placebo-controlled clinical trial. Maturitas 2005;51:397–404.
8. Pockaj BA, Gallagher JG, Loprinzi CL, et al. Phase III double-blind, randomized, placebo-controlled crossover trial of black cohosh in the management of hot flashes: NCCTG Trial N01CC. J Clin Oncol 2007;24:2836–2841.
9. Hernández Munoz G, Pluchino S. *Cimicifuga racemosa* for the treatment of hot flushes in women surviving breast cancer. Maturitas 2003;44(Suppl 1):S59–S65.
10. Jacobson JS, Troxel AB, Evans J, et al. Randomized trial of black cohosh for the treatment of hot flashes among women with a history of breast cancer. J Clin Oncol 2001;19:2739–2745.
11. Borrelli F, Ernst E. Black cohosh (*Cimicifuga racemosa*) for menopausal symptoms: a systematic review of its efficacy. Pharmacol Res 2008;58:8–14.
12. Palacio C, Masi G, Mooradian AD. Black cohosh for the management of menopausal symptoms. A systematic review of clinical trials. Drugs Aging 2009;26:23–36.
13. Shams T, Setia MS, Hemmings R, McCusker J, Sewitch Clampi A. Efficacy of black cohosh-containing preparations on menopausal symptoms: a meta-analysis. Altern Ther 2010;16:36–44.
14. Dinman S. Black cohosh [sic]: a contraindication in general anesthesia. Plast Surg Nurs 2006;26:42–43.
15. Borrelli F, Ernst E. Black cohosh (*Cimicifuga racemosa*): a systematic review of adverse events. Am J Obstet Gynecol 2008;199:455–456.

16. Setchell KD. Absorption and metabolism of soy isoflavones—from food to dietary supplements and adults to infants. J Nutr 2000;130:654S–655S.
17. Zand RS, Jenkins DJ, Diamandis EP. Steroid hormone activity of flavonoids and related compounds. Breast Cancer Res Treat 2000;62:35–49.
18. Duncan AM, Underhill KE, Xu X, et al. Modest hormonal effects of soy isoflavones in postmenopausal women. J Clin Endocrinol Metab 1999; 84:3479–3484.
19. Ginsburg J, Prelevic GM. Lack of significant hormonal effects and controlled trials of phyto-oestrogens. Lancet 2000;355:163–164.
20. Balk JL, Whiteside DA, Naus G, et al. A pilot study of the effects of phytoestrogen supplementation on postmenopausal endometrium. J Soc Gynecol Invest 2002;9:238–242.
21. Brown BD, Thomas W, Hutchins A, et al. Types of dietary fat and soy minimally affect hormones and biomarkers associated with breast cancer risk in premenopausal women. Nutr Cancer 2002;43:22–30.
22. Burke GL, Legault C, Anthony M, et al. Soy protein and isoflavone effects on vasomotor symptoms in per- and postmenopausal women: the soy estrogen alternative study. Menopause 2002;10:147–153.
23. Faure ED, Chantre P, Mares P. Effects of a standardized soy extract on hot flushes: a multicenter, double-blind, randomized, placebo-controlled study. Menopause 2002;9:329–334.
24. Secreto G, Chiechi LM, Amadori A, et al. Soy isoflavones and melatonin for the relief of climacteric symptoms: a multicenter, double-blind, randomized study. Maturitas 2004;47:11–20.
25. St. Germain A, Peterson CT, Robinson JG, Alekel L. Isoflavone-rich or isoflavone-poor soy protein does not reduce menopausal symptoms during 24 weeks of treatment. Menopause 2001;8:17–26.
26. Huntley AL, Ernst E. Soy for the treatment of perimenopausal symptoms—a systematic review. Maturitas 2004;47:1–9.
27. Krebs EE, Ensrud KE, MacDonald R, Wilt TJ. Phytoestrogens for treatment of menopausal symptoms: a systematic review. Obstet Gynecol 2004;104:824–836.
28. Jacobs A, Wegewitz U, Sommerfeld C, Grossklaus R. Efficacy of isoflavones in relieving vasomotor menopausal symptoms—a systematic review. Mol Nutr Food Res 2009;53:1084–1097.
29. Ma D-F, Qin L-Q, Wang P-Y, Katoh R. Soy isoflavone intake increases bone mineral density in the spine of menopausal women: meta-analysis of randomized controlled trials. Clin Nutr 2008;27:57–64.
30. Poulsen RC, Kruger MC. Soy phytoestrogens: impact on postmenopausal bone loss and mechanisms of action. Nutr Rev 2008;66:359–374.
31. Kwak HS, Park SY, Kim MG, et al. Marked individual variation in isoflavone metabolism after a soy challenge can modulate the skeletal effect of isoflavones in premenopausal women. J Korean Med Sci 2009;24:867–873.
32. Wu J, Oka J, Ezaki J, et al. Possible role of equol status in the effects of isoflavone on bone and fat mass in postmenopausal Japanese women: a double-blind, randomized, controlled trial. Menopause 2007;14:866–874.
33. Reynolds K, Chin A, Lees KA, et al. A meta-analysis of the effect of soy protein supplementation on serum lipids. Am J Cardiol 2006;98:633–640.
34. Divi RL, Chang HC, Doerge DR. Anti-thyroid isoflavones from soybean: isolation, characterization, and mechanisms of action. Biochem Pharmacol 1997;54:1087–1096.
35. Welty FK, Lee KS, Lew NS, et al. The association between soy nut consumption and decreased menopausal symptoms. J Womens Health 2007;6:361–369.

## CASE 97: BENIGN PROSTATIC HYPERPLASIA

### Pygeum africanum for BPH

*Clinical Course*

As the pharmacist on the team, you perform a literature search on the use of saw palmetto for BPH. You discover that there are reports of the dietary supplement both improving and worsening symptoms of erectile dysfunction (ED).[1,2] Because the patient's ED symptoms began while he was taking saw palmetto, you decide that it is plausible that saw palmetto could be contributing to ED symptoms. In addition, your readings indicate that saw palmetto should really only be used by patients with mild to moderate BPH. Based on this information, your recommendation is to stop the saw palmetto. However, because the patient is emphatic about wanting to continue a natural product, you search for alternative dietary supplements that may provide some benefit for this patient's BPH without contributing to ED. Would pygeum (African plum, *P. africanum*) be a reasonable option to consider?

### FOLLOW-UP QUESTIONS

1. What is the known or proposed mechanism of action?
2. How extensive or conclusive are the clinical trial data on effectiveness?
3. What is known about safety?
4. Does the product have any specific quality concerns?
5. Would this be an appropriate treatment choice in this particular patient?
6. If the patient is going to use the product, what counseling information will allow him to maximize any possible benefit and minimize any harm?

## REFERENCES

1. Boyle P, Robertson C, Lowe F, Roehrborn C. Updated meta-analysis of clinical trials of *Serenoa repens* extract in the treatment of symptomatic benign prostatic hyperplasia. BJU Int 2004;93:751–756.
2. Gerber G, Kuznetsov D, Johnson B, Burstein J. Randomized, double blind, placebo controlled trial of saw palmetto in men with lower urinary tract symptoms. Urology 2001;58:960–965.
3. McQueen CE, Bryant PJ. Pygeum for benign prostatic hypertrophy. Am J Health Syst Pharm 2000;58:120–123.
4. Levin RM, Das AK. A scientific basis for the therapeutic effects of *Pygeum africanum* and *Serenoa repens*. Urol Res 2000;28:201–209.
5. Boulbès D, Soustelle L, Costa P, et al. *Pygeum africanum* extract inhibits proliferation of human cultured prostatic fibroblasts and myofibroblasts. BJU Int 2006;98:1106–1113.
6. Breza J, Dzurny O, Borowka A, et al. Efficacy and acceptability of Tadenan® (*Pygeum africanum* extract) in the treatment of benign prostatic hyperplasia (BPH): a multicentre trial in central Europe. Curr Med Res Opin 1998;14:127–139.
7. Chatelain C, Autet W, Brackman F. Comparison of once and twice daily dosage forms of *Pygeum africanum* extract in patients with benign prostatic hyperplasia: a randomized, double-blind study, with long-term open label extension. Urology 1999;54:473–478.
8. Ishani A, MacDonald R, Nelson D, Rutks I, Wilt TJ. *Pygeum africanum* for the treatment of patients with benign prostatic hyperplasia: a systematic review and quantitative meta-analysis. Am J Med 2000;109:654–664.
9. Wilt T, Ishani A, MacDonald R, Rutks I, Stark G. *Pygeum africanum* for benign prostatic hyperplasia. Cochrane Database Syst Rev 2002;(1):CD001044.
10. Shenouda NS, Sakla MS, Newton LG, et al. Phytosterol *Pygeum africanum* regulates prostate cancer in vitro and in vivo. Endocrine 2007;31:72–81.

## CASE 107: ALLERGIC RHINITIS

### Butterbur Extract for Allergic Rhinitis

*Clinical Course*

Caleb's mother is quite concerned about drowsiness associated with prescription treatments for his symptoms because he has a tendency to nap when he is supposed to be doing homework. Mrs Thibodeaux uses butterbur extract for migraine prophylaxis and has heard that it is effective for allergy symptoms; she asks about using the same product for Caleb.

## FOLLOW-UP QUESTIONS

1. What is the known or proposed mechanism of action?
2. How extensive or conclusive are the clinical trial data on effectiveness?
3. What is known about safety?
4. Does the product have any specific quality concerns?
5. Would this be an appropriate treatment choice in this particular patient?
6. If the patient is going to use the product, what counseling information will allow him to maximize any possible benefit and minimize any harm?

## REFERENCES


1. Lee DKC, Haggart K, Robb FM, Lipworth BJ. Butterbur, a herbal remedy, confers complementary anti-inflammatory activity in asthmatic patients receiving inhaled corticosteroids. Clin Exp Allergy 2004;34:110–114.
2. Thomet OA, Schapowal A, Heinisch IV, et al. Anti-inflammatory activity of an extract of *Petasites hybridus* in allergic rhinitis. Int Immunopharmacol 2002;2:997–1006.
3. Giles M, Ulbricht C, Khalsa KP, Kirkwood CD, Park C, Basch E. Butterbur: an evidence-based systematic review by the Natural Standard Research Collaboration. J Herb Pharmacother 2005;5:119–143.
4. Schapowal A. Butterbur Ze 339 for the treatment of intermittent allergic rhinitis: dose-dependent efficacy in a prospective, randomized, double-bind, placebo-controlled study. Arch Otolaryngol Head Neck Surg 2004;130:1381–1386.
5. Schapowal A. Treating intermittent allergic rhinitis: a prospective, randomized, placebo and antihistamine-controlled study of butterbur extract Ze 339. Phytother Res 2005;19:530–537.
6. Kaufeler R, Polasek W, Brattstrom A, Koetter U. Efficacy and safety of butterbur herbal extract Ze 339 in seasonal allergic rhinitis: postmarketing surveillance study. Adv Ther 2006;23:373–384.
7. Schapowal A. Randomised controlled trial of butterbur and cetirizine for treating seasonal allergic rhinitis. BMJ 2002;324:144–146.
8. Lee DK, Gray RD, Robb FM, et al. A placebo-controlled evaluation of butterbur and fexofenadine on objective and subjective outcomes in perennial allergic rhinitis. Clin Exp Allergy 2004;34:646–649.
9. Lipton RB, Göbel H, Einhäupl KM, et al. *Petasites hybridus* root (butterbur) is an effective preventative treatment for migraine. Neurology 2004;63:2240–2244.
10. Anderson N, Meier T, Borlak J. Toxicogenomics applied to cultures of human hepatocytes enabled an identification of novel *Petasites hybridus* extracts for the treatment of migraine with improved hepatobiliary safety. Toxicol Sci 2009;112:507–520.
11. Wang YP, Yan J, Fu PP, Chou MW. Human liver microsomal reduction of pyrrolizidine alkaloid N-oxides to form the corresponding carcinogenic parent alkaloid. Toxicol Lett 2005;155:411–420.


## CASE 110: PSORIASIS

### Fish Oil/Omega-3 Fatty Acids for Psoriasis

*Clinical Course*

Because of Mr Kent's frustration with his increased psoriasis flare-ups despite his prescription treatments, he is very interested in trying anything to help decrease his symptoms. A friend who takes fish oil for eczema told him it might help the psoriasis, so he asks about the possibility of adding fish oil on a daily basis.

## FOLLOW-UP QUESTIONS

1. What is the known or proposed mechanism of action?
2. How extensive or conclusive are the clinical trial data on effectiveness?
3. What is known about safety?
4. Does the product have any specific quality concerns?
5. Would this be an appropriate treatment choice in this particular patient?
6. If the patient is going to use the product, what counseling information will allow him to maximize any possible benefit and minimize any harm?

## REFERENCES


1. Fetterman JW Jr, Zdanowicz MM. Therapeutic potential of *n*-3 polyunsaturated fatty acids in disease. Am J Health Syst Pharm 2009;66:1169–1179.
2. Grimm H, Mayer K, Mayser P, Eigenbrodt E. Regulatory potential of *n*-3 fatty acids in immunological and inflammatory processes. Br J Nutr 2002;87(Suppl 1):S59–S67.
3. Curtis CL, Hughes CE, Flannery CR, et al. *n*-3 fatty acids specifically modulate catabolic factors involved in articular cartilage degradation. J Biol Chem 2000;275:721–724.
4. Waitzberg DL, Torrinhas RS. Fish oil lipid emulsions and immune response: what clinicians need to know. Nutr Clin Pract 2009; 24:487–499.
5. Mayser P, Grimm H, Grimminger F. *n*-3 fatty acids in psoriasis. Br J Nutr 2002;87(Suppl 1):S77–S82.
6. Ziboh VA, Cohen KA, Ellis DN, et al. Effects of dietary supplementation of fish oil on neutrophil and epidermal fatty acids. Modulation of clinical course of psoriatic subjects. Arch Dermatol 1986;122:1277–1282.
7. Grimminger F, Mayser P, Papavassilis C, Thomas M, Schlotzer E, Heuer KU. A double-blind, randomized, placebo-controlled trial of *n*-3 fatty acid-based lipid infusion in acute, extended guttate psoriasis. Clin Invest 1993;71:634–643.
8. Frati C, Bevilacqua L, Apostolico V. Association of etretinate and fish oil in psoriasis therapy. Inhibition of hypertriglyceridemia resulting from retinoid therapy after fish oil supplementation. Acta Derm Venereol Suppl (Stockh) 1994;186:151–153.
9. Bittiner SB, Tucker WF, Cartwright I, Bleehen SS. A double-blind, randomised, placebo-controlled trial of fish in psoriasis. Lancet 1988;1:378–380.
10. Stoof TJ, Korstanje MJ, Bilo HJ, et al. Does fish oil protect renal function in cyclosporin-treated psoriasis patients? J Intern Med 1989;226:437–441.
11. Gupta AK, Ellis CN, Tellner DC, et al. Double-blind, placebo-controlled study to evaluate the efficacy of fish oil and low-dose UVB in the treatment of psoriasis. Br J Dermatol 1989;120:801–807.
12. Foran SE, Flood JG, Lewandrowski KB. Measurement of mercury levels in concentrated over-the-counter fish oil preparations: is fish oil healthier than fish? Arch Pathol Lab Med 2003;127: 1603–1605.
13. Smutna M, Kruzikova K, Marsalek P, Kopriva V, Svobodova Z. Fish oil and cod liver as safe and healthy food supplements. Neuroendocrinol Lett 2009;30(Suppl 1):156–162.

# APPENDIX A
# CONVERSION FACTORS AND ANTHROPOMETRICS*

## CONVERSION FACTORS

### SI Units

SI (*le Système International d'Unités*) units are used in many countries to express clinical laboratory and serum drug concentration data. Instead of employing units of mass (such as micrograms), the SI system uses moles (mol) to represent the amount of a substance. A molar solution contains 1 mol (the molecular weight of the substance in grams) of the solute in 1 L of solution. The following formula is used to convert units of mass to moles (mcg/mL to μmol/L or, by substitution of terms, mg/mL to mmol/L or ng/mL to nmol/L).

*Micromoles per Liter (μmol/L)*

$$\mu\text{mol/L} = \frac{\text{drug concentration (mcg/mL)} \times 1{,}000}{\text{molecular weight of drug (g/mol)}}$$

*Milliequivalents*

An equivalent weight of a substance is that weight which will combine with or replace 1 g of hydrogen; a milliequivalent is 1/1,000 of an equivalent weight.

**Milliequivalents per Liter (mEq/L)**

$$\text{mEq/L} = \frac{\text{weight of salt (g)} \times \text{valence of ion} \times 1{,}000}{\text{molecular weight of salt}}$$

$$\text{weight of salt (g)} = \frac{\text{mEq/L} \times \text{molecular weight of salt}}{\text{valence of ion} \times 1{,}000}$$

**Approximate Milliequivalents**

**Weights of Selected Ions**

| Salt | mEq/g Salt | mg Salt/mEq |
|---|---|---|
| Calcium carbonate ($CaCO_3$) | 20.0 | 50.0 |
| Calcium chloride ($CaCl_2 \cdot 2H_2O$) | 13.6 | 73.5 |
| Calcium gluceptate ($Ca[C_7H_{13}O_8]_2$) | 4.1 | 245.2 |
| Calcium gluconate ($Ca[C_6H_{11}O_7]_2 \cdot H_2O$) | 4.5 | 224.1 |
| Calcium lactate ($Ca[C_3H_5O_3]_2 \cdot 5H_2O$) | 6.5 | 154.1 |
| Magnesium gluconate ($Mg[C_6H_{11}O_7]_2 \cdot H_2O$) | 4.6 | 216.3 |
| Magnesium oxide (MgO) | 49.6 | 20.2 |
| Magnesium sulfate ($MgSO_4$) | 16.6 | 60.2 |
| Magnesium sulfate ($MgSO_4 \cdot 7H_2O$) | 8.1 | 123.2 |
| Potassium acetate ($K[C_2H_3O_2]$) | 10.2 | 98.1 |
| Potassium chloride (KCl) | 13.4 | 74.6 |
| Potassium citrate ($K_3[C_6H_5O_7] \cdot H_2O$) | 9.2 | 108.1 |
| Potassium iodide (KI) | 6.0 | 166.0 |
| Sodium acetate ($Na[C_2H_3O_2]$) | 12.2 | 82.0 |
| Sodium acetate ($Na[C_2H_3O_2] \cdot 3H_2O$) | 7.3 | 136.1 |
| Sodium bicarbonate ($NaHCO_3$) | 11.9 | 84.0 |
| Sodium chloride (NaCl) | 17.1 | 58.4 |
| Sodium citrate ($Na_3[C_6H_5O_7] \cdot 2H_2O$) | 10.2 | 98.0 |
| Sodium iodide (NaI) | 6.7 | 149.9 |
| Sodium lactate ($Na[C_3H_5O_3]$) | 8.9 | 112.1 |
| Zinc sulfate ($ZnSO_4 \cdot 7H_2O$) | 7.0 | 143.8 |

### Valences and Atomic Weights of Selected Ions

| Substance | Electrolyte | Valence | Molecular Weight |
|---|---|---|---|
| Calcium | $Ca^{2+}$ | 2 | 40.1 |
| Chloride | $Cl^-$ | 1 | 35.5 |
| Magnesium | $Mg^{2+}$ | 2 | 24.3 |
| Phosphate (pH = 7.4) | $HPO_4^-$ (80%)<br>$H2PO_4^-$ (20%) | 1.8 | 96.0[a] |
| Potassium | $K^+$ | 1 | 39.1 |
| Sodium | $Na^+$ | 1 | 23.0 |
| Sulfate | $SO_4^-$ | 2 | 96.0[a] |

[a]The molecular weight of phosphorus only is 31; that of sulfur only is 32.1.

*This appendix contains information from Appendices 1 and 2 of Anderson PO, Knoben JE, Troutman WG, et al (eds). *Handbook of Clinical Drug Data,* 10th ed. New York: McGraw-Hill, 2002:1053–1058, with permission.

## Anion Gap

The anion gap is the concentration of plasma anions not routinely measured by laboratory screening. It is useful in the evaluation of acid-base disorders. The anion gap is greater with increased plasma concentrations of endogenous species (e.g., phosphate, sulfate, lactate, and ketoacids) or exogenous species (e.g., salicylate, penicillin, ethylene glycol, ethanol, and methanol). The formulas for calculating the anion gap are as follows:

$$\text{Anion gap} = (Na^+ + K^+) - (Cl^- + HCO_3^-)$$

*or*

$$\text{Anion gap} = Na^+ - (Cl^- + HCO_3)$$

where the expected normal value for the first equation is 11 to 20 mmol/L, and the expected normal value for the second equation is 7 to 16 mmol/L. Note that there is a variation in the upper and lower limits of the normal range.

## Temperature

Fahrenheit to Centigrade: (°F – 32) × 5/9 = °C
Centigrade to Fahrenheit: (°C × 9/5) + 32 = °F
Centigrade to Kelvin: °C + 273 = °K

## Calories

1 calorie = 1 kilocalorie = 1,000 calories = 4.184 kilojoules (kJ)
1 kilojoule = 0.239 calories = 0.239 kilocalories = 239 calories

## Weights and Measures

### *Metric Weight Equivalents*

1 kilogram (kg) = 1,000 grams
1 gram (g) = 1,000 milligrams
1 milligram (mg) = 0.001 gram
1 microgram (mcg, μg) = 0.001 milligram
1 nanogram (ng) = 0.001 microgram
1 picogram (pg) = 0.001 nanogram
1 femtogram (fg) = 0.001 picogram

### *Metric Volume Equivalents*

1 liter (L) = 1,000 milliliters
1 deciliter (dL) = 100 milliliters
1 milliliter (mL) = 0.001 liter
1 microliter (μL) = 0.001 milliliter
1 nanoliter (nL) = 0.001 microliter
1 picoliter (pL) = 0.001 nanoliter
1 femtoliter (fL) = 0.001 picoliter

### *Apothecary Weight Equivalents*

1 scruple (℈) = 20 grains (gr)
60 grains (gr) = 1 dram (ʒ)
8 drams (ʒ) = 1 ounce (fl℥)
1 ounce (℥) = 480 grains
12 ounces (℥) = 1 pound (lb)

### *Apothecary Volume Equivalents*

60 minims (♏) = 1 fluidram (flʒ)
8 fluidrams (flʒ) = 1 fluid ounce (fl℥)
1 fluid ounce (ft℥) = 480 minims
16 fluid ounces (fl℥) = 1 pint (pt)

### *Avoirdupois Equivalents*

1 ounce (oz) = 437.5 grains
16 ounces (oz) = 1 pound (lb)

### *Weight/Volume Equivalents*

1 mg/dL = 10 mcg/mL
1 mg/dL = 1 mg%
1 ppm = 1 mg/L

### *Conversion Equivalents*

1 gram (g) = 15.43 grains
1 grain (gr) = 64.8 milligrams
1 ounce (℥) = 31.1 grams
1 ounce (oz) = 28.35 grams
1 pound (lb) = 453.6 grams
1 kilogram (kg) = 2.2 pounds
1 milliliter (mL) = 16.23 minims
1 minim (♏) = 0.06 milliliter
1 fluid ounce (fl oz) = 29.57 milliliter
1 pint (pt) = 473.2 milliliter
0.1 milligram = 1/600 grain
0.12 milligram = 1/500 grain
0.15 milligram = 1/400 grain
0.2 milligram = 1/300 grain
0.3 milligram = 1/200 grain
0.4 milligram = 1/150 grain
0.5 milligram = 1/120 grain
0.6 milligram = 1/100 grain
0.8 milligram = 1/80 grain
1 milligram = 1/65 grain

### *Metric Length Equivalents*

2.54 cm = 1 inch
30.48 cm = 1 foot
1.6 km = 1 mile

# ANTHROPOMETRICS

## Creatinine Clearance Formulas

### *Formulas for Estimating Creatinine Clearance in Patients with Stable Renal Function*

**Cockroft-Gault Formula**

Adults (age 18 years and older)[1]:

$$\text{CLcr (males)} = \frac{(140 - \text{age}) \times \text{weight}}{Cr_s \times 72}$$

$$\text{CLcr (females)} = 0.85 \times \text{above value}^*$$

where CLcr is creatinine clearance (in mL/minute), $Cr_s$ is serum creatinine (in mg/dL), age is in years, and weight is in kilograms.

*Some studies suggest that the predictive accuracy of this formula for women is better *without* the correction factor of 0.85.

Children (age 1 to 18 years)[2]:

$$\text{CLcr} = \frac{0.48 \times \text{height} \times \text{BSA}}{Cr_s \times 1.73}$$

where BSA is body surface area (in $m^2$), CLcr is creatinine clearance (in mL/minute), $Cr_s$ is serum creatinine (in mg/dL), and height is in centimeters.

*Formula for Estimating Creatinine Clearance from a Measured Urine Collection*

$$\text{CLcr (mL/minute)} = \frac{U \times V^*}{P \times T}$$

where $U$ is the concentration of creatinine in a urine specimen (in same units as $P$), $V$ is the volume of urine (in mL), $P$ is the concentration of creatinine in serum at the midpoint of the urine collection period (in same units as $U$), and $T$ is the time of the urine collection period in minutes (e.g., 6 hours = 360 minutes; 24 hours = 1,440 minutes).

*The product of $U \times V$ equals the production of creatinine during the collection period and, at steady state, should equal 20 to 25 mg/kg per day for ideal body weight (IBW) in males and 15 to 20 mg/kg per day for IBW in females. If it is less than this, inadequate urine collection may have occurred, and CLcr will be underestimated.

*MDRD Formula for Estimating Glomerular Filtration Rate (from the Modification of Diet in Renal Disease Study)*[3]

Conventional calibration MDRD equation (used only with those creatinine methods that have not been recalibrated to be traceable to isotope dilution mass spectrometry [IDMS]).

For creatinine in mg/dL:

$$X = 186\ \text{creatinine}^{-1.154} \times \text{age}^{-0.203} \times \text{constant}$$

For creatinine in μmol/L:

$$X = 32{,}788 \times \text{creatinine}^{-1.154} \times \text{age}^{-0.203} \times \text{constant}$$

where $X$ is the glomerular filtration rate (GFR), constant for white males is 1 and for females is 0.742, and constant for African Americans is 1.21. Creatinine levels in μmol/L can be converted to mg/dL by dividing by 88.4.

*IDMS-Traceable MDRD Equation (Used Only with Creatinine Methods That Have Been Recalibrated to Be Traceable to IDMS)*

For creatinine in mg/dL:

$$X = 175 \times \text{creatinine}^{-1.154} \times \text{age}^{-0.203} \times \text{constant}$$

For creatinine in μmol/L:

$$X = 175 \times (\text{creatinine}/88.4)^{-1.154} \times \text{age}^{-0.203} \times \text{constant}$$

where $X$ is the glomerular filtration rate (GFR), constant for white males is 1 and for females is 0.742, and constant for African Americans is 1.21.

## Ideal Body Weight (IBW)

IBW is the weight expected for a nonobese person of a given height. The IBW formulas below and various life insurance tables can be used to estimate IBW. Dosing methods described in the literature may use IBW as a method in dosing obese patients.

Adults (age 18 years and older)[4]:

$$\text{IBW (males)} = 50 + (2.3 \times \text{height in inches over 5 ft})$$

$$\text{IBW (females)} = 45.5 + (2.3 \times \text{height in inches over 5 ft})$$

where IBW is in kilograms.

Children (age 1 to 18 years)[2]:

Under 5 feet tall:

$$\text{IBW} = \frac{\text{height}^2 \times 1.65}{1{,}000}$$

where IBW is in kilograms and height is in centimeters.

Five feet or taller:

$$\text{IBW (males)} = 39 + (2.27 \times \text{height in inches over 5 ft})$$

$$\text{IBW (females)} = 42.2 + (2.27 \times \text{height in inches over 5 ft})$$

where IBW is in kilograms.

## REFERENCES

1. Cockcroft DW, Gault MH. Prediction of creatinine clearance from serum creatinine. Nephron 1976;16:31–41.
2. Traub SI, Johnson CE. Comparison of methods of estimating creatinine clearance in children. Am J Hosp Pharm 1980;37:195–201.
3. Levey AS, Bosch JP, Lewis JB, et al. A more accurate method to estimate glomerular filtration rate from serum creatinine: A new prediction equation. Modification of Diet in Renal Disease Study Group. Ann Intern Med 1999;130:461–470.
4. Devine BJ. Gentamicin therapy. Drug Intell Clin Pharm 1974;8:650–655.

# APPENDIX B
# COMMON LABORATORY TESTS

The following table is an alphabetical listing of some common laboratory tests and their reference ranges for adults as measured in plasma or serum (unless otherwise indicated). Reference values differ among laboratories, so readers should refer to the published reference ranges used in each institution. For some tests, both SI units and conventional units are reported.

| Laboratory | Conventional Units | Conversion Factor | SI Units |
|---|---|---|---|
| Acid phosphatase | | | |
| Male | 2–12 units/L | 16.7 | 33–200 nkat/L |
| Female | 0.3–9.2 units/L | 16.7 | 5–154 nkat/L |
| Activated partial thromboplastin time (aPTT) | 25–40 s | | |
| Adrenocorticotropic hormone (ACTH) | 15–80 pg/mL or ng/L | 0.2202 | 3.3–17.6 pmol/L |
| Alanine aminotransferase (ALT, SGPT) | 7–53 IU/L | 0.01667 | 0.12–0.88 μkat/L |
| Albumin | 3.5–5.0 g/dL | 10 | 35–50 g/L |
| Albumin:creatinine ratio (urine) | | | |
| Normal | Less than 30 mg/g creatinine | | |
| Microalbuminuria | 30–300 mg/g creatinine | | |
| Proteinuria | Greater than 300 mg/g creatinine | | |
| or | or | | |
| Normal | | | |
| Male | Less than 2.0 mg/mmol creatinine | | |
| Female | Less than 2.8 mg/mmol creatinine | | |
| Microalbuminuria | | | |
| Male | 2.0–20 mg/mmol creatinine | | |
| Female | 2.8–28 mg/mmol creatinine | | |
| Proteinuria | | | |
| Male | Greater than 20 mg/mmol creatinine | | |
| Female | Greater than 28 mg/mmol creatinine | | |
| Aldosterone | | | |
| Supine | Less than 16 ng/dL | 27.7 | Less than 444 pmol/L |
| Upright | Less than 31 ng/dL | 27.7 | Less than 860 pmol/L |
| Alkaline phosphatase | | | |
| 10–15 years | 130–550 IU/L | 0.01667 | 2.17–9.17 μkat/L |
| 16–20 years | 70–260 IU/L | 0.01667 | 1.17–4.33 μkat/L |
| Greater than 20 years | 38–126 IU/L | 0.01667 | 0.13–2.10 μkat/L |
| Alpha-fetoprotein (AFP) | Less than 15 ng/mL | 1 | Less than 15 mcg/L |
| Alpha$_1$-antitrypsin | 80–200 mg/dL | 0.01 | 0.8–2.0 g/L |
| Amikacin, therapeutic | 15–30 mg/L peak | 1.71 | 25.6–51.3 μmol/L peak |
| | Less than or equal to 8 mg/L trough | | Less than or equal to 13.7 μmol/L trough |
| Amitriptyline | 80–200 ng/mL or mcg/L | 3.4 | 272–680 nmol/L |
| Ammonia (plasma) | 15.33–56.20 mcg $NH_3$/dL | 0.5872 | 9–33 μmol $NH_3$/L |
| Amylase | 25–115 IU/L | 0.01667 | 0.42–1.92 μkat/L |
| Androstenedione | 50–250 ng/dL | 0.0349 | 1.7–8.7 nmol/L |
| Angiotensin-converting enzyme | 15–70 units/L | 16.67 | 250–1,167 nkat/L |
| Anion gap | 7–16 mEq/L | 1 | 7–16 mmol/L |
| Anti–double-stranded DNA (anti-ds DNA) | Negative | | |
| Anti-HAV | Negative | | |
| Anti-HBc | Negative | | |
| Anti-HBs | Negative | | |
| Anti-HCV | Negative | | |
| Anti-Sm antibody | Negative | | |
| Antinuclear antibody (ANA) | Negative | | |
| Apolipoprotein A-1 | | | |
| Male | 95–175 mg/dL | 0.01 | 0.95–1.75 g/L |
| Female | 100–200 mg/dL | 0.01 | 1.0–2.0 g/L |

*(continued)*

| Laboratory | Conventional Units | Conversion Factor | SI Units |
| --- | --- | --- | --- |
| Apolipoprotein B | | | |
| Male | 50–110 mg/dL | 0.01 | 0.5–1.10 g/L |
| Female | 50–105 mg/dL | 0.01 | 0.5–1.05 g/L |
| Aspartate aminotransferase (AST, SGOT) | 11–47 IU/L | 0.01667 | 0.18–0.78 μkat/L |
| Beta$_2$-microglobulin | Less than 0.2 mg/dL | 10 | 2 mg/L |
| Bicarbonate | 22–26 mEq/L | 1 | 22–26 mmol/L |
| Bilirubin | | | |
| Total | 0.3–1.1 mg/dL | 17.1 | 5.13–18.80 μmol/L |
| Direct | 0–0.3 mg/dL | 17.1 | 0–5.1 μmol/L |
| Indirect | 0.1–1.0 mg/dL | 17.1 | 1.71–17.1 μmol/L |
| Bleeding time | 3–7 min | | |
| Blood gases (arterial) | | | |
| pH | 7.35–7.45 | 1 | 7.35–7.45 |
| $Po_2$ | 80–105 mm Hg | 0.133 | 10.6–14.0 kPa |
| $Pco_2$ | 35–45 mm Hg | 0.133 | 4.7–6.0 kPa |
| $HCO_3$ | 22–26 mEq/L | 1 | 22–26 mmol/L |
| $O_2$ saturation | Greater than or equal to 95% | 0.01 | 0.95 |
| Blood urea nitrogen | 8–25 mg/dL | 0.357 | 2.9–8.9 mmol/L |
| B-type natriuretic peptide (BNP) | 0–99 pg/mL | 1 | 0–99 ng/L |
| BUN-to-creatinine ratio | 10:1 to 20:1 | | |
| C-peptide | 0.51–2.70 ng/mL | 330<br>0.33 | 170–900 pmol/L or<br>0.172–0.900 nmol/L |
| C-reactive protein | Less than 0.8 mg/dL | 10 | Less than 8 mg/L |
| CA-125 | Less than 35 units/mL | 1 | Less than 35 kilounits/L |
| CA 15-3 | Less than 30 units/mL | 1 | Less than 30 kilounits/L |
| CA 19-9 | Less than 37 units/mL | 1 | Less than 37 kilounits/L |
| CA 27-29 | Less than 38 units/mL | 1 | Less than 38 kilounits/L |
| Calcium | | | |
| Total | 8.6–10.3 mg/dL<br>4.3–5.16 mEq/L | 0.25<br>0.50 | 2.15–2.58 mmol/L<br>2.15–2.58 mmol/L |
| Ionized | 4.5–5.1 mg/dL<br>2.26–2.56 mEq/L | 0.25<br>0.50 | 1.13–1.28 mmol/L<br>1.13–1.28 mmol/L |
| Carbamazepine, therapeutic | 4–12 mg/L | 4.23 | 17–51 μmol/L |
| Carboxyhemoglobin (nonsmoker) | Less than 2% | 0.01 | Less than 0.02 |
| Carcinoembryonic antigen (CEA) | | | |
| Nonsmoker | Less than 2.5 ng/mL | 1 | Less than 2.5 mcg/L |
| Smoker | Less than 5 ng/mL | | Less than 5 mcg/L |
| Cardiac troponin I (see troponin I) | Variable ng/mL | 1 | Variable mcg/L |
| CD4 lymphocyte count | 31–61% of total lymphocytes | | |
| CD8 lymphocyte count | 18–39% of total lymphocytes | | |
| Cerebrospinal fluid (CSF) | | | |
| Pressure | 75–175 mm $H_2O$ | | |
| Glucose | 40–70 mg/dL | 0.0555 | 2.2–3.9 mmol/L |
| Protein | 15–45 mg/dL | 0.01 | 0.15–0.45 g/L |
| WBC | Less than 10/mm$^3$ | | |
| Ceruloplasmin | 18–45 mg/dL | 10<br>0.063 | 180–450 mg/L<br>1.1–2.8 μmol/L |
| Chloride | 97–110 mEq/L | 1 | 97–110 mmol/L |
| Cholesterol | | | |
| Desirable | Less than 200 mg/dL | 0.0259 | Less than 5.18 mmol/L |
| Borderline high | 200–239 mg/dL | 0.0259 | 5.18–6.19 mmol/L |
| High | Greater than or equal to 240 mg/dL | 0.0259 | Greater than or equal to 6.2 mmol/L |
| Chorionic gonadotropin (β-hCG) | Less than 5 milliunits/mL | 1 | Less than 5 units/L |
| Clozapine | Minimum trough 300–350 ng/mL or mcg/L | 3.06 | 918–1,071 nmol/L |
| $CO_2$ content | 22–30 mEq/L | 1 | 22–30 mmol/L |
| Complement component 3 (C3) | 70–160 mg/dL | 0.01 | 0.7–1.6 g/L |
| Complement component 4 (C4) | 20–40 mg/dL | 0.01 | 0.2–0.4 g/L |
| Copper | 70–150 mcg/dL | 0.157 | 11–24 μmol/L |
| Cortisol (fasting, morning) | 5–25 mcg/dL | 27.6 | 138–690 nmol/L |
| Cortisol (free, urinary) | 10–100 mcg/day | 2.76 | 28–276 nmol/day |
| Creatine kinase | | | |
| Male | 30–200 IU/L | 0.01667 | 0.50–3.33 μkat/L |
| Female | 20–170 IU/L | 0.01667 | 0.33–2.83 μkat/L |
| MB fraction | 0–7 IU/L | 0.01667 | 0.0–0.12 μkat/L |
| Creatinine clearance (CLcr) (urine) | 85–135 mL/min/1.73 m$^2$ | 0.00963 | 0.82–1.3 mL/s/m$^2$ |

*(continued)*

| Laboratory | Conventional Units | Conversion Factor | SI Units |
|---|---|---|---|
| Creatinine | | | |
| Male 4–20 years | 0.2–1.0 mg/dL | 88.4 | 18–88 μmol/L |
| Female 4–20 years | 0.2–1.0 mg/dL | 88.4 | 18–88 μmol/L |
| Male (adults) | 0.7–1.3 mg/dL | 88.4 | 62–115 μmol/L |
| Female (adults) | 0.6–1.1 mg/dL | 88.4 | 53–97 μmol/L |
| Cyclosporine | | | |
| Renal transplant | 100–300 ng/mL or mcg/L | 0.832 | 83–250 nmol/L |
| Cardiac, liver, or pancreatic transplant | 200–350 ng/mL or mcg/L | 0.832 | 166–291 nmol/L |
| Cryptococcal antigen | Negative | | |
| D-dimers | Less than 250 ng/mL | 1 | Less than 250 mcg/L |
| Desipramine | 75–300 ng/mL or mcg/L | 3.75 | 281–1,125 mmol/L |
| Dexamethasone suppression test (DST) (overnight) | 8:00 AM cortisol less than 5 mcg/dL | 0.0276 | Less than 0.14 μmol/L |
| DHEAS | | | |
| Male | 170–670 mcg/dL | 0.0271 | 4.6–18.2 μmol/L |
| Female | | | |
| Premenopausal | 50–540 mcg/dL | 0.0271 | 1.4–14.7 μmol/L |
| Postmenopausal | 30–260 mcg/dL | 0.0271 | 0.8–7.1 μmol/L |
| Digoxin, therapeutic | 0.5–1.0 ng/mL or mcg/L | 1.28 | 0.6–1.3 nmol/L |
| Erythrocyte count (blood) See under red blood cell count | | | |
| Erythrocyte sedimentation rate (ESR) | | | |
| Westergren | | | |
| Male | 0–20 mm/hour | | |
| Female | 0–30 mm/hour | | |
| Wintrobe | | | |
| Male | 0–9 mm/hour | | |
| Female | 0–15 mm/hour | | |
| Erythropoietin | 2–25 mIU/mL | 1 | 2–25 IU/L |
| Estradiol | | | |
| Male | 10–36 pg/mL | 3.67 | 37–132 pmol/L |
| Female | 34–170 pg/mL | 3.67 | 125–624 pmol/L |
| Ethanol, legal intoxication | Greater than or equal to 50–100 mg/dL | 0.217 | 10.9–21.7 mmol/L |
| | Greater than or equal to 0.05–0.1% | 217 | |
| Ethosuccimide, therapeutic | 40–100 mg/L or mcg/mL | 7.08 | 283–708 μmol/L |
| Factor VIII or factor IX | | | |
| Severe hemophilia | Less than 1 IU/dL | 0.01 | Less than 0.01 units/mL |
| Moderate hemophilia | 1–5 IU/dL | 0.01 | 0.01–0.05 units/mL |
| Mild hemophilia | Greater than 5 IU/dL | 0.01 | Greater than 0.05 units/mL |
| Usual adult levels | 60–140 IU/dL | 0.01 | 0.60–1.40 units/mL |
| Ferritin | | | |
| Male | 20–250 ng/mL | 1 | 20–250 mcg/L |
| Female | 10–150 ng/mL | 1 | 10–150 mcg/L |
| Fibrin degradation products (FDP) | 2–10 mg/L | | |
| Fibrinogen | 200–400 mg/dL | 0.01 | 2.0–4.0 g/L |
| Folate (plasma) | 3.1–12.4 ng/mL | 2.266 | 7.0–28.1 nmol/L |
| Folic acid (RBC) | 125–600 ng/mL | 2.266 | 283–1,360 nmol/L |
| Follicle-stimulating hormone (FSH) | | | |
| Male | 1–7 mIU/mL | 1 | 1–7 IU/L |
| Female | | | |
| Follicular phase | 1–9 mIU/mL | 1 | 1–9 IU/L |
| Midcycle | 6–26 mIU/mL | 1 | 6–26 IU/L |
| Luteal phase | 1–9 mIU/mL | 1 | 1–9 IU/L |
| Postmenopausal | 30–118 mIU/mL | 1 | 30–118 IU/L |
| Free thyroxine index ($FT_4I$) | 6.5–12.5 | | |
| Gamma glutamyl transferase (GGT) | 0–30 IU/L | 0.01667 | 0–0.5 μkat/L |
| Gastrin (fasting) | 0–130 pg/mL | 1 | 0–130 ng/L |
| Gentamicin, therapeutic | 4–10 mg/L peak | 2.09 | 8.4–21.0 μmol/L peak |
| | Less than or equal to 2 mg/L trough | | Less than or equal to 4.2 μmol/L trough |
| Globulin | 2.3–3.5 g/dL | 10 | 23–35 g/L |
| Glucose (fasting, plasma) | 65–109 mg/dL | 0.0555 | 3.6–6.0 mmol/L |
| Glucose, two hour postprandial blood (PPBG) | Less than 140 mg/dL | 0.0555 | Less than 7.8 mmol/L |
| Granulocyte count | $1.8–6.6 \times 10^3/\mu L$ | $10^6$ | $1.8–6.6 \times 10^9/L$ |
| Growth hormone (fasting) | | | |
| Male | Less than 5 ng/mL | 1 | Less than 5 mcg/L |
| Female | Less than 10 ng/mL | 1 | Less than 10 mcg/L |
| Haptoglobin | 60–270 mg/dL | 0.01 | 0.6–2.7 g/L |
| HBeAg | Negative | | |

*(continued)*

| Laboratory | Conventional Units | Conversion Factor | SI Units |
|---|---|---|---|
| HbsAg | Negative | | |
| HBV DNA | Negative | | |
| Hematocrit | | | |
| Male | 40.7–50.3% | 0.01 | 0.407–0.503 |
| Female | 36.1–44.3% | 0.01 | 0.361–0.443 |
| Hemoglobin (blood) | | | |
| Male | 13.8–17.2 g/dL | 10 | 138–172 g/L |
| | | Alternate SI: 0.62 | 8.56–10.67 mmol/L |
| Female | 12.1–15.1 g/dL | 10 | 121–151 g/L |
| | | Alternate SI: 0.62 | 7.5–9.36 mmol/L |
| Hemoglobin A1C | 4.0–6.0% | 0.01 | 0.04–0.06 |
| Heparin | | | |
| Via protamine titration method | 0.2–0.4 mcg/mL | | |
| Via anti-factor Xa assay | 0.3–0.7 mcg/mL | | |
| High-density lipoprotein (HDL) cholesterol | Greater than 35 mg/dL | 0.0259 | Greater than 0.91 mmol/L |
| Homocysteine | 3.3–10.4 μmol/L | | |
| Ibuprofen | | | |
| Therapeutic | 10–50 mcg/mL | 4.85 | 49–243 μmol/L |
| Toxic | 100–700 mcg/mL or more | 4.85 | 485–3,395 μmol/L or more |
| Imipramine, therapeutic | 100–300 ng/mL or mcg/L | 3.57 | 357–1071 nmol/L |
| Immunoglobulin A (IgA) | 85–385 mg/dL | 0.01 | 0.85–3.85 g/L |
| Immunoglobulin G (IgG) | 565–1,765 mg/dL | 0.01 | 5.65–17.65 g/L |
| Immunoglobulin M (IgM) | 53–375 mg/dL | 0.01 | 0.53–3.75 g/L |
| Insulin (fasting) | 2–20 microunits/mL or milliunits/L | 7.175 | 14.35–143.5 pmol/L |
| International normalized ratio (INR), therapeutic | 2.0–3.0 (2.5–3.5 for some indications) | | |
| Iron | | | |
| Male | 45–160 mcg/dL | 0.179 | 8.1–31.3 μmol/L |
| Female | 30–160 mcg/dL | 0.179 | 5.4–31.3 μmol/L |
| Iron binding capacity (total) | 220–420 mcg/dL | 0.179 | 39.4–75.2 μmol/L |
| Iron saturation | 15–50% | 0.01 | 0.15–0.50 |
| Lactate (plasma) | 0.7–2.1 mEq/L | 1 | 0.7–2.1 mmol/L |
| | 6.3–18.9 mg/dL | 0.111 | |
| Lactate dehydrogenase | 100–250 IU/L | 0.01667 | 1.67–4.17 μkat/L |
| Lead | Less than 25 mcg/dL | 0.0483 | Less than 1.21 μmol/L |
| Leukocyte count | 3.8–9.8 × $10^3/\mu L$ | $10^6$ | 3.8–9.8 × $10^9/L$ |
| Lidocaine, therapeutic | 1.5–6.0 mcg/mL or mg/L | 4.27 | 6.4–25.6 μmol/L |
| Lipase | Less than 100 IU/L | 0.01667 | 1.7 μkat/L |
| Lithium, therapeutic | 0.5–1.25 mEq/L | 1 | 0.5–1.25 mmol/L |
| Low-density lipoprotein (LDL) cholesterol | | | |
| Desirable | Less than 130 mg/dL | 0.0259 | Less than 3.36 mmol/L |
| Borderline high risk | 130–159 mg/dL | 0.0259 | 3.36–4.11 mmol/L |
| High risk | Greater than or equal to 160 mg/dL | 0.0259 | Greater than or equal to 4.13 mmol/L |
| Luteinizing hormone (LH) | | | |
| Male | 1–8 milliunits/mL | 1 | 1–8 units/L |
| Female | | | |
| Follicular phase | 1–12 milliunits/mL | 1 | 1–12 units/L |
| Midcycle | 16–104 milliunits/mL | 1 | 16–104 units/L |
| Luteal phase | 1–12 milliunits/mL | 1 | 1–12 units/L |
| Postmenopausal | 16–66 milliunits/mL | 1 | 16–66 units/L |
| Lymphocyte count | 1.2–3.3 × $10^3/\mu L$ | 106 | 1.2–3.3 × $10^9/L$ |
| Magnesium | 1.3–2.2 mEq/L | 0.5 | 0.65–1.10 mmol/L |
| | 1.58–2.68 mg/dL | 0.411 | 0.65–1.10 mmol/L |
| Mean corpuscular volume | 80.0–97.6 $\mu m^3$ | 1 | 80.0–97.6 fL |
| Mononuclear cell count | 0.2–0.7 × $10^3/\mu L$ | 106 | 0.2–0.7 × $10^9/L$ |
| Nortriptyline, therapeutic | 50–150 ng/mL or mcg/L | 3.8 | 190–570 nmol/L |
| NT-ProBNP (see Pro-BNP) | | | |
| Osmolality (serum) | 275–300 mOsm/kg | 1 | 275–300 mmol/kg |
| Osmolality (urine) | 250–900 mOsm/kg | 1 | 250–900 mmol/kg |
| Parathyroid hormone (PTH), intact | 10–60 pg/mL or ng/L | 0.107 | 1.1–6.4 pmol/L |
| Parathyroid hormone (PTH), N-terminal | 8–24 pg/mL or ng/L | | |
| Parathyroid hormone (PTH), C-terminal | 50–330 pg/mL or ng/L | | |
| Phenobarbital, therapeutic | 15–40 mcg/mL or mg/L | 4.31 | 65–172 μmol/L |
| Phenytoin, therapeutic | 10–20 mcg/mL or mg/L | 3.96 | 40–79 μmol/L |
| Phosphate | 2.5–4.5 mg/dL | 0.323 | 0.81–1.45 mmol/L |
| Platelet count | 140–440 × $10^3/\mu L$ | $10^6$ | 140–440 × $10^9/L$ |
| Potassium (plasma) | 3.3–4.9 mEq/L | 1 | 3.3–4.9 μmol/L |
| Prealbumin (adult) | 19.5–35.8 mg/dL | 10 | 195–358 mg/L |
| Primidone, therapeutic | 5–12 mcg/mL or mg/L | 4.58 | 23–55 μmol/L |

*(continued)*

| Laboratory | Conventional Units | Conversion Factor | SI Units |
|---|---|---|---|
| ProBNP | Less than 125 pg/mL or ng/L | 0.118 | Less than 14.75 pmol/L |
| Procainamide, therapeutic | 4–10 mcg/mL or mg/L | 4.23 | 17–42 μmol/L |
| Progesterone | | | |
| Male | 13–97 ng/dL | 0.0318 | 0.4–3.1 nmol/L |
| Female | | | |
| Follicular phase | 15–70 ng/dL | | 0.5–2.2 nmol/L |
| Luteal phase | 200–2,500 ng/dL | | 6.4–79.5 nmol/L |
| Prolactin | Less than 20 ng/mL | 1 | Less than 20 mcg/L |
| Prostate-specific antigen (PSA) | Less than 4 ng/mL | 1 | Less than 4 mcg/L |
| Protein, total | 6.0–8.0 g/dL | 10 | 60–80 g/L |
| Prothrombin time (PT) | 10–12 sec | | |
| Quinidine, therapeutic | 2–5 mcg/mL or mg/L | 3.08 | 6.2–15.4 μmol/L |
| Radioactive iodine uptake (RAIU) | Less than 6% in 2 hours | | |
| Red blood cell (RBC) count (blood) | | | |
| Male | $4–6.2 \times 10^6/\mu L$ | $10^6$ | $4–6.2 \times 10^{12}/L$ |
| Female | $4–6.2 \times 10^6/\mu L$ | $10^6$ | $4–6.2 \times 10^{12}/L$ |
| Pregnant | | | |
| Trimester 1 | $4–5 \times 10^6/\mu L$ | $10^6$ | $4–5 \times 10^{12}/L$ |
| Trimester 2 | $3.2–4.5 \times 10^6/\mu L$ | $10^6$ | $3.2–4.5 \times 10^{12}/L$ |
| Trimester 3 | $3.0–4.9 \times 10^6/\mu L$ | $10^6$ | $3.0–4.9 \times 10^{12}/L$ |
| Postpartum | $3.2–5 \times 10^6/\mu L$ | $10^6$ | $3.2–5.0 \times 10^6/L$ |
| Red blood cell distribution width (RDW) | 11.5–14.5% | 0.01 | 0.115–0.145 |
| Reticulocyte count | | | |
| Male | 0.5–1.5% of total RBC count | 0.01 | 0.005–0.015 |
| Female | 0.5–2.5% of total RBC count | 0.01 | 0.005–0.025 |
| Retinol-binding protein (RBP) | 2.7–7.6 mg/dL | 10 | 27–76 mg/L |
| Rheumatoid factor (RF) titer | Negative | | |
| Salicylate, therapeutic | 150–300 mcg/mL or mg/L | 0.00724 | 1.09–2.17 mmol/L |
| | 15–30 mg/dL | 0.0724 | |
| Sodium | 135–145 mEq/L | 1 | 135–145 mmol/L |
| Tacrolimus | | | |
| Renal transplant | 6–12 ng/mL or mcg/L | | |
| Liver transplant | 4–10 ng/mL or mcg/L | | |
| Pancreatic transplant | 10–18 ng/mL or mcg/L | | |
| Bone marrow transplant | 10–20 ng/mL or mcg/L | | |
| Testosterone (total) | | | |
| Men | 300–950 ng/dL | 0.0347 | 10.4–33.0 nmol/L |
| Women | 20–80 ng/dL | | 0.7–2.8 nmol/L |
| Testosterone (free) | | | |
| Men | 9–30 ng/dL | 0.0347 | 0.31–1.04 nmol/L |
| Women | 0.3–1.9 ng/dL | | 0.01–0.07 nmol/L |
| Theophylline | | | |
| Therapeutic | 5–15 mcg/mL or mg/L | 5.55 | 28–83 μmol/L |
| Toxic | 20 or more mcg/mL or mg/L | 5.55 | 111 or more μmol/L |
| Thrombin time | 20–24 sec | | |
| Thyroglobulin | Less than 42 ng/mL | 1 | Less than 42 mcg/L |
| Thyroglobulin antibodies | Negative | | |
| Thyroxine-binding globulin (TBG) | 1.2–2.5 mg/dL | 10 | 12–25 mcg/L |
| Thyroid-stimulating hormone (TSH) | 0.35–6.20 microunits/mL | 1 | 0.35–6.20 milliunits/L |
| TSH receptor antibodies (TSH Rab) | 0–1 unit/mL | | |
| Thyroxine ($T_4$) | | | |
| Total | 4.5–12.0 mcg/dL | 12.87 | 58–155 nmol/L |
| Free | 0.7–1.9 ng/dL | 12.87 | 9.0–24.5 pmol/L |
| Thyroxine index, free ($FT_4I$) | 6.5–12.5 | | |
| TIBC See Iron-binding capacity (total) | | | |
| Tobramycin, therapeutic | 4–10 mcg/mL or mg/L peak | 2.14 | 8.6–21.4 μmol/L |
| | Less than or equal to 2 mcg/mL mg/L trough | 2.14 | Less than or equal to 4.28 μmol/L |
| Transferrin | 200–430 mg/dL | 0.01 | 2.0–4.3 g/L |
| Transferrin saturation | 30–50% | 0.01 | 0.30–0.50 |
| Triglycerides (fasting) | Less than 160 mg/dL | 0.0113 | Less than 1.8 mmol/L |
| Triiodothyronine ($T_3$) | 45–132 ng/dL | 0.0154 | 0.91–2.70 nmol/L |
| Triiodothyronine ($T_3$) resin uptake | 25–35% | | |
| Troponin I | Less than 0.6 ng/mL | 1 | Less than 0.6 μg/L |
| Uric acid | 3–8 mg/dL | 59.48 | 179–476 μmol/L |
| Urinalysis (urine) | | | |
| pH | 4.8–8.0 | | |
| Specific gravity | 1.005–1.030 | | |

*(continued)*

| Laboratory | Conventional Units | Conversion Factor | SI Units |
|---|---|---|---|
| Protein | Negative | | |
| Glucose | Negative | | |
| Ketones | Negative | | |
| RBC | 1–2 per low-power field | | |
| WBC | 3–4 per low-power field | | |
| Valproic acid, therapeutic | 50–100 mcg/mL or mg/L | 6.93 | 346–693 μmol/L |
| Vancomycin, therapeutic trough for CNS infections | 20–40 mcg/mL or mg/L peak | 0.690 | 14–28 μmol/L peak |
| | 5–20 mcg/mL or mg/L trough | 0.690 | 3–14 μmol/L trough |
| | 15–20 mcg/mL or mg/L trough | 0.690 | 10–14 μmol/L trough |
| Vitamin A (retinol) | 30–95 mcg/dL | 0.0349 | 1.05–3.32 μmol/L |
| Vitamin $B_{12}$ | 180–1,000 pg/mL | 0.738 | 133–738 pmol/L |
| Vitamin $D_3$, 1, 25-dihydroxy | 20–76 pg/m | 2.4 | 48–182 pmol/L |
| Vitamin $D_3$, 25-hydroxy | 10–50 ng/mL | 2.496 | 25–125 nmol/L |
| Vitamin E (alpha tocopherol) | 0.5–2.0 mg/dL | 23.22 | 12–46 μmol/L |
| WBC count | 4–10 × $10^3$/μL or 4–10 × $10^3$/mm$^3$ | $10^6$ | 4–10 × $10^9$/L |
| WBC differential (peripheral blood) | | | |
| Polymorphonuclear neutrophils (PMNs) | 50–65% | | |
| Bands | 0–5% | | |
| Eosinophils | 0–3% | | |
| Basophils | 1–3% | | |
| Lymphocytes | 25–35% | | |
| Monocytes | 2–6% | | |
| WBC differential (bone marrow) | | | |
| Polymorphonuclear neutrophils (PMNs) | 3–11% | | |
| Bands | 9–15% | | |
| Metamyelocytes | 9–25% | | |
| Myelocytes | 8–16% | | |
| Promyelocytes | 1–8% | | |
| Myeloblasts | 0–5% | | |
| Eosinophils | 1–5% | | |
| Basophils | 0–1% | | |
| Lymphocytes | 11–23% | | |
| Monocytes | 0–1% | | |
| Zinc | 60–150 mcg/dL | 0.153 | 9.2–23.0 μmol/L |

*This table was reprinted with permission from: Chisholm-Burns MA, Wells BG, Schwinghammer TL, et al. (eds). Pharmacotherapy Principles and Practice. New York: McGraw-Hill, 2008.*

# APPENDIX C
# PART I: Common Medical Abbreviations

*Note:* Many of the medical abbreviations contained in Part I of this appendix are used in the casebook. A more extensive list of abbreviations is available on the internet at *www.pharma-lexicon.com.*

| | |
|---|---|
| A & O | Alert and oriented |
| A & P | Auscultation and percussion; anterior and posterior; assessment and plan |
| A & W | Alive and well |
| A1C | Hemoglobin A1C |
| aa | Of each (*ana*) |
| AA | Aplastic anemia; Alcoholics Anonymous |
| AAA | Abdominal aortic aneurysm |
| AAL | Anterior axillary line |
| AAO | Awake, alert, and oriented |
| ABC | Absolute band count; absolute basophil count; aspiration, biopsy, and cytology; artificial beta cells |
| Abd | Abdomen |
| ABG | Aterial blood gases |
| ABP | Arterial blood pressure |
| ABW | Actual body weight |
| ABx | Antibiotics |
| AC | Before meals (*ante cibos*) |
| ACE | Angiotensin-converting enzyme |
| ACEI | Angiotensin-converting enzyme inhibitor |
| ACL | Anterior cruciate ligament |
| ACLS | Advanced cardiac life support |
| ACS | Acute coronary syndrome |
| ACT | Activated clotting time |
| ACTH | Adrenocorticotropic hormone |
| AD | Alzheimer's disease, right ear (*auris dextra*) |
| ADA | American Diabetes Association; adenosine deaminase |
| ADE | Adverse drug effect (or event) |
| ADH | Antidiuretic hormone |
| ADHD | Attention-deficit hyperactivity disorder |
| ADL | Activities of daily living |
| ADR | Adverse drug reaction |
| AED | Antiepileptic drug(s) |
| AF | Atrial fibrillation |
| AFB | Acid-fast bacillus; aortofemoral bypass; aspirated foreign body |
| Afeb | Afebrile |
| AFP | $\alpha$-Fetoprotein |
| A/G | Albumin-globulin ratio |
| AI | Aortic insufficiency |
| AIDS | Acquired immunodeficiency syndrome |
| AKA | Above-knee amputation; alcoholic ketoacidosis; all known allergies; also known as |
| AKI | Acute kidney injury |
| ALD | Alcoholic liver disease |
| ALFT | Abnormal liver function test |
| ALL | Acute lymphocytic leukemia; acute lymphoblastic leukemia |
| ALP | Alkaline phosphatase |
| ALS | Amyotrophic lateral sclerosis |
| ALT | Alanine aminotransferase |
| AMA | Against medical advice; American Medical Association; antimitochondrial antibody |
| AMI | Acute myocardial infarction |
| AML | Acute myelogenous leukemia |
| Amp | Ampule |
| ANA | Antinuclear antibody |
| ANC | Absolute neutrophil count |
| ANLL | Acute nonlymphocytic leukemia |
| AODM | Adult onset diabetes mellitus |
| A & O × 3 | Awake and oriented to person, place, and time |
| A & O × 4 | Awake and oriented to person, place, time, and situation |
| AOM | Acute otitis media |
| AP | Anteroposterior |
| APACHE | Acute Physiology and Chronic Health Evaluation |
| APAP | Acetaminophen (*N*-acetyl-*p*-aminophenol) |
| aPTT | Activated partial thromboplastin time |
| ARC | AIDS-related complex |
| ARDS | Adult respiratory distress syndrome |
| ARF | Acute renal failure; acute respiratory failure; acute rheumatic fever |
| AROM | Active range of motion |
| AS | Left ear (*auris sinistra*) |
| ASA | Aspirin (acetylsalicylic acid) |
| ASCVD | Arteriosclerotic cardiovascular disease |
| ASD | Atrial septal defect |
| ASH | Asymmetric septal hypertrophy |
| ASHD | Arteriosclerotic heart disease |
| AST | Aspartate aminotransferase |
| ATG | Antithymocyte globulin |
| ATN | Acute tubular necrosis |
| AU | Each ear (*auris uterque*) |
| AV | Arteriovenous; atrioventricular |
| AVM | Arteriovenous malformation |
| AVR | Aortic valve replacement |
| AWMI | Anterior wall myocardial infarction |
| BAC | Blood alcohol concentration |
| BAL | Bronchioalveolar lavage |
| BBB | Bundle branch block; blood-brain barrier |
| BC | Blood culture |
| BCG | Bacillus Calmette Guerin |
| BCNP | Board Certified Nuclear Pharmacist |
| BCNSP | Board Certified Nutrition Support Pharmacist |
| BCNU | Carmustine |
| BCOP | Board Certified Oncology Pharmacist |
| BCP | Birth control pill |

| | |
|---|---|
| BCPP | Board Certified Psychiatric Pharmacist |
| BCPS | Board Certified Pharmacotherapy Specialist |
| BE | Barium enema |
| BID | Twice daily (*bis in die*) |
| BKA | Below-knee amputation |
| BM | Bone marrow; bowel movement |
| BMC | Bone marrow cells |
| BMD | Bone mineral density |
| BMR | Basal metabolic rate |
| BMT | Bone marrow transplantation |
| BNP | Brain natriuretic peptide |
| BP | Blood pressure |
| BPD | Bronchopulmonary dysplasia |
| BPH | Benign prostatic hyperplasia |
| bpm | Beats per minute |
| BPRS | Brief Psychiatric Rating Scale |
| BR | Bedrest |
| BRBPR | Bright red blood per rectum |
| BRM | Biological response modifier |
| BRP | Bathroom privileges |
| BS | Bowel sounds; breath sounds; blood sugar |
| BSA | Body surface area |
| BSO | Bilateral salpingo-oophorectomy |
| BTFS | Breast tumor frozen section |
| BUN | Blood urea nitrogen |
| BV | Bacterial vaginosis |
| Bx | Biopsy |
| C & S | Culture and sensitivity |
| CA | Cancer; calcium |
| CABG | Coronary artery bypass graft |
| CAD | Coronary artery disease |
| CAH | Chronic active hepatitis |
| CAM | Complementary and alternative medicine |
| CAPD | Continuous ambulatory peritoneal dialysis |
| CBC | Complete blood count |
| CBD | Common bile duct |
| CBG | Capillary blood gas; corticosteroid binding globulin |
| CBT | Cognitive-behavioral therapy |
| CC | Chief complaint |
| CCA | Calcium channel antagonist |
| CCB | Calcium channel blocker |
| CCE | Clubbing, cyanosis, edema |
| CCK | Cholecystokinin |
| CCMS | Clean catch midstream |
| CCNU | Lomustine |
| CCPD | Continuous cycling peritoneal dialysis |
| CCU | Coronary care unit |
| CDAD | *Clostridium difficile*–associated diarrhea |
| CEA | Carcinoembryonic antigen |
| CF | Cystic fibrosis |
| CFS | Chronic fatigue syndrome |
| CFU | Colony-forming unit |
| CHD | Coronary heart disease |
| CHF | Congestive heart failure |
| CHO | Carbohydrate |
| CHOP | Cyclophosphamide, hydroxydaunorubicin (doxorubicin), Oncovin (vincristine), prednisone |
| CI | Cardiac index |
| CK | Creatine kinase |
| CKD | Chronic kidney disease |
| CLcr | Creatinine clearance |
| CLL | Chronic lymphocytic leukemia |
| CM | Costal margin |
| CMG | Cystometrogram |
| CML | Chronic myelogenous leukemia |
| CMV | Cytomegalovirus |
| CN | Cranial nerve |
| CNS | Central nervous system |
| c/o | Complains of |
| CO | Cardiac output; carbon monoxide |
| COLD | Chronic obstructive lung disease |
| COPD | Chronic obstructive pulmonary disease |
| CP | Chest pain; cerebral palsy |
| CPA | Costophrenic angle |
| CPAP | Continuous positive airway pressure |
| CPK | Creatine phosphokinase |
| CPP | Cerebral perfusion pressure |
| CPR | Cardiopulmonary resuscitation |
| CR | Complete remission |
| CRF | Chronic renal failure; corticotropin-releasing factor |
| CRH | Corticotropin-releasing hormone |
| CRI | Chronic renal insufficiency; catheter-related infection |
| CRNA | Certified Registered Nurse Anesthetist |
| CRNP | Certified Registered Nurse Practitioner |
| CRP | C-reactive protein |
| CRTT | Certified Respiratory Therapy Technician |
| CS | Central Supply |
| CSA | Cyclosporine |
| CSF | Cerebrospinal fluid; colony-stimulating factor |
| CT | Computed tomography; chest tube |
| CTB | Cease to breathe |
| cTnI | Cardiac troponin I |
| CTZ | Chemoreceptor trigger zone |
| CV | Cardiovascular |
| CVA | Cerebrovascular accident |
| CVAT | Costovertebral angle tenderness |
| CVC | Central venous catheter |
| CVP | Central venous pressure |
| Cx | Culture; cervix |
| CXR | Chest x-ray |
| D & C | Dilatation and curettage |
| d4T | Stavudine |
| $D_5W$ | 5% Dextrose in water |
| DBP | Diastolic blood pressure |
| D/C | Discontinue; discharge |
| DCC | Direct current cardioversion |
| ddC | Zalcitabine |
| ddI | Didanosine |
| DES | Diethylstilbestrol |
| DI | Diabetes insipidus |
| DIC | Disseminated intravascular coagulation |
| Diff | Differential |
| DIP | Distal interphalangeal |
| DJD | Degenerative joint disease |
| DKA | Diabetic ketoacidosis |
| dL | Deciliter |
| DM | Diabetes mellitus |
| DMARD | Disease-modifying antirheumatic drug |

| | |
|---|---|
| DNA | Deoxyribonucleic acid |
| DNR | Do not resuscitate |
| DO | Doctor of Osteopathy |
| DOA | Dead on arrival; date of admission; duration of action |
| DOB | Date of birth |
| DOE | Dyspnea on exertion |
| DOT | Directly observed therapy |
| DP | Dorsalis pedis |
| DPGN | Diffuse proliferative glomerulonephritis |
| DRE | Digital rectal examination |
| DRG | Diagnosis-related group |
| DS | Double strength |
| DSHEA | Dietary Supplement Health and Education Act (1994) |
| DST | Dexamethasone suppression test |
| DTIC | Dacarbazine |
| DTP | Diphtheria-tetanus-pertussis |
| DTR | Deep-tendon reflex |
| DVT | Deep-vein thrombosis |
| Dx | Diagnosis |
| EBV | Epstein-Barr virus |
| EC | Enteric-coated |
| ECF | Extended care facility |
| ECG | Electrocardiogram |
| ECMO | Extracorporeal membrane oxygenator |
| ECOG | Eastern Cooperative Oncology Group |
| ECT | Electroconvulsive therapy |
| ED | Emergency Department |
| EEG | Electroencephalogram |
| EENT | Eyes, ears, nose, throat |
| EF | Ejection fraction |
| EGD | Esophagogastroduodenoscopy |
| EIA | Enzyme immunoassay |
| EKG | Electrocardiogram |
| EMG | Electromyogram |
| EMT | Emergency medical technician |
| Endo | Endotracheal; endoscopy |
| EOMI | Extraocular movements (or muscles) intact |
| EPO | Erythropoietin |
| EPS | Extrapyramidal symptoms |
| EPT | Early pregnancy test; expedited partner therapy |
| ER | Estrogen receptor; emergency room |
| ERCP | Endoscopic retrograde cholangiopancreatography |
| ERT | Estrogen replacement therapy |
| ESLD | End-stage liver disease |
| ESR | Erythrocyte sedimentation rate |
| ESRD | End-stage renal disease |
| ESWL | Extracorporeal shockwave lithotripsy |
| ET | Endotracheal |
| ETOH | Ethanol |
| FB | Finger-breadth; foreign body |
| FBS | Fasting blood sugar |
| FDA | Food and Drug Administration |
| FDP | Fibrin degradation products |
| FEF | Forced expiratory flow (rate) |
| FEM-POP | Femoral-popliteal |
| $FEV_1$ | Forced expiratory volume in 1 second |
| FFP | Fresh frozen plasma |
| FH | Family history |
| $FiO_2$ | Fraction of inspired oxygen |
| fL | Femtoliter |
| FM | Face mask |
| FOBT | Fecal occult blood test |
| FOC | Fronto-occipital circumference |
| FPG | Fasting plasma glucose |
| FPIA | Fluorescence polarization immunoassay |
| FSH | Follicle-stimulating hormone |
| FTA | Fluorescent treponemal antibody |
| f/u | Follow-up |
| FUDR | Floxuridine |
| FUO | Fever of unknown origin |
| Fx | Fracture |
| G6PD | Glucose-6-phosphate dehydrogenase |
| GABHS | Group A beta-hemolytic streptococcus |
| GAD | Generalized anxiety disorder |
| GB | Gallbladder |
| GBS | Group B *Streptococcus*; Guillain-Barré syndrome |
| GC | Gonococcus |
| G-CSF | Granulocyte colony-stimulating factor |
| GDM | Gestational diabetes mellitus |
| GE | Gastroesophageal; gastroenterology |
| GERD | Gastroesophageal reflux disease |
| GFR | Glomerular filtration rate |
| GGT | $\gamma$-Glutamyltransferase |
| GGTP | $\gamma$-Glutamyl transpeptidase |
| GI | Gastrointestinal |
| GM-CSF | Granulocyte-macrophage colony-stimulating factor |
| GN | Glomerulonephritis; graduate nurse |
| gr | Grain |
| GT | Gastrostomy tube |
| gtt | Drops (*guttae*) |
| GTT | Glucose tolerance test |
| GU | Genitourinary |
| GVHD | Graft-versus-host disease |
| GVL | Graft-versus-leukemia |
| Gyn | Gynecology |
| H & H | Hemoglobin and hematocrit |
| H & P | History and physical examination |
| H/A | Headache |
| HAART | Highly active antiretroviral therapy |
| HAM-D | Hamilton Rating Scale for Depression |
| HAV | Hepatitis A virus |
| Hb, hgb | Hemoglobin |
| $HbA_{1C}$ | Hemoglobin A1C |
| HBIG | Hepatitis B immune globulin |
| HBP | High blood pressure |
| HBsAg | Hepatitis B surface antigen |
| HBV | Hepatitis B virus |
| HC | Hydrocortisone; home care |
| HCG | Human chorionic gonadotropin |
| $HCO_3$ | Bicarbonate |
| Hct | Hematocrit |
| HCTZ | Hydrochlorothiazide |
| HCV | Hepatitis C virus |
| Hcy | Homocysteine |
| HD | Hodgkin's disease; hemodialysis |
| HDL | High-density lipoprotein |
| HEENT | Head, eyes, ears, nose, and throat |
| HEPA | High-efficiency particulate air |

| | |
|---|---|
| HF | Heart failure |
| H flu | *Haemophilus influenzae* |
| HGH | Human growth hormone |
| HH | Hiatal hernia |
| HHS | Hyperosmolar hyperglycemic state |
| Hib | *Haemophilus influenzae* type b |
| HIV | Human immunodeficiency virus |
| HJR | Hepatojugular reflux |
| HLA | Human leukocyte antigen; human lymphocyte antigen |
| HMG-CoA | Hydroxy-methylglutaryl coenzyme A |
| H/O | History of |
| HOB | Head of bed |
| HPA | Hypothalamic-pituitary axis |
| hpf | High-power field |
| HPI | History of present illness |
| HPV | Human papilloma virus |
| HR | Heart rate |
| HRT | Hormone replacement therapy |
| HS | At bedtime (*hora somni*) |
| HSCT | Hematopoietic stem cell transplantation |
| HSM | Hepatosplenomegaly |
| HSV | Herpes simplex virus |
| HTN | Hypertension |
| Hx | History |
| I & D | Incision and drainage |
| I & O | Intake and output |
| IABP | Intra-arterial balloon pump |
| IBD | Inflammatory bowel disease |
| IBW | Ideal body weight |
| ICD | Implantable cardioverter defibrillator |
| ICP | Intracranial pressure |
| ICS | Intercostal space |
| ICU | Intensive care unit |
| ID | Identification; infectious disease |
| IDDM | Insulin-dependent diabetes mellitus |
| IFN | Interferon |
| Ig | Immunoglobulin |
| IgA | Immunoglobulin A |
| IgD | Immunoglobulin D |
| IHD | Ischemic heart disease |
| IJ | Internal jugular |
| IM | Intramuscular; infectious mononucleosis |
| IMV | Intermittent mandatory ventilation |
| INH | Isoniazid |
| INR | International normalized ratio |
| IOP | Intraocular pressure |
| IP | Intraperitoneal |
| IPG | Impedance plethysmography |
| IPI | International prognostic index |
| IPN | Interstitial pneumonia |
| IPPB | Intermittent positive pressure breathing |
| IPS | Idiopathic pneumonia syndrome |
| IRB | Institutional Review Board |
| ISA | Intrinsic sympathomimetic activity |
| ISDN | Isosorbide dinitrate |
| ISH | Isolated systolic hypertension |
| ISMN | Isosorbide mononitrate |
| IT | Intrathecal |
| ITP | Idiopathic thrombocytopenic purpura |
| IU | International unit |
| IUD | Intrauterine device |
| IV | Intravenous; Roman numeral IV; symbol for Class 4 controlled substances |
| IVC | Inferior vena cava; intravenous cholangiogram |
| IVDA | Intravenous drug abuse |
| IVF | Intravenous fluids |
| IVIG | Intravenous immunoglobulin |
| IVP | Intravenous pyelogram; intravenous push |
| IVSS | Intravenous Soluset |
| IWMI | Inferior wall myocardial infarction |
| JODM | Juvenile-onset diabetes mellitus |
| JRA | Juvenile rheumatoid arthritis |
| JVD | Jugular venous distention |
| JVP | Jugular venous pressure |
| K | Potassium |
| kcal | Kilocalorie |
| KCL | Potassium chloride |
| KOH | Potassium hydroxide |
| KUB | Kidney, ureters, bladder |
| KVO | Keep vein open |
| L | Liter |
| LAD | Left anterior descending; left axis deviation |
| LAO | Left anterior oblique |
| LAP | Leukocyte alkaline phosphatase |
| LBBB | Left bundle branch block |
| LBP | Low back pain |
| LCM | Left costal margin |
| LDH | Lactate dehydrogenase |
| LDL | Low-density lipoprotein |
| LE | Lower extremity |
| LES | Lower esophageal sphincter |
| LFT | Liver function test |
| LHRH | Luteinizing hormone-releasing hormone |
| LIMA | Left internal mammary artery |
| LLE | Left lower extremity |
| LLL | Left lower lobe |
| LLQ | Left lower quadrant (abdomen) |
| LLSB | Left lower sternal border |
| LMD | Local medical doctor |
| LMP | Last menstrual period |
| LOC | Loss of consciousness; laxative of choice |
| LOS | Length of stay |
| LP | Lumbar puncture |
| LPN | Licensed Practical Nurse |
| LPO | Left posterior oblique |
| LPT | Licensed Physical Therapist |
| LR | Lactated Ringer's |
| LS | Lumbosacral |
| LTCF | Long-term care facility |
| LUE | Left upper extremity |
| LUL | Left upper lobe |
| LUQ | Left upper quadrant |
| LVH | Left ventricular hypertrophy |
| MAP | Mean arterial pressure |
| MAR | Medication administration record |
| mcg | Microgram |
| MCH | Mean corpuscular hemoglobin |
| MCHC | Mean corpuscular hemoglobin concentration |

| | |
|---|---|
| MCL | Midclavicular line |
| MCP | Metacarpophalangeal |
| MCV | Mean corpuscular volume |
| MD | Medical Doctor |
| MDI | Metered-dose inhaler |
| MEFR | Maximum expiratory flow rate |
| mEq | Milliequivalent |
| mg | Milligram |
| MHC | Major histocompatibility complex |
| MI | Myocardial infarction; mitral insufficiency |
| MIC | Minimum inhibitory concentration |
| MICU | Medical intensive care unit |
| mL | Milliliter |
| MM | Multiple myeloma |
| MMA | Methylmalonic acid |
| MMEFR | Maximal midexpiratory flow rate |
| MMR | Measles-mumps-rubella |
| MMSE | Mini Mental State Examination |
| MOM | Milk of magnesia |
| MPV | Mean platelet volume |
| MRG | Murmur/rub/gallop |
| MRI | Magnetic resonance imaging |
| MRSA | Methicillin-resistant *Staphylococcus aureus* |
| MRSE | Methicillin-resistant *Staphylococcus epidermidis* |
| MS | Mental status; mitral stenosis; musculoskeletal; multiple sclerosis; morphine sulfate |
| MSE | Mental Status Exam |
| MSM | Men who have sex with men |
| MSW | Master of Social Work |
| MTD | Maximum tolerated dose |
| MTP | Metatarsophalangeal |
| MTX | Methotrexate |
| MUD | Matched unrelated donor |
| MUGA | Multiple gated acquisition |
| MVA | Motor vehicle accident |
| MVI | Multivitamin |
| MVR | Mitral valve replacement; mitral valve regurgitation |
| MVS | Mitral valve stenosis; motor, vascular, and sensory |
| NAAT | Nucleic acid amplification test |
| NAD | No acute (or apparent) distress |
| N/C | Non-contributory; nasal cannula |
| NC/AT | Normocephalic/atraumatic |
| NG | Nasogastric |
| NGT | Nasogastric tube |
| NGTD | No growth to date (on culture) |
| NHL | Non-Hodgkin's lymphoma |
| NIDDM | Non–insulin-dependent diabetes mellitus |
| NIH | National Institutes of Health |
| NKA | No known allergies |
| NKDA | No known drug allergies |
| NL | Normal |
| NNRTI | Non-nucleoside reverse transcriptase inhibitor |
| NOS | Not otherwise specified |
| NPH | Neutral protamine Hagedorn; normal pressure hydrocephalus |
| NPN | Non-protein nitrogen |
| NPO | Nothing by mouth (*nil per os*) |
| NRTI | Nucleoside reverse transcriptase inhibitor |
| NS | Neurosurgery; normal saline |
| NSAID | Nonsteroidal anti-inflammatory drug |
| NSCLC | Non-small cell lung cancer |
| NSR | Normal sinus rhythm |
| NSS | Normal saline solution |
| NSVD | Normal spontaneous vaiginal delivery |
| NTG | Nitroglycerin |
| NT/ND | Non-tender/non-distended |
| N/V | Nausea and vomiting |
| NVD | Nausea/vomiting/diarrhea; neck vein distention; nonvalvular disease; neovascularization of the disk |
| NYHA | New York Heart Association |
| O & P | Ova and parasites |
| OA | Osteoarthritis |
| OB | Obstetrics |
| OBS | Organic brain syndrome |
| OCD | Obsessive-compulsive disorder |
| OCG | Oral cholecystogram |
| OD | Right eye (*oculus dexter*); overdose; Doctor of Optometry |
| OGT | Oral glucose tolerance test |
| OHTx | Orthotopic heart transplantation |
| OLTx | Orthotopic liver transplantation |
| OME | Otitis media with effusion |
| OOB | Out of bed |
| OPD | Outpatient department |
| OPG | Ocular plethysmography |
| OPV | Oral poliovirus vaccine |
| OR | Operating room |
| OS | Left eye (*oculus sinister*) |
| OSA | Obstructive sleep apnea |
| OT | Occupational therapy |
| OTC | Over-the-counter |
| OU | Each eye (*oculus uterque*) |
| P | Pulse, plan, percussion, pressure |
| P & A | Percussion and auscultation |
| P & T | Peak and trough |
| PA | Physician Assistant; posterior-anterior; pulmonary artery |
| PAC | Premature atrial contraction |
| $Paco_2$ | Arterial carbon dioxide tension |
| $Pao_2$ | Arterial oxygen tension |
| PAOP | Pulmonary artery occlusion pressure |
| PAT | Paroxysmal atrial tachycardia |
| PBI | Protein-bound iodine |
| PBSCT | Peripheral blood stem cell transplantation |
| PC | After meals (*post cibum*) |
| PCA | Patient-controlled analgesia |
| PCI | Percutaneous coronary intervention |
| PCKD | Polycystic kidney disease |
| PCN | Penicillin |
| PCOS | Polycystic ovarian syndrome |
| PCP | *Pneumocystis carinii* pneumonia; phencyclidine |
| PCWP | Pulmonary capillary wedge pressure |
| PDA | Patent ductus arteriosus |
| PDE | Phosphodiesterase |
| PE | Physical examination; pulmonary embolism |
| PEEP | Positive end-expiratory pressure |
| PEFR | Peak expiratory flow rate |
| PEG | Percutaneous endoscopic gastrostomy; polyethylene glycol |

| | |
|---|---|
| PERLA | Pupils equal, react to light and accommodation |
| PERRLA | Pupils equal, round, and reactive to light and accommodation |
| PET | Positron emission tomography |
| PFT | Pulmonary function test |
| pH | Hydrogen ion concentration |
| PharmD | Doctor of Pharmacy |
| PI | Principal investigator; protease inhibitor |
| PICC | Peripherally inserted central catheter |
| PID | Pelvic inflammatory disease |
| PIP | Proximal interphalangeal |
| PKU | Phenylketonuria |
| PMD | Private medical doctor |
| PMH | Past medical history |
| PMI | Point of maximal impulse |
| PMN | Polymorphonuclear leukocyte |
| PMS | Premenstrual syndrome |
| PNC-E | Postnecrotic cirrhosis-ethanol |
| PND | Paroxysmal nocturnal dyspnea |
| PNH | Paroxysmal nocturnal hemoglobinuria |
| po | By mouth (*per os*) |
| $po_2$ | Partial pressure of oxygen |
| POAG | Primary open-angle glaucoma |
| POD | Postoperative day |
| POS | Polycystic ovarian syndrome |
| PP | Patient profile |
| PPBG | Postprandial blood glucose |
| ppd | Packs per day |
| PPD | Purified protein derivative |
| PPH | Past psychiatric history |
| PPI | Proton pump inhibitor |
| PPN | Peripheral parenteral nutrition |
| pr | Per rectum |
| PR | Progesterone receptor; partial remission |
| PRA | Panel-reactive antibody; plasma renin activity |
| PRBC | Packed red blood cells |
| PRN | When necessary; as needed (*pro re nata*) |
| PSA | Prostate-specific antigen |
| PSCT | Peripheral stem cell transplant |
| PSE | Portal systemic encephalopathy |
| PSH | Past surgical history |
| PSVT | Paroxysmal supraventricular tachycardia |
| PT | Prothrombin time; physical therapy; patient; posterior tibial |
| PTA | Prior to admission |
| PTCA | Percutaneous transluminal coronary angioplasty |
| PTE | Pulmonary thromboembolism |
| PTH | Parathyroid hormone |
| PTSD | Posttraumatic stress disorder |
| PTT | Partial thromboplastin time |
| PTU | Propylthiouracil |
| PUD | Peptic ulcer disease |
| PVC | Premature ventricular contraction |
| PVD | Peripheral vascular disease |
| Q | Every (*quaque*) |
| QA | Quality assurance |
| QD | Every day (*quaque die*) |
| QI | Quality improvement |
| QID | Four times daily (*quater in die*) |
| QNS | Quantity not sufficient |
| QOD | Every other day |
| QOL | Quality of life |
| QS | Quantity sufficient |
| R & M | Routine and microscopic |
| RA | Rheumatoid arthritis; right atrium |
| RADT | Rapid antigen detection test |
| RAIU | Radioactive iodine uptake |
| RAO | Right anterior oblique |
| RBBB | Right bundle branch block |
| RBC | Red blood cell |
| RCA | Right coronary artery |
| RCM | Right costal margin |
| RDA | Recommended daily allowance |
| RDP | Random donor platelets |
| RDS | Respiratory distress syndrome |
| RDW | Red cell distribution width |
| REM | Rapid eye movement |
| RES | Reticuloendothelial system |
| RF | Rheumatoid factor; renal failure; rheumatic fever |
| Rh | Rhesus factor in blood |
| RHD | Rheumatic heart disease |
| RLE | Right lower extremity |
| RLL | Right lower lobe |
| RLQ | Right lower quadrant (abdomen) |
| RML | Right middle lobe |
| RN | Registered nurse |
| RNA | Ribonucleic acid |
| R/O | Rule out |
| ROM | Range of motion |
| ROS | Review of systems |
| RPGN | Rapidly progressive glomerulonephritis |
| RPh | Registered Pharmacist |
| RPR | Rapid plasma reagin |
| RR | Respiratory rate; recovery room |
| RRR | Regular rate and rhythm |
| RRT | Registered Respiratory Therapist |
| RSV | Respiratory syncytial virus |
| RT | Radiation therapy |
| RTA | Renal tubular acidosis |
| RTC | Return to clinic |
| RT-PCR | Reverse transcriptase-polymerase chain reaction |
| RUE | Right upper extremity |
| RUL | Right upper lobe |
| RUQ | Right upper quadrant (abdomen) |
| RVH | Right ventricular hypertrophy |
| $S_1$ | First heart sound |
| $S_2$ | Second heart sound |
| $S_3$ | Third heart sound (ventricular gallop) |
| $S_4$ | Fourth heart sound (atrial gallop) |
| SA | Sinoatrial |
| SAD | Seasonal affective disorder |
| SAH | Subarachnoid hemorrhage |
| $Sao_2$ | Arterial oxygen percent saturation |
| SBE | Subacute bacterial endocarditis |
| SBFT | Small bowel follow-through |
| SBGM | Self blood glucose monitoring |
| SBO | Small bowel obstruction |
| SBP | Systolic blood pressure; spontaneous bacterial peritonitis |
| SC | Subcutaneous; subclavian |
| SCID | Severe combined immunodeficiency |
| SCLC | Small cell lung cancer |
| SCr | Serum creatinine |

| | |
|---|---|
| SDP | Single donor platelets |
| SEM | Systolic ejection murmur |
| SG | Specific gravity |
| SGOT | Serum glutamic oxaloacetic transaminase |
| SCT | Stem cell transplantation |
| SGPT | Serum glutamic pyruvic transaminase |
| SH | Social history |
| SIADH | Syndrome of inappropriate antidiuretic hormone secretion |
| SIDS | Sudden infant death syndrome |
| SIMV | Synchronized intermittent mandatory ventilation |
| SIRS | Systemic inflammatory response syndrome |
| SJS | Stevens-Johnson syndrome |
| SL | Sublingual |
| SLE | Systemic lupus erythematosus |
| SMBG | Self-monitoring of blood glucose |
| SNF | Skilled nursing facility |
| SNRI | Serotonin-norepinephrine reuptake inhibitor |
| SNS | Sympathetic nervous system |
| SOS | Sinusoidal obstruction syndrome |
| SOB | Shortness of breath; side of bed |
| S/P | Status post |
| SPEP | Serum protein electrophoresis |
| SPF | Sun protection factor |
| SRI | Serotonin reuptake inhibitor |
| SSKI | Saturated solution of potassium iodide |
| SSRI | Selective serotonin reuptake inhibitor |
| STAT | Immediately; at once |
| STD | Sexually transmitted disease |
| STI | Sexually transmitted infection |
| SV | Stroke volume |
| SVC | Superior vena cava |
| SVR | Supraventricular rhythm; systemic vascular resistance |
| SVRI | Systemic vascular resistance index |
| SVT | Supraventricular tachycardia |
| SW | Social worker |
| SWI | Surgical wound infection |
| Sx | Symptoms |
| T | Temperature |
| T & A | Tonsillectomy and adenoidectomy |
| T & C | Type and crossmatch |
| TAH | Total abdominal hysterectomy |
| TB | Tuberculosis |
| TBG | Thyroid-binding globulin |
| TBI | Total body irradiation; traumatic brain injury |
| T. bili | Total bilirubin |
| T/C | To consider |
| TCA | Tricyclic antidepressant |
| TCN | Tetracycline |
| TED | Thromboembolic disease |
| TEE | Transesophageal echocardiogram |
| TEN | Toxic epidermal necrolysis |
| TENS | Transcutaneous electrical nerve stimulation |
| TFT | Thyroid function test |
| TG | Triglyceride |
| THA | Total hip arthroplasty |
| THC | Tetrahydrocannabinol |
| TIA | Transient ischemic attack |
| TIBC | Total iron-binding capacity |
| TID | Three times daily (*ter in die*) |
| TIH | Tumor-induced hypercalcemia |
| TIPS | Transjugular intrahepatic portosystemic shunt |
| TLC | Therapeutic lifestyle changes |
| TLI | Total lymphoid irradiation |
| TLS | Tumor lysis syndrome |
| TM | Tympanic membrane |
| TMJ | Temporomandibular joint |
| TMP/SMX | Trimethoprim-sulfamethoxazole |
| TnI | Troponin I (cardiac) |
| TnT | Troponin T |
| TNTC | Too numerous to count |
| TOD | Target organ damage |
| TPN | Total parenteral nutrition |
| TPR | Temperature, pulse, respiration |
| T. prot | Total protein |
| TSH | Thyroid-stimulating hormone |
| TSS | Toxic shock syndrome |
| TTP | Thrombotic thrombocytopenic purpura |
| TUIP | Transurethral incision of the prostate |
| TURP | Transurethral resection of the prostate |
| Tx | Treat; treatment |
| UA | Urinalysis; uric acid |
| UC | Ulcerative colitis |
| UCD | Usual childhood diseases |
| UE | Upper extremity |
| UFC | Urinary free cortisol |
| UGI | Upper gastrointestinal |
| UOQ | Upper outer quadrant |
| UPT | Urine Pregnancy Test |
| URI | Upper respiratory infection |
| USP | United States Pharmacopeia |
| UTI | Urinary tract infection |
| UV | Ultraviolet |
| VA | Veterans' Affairs |
| VAMC | Veterans' Affairs Medical Center |
| VDRL | Venereal Disease Research Laboratory |
| VF | Ventricular fibrillation |
| VL | Viral load |
| VLDL | Very low-density lipoprotein |
| VNA | Visiting Nurses' Association |
| VO | Verbal order |
| VOD | Veno-occlusive disease |
| VP-16 | Etoposide |
| $V_A/Q$ | Ventilation/perfusion |
| VRE | Vancomycin-resistant *Enterococcus* |
| VS | Vital signs |
| VSS | Vital signs stable |
| VT | Ventricular tachycardia |
| VTE | Venous thromboembolism |
| WA | While awake |
| WBC | White blood cell |
| W/C | Wheelchair |
| WDWN | Well-developed, well-nourished |
| WHO | World Health Organization |
| WNL | Within normal limits |
| W/U | Work-up |
| Y-BOCS | Yale-Brown Obsessive-Compulsive Scale |
| yo | Year-old |
| yr | Year |
| ZDV | Zidovudine |

# PART II: Prevent Medication Errors by Avoiding These Dangerous Abbreviations or Dose Designations

| Abbreviation or Dose Expression | Intended Meaning | Misinterpretation | Correction |
|---|---|---|---|
| Apothecary symbols | dram, minim | Misunderstood or misread (symbol for dram misread for "3" and minim misread "mL"). | Use the metric system. |
| AU | aurio uterque (each ear) | Mistaken for OU (oculo uterque—each eye). | Don't use this abbreviation. |
| D/C | discharge, discontinue | Premature discontinuation of medications when D/C (intended to mean "discharge") has been misinterpreted as "discontinued" when followed by a list of drugs. | Use "discharge" and "discontinue." |
| *Drug names* | | | |
| ARA-A | vidarabine | cytarabine (ARA-C) | Use the complete spelling for drug names. |
| AZT | zidovudine (RETROVIR) | azathioprine | |
| CPZ | COMPAZINE (prochlorperazine) | chlorpromazine | |
| DPT | DEMEROL-PHENERGAN-THORAZINE | diphtheria-pertussis-tetanus (vaccine) | |
| HCl | hydrochloric acid | potassium chloride (the "H" is misinterpreted as "K") | |
| HCT | hydrocortisone | hydrochlorothiazide | |
| HCTZ | hydrochlorothiazide | hydrocortisone (seen as HCT250 mg) | |
| $MgSO_4$ | magnesium sulfate | morphine sulfate | |
| $MSO_4$ | morphine sulfate | magnesium sulfate | |
| MTX | methotrexate | mitoxantrone | |
| TAC | triamcinolone | tetracaine, ADRENALIN, cocaine | |
| $ZnSO_4$ | zinc sulfate | morphine sulfate | |
| *Stemmed names* | | | |
| "Nitro" drip | nitroglycerin infusion | sodium nitroprusside infusion | |
| "Norflox" | norfloxacin | NORFLEX (orphenadrine) | |
| μg | microgram | Mistaken for "mg" when *handwritten*. | Use mcg. |
| o.d. or OD | once daily | Misinterpreted as "right eye" (OD—oculus dexter) and administration of oral medications in the eye. | Use "daily." |
| TIW or tiw | three times a week | Mistaken as "three times a day." | Don't use this abbreviation. |
| per os | orally | The "os" can be mistaken for "left eye." | Use "PO," "by mouth," or "orally." |
| q.d. or QD | every day | Mistaken as q.i.d., especially if the period after the "q" or the tail of the "q" is misunderstood as an "i." | Use "daily" or "every day." |
| qn | nightly or at bedtime | Misinterpreted as "qh" (every hour). | Use "nightly." |
| qhs | nightly at bedtime | Misread as every hour. | Use "nightly." |
| q6PM, etc. | every evening at 6 PM | Misread as every 6 hours. | Use 6 PM "nightly." |
| q.o.d. or QOD | every other day | Misinterpreted as "q.d." (daily) or "q.i.d." (four times daily) if the "o" is poorly written. | Use "every other day." |
| sub q | subcutaneous | The "q" has been mistaken for "every" (e.g., one heparin dose ordered "sub q 2 hours before surgery" misunderstood as every 2 hours before surgery). | Use "subcut." or write "subcutaneous." |
| SC | subcutaneous | Mistaken for SL (sublingual). | Use "subcut." or write "subcutaneous." |
| U or u | unit | Read as a zero (0) or a four (4), causing a 10-fold overdose or greater (4U seen as "40" or 4u seen as 44"). | "Unit" has no acceptable abbreviation. Use "unit." |
| IU | international unit | Misread as IV (intravenous). | Use "units." |
| cc | cubic centimeters | Misread as "U" (units). | Use "mL." |
| x3d | for 3 days | Mistaken for "three doses." | Use "for 3 days." |
| BT | bedtime | Mistaken as "BID" (twice daily). | Use "hs." |
| ss | sliding scale (insulin) or 1/2 (apothecary) | Mistaken for "55." | |
| > and < | greater than and less than | Mistakenly used opposite of intended. | Use "greater than" or "less than." |
| / (slash mark) | separates two doses or indicates "per" | Misunderstood as the number 1 ("25 unit/10 units" read as "110" units. | Do not use a slash mark to separate doses. Use "per." |
| Name letters and dose numbers run together (e.g., Inderal40 mg) | Inderal 40 mg | Misread as Inderal 140 mg. | Always use space between drug name, dose, and unit of measure. |
| Zero after decimal point (1.0) | 1 mg | Misread as 10 mg if the decimal point is not seen. | Do not use terminal zeros for doses expressed in whole numbers. |
| No zero before decimal dose (.5 mg) | 0.5 mg | Misread as 5 mg. | Always use zero before a decimal when the dose is less than a whole unit. |


To report real or potential medication errors, contact the ISMP by telephone (215-947-7797), fax (215-914-1492), or e-mail (*ismpinfo@ismp.org*).

# APPENDIX D
# SAMPLE RESPONSES TO CASE QUESTIONS

## 42

## PEDIATRIC GASTROENTERITIS

One Thing You *Should* Try at Home. . . . . . . . Level II

**William McGhee, PharmD**

**Laura Panko, MD, FAAP**

### CASE SUMMARY

A 3-day history of vomiting, diarrhea, and other symptoms causes a young mother to seek medical attention at the emergency department for her 9-month-old daughter. The patient has signs of moderate dehydration on physical and laboratory examination. The presumed diagnosis is viral gastroenteritis probably caused by rotavirus. Students should understand that replacement of fluid and electrolyte losses is critical to the effective treatment of acute diarrhea. Oral rehydration therapy (ORT) with carbohydrate-based solutions is the primary treatment for diarrhea in children with mild to moderate dehydration. When caregivers are properly instructed, therapy can begin at home. IV fluids may be needed for cases of severe dehydration. Continuing fluid losses should be replenished, and early refeeding with age-appropriate diets is essential to reduce stool volume after completion of rehydration therapy. Although antidiarrheal and antiemetic products are available, they have limited effectiveness, can cause adverse effects, and, most importantly, may divert attention from appropriate fluid and electrolyte replacement. Ondansetron may have a limited role in patients with intractable vomiting who present to the ED after failed attempts at ORT. Families should have a commercially available oral rehydration solution (ORS) at home to start treatment as soon as diarrhea begins. The availability of two rotavirus vaccines is expected to dramatically reduce the morbidity and mortality of rotavirus-induced diarrhea worldwide.

### QUESTIONS

#### Problem Identification

**1.a. Create a list of the patient's drug therapy problems.**

- This patient has typical viral gastroenteritis and diarrhea, a common pediatric problem in the United States, where it is estimated that 16.5 million children younger than 5 years of age experience 21–37 million episodes of diarrhea annually. Peak incidence is in the 6- to 24-month age group. Every year, it accounts for approximately 150,000 hospital admissions (10% of hospitalizations in children between 1 and 5 years of age), 3.7 million physician visits, and 300 deaths in children younger than age 5 in the United States.[1,2] Worldwide, diarrhea accounts for 1.4–2.5 million deaths per year.[2] Viral gastroenteritis is usually caused by rotavirus infection, which is characterized by the acute onset of emesis, progressing to watery diarrhea with diminishing emesis. Rotavirus is the most common cause of pediatric gastroenteritis in the United States, accounting for 49% of pediatric cases presenting to the emergency department with acute gastroenteritis.[3] Other common viruses include Norwalk-like viruses and adenovirus.[4] For children treated in the ED, the estimated direct median cost is $867, and for those hospitalized with rotavirus, the estimated median direct cost of care is $4,565.[3]
- Rotavirus is transmitted by the fecal–oral route, and spread of the virus is common in hospitals and similar settings such as daycare. Infection occurs when ingested virus infects enterocytes in the small intestine, leading to cell damage or death and loss of brush border digestive enzymes. Approximately 48 hours after exposure, infected children develop fever, vomiting, and watery diarrhea. Fever and vomiting usually subside in 1–2 days, but diarrhea can continue for several days, leading to significant dehydration. Dehydration, along with the corresponding electrolyte losses, is the primary cause of morbidity in gastroenteritis. Children with poor nutrition also are at risk for complications.[1] Approximately 65% of hospitalizations and 85% of diarrhea-related deaths occur in the first year of life.
- The patient has moderate dehydration (acute weight loss of 9%, from 9.0 kg [19.8 lb] to 8.2 kg [18.0 lb]) as well as clinical and laboratory evidence of dehydration with metabolic acidosis.

**1.b. What information (signs, symptoms, laboratory values) indicates the presence or severity of gastroenteritis?**

- The most accurate indicator of the degree of dehydration is actual weight loss. Fortunately for the patient, she had a physician's office visit 5 days earlier, during which she was weighed and an actual weight loss of 0.8 kg (1.8 lb, or 9%) was documented.
- By history, the patient had a 3-day history of fever, vomiting, and diarrhea of acute onset; she had a reported decrease in the number of wet diapers; and her lips and tongue appeared to be dry.
- She has a social history of daycare attendance, where several of her daycare mates had similar illnesses recently. Attendance at daycare is part of a typical history in pediatric gastroenteritis. Children can be infected but asymptomatic and transmit the infection unknowingly. In addition, on the day she presented to the emergency room (ER), her mother developed abdominal discomfort and loose stools.
- On physical examination, she was sleepy but arousable, and her mental status was normal. Her skin turgor had mild "tenting," and the capillary refill was increased, at 2–3 seconds. Her tongue and lips were dry, and there were scant tears. Her eyes were moderately sunken and the anterior fontanelle was sunken. She was tachypneic and tachycardic.

**TABLE 42-1 Clinical Assessment Guidelines for Dehydration in Children of All Ages**

| Parameter | Mild | Moderate | Severe |
|---|---|---|---|
| Weight loss (%) | 3–5 | 6–9 | ≥10 |
| Body fluid loss (mL/kg) | 30–50 | 50–100 | >100 |
| Stage of shock | Impending | Compensated | Uncompensated |
| Heart rate | Normal | Increased | Increased |
| Blood pressure | Normal | Normal | Normal to reduced |
| Respiratory rate | Normal | Normal | Increased |
| Skin turgor | Normal | Decreased | "Tenting" |
| Anterior fontanelle | Normal | Sunken | Sunken |
| Capillary refill (sec) | <2 | 2–3 | >3 |
| Mucous membranes | Slightly dry | Dry | Dry |
| Tearing | Normal/absent | Absent | Absent |
| Eye appearance | Normal | Sunken orbits | Deeply sunken orbits |
| Mental status | Normal | Normal to listless | Normal to lethargic to comatose |
| Urine volume (mL/kg/h) | Slightly decreased | <1 | <1 |
| Urine specific gravity | 1.020 | 1.025 | >1.035 |
| BUN | Upper normal | Elevated | High |
| Blood pH | 7.40–7.22 | 7.30–6.92 | 7.10–6.8 |
| Thirst | Slightly increased | Moderately increased | Very thirsty or too lethargic to indicate |

- Her labs indicated metabolic acidosis (total carbon dioxide [$CO_2$] 14 mEq/L and Cl 113 mEq/L), and her urinalysis showed a specific gravity of 1.029 (indicating moderate dehydration). Ketones were 2+ in the urine, indicating fat breakdown in a hypocaloric diet. Her serum sodium was 137 mEq/L, indicating isotonic dehydration (defined as serum sodium between 130 and 150 mEq/L), and her BUN was slightly high, at 23 mg/dL.
- Table 42-1 is a dehydration assessment tool to help categorize the degree of dehydration. Dehydration is categorized clinically into mild, moderate, and severe, but rarely does a child fall entirely into one category or another. When a child does not fit into one category, the category with the most signs should be used. In assessing the degree of dehydration, changes in mental status, skin turgor, mucous membranes, and eyes are important assessment tools because they correlate with the degree of dehydration better than other signs and symptoms.

## Desired Outcome

**2. What are the goals of pharmacotherapy in this case?**

- The goals of appropriate pharmacotherapy of dehydration include reversing dehydration, restoring normal urine output, and maintaining adequate nutrition.
- Replacement of fluid and electrolyte losses is the critical element of effective treatment. This is necessary to prevent excessive water, electrolyte, and acid–base disturbances.
- Reinstitution of an age-appropriate diet is essential to ensure adequate nutrition and to reduce stool volume. Further morbidity and unnecessary hospitalization may be prevented.
- Other secondary goals may include providing symptomatic relief and treating any curable causes of diarrhea.

## Therapeutic Alternatives

**3.a. What nondrug therapies might be useful for this patient?**

- ORT with carbohydrate-based solutions is the mainstay of treatment of fluid and electrolyte losses caused by diarrhea in children with mild to moderate dehydration. It can be used regardless of the patient's age, causative pathogen, or initial serum sodium concentration. The basis for the effectiveness of ORT is the phenomenon of glucose–sodium cotransport, where sodium ions given orally are absorbed along with glucose (and other organic molecules) from the lumen of the intestine into the bloodstream.[4] Once these molecules are absorbed, free water naturally follows. Any of the commercially available ORSs can be used successfully to rehydrate otherwise healthy children with mild to moderate dehydration. These products are formulated on physiologic principles and should be close to isotonic to avoid unnecessary shifts in fluid. They are to be distinguished from other nonphysiologic clear liquids that are commonly but inappropriately used to treat dehydration. Clear liquids to be avoided include colas, ginger ale, apple juice, chicken broth, and sports beverages. This patient was inappropriately treated because in addition to an ORS (Pedialyte®), she received a variety of clear liquids including water, cola, and diluted apple juice. These liquids have unacceptably low electrolyte concentrations, and cola beverages are hypertonic because of the high glucose concentrations, with osmolalities greater than 700 mOsm.
- *Early feeding of age-appropriate foods.* Although carbohydrate-based ORT is highly effective in replacing fluid and electrolyte losses, it has no effect on stool volume or duration of diarrhea, which can be discouraging to parents. To overcome this limitation, cereal-based ORT (e.g., rice flour–based ORT) has been used investigationally and can reduce stool volume by 20–30%. However, no commercial products are available in the United States. Another ORT product based on rice syrup solids (Infalyte®) is equivalent in efficacy to carbohydrate-based ORT. Nonetheless, early feeding of patients as soon as oral rehydration is completed may provide similar reductions in stool volume.[5] Therefore, children with diarrhea requiring rehydration should be fed with age-appropriate diets immediately after completing ORT. Optimal ORT incorporates early feeding of age-appropriate foods. Unrestricted diets generally do not worsen the symptoms of mild or moderate diarrhea and decrease the stool output compared with ORT alone. For breastfed infants, there is no need to stop breastfeeding. Supplementation with ORT between regular feedings should be considered to ensure adequate intake. In addition, most children being fed milk-based formulas tolerate them well. Children who do not tolerate them, however, can be changed to a soy-based formula for the duration of diarrhea. Older children can resume a normal diet for their age once ORT is complete.
- ORT is well established as the appropriate therapy for preventing and treating diarrhea with mild to moderate dehydration associated with pediatric gastroenteritis. The principles of ORT include two phases of treatment: (1) a rehydration phase in which water and electrolytes are administered with an appropriate ORS; and (2) reintroduction of age-appropriate diets as soon as rehydration is complete (replacement of ongoing fluid losses from diarrhea and vomiting is necessary with the ORS). As simple as this sounds, many health care providers, contrary to the guidelines of the AAP and the recommendations of the

Centers for Disease Control and Prevention (CDC), overuse IV hydration, prolong rehydration, delay reintroduction of age-appropriate diets, and withhold ORT inappropriately, especially in children who are vomiting. Continuing education of health care workers and reemphasizing the value of oral rehydration versus IV rehydration is essential for the success of ORT.

**3.b. What feasible pharmacotherapeutic alternatives are available for treating this patient's diarrhea?**

- Antidiarrheal compounds have been used to treat pediatric gastroenteritis. Their purpose is to shorten the course of diarrhea and to relieve discomfort by reducing stool output and electrolyte losses. However, despite a large number of antidiarrheal compounds available, none has found a place in the routine treatment of acute diarrhea associated with pediatric gastroenteritis. Their usefulness remains to be proven, and evidence-based guidelines do not recommend their use.[6] These agents have a variety of proposed mechanisms; their possible benefits and limitations are outlined below.

  ✓ *Antimotility agents (opioids and opioid/anticholinergic combination products)* delay GI transit and increase gut capacity and fluid retention. *Loperamide* with ORT significantly reduces the volume of stool losses, but this reduction is not clinically significant. Loperamide also may have an unacceptable rate of side effects (lethargy, respiratory depression, altered mental status, ileus, abdominal distention). *Anticholinergic agents* (e.g., atropine or mepenzolate bromide) may cause dry mouth that can alter the clinical evaluation of dehydration. Infants and children are especially susceptible to toxic effects of anticholinergics. Antimotility agents can worsen the course of diarrhea in shigellosis, antibiotic-associated pseudomembranous colitis, and *Escherichia coli* O157:H7–induced diarrhea. *Most important, reliance on antidiarrheal compounds may shift the focus of treatment away from appropriate ORT and the early feeding of the child.* They are not recommended by the AAP to treat acute diarrhea in children because of the modest clinical benefit, limited scientific evidence of efficacy, and concern for toxic effects.

  ✓ *Antisecretory agents (bismuth subsalicylate)* may have an adjunctive role for acute diarrhea. Bismuth subsalicylate decreases intestinal secretions secondary to cholera and *E. coli* toxins, decreases frequency of unformed stools, decreases total stool output, and reduces the need for ORT. However, the benefit is modest, and it requires dosing every 4 hours. Also, pediatric patients may absorb salicylate (but the effect on Reye's syndrome is unknown). This treatment is not recommended by the AAP because of modest benefit and concern for toxicity.

  ✓ *Adsorbent drugs (polycarbophil)* may bind bacterial toxins and water, but their effectiveness remains unproved. There is no conclusive evidence of decreased duration of diarrhea, number of stools, or total stool output. Major toxicity is not a concern with these products, but they may adsorb nutrients, enzymes, and drugs. These products are not recommended by the AAP because of lack of efficacy.

  ✓ *Probiotics* are defined as beneficial species of bacteria that when ingested, colonize and replicate in the intestine, producing a beneficial effect in the host. The rationale for using them in pediatric gastroenteritis is that they act against intestinal pathogens. Their exact mechanism is unknown, but they may act by producing antimicrobial substances, decreasing adhesion of pathogens to enterocytes, decreasing toxin production, and/or stimulating specific immune responses to pathogens. Multiple meta-analyses indicate significant but modest benefit from the use of probiotics, shortening the duration of diarrhea by approximately 1 day. This effect was especially seen in young children with rotavirus infections who were administered probiotics early in the course of the illness. (The most consistent effect was seen with use of *Lactobacillus* GG, a bacterial strain isolated in humans in the 1980s by Drs Gorbach and Goldin, thus the name *Lactobacillus* GG.) Based on the results of four meta-analyses, the recently published ESPGHAN/ESPID guidelines concluded that "probiotics may be an effective adjunct to the management of diarrhea."[6] However, since there is little or no evidence of efficacy for many products tested, the guidelines suggested the use of "probiotic strains with proven efficacy and in appropriate doses for the management of children with acute gastroenteritis as an adjunct to rehydration therapy."[6] Notwithstanding this most recent recommendation, probiotics have not been generally recommended in the treatment of pediatric gastroenteritis. Most published studies have methodological limitations, and there was wide variation in the probiotics evaluated and doses utilized. Many of the studies were performed in developing countries where response to probiotics may be different from industrialized countries.[7] Although they generally are considered safe, there are reports of bacteremia and fungemia occurring in immunosuppressed patients. Because they are categorized as nutraceuticals, the FDA has no authority to regulate or standardize the production or the purity of these products. There is great variability in product content, and some formulations have even contained no bacteria when tested. Because of these concerns, the use of probiotics routinely for the treatment of pediatric gastroenteritis is premature and their use, similar to antimotility agents, *may shift the focus of treatment away from appropriate ORT and the early feeding of the child.* However, the future availability of standardized products and accepted dosage and treatment regimens along with the full understanding that their usefulness is limited (to shorten the duration of diarrhea only) may make a future role in acute gastroenteritis possible.

  ✓ *Antiemetic drugs* have been used in dehydrated patients who are vomiting, but their use is generally discouraged. They are used with the intent of reducing the rate of dehydration and improving the efficiency of ORT. However, the possible benefits of antiemetics must be weighed against side effects that can interfere with the evaluation of the patient such as lethargy and drowsiness (e.g., *promethazine*), dystonic reactions (*metoclopramide*), or prolonged diarrhea (*ondansetron*).

Several studies have examined the usefulness of *ondansetron* in ED settings. Although there is less emesis, an increase in the amount of diarrhea may be experienced during the first 24–48 hours after use. Nonetheless, it has been used safely in children as young as 1 month of age for treatment of postoperative or chemotherapy-related nausea and vomiting. A recent meta-analysis of six randomized, double-blind, placebo-controlled trials of ondansetron indicated that it appears to have a role in the treatment of acute gastroenteritis. In these trials, children who were administered IV or PO ondansetron were less likely to have persistent vomiting, be prescribed IV fluids, or be admitted to the hospital from the ED.[8] On follow-up, patients treated with ondansetron consistently demonstrated an increase in diarrhea. However, this did not result in an increased requirement for further health care or return to the ED. Although there is insufficient evidence to justify ondansetron's routine use in children with mild to moderate gastroenteritis and no published guidelines recommend its general use, the authors of this meta-analysis concluded that "future treatment guidelines should incorporate ondansetron therapy for select children with gastroenteritis."[8] Perhaps ondansetron should be reserved for patients with mild to moderate gastroenteritis with intractable vomiting who cannot tolerate ORT, where avoidance of hospitalization might be possible.

✓ *Zinc supplementation* is recommended for treating acute diarrhea in malnourished children in developing countries. In those areas, zinc deficiency occurs in children not only because of increased stool losses with diarrhea, but also because of prior reduced intake of animal foods, excess dietary phytates that decrease zinc absorption, and poor food intake.[9] Oral zinc has ion absorption and antisecretory effects that result in reduced duration and severity of diarrhea as determined by stool output and frequency. Because of these benefits, in May 2004 both UNICEF and WHO jointly recommended that all children with diarrhea in developing countries be treated with zinc in addition to ORT. It has been estimated that if the UNICEF/WHO recommendations were implemented worldwide, zinc administration could save 400,000 lives annually. There is insufficient evidence to justify the use of zinc for well-nourished children with gastroenteritis.[7]

## Optimal Plan

**4.a. What drug(s), dosage forms, schedule, and duration of therapy are best for this patient?**

- Treatment of a child with dehydration is directed primarily by the degree of dehydration present.[4] This patient had diarrhea with moderate dehydration (6–9% loss of body weight). There are four potential treatment situations.

  ✓ *Diarrhea without dehydration.* ORT may be given in doses of 10 mL/kg to replace ongoing stool losses. Some children may not take the ORT because of its salty taste. For these few patients, freezer pops are available in a variety of flavors. ORT may not be necessary if fluid consumption and age-appropriate feeding continues. Infants should continue to breastfeed or take regular-strength formula. Older children can usually drink full-strength milk.

  ✓ *Diarrhea with mild dehydration (3–5% weight loss).* Correct dehydration with ORT, 50 mL/kg over a 4-hour period. Reassess the status of dehydration and volume of ORT at 2-hour intervals. Concomitantly replace continuing losses from stool or emesis at 10 mL/kg for each stool; estimate emesis loss and replace with fluid. Children with emesis can usually tolerate ORT, but it is necessary to administer ORT in small 5- to 10-mL aliquots (one to two teaspoonfuls) every 1–2 minutes. Feeding should start immediately after rehydration is complete, using the feeding guidelines described previously.

  ✓ *Diarrhea with moderate dehydration (6–9% weight loss).* Although the patient presented to the emergency department, ORT is still the initial treatment of choice to reverse moderate dehydration, and it can usually be performed at home.[5] Compared with IV rehydration, oral rehydration can be initiated more quickly and is equally effective. To correct the dehydration, administer ORT, 100 mL/kg, plus replacement of ongoing losses (10 mL/kg for each stool, plus estimated losses from emesis as above) during the first 4 hours. Assess rehydration status hourly and adjust the amount of ORT accordingly. Close supervision is required, but this can be done at home. Rapid restoration of blood volume helps to correct acidosis and to increase tissue perfusion. Resume feeding of age-appropriate diet as soon as rehydration is completed.

  ✓ *Diarrhea with severe dehydration (≥10% weight loss).* Severe dehydration and uncompensated shock should be treated aggressively with IV isotonic fluids to restore intravascular volume. Poorly treated pediatric gastroenteritis, especially in infants, can cause life-threatening severe dehydration and should be considered a medical emergency. The patient may be in shock and should be referred to an emergency department. Administer 20 mL/kg aliquots of normal saline or Ringer's lactated solution over 15–30 minutes (even faster in uncompensated shock). Reassess the patient's status after each completed fluid bolus. Repeat boluses of up to 80 mL/kg total fluid may be used. Isotonic fluid replacement may be discontinued when blood pressure is restored, heart rate is normalized, peripheral pulses are strong, and skin perfusion is restored. Urine output is the best indicator of restored intravascular volume and should be at least 1 mL/kg/h. If the patient does not respond to rapid IV volume replacement, other underlying disorders should be considered, including septic shock, toxic shock syndrome, myocarditis, cardiomyopathy, pericarditis, and other underlying diseases. ORT may be instituted to complete rehydration when the patient's status is satisfactory. Estimate the degree of remaining dehydration and treat according to the above guidelines. IV access should be maintained until it is certain that IV therapy will not be reinstituted. After ORT is complete, resume age-appropriate feeding following the guidelines outlined previously.

**4.b. What is the efficacy and safety record of the available rotavirus vaccines, and what impact are they expected to have on preventing rotavirus-induced diarrhea?**

- Because rotavirus-induced disease kills approximately 440,000 children each year in developing countries and accounts for one third of hospitalizations for diarrhea worldwide, preventing it is the most effective way to lower its impact throughout the world. A decade ago, efforts to reduce the tremendous worldwide health burden of gastroenteritis suffered a setback when the available licensed rotavirus vaccine (Rotashield®) was removed from the market because of the rare side effect of intussusception. Since then, two oral rotavirus vaccines have been approved for use in the United States.

  ✓ RotaTeq® (RV5), a live oral human–bovine rotavirus vaccine, became available in 2006. It contains five live reassortant rotavirus strains active against rotavirus gastroenteritis caused by G1, G2, G3, and G4 serotypes and has proven to be highly successful in preventing rotavirus-induced diarrhea caused by these common serotypes. It is given as a three-dose series at 2, 4, and 6 months of age (the first dose can be given as early as 6 weeks, but the series needs to be initiated by 14 weeks, 6 days; the maximum age for the last dose is 8 months, 0 days). It is a liquid formulation requiring no reconstitution and is supplied as a single 2-mL dose in a squeezable plastic tube.

  ✓ Rotarix® (RV1) became available in the United States in 2008. It contains a single human rotavirus strain (RIX4414) active against G1, G2, G3, and G9 serotypes. It is given to infants as a two-dose series at 2 and 4 months (it can be initiated as early as 6 weeks with the second dose given as late as 8 months, 0 days). It is available as a vial of lyophilized vaccine with a prefilled oral applicator of diluent. It has latex in the tip and should be avoided in persons with a latex allergy.

The safety and efficacy of RV5 and RV1 were determined from 11 randomized, controlled trials in 146,000 infants including 3 trials for RV5 and 7 trials for RV1.[10] An increased risk of intussusception was not associated with either vaccine. Efficacy against any rotavirus gastroenteritis ranged from 74% to 87%, and efficacy against severe disease ranged from 85% to 98%.[10] Both vaccines reduced hospitalizations, emergency department visits, and physician visits. The AAP recommends routine immunization of infants in the United States with rotavirus vaccine and does not express a preference for either RV5 or RV1. The vaccine series can be completed by using a combination of the two vaccines if one is unavailable but requires a three-dose series if one dose was RV5. Either vaccine can be substituted to complete the vaccine series. In 2009, the WHO recommended worldwide use of rotavirus vaccines.[7]

## Outcome Evaluation

**5. What clinical and laboratory parameters should be monitored to evaluate therapy for achievement of the desired therapeutic outcome?**

- Vital signs should normalize with appropriate therapy, but they may be unreliable in patients with fever, agitation, pain, or respiratory illnesses. Tachycardia is usually the first sign of mild dehydration (see Table 42-1). With increasing acidosis and fluid loss, the respiratory rate increases and breathing becomes deeper (hyperpnea). Hypotension is usually a sign of severe dehydration.
- Any existing central nervous system (CNS) alterations should be reversed. No CNS changes occur in mild dehydration; some patients may appear listless with moderate dehydration, and severely dehydrated patients appear quite ill with lethargy or irritability.
- Skin changes should be normalized. Mucous membranes should appear moist (previously dry in all degrees of dehydration). Capillary refill is normally <2 seconds and usually is not altered in mild dehydration. Capillary refill in moderately dehydrated patients is 2–3 seconds and >3 seconds in severe dehydration. Skin turgor (elasticity) should be normal. There is no change in mild dehydration, but it decreases in moderate dehydration, with "tenting" occurring in patients with severe dehydration. The anterior fontanelle should no longer be sunken, which is seen in moderate to severe dehydration.
- The eyes should appear normal. No change occurs in mild dehydration, but in moderate to severe dehydration, tearing will be absent and the eyes will appear sunken.
- Laboratory tests should be assessed appropriately. Most dehydration occurring with pediatric gastroenteritis is isotonic, and serum electrolyte determinations are unnecessary. However, some patients with moderate dehydration (those whose histories and physical examinations are inconsistent with routine gastroenteritis), those with prolonged inappropriate intake of hypotonic or hypertonic solutions, and all severely dehydrated patients should have serum electrolytes determined and corrected.
- Urine volume and specific gravity should be normalized. Progressive decreases in urine volume and increases in specific gravity are expected with increasing severity of dehydration. Urine output will be decreased to <1 mL/kg/h in both moderate and severe dehydration (see Table 42-1). Specific gravity is 1.020 in mild dehydration, 1.025 in moderate dehydration, and maximal in patients with severe dehydration. Adequate rehydration should normalize both urine output and specific gravity. During rehydration, lung sounds should be assessed periodically to determine if continued fluid administration is warranted. Lung sounds should remain clear. The development of crackles requires careful evaluation and the temporary stopping of further fluid administration until the evaluation is complete.

## Patient Education

**6. What information should be provided to the child's parents to enhance compliance, ensure successful therapy, and minimize adverse effects?**

- Treatment of diarrhea due to gastroenteritis in your child should begin at home. It is a good idea for you to keep ORT at home at all times (especially in rural areas and poor urban neighborhoods where access to health care may be delayed), and to use it as instructed by your doctor. Sometimes doctors instruct new parents about this treatment at the first newborn visit. Be careful of information obtained from sources on the Internet. Much of the information available is not consistent with the accepted medical guidelines for the use of ORT in pediatric gastroenteritis.
- However, infants with diarrhea should receive a medical evaluation for diarrhea. Additionally, any child with diarrhea and fever should be evaluated to rule out serious illness.
- Early home management with ORT results in fewer complications such as severe dehydration and poor nutrition, as well as fewer office or ER visits.
- Any of the commercial ORSs can be used to effectively rehydrate your child. However, rehydration alone does not reduce the duration of diarrhea or the volume of stool output. Early feeding after rehydration is necessary and can reduce the duration of diarrhea by as much as one half day.
- Effective oral rehydration always combines early feeding with an age-appropriate diet after rehydration. This corrects dehydration, improves nutritional status, and reduces the volume of stool output.
- Vomiting usually does not preclude the use of oral rehydration. Consistent administration of small amounts (one to two teaspoonfuls) of an ORS every 1–2 minutes can provide as much as 10 oz/h of rehydration fluid. Parents must resist the child's desires for larger amounts of liquid. Otherwise, further vomiting may occur.
- If the child does not stop vomiting after the appropriate administration of oral rehydration (as above) and appears to be severely dehydrated, contact your doctor, who may refer you to the ER for IV rehydration therapy.
- Oral rehydration is insufficient therapy for bloody diarrhea (dysentery). Contact your doctor if this occurs.
- Additional treatments, including antidiarrheal compounds, antiemetics, probiotics, and antimicrobial therapy, are almost never necessary in the treatment of pediatric gastroenteritis. Most children can be successfully rehydrated with ORS without the use of antiemetic medication.

- Proper hand-washing technique, diaper-changing practices, and personal hygiene can help to prevent spread of the disease to other family members.
- The child should be kept out of daycare until the diarrhea stops.

## REFERENCES


1. Elliot EJ. Acute gastroenteritis in children. BMJ 2007;334:35–40.
2. Kosek M, Bern C, Guerrant RL. The global burden of diarrhoeal disease, as estimated from studies published between 1992 and 2000. Bull World Health Organ 2003;81:197–204.
3. Mast TC, Walter EB, Bulotsky M, et al. Burden of childhood rotavirus disease on health systems in the United States. Pediatr Infect Dis J 2010;29:e19–e25.
4. Duggan C, Santosham M, Glass RI. The management of acute diarrhea in children: oral rehydration, maintenance, and nutritional therapy. MMWR Morb Mortal Wkly Rep 1992;41(RR-16):1–20.
5. Spandorfer PR, Alessandrini EA, Joffe MD, et al. Oral versus intravenous rehydration of moderately dehydrated children: a randomized, controlled trial. Pediatrics 2005;115:295–301.
6. Guarino A, Albano F, Ashkenazi S, et al. European Society for Paediatric Gastroenterology, Hepatology, and Nutrition/European Society for Paediatric Infectious Diseases evidence-based guidelines for the management of acute gastroenteritis in children in Europe. J Pediatr Gastroenterol Nutr 2008;46(Suppl 2):S81–S122.
7. Szajewska H, Dziechciarz P. Gastrointestinal infections in the pediatric population. Curr Opin Gastroenterol 2010;26:36–44.
8. DeCamp LR, Byerley JS, Doshi N, et al. Use of antiemetic agents in acute gastroenteritis: a systematic review and meta-analysis. Arch Pediatr Adolesc Med 2008;162:858–865.
9. Bhatnagar S, Bahl R, Sharma PK, et al. Zinc with oral rehydration therapy reduces stool output and duration of diarrhea in hospitalized children: a randomized controlled trial. J Pediatr Gastroenterol Nutr 2004:38:34–40.
10. Committee on Infectious Diseases, American Academy of Pediatrics. Prevention of rotavirus disease: updated guidelines for use of rotavirus vaccine. Pediatrics 2009;123:1412–1420.


# 126

# DIABETIC FOOT INFECTION

Let's Nail That Infection . . . . . . . . . . . . . . . . . . Level II


**Renee-Claude Mercier, PharmD, BCPS, PhC**

**Paulina Deming, PharmD, PhC**


## CASE SUMMARY

In this 67-year-old Hispanic man with poorly controlled type 2 diabetes mellitus and several comorbid conditions, an ingrown toenail has become infected, causing significant erythema and swelling of the right foot with purulent discharge from the wound. Physical and laboratory findings, including an elevated WBC, ESR, and fever, suggest a potential systemic infection secondary to cellulitis. The patient undergoes incision and drainage of the lesion, and tissue is submitted to the laboratory for culture. Empiric antimicrobial treatment must be initiated before results of wound culture and sensitivity testing are known. Because of this patient's comorbidities and the size and severity of the wound, parenteral antibiotic therapy should be initiated. Because this is an acutely infected wound, aerobic gram-positive bacteria (especially *S. aureus*) are the most likely causative organisms. However, broad-spectrum coverage for gram-negative and anaerobic bacteria should also be instituted due to the location of the wound (bottom of foot), its size and severity, foul-smelling drainage, and the patient's diabetes. This patient does have risk factors for hospital-acquired MRSA (HA-MRSA) infection (i.e., recent hospitalization, existing chronic illnesses), and empiric coverage of this organism should be considered. When tissue cultures are reported as positive for *S. aureus* (MRSA) and *B. fragilis*, the reader is asked to narrow to more specific therapy, which includes parenteral vancomycin or either oral or parenteral linezolid with anaerobic coverage (metronidazole or clindamycin). Second-line agents include dalfopristin/quinupristin, daptomycin, or telavancin all in combination with a drug with anaerobic coverage (metronidazole or clindamycin) or tigecycline as a single agent. This infection will require 2–4 weeks of therapy, so the patient will most likely be discharged on outpatient antibiotic therapy. Although parenteral therapy using any of a variety of agents, or oral linezolid, may be completed as an outpatient, attention must be given to the patient's social and economic situation. Better glycemic control and education regarding techniques for proper foot care are important components of a comprehensive treatment plan for this patient.

## QUESTIONS

### Problem Identification

**1.a. Create a list of the patient's drug therapy problems.**

- Cellulitis and infection of the right foot in a patient with diabetes, requiring treatment.
- Poorly controlled type 2 diabetes mellitus, as evidenced by an A1C of 11.8% (goal <7%) and recent episode of hyperglycemic hyperosmolar state (HHS). Metformin is contraindicated in this patient due to his SCr of 2.1 mg/dL. However, his renal function may improve with hydration, and this should be monitored.
- Nonadherence with medication administration and home glucose monitoring.
- Renal insufficiency secondary to diabetic nephropathy, appropriately treated with lisinopril, may necessitate dosing adjustment of antimicrobial agents.
- Coronary artery disease, post-MI w/percutaneous coronary intervention and stenting; treatment with a β-blocker should be considered, and dual antiplatelet therapy with aspirin and clopidogrel is appropriate since the patient is within 1 year of surgery.
- Hyperlipidemia, appropriately treated with simvastatin.
- History of alcohol abuse; patient may have liver dysfunction, and the use of metronidazole should elicit discussion on the potential for a disulfiram drug reaction.
- Fungal infection of toenails, requiring treatment.
- Language barrier requiring additional resources (i.e., translator) to optimize patient education.
- Recent travel abroad in Mexico where antibiotics are not controlled and antibiotic resistance is much higher. Patient could have been self-treating his infection or could have acquired more resistant pathogens.

**1.b. What signs, symptoms, or laboratory values indicate the presence of an infection?**

- Swollen, sore, and red foot.
- Purulent drainage with cellulitis.

- 2+ edema of the foot increasing in amplitude.
- Elevated WBC count elevated ($17.3 \times 10^3/mm^3$).
- X-ray showing tissue swelling from first metatarsal to midfoot consistent with cellulitis.

**1.c. What risk factors for infection does the patient have?**

- Patient with ingrown toenail; attempted self-treatment.
- He is a patient with poorly controlled diabetes.
- Vascular calcifications in the foot per x-ray indicate a decreased blood supply.
- He has decreased sensation of bilateral lower extremities.
- Poor foot care (presence of fungus and overgrown toenails).
- Recent hospitalization and recent travel to Mexico.

**1.d. What organisms are most likely involved in this infection?**

- Aerobic isolates: *S. aureus, Streptococcus* spp., *Enterococcus* spp., *Proteus mirabilis, Escherichia coli, Klebsiella* spp., and *Pseudomonas aeruginosa.*
- Anaerobic isolates: *Peptostreptococcus* and B. *fragilis.*[1]

## Desired Outcome

**2. What are the therapeutic goals for this patient?**

- Eradicate the bacteria.
- Prevent the development of osteomyelitis and the need for amputation.
- Preserve as much normal limb function as possible.
- Improve control of diabetes mellitus.
- Prevent infectious complications.

## Therapeutic Alternatives

**3.a. What nondrug therapies might be useful for this patient?**

- Deep culture of the wound for both anaerobes and aerobes.
- Appropriate wound care by experienced podiatrists (incision and drainage, debridement of the wound, toenail clipping), nurses (wound care, dressing changes of wound, foot care teaching), and physical therapists (whirlpool treatments, wound debridement, teaching about minimal weight-bearing with a walker or crutches).
- Bed rest, minimal weight-bearing, leg elevation, and control of edema.
- Proper education about wound care and the importance of good diabetes control, glucometer use, adherence to the medication regimens, and foot care in this patient with diabetes.

**3.b. What feasible pharmacotherapeutic alternatives are available for the empiric treatment of diabetic foot infection?**

- Diabetic foot infections are classified into two categories:
  - ✓ *Non–limb-threatening infections.* Superficial, no systemic toxicity, cellulitis extending less than 2 cm from portal of entry, ulceration not extending fully through skin, and no significant ischemia.
  - ✓ *Limb-threatening infections.* More extensive cellulitis, lymphangitis, and ulcers penetrating through skin into subcutaneous tissues; prominent ischemia.
- Oral antimicrobial therapy may be used in mild, uncomplicated diabetic foot infections *only.*[2] Suggested regimens include:
  - ✓ *Amoxicillin/clavulanate monotherapy*; or
  - ✓ Either *ciprofloxacin* or *levofloxacin in combination with clindamycin.*

  Although these regimens cover the most likely causative organisms, it is important to note that amoxicillin/clavulanate does not cover *P. aeruginosa.*
- Treatment of limb-threatening infections must include IV antibiotic therapy.[1] IV monotherapy may be used with:
  - ✓ *Piperacillin/tazobactam*;
  - ✓ *Ticarcillin/clavulanate*;
  - ✓ *Imipenem/cilastatin*;
  - ✓ *Meropenem*; or
  - ✓ *Doripenem.*

  These agents cover all of the most likely causative organisms, including anaerobes and *P. aeruginosa.* However, imipenem/cilastatin is a potent β-lactamase inducer, so therapy with the other agents may be preferable.
- The following agents could also be used as IV therapy, but they do not cover *P. aeruginosa*:
  - ✓ *Ampicillin/sulbactam*
  - ✓ *Ertapenem*
  - ✓ *Cefoxitin or cefotetan*
  - ✓ Third-generation cephalosporin *(ceftriaxone/cefotaxime) plus IV clindamycin combination*
- *Clindamycin IV plus either aztreonam or an oral or IV fluoroquinolone* could be used in patients with limb-threatening infections who are allergic to penicillin.
- MRSA may be a suspected causative organism in some cases. There are two genetically distinct types of MRSA that can be of concern in diabetic foot infections: community-acquired MRSA (CA-MRSA) and HA-MRSA. While acquisition of HA-MRSA is associated with well-defined risk factors (history of prolonged hospital or nursing home stay, past antimicrobial use, indwelling catheters, pressure sores, surgery, or dialysis), risk factors for acquisition of CA-MRSA are not as well established. CA-MRSA is susceptible to more antibiotics than HA-MRSA.[3]
- *Vancomycin IV or linezolid oral or IV* may be used if HA-MRSA is a suspected causative organism. Persons who are at high risk for HA-MRSA wound infection include those who: (a) have a previous history of HA-MRSA infection/colonization, (b) have positive nasal cultures for HA-MRSA, (c) have a recent history (within the last year) of prolonged hospitalization or intensive care unit stay, or (d) receive frequent and/or prolonged courses of broad-spectrum antibiotics.[4–6] Should vancomycin or linezolid be used empirically, gram-negative and anaerobic coverage will need to be added to provide adequate empiric coverage.
- Should CA-MRSA be more of a concern (e.g., in a patient with no HA-MRSA risk factors who is admitted from an area where the CA-MRSA rate is relatively high), the antibiotic regimen should include any of those agents active against HA-MRSA or *clindamycin, sulfamethoxazole/trimethoprim,* or *doxycycline* or *minocycline.*[3]
- Aminoglycosides should be avoided in diabetic patients as they are at increased risk for the development of diabetic nephropathy and renal failure.
- *Becaplermin 0.01% gel (Regranex)* is approved by the FDA for the treatment of diabetic ulcers on the lower limbs and feet. Becaplermin is a genetically engineered form of platelet-derived growth factor, a naturally occurring protein in the body that stimulates diabetic ulcer healing. It is to be used as adjunctive therapy, *in addition* to infection control and wound care. In one clinical trial, becaplermin applied once daily in combination

with good wound care significantly increased the incidence of complete healing when compared to placebo gel (50% vs. 35%, respectively). Becaplermin gel also significantly decreased the time to complete healing of diabetic ulcers by 32% (about 6 weeks faster). The incidence of adverse events, including infection and cellulitis, was similar in patients treated with becaplermin gel, placebo gel, or good diabetic wound care alone.[7] Further studies are needed to assess which patients might best benefit from becaplermin use, particularly considering its cost (average wholesale price $665 per 15 GM tube at the time of this writing).

**3.c. What economic and social considerations are applicable to this patient?**

- A simplified drug regimen (monotherapy and less frequent dosing, whenever possible) should be selected because of his history of poor medication adherence.
- The patient receives his health care primarily at First Choice Clinic. This may become an important consideration in selecting his future therapeutic plan.
- For this patient to receive appropriate wound care and home IV therapy if judged necessary, the health care team must establish that his family or a home health care nurse will be able to provide assistance.

## Optimal Plan

**4. Outline a drug regimen that would provide optimal initial empiric therapy for the infection.**

- This diabetic foot infection has significant involvement of the skin and skin structures with deep tissue involvement. Moreover, the area of cellulitis and induration exceeds 2 cm (4 cm × 5 cm). Because this is an acutely infected wound, aerobic gram-positive bacteria (especially *S. aureus*) are the most likely causative organisms.[1] However, broad-spectrum coverage for gram-negative and anaerobic bacteria should also be instituted due to the location of the wound (bottom of foot), foul-smelling discharge, its size and severity, and the patient's diabetes. This patient does have risk factors for HA-MRSA infection (i.e., recent hospitalizations, existing chronic illnesses), and empiric coverage of this organism should be considered as well. Initial empiric IV therapy is appropriate in serious, limb-threatening diabetic foot infections such as this one.
- A number of treatment options are appropriate for empiric therapy of diabetic foot infection in this patient. The antimicrobial therapy selection may be based on institutional cost and drug availability through the formulary system. It should also be adjusted for the patient's renal function. This patient's calculated creatinine clearance, based on total body weight (patient's weight is below ideal body weight), is 29 mL/min.
- The only parenteral monotherapy agent available to adequately cover all of these potential causative organisms is tigecycline 100 mg IV loading dose, followed by 50 mg IV Q 12 h. However, tigecycline is not yet approved for diabetic foot infection, and does not cover *P. aeruginosa*. Because this infection is moderate in severity and the patient does not have risk factors for pseudomonal infection (i.e., previous history of pseudomonal infection, corticosteroid use, frequent broad-spectrum antibiotic use, or nursing home residence), it is not necessary to empirically cover *Pseudomonas*. An advantage of using this drug is that it does not need to be dose adjusted for renal dysfunction and is the only monotherapy option. A drawback is that it is associated with a high rate of nausea (≥20%).
- All other antibiotic regimens appropriate for this patient include two or more antibiotics (one to cover HA-MRSA and other gram-positive bacteria, and one or two to cover gram-negative and anaerobic bacteria). It would be best to limit therapy to no more than two antibiotics to optimize nursing ease and patient adherence and to minimize drug costs and toxicity.
- To cover HA-MRSA, one of the following agents would be preferred:
  - ✓ Vancomycin 1 g IV Q 48 h (or other dosing regimen to achieve vancomycin trough of 10–15 mg/L);
  - ✓ Linezolid 600 mg po Q 12 h; or
  - ✓ Daptomycin 240 mg IV Q 24 h is a second-line option.
  - ✓ Telavancin (10 mg/kg [600 mg] Q 48 h) is also a second-line option.
- To cover gram-negative bacteria and anaerobes, one of the following agents would be preferred (dosed for renal dysfunction when indicated):
  - ✓ Piperacillin/tazobactam 2.25 g IV Q 6 h;
  - ✓ Ticarcillin/clavulanate 2.0 g IV Q 6 h;
  - ✓ Ampicillin/sulbactam 3 g IV Q 8 h;
  - ✓ Ertapenem 500 mg IV Q 24 h;
  - ✓ Imipenem/cilastatin 250 mg IV Q 6 h;
  - ✓ Meropenem 1 g IV Q 12 h; or
  - ✓ Doripenem 250 mg IV Q 8 h.
- Other acceptable IV alternatives for gram-negative and anaerobic coverage, with dose adjustments appropriate for Mr Chavez's renal function, include the combination of either clindamycin or metronidazole plus either a third-generation cephalosporin, aztreonam, or a fluoroquinolone. However, this would cause the patient to be on a three-drug empiric regimen (including the antibiotic active against HA-MRSA), which may be more costly, inconvenient, and associated with more adverse drug reactions than monotherapy or dual therapy options (e.g., clindamycin and cephalosporins are more highly associated with *Clostridium difficile* colitis than other antibiotics).

## Outcome Evaluation

**5.a. What clinical and laboratory parameters are necessary to evaluate your therapy for achievement of the desired therapeutic outcomes and monitoring for adverse effects?**

- Regardless of the drug chosen, improvement in the signs and symptoms of infection and healing of the wound with prevention of limb amputation are the primary endpoints.
- Observe for decreased swelling, induration, and erythema. Improvement should be observed after 72–96 hours of appropriate antimicrobial therapy and surgical debridement.
- A decrease in cloudy drainage and formation of new scar tissue are signs of positive response to therapy that may take as long as 7–14 days to be seen.
- Obtain a WBC count and differential every 48–72 hours for the first week or until normalization if less than 1 week, and weekly thereafter until the end of therapy. Continue monitoring until therapy is completed because neutropenia is associated with many antibiotics (e.g., ampicillin/sulbactam, vancomycin).
- Vancomycin used at high dose has been associated with higher incidence of renal dysfunction, and Mr Chavez already has an impaired renal function that increases the risk. Routine weekly SCr levels may be recommended to prevent vancomycin-

associated nephrotoxicity and ototoxicity that can develop with accumulation of the drug should the patient's renal function worsen. It would be reasonable to order a weekly vancomycin trough level also to ensure that an adequate trough level (~10–15 mg/L) is being achieved.

- Question the patient to detect any unusual side effects related to the drug or infusion (e.g., rash, nausea, vomiting, diarrhea) daily for the first 3–5 days and then weekly thereafter.

**5.b. What therapeutic alternatives are available for treating this patient once results of cultures are known to contain MRSA and *B. fragilis*?**

- Once the culture results are available and the involved organism(s) is (are) considered pathogenic and responsible for the infectious process, therapy should be targeted at the specific organism(s).
  - ✓ *Vancomycin* given IV is often considered the drug of choice for skin and soft tissue infections caused by MRSA, as it has established efficacy, is generally well tolerated, and is inexpensive.
  - ✓ *Linezolid* is at least as effective as vancomycin in MRSA skin and soft tissue infections and has the advantage of oral administration, but it is expensive.[8] A weekly CBC must be obtained from patients receiving linezolid as it carries a significant risk of thrombocytopenia that may require treatment discontinuation (0.3–10.0%).
  - ✓ *Quinupristin/dalfopristin* is another alternative, but it has the drawback of being associated with significant side effects, including severe infusion site reactions and myalgias/arthralgias.
  - ✓ *Daptomycin* is a lipopeptide antibiotic approved for the treatment of complicated skin and soft tissue infections due to susceptible organisms including MRSA. It is expensive and its use is generally restricted to prevent the development of resistance.
  - ✓ *Telavancin* is the newest antibiotic to have been approved for the treatment of complicated skin and soft tissue infections due to susceptible organisms including MRSA. It is fairly expensive, has been associated with renal dysfunction, and should be reserved for resistant bacteria or failure of first-line therapy.
- None of the above agents have anaerobic coverage, and, therefore, *metronidazole* or *clindamycin* will need to be added. Either agent could be used orally or parenterally. Metronidazole may be associated with a disulfiram reaction if the patient consumes alcohol again. Clindamycin has an increased risk of *C. difficile* colitis.
  - ✓ *Tigecycline* is also effective against MRSA, and it would provide excellent activity against *B. fragilis*. This is the only option that could be used as a single agent.

**5.c. Design an optimal drug treatment plan for treating the mixed infection while he remains hospitalized.**

- The patient's therapy should be narrowed to vancomycin 1 g IV Q 48 h. After the third dose, a vancomycin trough level should be recommended and therapy adjusted to maintain a trough ≥10 mg/L. Metronidazole 500 mg po Q 8 h should be initiated to cover the *B. fragilis*.
- The patient's infection should be assessed daily for changes in swelling, induration, and erythema. Temperature should be assessed at least twice daily and a WBC obtained daily if it was initially increased. Improvements in these physical signs and laboratory parameters should be observed after 72–96 hours of appropriate antimicrobial therapy and surgical debridement. If the area of swelling and erythema increases, or if response to therapy appears inadequate, it may be necessary to broaden therapy so that gram-negative bacteria are covered as well. Response to therapy is often patient dependent, and in some cases improvement may not be seen until after 7–10 days of treatment.
- The duration of therapy is controversial and based on the patient's personal situation. Therapy should be continued until all signs and symptoms disappear and for at least 2–4 weeks total. Some patients require longer therapy, and wound healing in diabetic patients is often very slow.
- The patient should remain hospitalized until he is afebrile for 24–48 hours, has signs of improvement and positive response to therapy (decreased swelling, redness, purulent drainage; normalization of the WBC), and outpatient wound care has been established, either by proper teaching to the patient (and his family) or through home health care services.

**5.d. Design an optimal pharmacotherapeutic plan for completion of his treatment after he is discharged from the hospital.**

- The decision about completion of therapy with IV versus oral therapy is often based on clinical experience because few clinical trials have been performed on long-term treatment of diabetic foot infections.
- In this patient, continued use of IV vancomycin would probably be the best choice. Either the drug could be infused at home, most likely with the wife's or daughter's assistance and frequent nursing care visits, or the patient may be required to visit a home infusion clinic to receive therapy, depending on what is economically feasible. Discharge planning should be involved in this case to ensure a smooth transition to outpatient therapy.
- The patient should be seen in clinic at least once weekly while on therapy to assess therapeutic efficacy and safety. At each visit, a CBC should be obtained to evaluate for vancomycin-associated neutropenia or thrombocytopenia. An SCr should be obtained as well, and, if any significant changes in renal function are observed, the vancomycin dose should be adjusted or the drug stopped and changed to a non-nephrotoxic agent.

## Patient Education

**6. What information should be provided to the patient to enhance adherence, ensure successful therapy, and minimize adverse effects with IV vancomycin and oral metronidazole?**

- We will need to see you in the clinic each week to make sure the antibiotic is working. At these visits, we will draw some blood so that we can check for side effects of the medication.
- Vancomycin will be infused slowly, over 1–2 hours, to prevent flushing and blood pressure decreases that are associated with rapid infusion.
- Contact your physician or me if any unusual side effects, such as rash, shortness of breath, diminished hearing or ringing in the ears, or decreased urine production, occur while receiving this medicine.
- Contact your home health care provider if pain, redness, or swelling is observed at the IV site.
- Avoid alcohol intake as you may experience a significant drug interaction with metronidazole that could be characterized by intense flushing, breathlessness, headache, increased or irregular heart rate, low blood pressure, nausea, and vomiting.

- *Note*: The patient needs to be made aware that osteomyelitis and limb amputation are possible consequences of these infections in diabetic patients. He also needs to be provided with personnel resources (telephone numbers, addresses) to contact if unusual reactions occur while on therapy, if infection worsens, or if he has questions or concerns. Adherence to outpatient clinic follow-up visits is of prime importance for success in this case.

## REFERENCES


1. Lipsky BA, Berendt AR, Deery G, et al. Diagnosis and treatment of diabetic foot infections. Clin Infect Dis 2004;39:885–910.
2. Levin ME. Management of the diabetic foot: preventing amputation. South Med J 2002;95:10–20.
3. Rybak JM, LaPlante KL. Community-associated methicillin-resistant *Staphylococcus aureus*: a review. Pharmacotherapy 2005;25:74–85.
4. Lipsky BA, Tabak YP, Johannes RS, Vo L, Hyde L, Weigelt JA. Skin and soft tissue infections in hospitalised patients with diabetes: culture isolates and risk factors associated with mortality, length of stay and cost. Diabetologia 2010;53:914–923.
5. Herwaldt LA. Control of methicillin-resistant *Staphylococcus aureus* in the hospital setting. Am J Med 1999;106:11S–18S [discussion 48S–52S].
6. Asensio A, Guerrero A, Quereda C, Lizán M, Martinez-Ferrer M. Colonization and infection with methicillin-resistant *Staphylococcus aureus*: associated factors and eradication. Infect Control Hosp Epidemiol 1996;17:20–28.
7. Wieman TJ, Smiell JM, Su Y. Efficacy and safety of a topical gel formulation of recombinant human platelet-derived growth factor-B (becaplermin) in patients with chronic neuropathic diabetic ulcers. A phase III randomized, placebo-controlled, double-blind study. Diabetes Care 1998;21:822–827.
8. Weigelt J, Itani K, Stevens D, Lau W, Dryden M, Knirsch C. Linezolid versus vancomycin in the treatment of complicated skin and soft tissue infections. Antimicrob Agents Chemother 2005;46:2260–2266.
9. Nicolau DP, Stein GE. Therapeutic options for diabetic foot infections: a review with an emphasis on tissue penetration characteristics. J Am Podiatr Med Assoc 2010;100:52–63.
10. Cruciani M, Lipsky BA, Mengoli C, de Lalla F. Granulocyte-colony stimulating factors as adjunctive therapy for diabetic foot infections. Cochrane Database Syst Rev 2009;3:CD006810.